SARAH

P9-CEH-604

NSC
Advanced First Aid, CPR & AED
TEXTBOOK

6M0414

Interior design, layout and composition and cover design: Bending Design Inc.

Photo Credits: Cover: © George Doyle & Ciaran Griffin/Stockbyte; © iStockphoto, © George Doyle/Stockbyte; Page 139 (a): Collection: Hemera/Thinkstock; Page 139 (b): iStockphoto.com/ia_64; Page 140 (a): © Dr. P. Marazzi/ Photo Researchers; Page 140 (b): © Drew Domkus; Page 141 (b): iStockphoto; Page 168: © Dr. P. Marazzi/Photo Researchers; Page 169: © Dr. P. Marazzi/Photo Researchers; Page 170: © Image courtesy Bradley R. Davis; Page 171: © Gilbert Grant/Photo Researchers; Page 175: © Mediscan; Page 220: © Mediscan; Page 224: © Mediscan; Page 280: © Bill Beatty/Visuals Unlimited; Page 281 (a): www.poison-ivy.org; Page 281 (b): Courtesy M.D. Vaden, Certified Arborist, Oregon; Page 281 (c): © Gilbert Grant/Photo Researchers; Page 303: (a) © Tom McHugh/Photo Researchers; Page 303 (b): © Jupiterimages/Thinkstock; Page 303 (c): Thinkstock; Page 303 (d): © Suzanne L. Collins/Photo Researchers; Page 303 (e): © Tom Brakefield/Thinkstock; Page 303 (f): Thinkstock; Page 306 (a): Centers for Disease Control and Prevention; Page 306 (b): © Robert Noonan/Photo Researchers; Page 309 (a): © Brad Morgen/Visuals Unlimited; Page 309 (b): photo by Scott Bauer, Agricultural Research Service, USDA; Page 311: © Caliendo/Custom Medical Stock; Page 313: © Getty Images; Page 315: © A.N.T.i/Photo Researchers; Page 325 (a): © Mediscan; Page 325 (b): © Mediscan; Page 332: © Image Courtesy Robb S. Rehberg; Page 369: © Image courtesy Karol-Lee Trakalo; Page 381: © iStockphoto/Thinkstock; Page 413: © Image courtesy NOAA Photo Library. All other photographs © National Safety Council/Rick Brady, photographer.

COPYRIGHT, WAIVER OF FIRST SALE DOCTRINE

National Safety Council materials are fully protected by the United States copyright laws and are solely for the noncommercial, internal use of the purchaser. Without the prior written consent of the National Safety Council, purchaser agrees that such materials shall not be rented, leased, loaned, sold, transferred, assigned, broadcast in any media form, publicly exhibited or used outside the organization of the purchaser or reproduced, stored in a retrieval system or transmitted in any form or by any means, electronic, mechanical, photocopying, recording or otherwise. Use of these materials for training for which compensation is received is prohibited, unless authorized by the National Safety Council in writing.

DISCLAIMER

Although the information and recommendations contained in this publication have been compiled from sources believed to be reliable, the National Safety Council makes no guarantee as to, and assumes no responsibility for, the correctness, sufficiency or completeness of such information or recommendations. Other or additional safety measures may be required under particular circumstances.

NATIONAL SAFETY COUNCIL MISSION STATEMENT

The National Safety Council saves lives by preventing injuries and deaths at work, in homes and communities and on the roads, through leadership, research, education and advocacy.

nsc.org

© 2011 National Safety Council
All Rights Reserved
Printed in the U.S.A.

ISBN: 978-0-87912-307-9

About The National Safety Council

The National Safety Council® is a nonprofit organization whose mission is to save lives by preventing injuries and deaths at work, in homes and communities and on the road through leadership, research, education and advocacy. NSC advances this mission by partnering with businesses, government agencies, elected officials and the public to make an impact where the most preventable injuries and deaths occur, in areas such as distracted driving, teen driving, workplace safety and beyond the workplace, particularly in and near our homes.

Founded in 1913 and chartered by the U.S. Congress, the National Safety Council relies on research to determine optimal solutions to safety issues and directs its educational efforts to build awareness, provide training and share best practices. The Council recognizes organizations that have focused on safety as a critical part of their operational excellence with the Robert W. Campbell Award®, safety's most prestigious honor. NSC Congress & Expo the world's largest annual event dedicated to safety, and Safety+Health® magazine is a ing source of occupational safety information. The World Health Organization named NSC ignated U.S. certification center for its Safe Communities America® Program. Each Green Cross for Safety® Medal from NSC salutes a company with an outstanding d for its leadership in responsible citizenship and community service. Offering rning options, NSC is a leader in First Aid and Workplace Safety training and nsive driving course category where it remains the chief innovator.

Council is committed to helping its members prevent unintentional providing knowledge and resources that enable them to reduce risks, asure progress and continuously improve their safety management ers and global networks, NSC is the leading advocate for safety and Safety Month.

Author Acknowledgements

Many National Safety Council staff and affiliates have contributed to the production of this book, and we would like to acknowledge the following people for their assistance:

Paul Satterlee, MD, for reviewing and providing oversight of content.

Tom Lochhaas, for providing technical writing services.

Goodman Research Inc., for program evaluation and recommendations for improvement.

Donna M. Siegfried, Senior Director, First Aid Programs, for providing vision and support.

Barbara Caracci, Director, Program Development and Training, for providing oversight of content, development and production.

Donna Fredenhagen, Product Manager, for providing marketing support.

Kathy Safranek, Project Administrator, for providing day-to-day assistance.

Roseann Solak, Manager, Product Development, for oversight management of development processes and design teams.

Pauline DePinto, Product Coordinator, for coordinating development and production.

Alice Spencer, Project Manager, for coordinating development and production.

The council also recognizes with appreciation the many other NSC employees who devoted time to this project.

Reviewer Acknowledgements

Rebecca Gribben, BS, NREMT
Training Director
Advent Resource Management
Houston, TX

Deb Kaye, BS, NREMT
Director/Instructor EMS
Dakota County Technical College
Rosemount, MN

David Morgan, EMT, BS
Principal Trainer
Safety First
Newark, NJ

Robb Rehberg, PhD, ATC CSCS, NREMT
Coordinator of Athletic Training Clinical Education
William Paterson University
Wayne, NJ

Table of Contents

Chapter 1 • Preparing to Act

Chapter Preview

- What Is First Aid?
- The Need for First Aid
- Deciding to Help
- Staying Prepared
- The Emergency Medical Services System
- Legal Concepts in First Aid

You are staying late at work to catch up on a project, when a co-worker returns to the office to pick up something she forgot. While she is in her office, her young son, whom she left in the reception area, is running around. He falls and hurts his arm, and you hear him crying and come out to see if you can help. His mother calms him while you get a first aid kit.

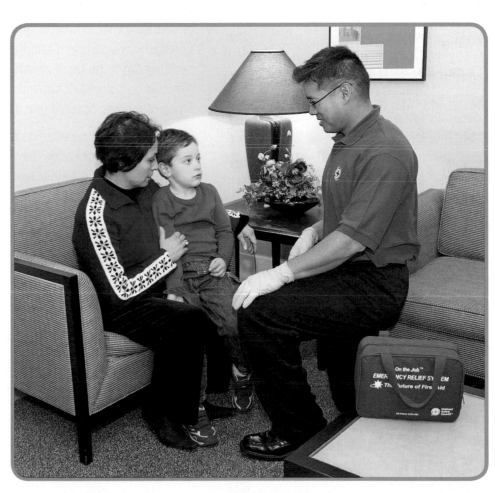

First aid training is important because injuries and sudden illness occur frequently. People of all ages, in all places, may experience an injury or sudden illness requiring immediate attention when a doctor or medical professional is not present. Often the person needing first aid is a family member or loved one. In many cases the victim's life or well-being depends on actions that first aiders take during the first few minutes before emergency responders take over.

This chapter will help you become prepared to act in an emergency. It explains the need for first aid and how to decide to help when you recognize an emergency. You will also learn what it means to be prepared, your role in the Emergency Medical Services (EMS) system and relevant legal issues in first aid.

What Is First Aid?

First aid is the immediate help given to a victim of injury or sudden illness until appropriate medical help arrives or the victim is seen by a health care provider. First aid is typically given by a friend or family member, a co-worker or a bystander at the scene with minimal or no medical equipment. First aid is generally not all the treatment the person needs, but it helps the victim for the usually short time until advanced care begins. First aid can also be simple care given when medical attention is not needed, such as caring for a small wound.

The primary goals of first aid are to:

- Keep the victim alive until he or she receives medical care

- Prevent the victim's condition from getting worse

- Help promote early recovery from the injury or illness

- Ensure the victim receives appropriate medical care

Other goals include reassuring the victim and providing comfort until medical care is provided.

Most first aid does not require extensive training or equipment. With the first aid training in this course and a basic first aid kit, you can perform first aid in most situations.

The Need For First Aid

In the United States every year:

- Heart disease remains the most common cause of death, resulting in about 616,000 deaths a year.[1]

- More than 1,250,000 heart attacks occur,[2] resulting in more than 132,000 deaths.[3]

- About 795,000 people a year have a stroke, resulting in about 136,000 deaths.[4]

- About 124,200 people die from unintentional injuries.[5]

- About 39 million visits are made to emergency departments every year because of injuries.[6]

Tables 1-1 and **1-2** list the most common causes of injuries for which the victim goes to a hospital emergency department and the annual deaths resulting from the most common types of injuries. **Figures 1-1** and **1-2** show the most common types of injuries occurring in the workplace.

In many cases these deaths could have been prevented. In other cases the victim might have lived if a trained first aider had been present to give help until medical help arrived. This text describes both injury and illness prevention and the care to give until help arrives. With what you learn in this first aid course, you can help make a difference and perhaps save a life.

[1]*National Safety Council. (2011). Injury Facts®, 2011 Edition. Itasca, IL: Author.*

[2]*Centers for Disease Control and Prevention. http://www. cdc.gov/heartdisease/facts.htm Accessed March 29, 2011.*

[3]*Centers for Disease Control and Prevention. http:// www.cdc.gov/NCHS/data/nvsr/nvsr58/nvsr58_19.pdf. Accessed March 29, 2011.*

[4]*American Heart Association, http://circ.ahajournals.org/cgi/ reprint/CIR.0b013e3182009701 Accessed March 29, 2011.*

[5]*National Safety Council. (2011). Injury Facts®, 2011 Edition. Itasca, IL: Author.*

[6]*National Safety Council. (2011). Injury Facts®, 2011 Edition. Itasca, IL: Author.*

Table 1-1: Unintentional Injuries Treated in Hospital Emergency Departments in 2008

Falls	8,551,037
Struck by or against object	4,492,287
Overexertion	3,278,300
Motor vehicle occupants	2,581,605
Cut or pierced by object	2,072,604
Other specified*	1,109,782
Bites and stings (other than dog bites)	993,923
Unknown/unspecified	806,819
Poisoning (includes drug overdose)	732,316
Other transport**	620,386

Source: National Safety Council, Injury Facts 2011; data from NEISS All Injury Program, Office of Statistics and Programming, National Center for Injury Prevention and Control, CDC and Consumer Product Safety Commission.
* Includes electric current, explosions, fireworks, radiation, animal scratch, etc.; excludes all causes listed in the table and bb/pellet gunshot, drowning and near drowning, firearm gunshot, suffocation, machinery, natural and environmental conditions, pedestrians, and motorcyclists.
** Includes occupant of any transport vehicle other than a motor vehicle or motorcycle (e.g., airplane, rail car, boat, ATV, animal rider).

Table 1-2: Deaths Due to Unintentional Injuries in 2009

Poisoning (includes drug overdose)	39,000
Motor vehicle crashes	35,900
Falls	26,100
Choking	4,600
Drowning	3,700
Fires, flames and smoke	3,200
Mechanical suffocation	1,800
All other unintentional injuries*	13,900

Source: National Safety Council, Injury Facts 2011; National Safety Council analysis of National Center for Health Statistics mortality data and Bureau of the Census population data.
* Includes natural heat and cold; firearms; struck by or against object; machinery; electric current; and air, water and rail transport.

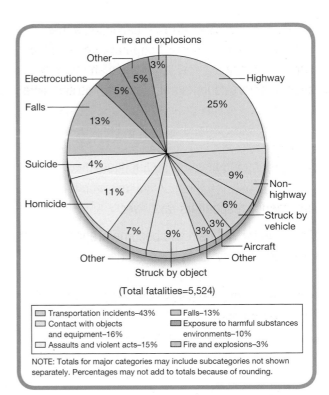

Figure 1-1 *The manner in which workplace fatalities occurred. (Source: U.S. Department of Labor, Bureau of Labor Statistics. Census of Fatal Occupational Injuries, 2002.)*

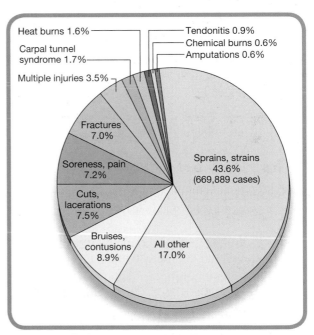

Figure 1-2 *Occupational injuries and illnesses involving days away from work. (Source: Bureau of Labor Statistics, U.S. Department of Labor. Survey of Occupational Injuries and Illnesses, 2001.)*

Learning Checkpoint 1

1. True or False: When first aid is given, the victim does not need further medical attention.

2. True or False: First aid given promptly can save lives and reduce the severity of injuries.

Deciding To Help

Recognizing the need for first aid and knowing what first aid to give are the first steps in preparedness, but you also need to make the conscious decision to help in an emergency. This is not always an easy decision. You may hesitate to act because of any of the following common concerns:

- **You may be worried about not doing the right thing**. Remember that you have first aid training. This course will teach you all you need to know to be able to help. Once you call for help, professionals will arrive very soon. Usually you are needed to help only for a few minutes.

- **You may think someone else would provide better care**. Do not delay giving first aid because you hope someone else will do it. Many people are naturally shy about stepping forward in an emergency, but unless someone else has already begun to help the victim and is obviously trained in what to do, it is up to you to help the victim. People without first aid training can assist you, such as by calling 9-1-1, going to get first aid supplies or helping calm a victim they know. But do not let precious minutes pass while waiting to see if someone else will help.

- **You may not be sure it is an emergency**. This first aid course will teach you the signs of an emergency when an injured or suddenly ill person needs help right away. When in doubt, call 9-1-1 and tell the dispatcher what you see. It is better to make the call and find out later the victim's condition was not serious, than to not call and allow a victim's condition to deteriorate before seeking care for the victim.

- **You may be upset by the sight of blood or the injury**. Some injuries can be very upsetting, especially those involving blood, badly burned skin, vomiting and other factors. You may have to muster your self-control. Try to focus on the immediate tasks at hand to prevent the experience from overwhelming you. You may need to look away and take a deep breath. You may need to ask others to help. People who are easily upset may gain from learning stress-reduction techniques along with first aid to stay in control in an emergency. If you react strongly to photographs of severe injuries such as those in this text and if you believe you might have difficulty acting in an emergency because of such factors, talk with your instructor about relaxation techniques that may be appropriate for you.

- **You may be worried about catching a disease from the victim**. Most of us would not worry about helping a family member or friend because of a fear of disease, but we may be reluctant to touch a stranger. Because some diseases can be transmitted through contact with another person's blood or other body fluids, this is – and should be – a concern. As discussed in **Chapter 2**, you should take steps in any emergency to prevent disease transmission. When you give first aid using the precautions you will learn in this course, you will not face a higher risk of contracting a disease.

Staying Prepared

An emergency can occur at any time in any place and most emergencies occur without warning. One moment you are enjoying dinner with friends, and the next moment someone at the table is choking on food and unable to breathe.

A child running through a playground falls on broken glass and suddenly is bleeding severely. A co-worker abruptly clutches his chest and collapses. In each of these cases you need to act immediately, for the victim may have only minutes to live unless you give first aid. Therefore it is essential to always be prepared to act as needed.

Being prepared means knowing what to do – but it also means feeling ready and taking steps to ensure you do not lose precious time when responding to an emergency:

- **Know the appropriate first aid techniques**. This first aid course will teach you what to do in all emergencies involving injury or sudden illness.

- **Be confident in your skills**. Sometimes people at the scene of an emergency are hesitant to help. Remember that you have first aid training, and you should feel confident that you can help the victim. Never hesitate or wait for others to act – remember that the victim's life may depend on acting quickly.

Table 1-3: Locations of Nonfatal Injuries

Place of Occurrence	Number of Injury Episodes
Home (inside)	8,344,000
Home (outside)	5,925,000
School/child care center/ preschool	3,361,000
Hospital/residential institution	570,000*
Street/highway/parking lot	4,665,000
Sport facility/recreation area/ lake/river/pool	4,172,000
Industrial/construction/farm	922,000
Trade/service area	1,661,000
Other public building	449,000*
Other (unspecified)	3,165,000

Source: National Safety Council. (2011). Injury Facts®, 2011 Edition. Itasca, IL: Author.
  * Estimate does not meet standard of reliability or precision and should be used with caution.

- **Have a personal first aid kit at home and in your car**. Be sure first aid kits are well stocked with the right supplies. Keep emergency phone numbers, such as EMS, the Poison Control Center and other emergency agencies, in a handy place.

- **Know whether your community uses 9-1-1 or a different emergency telephone number**. Note that this text says "Call 9-1-1" throughout. If your community does not use the 9-1-1 system, call your local emergency number instead. Some companies have an internal emergency number employees are expected to call (that department will then call EMS).

- **When teaching children to call 9-1-1, say "nine-one-one" and never "nine-eleven."** Young children are known to lose valuable time searching for an "eleven" button on the telephone keypad.

- **If you or your significant others have a medical condition, be sure that information is available to others in an emergency**. Information should include the telephone numbers of health care providers, allergies and any prescription medications. People with certain medical conditions such as diabetes, epilepsy and severe allergies are advised to wear a medical alert bracelet or necklace to alert others in an emergency **(Figure 1-3)**.

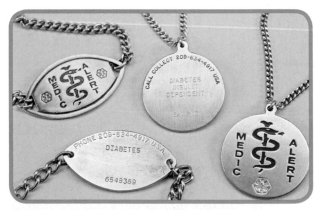

Figure 1-3 *Medical alert jewelry.*

People with certain illnesses or conditions may also carry medications for emergency use. For example, people with severe allergies may carry an epinephrine auto-injector such as an EpiPen, and some people with heart conditions may carry nitroglycerine tablets.

Most accidental injury deaths occur as a result of injuries in the home, followed by injuries in motor vehicle crashes, and injuries in public places and at work **(Figure 1-4)**. First aiders therefore need to be prepared to give first aid in any place at any time. As **Figure 1-5** shows, home and community unintentional injury deaths have continued to rise in the last decade. **Table 1-3** shows the locations of nonfatal injuries that typically require first aid.

Your First Aid Kit

Keep a well-stocked first aid kit in your home and vehicle, and know where one is kept at work or at school. Take one with you on recreational activities. A cell phone is also helpful in most emergencies.

Make sure your first aid kit includes the items shown in **Figure 1-6**. Note that you may not necessarily use all items in a kit just because they are there.

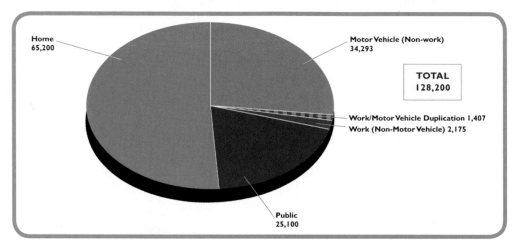

Figure 1-4 *Unintentional injury deaths by class, United States, 2009. National Safety Council. (2011). Injury Facts®, 2011 Edition. Itasca, IL: Author.*

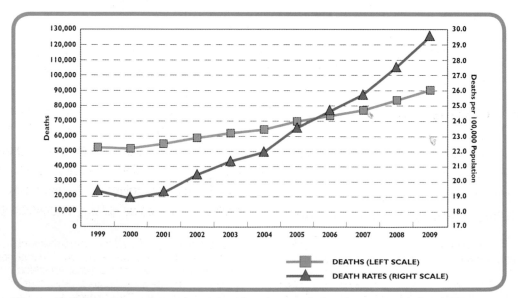

Figure 1-5 *Home and community deaths and death rates, United States 1999-2009. (National Safety Council, Injury Facts®, 2011 Edition.)*

Learning Checkpoint 2

1. Being prepared for an emergency means –

    a. knowing what to do.

    b. being ready to act anytime, anywhere.

    c. knowing how to get medical care for a victim.

    d. All of the above

2. It is a good idea to have a first aid kit –

    a. in your home.

    b. in your car.

    c. on recreational outings.

    d. All of the above

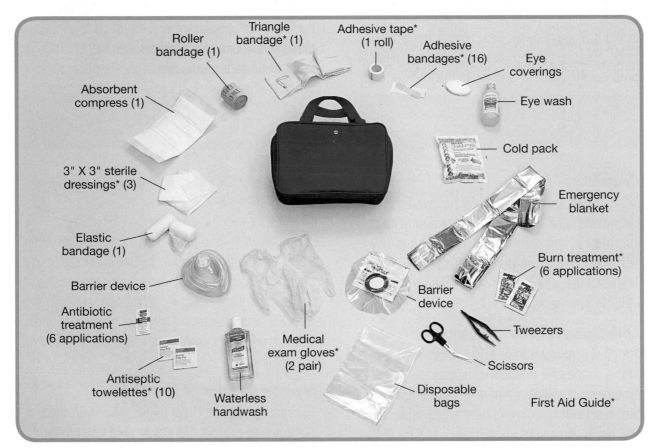

Figure 1-6 *Components of a first aid kit (*denotes minimum requirements for workplace first aid kits). Include optional supplies based on specific hazards in a particular work environment.*

The Emergency Medical Services System

People trained in first aid are the first link in the **Emergency Medical Services (EMS)** system. The EMS system in the United States is a comprehensive network of professionals linked together to provide appropriate levels of medical care for victims of injury or sudden illness.[1] As a first aider, your role in the system, in addition to giving the victim first aid until he or she is seen by advanced caregivers, is to make sure the EMS system responds as quickly as possible to help the

[1]*The term **sudden illness** is generally used to describe medical conditions that occur suddenly and require first aid until the person can be seen by a medical professional. This term will be used throughout this text. "Sudden" illness is generally different from other illness situations in which the sick person is already under the care of a health care professional or has time to see a* health care professional for a nonemergency condition. Note that in some cases a person with a nonemergency chronic illness, such as diabetes or asthma, may suddenly experience an emergency situation as a result of that illness. If so, that immediate emergency situation, such as a person with asthma having an attack and not being able to breathe, is then called sudden illness.

victim, by calling 9-1-1. In most communities help will arrive within minutes.

The Emergency Medical Services system includes a number of different professionals with different levels of training and responsibilities **(Box 1-1)**.

When to Call EMS

Call 9-1-1 immediately if you recognize a life-threatening injury or illness. A life-threatening emergency is one in which a problem threatens the victim's breathing or circulation of blood (i.e., cardiac arrest or severe bleeding), as described in later chapters. If you are alone with the victim and not near a telephone, shout for help and ask someone to call 9-1-1. Do not try to transport a victim to the emergency department yourself. Movement may worsen his or her condition, or the victim may suddenly need additional care on the way. An ambulance also can usually reach the emergency department faster than you can, and the EMTs can provide care as needed on the way. If you are not sure whether a situation is serious enough to call, do not hesitate – call 9-1-1. It is better to be safe than sorry.

BOX 1-1: EMS PROFESSIONALS

Dispatcher

A 9-1-1 call for help is usually received by an EMS dispatcher. This person is trained in obtaining information and determining what emergency personnel and equipment will likely be needed. The EMS dispatcher then sends the appropriate EMS unit to the scene.

Emergency Medical Responder (EMR)

The first professional with BLS training to arrive at the scene of a medical emergency is often an emergency medical responder (formerly called a first responder). You may be the first professional rescuer if you are close to the scene. The EMR generally takes over care of the victim from a lay person who may be giving first aid or from anyone with less training. The EMR also gathers any information concerning the victim, may control the scene or direct others to do so, and in some instances prepares for the arrival of an ambulance. In a health care setting a professional rescuer may provide emergency care until a physician, nurse or other health care professional with a higher level of training takes over. In an out-of-hospital setting, emergency care may be given until emergency medical technicians arrive with an ambulance.

Emergency Medical Technicians (EMT) and Paramedics

In an out-of-hospital emergency, EMTs and/or advanced EMTs and paramedics usually arrive in an ambulance. They take over the medical care of the victim, give necessary medical care at the scene and transport the victim for advanced medical care. EMTs with different levels of training perform different medical treatments. Paramedics have the highest level of training.

Medical Director

The medical director is a physician within the EMS system who oversees the care given by EMTs and some EMRs. The medical director establishes protocols for medical care to be given to victims at the scene and is available for consultation by radio or telephone to EMTs giving care.

Hospitals and Specialized Centers

EMRs and EMTs provide prehospital care before and during the transport of the victim to a hospital. Depending on the medical care needed and facilities in the area, the victim receives care from physicians in a hospital emergency department or a specialized center such as a trauma center, burn center or pediatric center.

If the victim is responsive and may not be seriously injured or ill, go on to the next step and check the victim further before calling 9-1-1, and then call 9-1-1 or a health care provider if needed.

Always call 9-1-1 when:

- The victim may have a life-threatening condition
- The victim is unresponsive (not talking, moving or responding to you)
- The victim's condition may become life-threatening
- Moving the victim could make his or her condition worse *Don't transport yourself.*

Box 1-2 lists serious conditions for which to call 9-1-1. Later chapters also describe when to call 9-1-1 for other specific problems.

Note that victims may say their condition is not all that serious. For example, heart attack victims often say they have "indigestion" even when they have clear heart attack signs and symptoms. You should call 9-1-1 anyway and let the dispatcher decide if the situation is an emergency.

In addition to calling 9-1-1 for injury or illness, call in these situations:

- Fire or explosion
- Vehicle crash
- Downed electrical wire
- Chemical spill, gas leak or the presence of any unknown substances
- Swiftly moving or rapidly rising water

How to Call EMS

When you call 9-1-1 or your local emergency number, be ready to give the following information. (If, however, this information is not readily available, do not delay making the call.)

- Your name
- The phone number you are using
- The location and number of victims – specific enough for the arriving crew to be able to find them
- What happened to the victim(s) and any special circumstances or conditions that may require special rescue or medical equipment
- The victim's condition. For example, is the victim responsive? Breathing? Bleeding?
- The victim's approximate age and sex
- What is being done for the victim(s). For example, is anyone on the scene able and willing to give CPR, is an AED present, etc.

It is important not to hang up until the dispatcher instructs you to do so because you may be given advice on how to care for the victim.

If another responsible person is present, tell him or her to call 9-1-1 while you go on to check the victim and give first aid **(Figure 1-7)**. Tell the other person to give the dispatcher the information listed previously.

BOX 1-2: WHEN TO CALL 9-1-1

- Unresponsiveness or altered mental status (dizzy, confused, disoriented, etc.)
- Not breathing normally, difficulty breathing
- Chest pain or pressure that does not go away
- Severe bleeding
- Head or spine injuries
- Poisoning, drug overdose
- Vomiting blood
- Seizures
- Severe burn
- Drowning or near drowning
- Threatened suicide
- Imminent childbirth

Many communities have an **enhanced 9-1-1** system that automatically provides the dispatcher with the caller's phone number and the location of telephone landlines. This information can be life-saving if the call is interrupted, but do not depend on the dispatcher already knowing your location. The location of a cell phone may not be known, and even when using a landline you may need to specify where you are (such as to say you are with the victim in the yard behind the house), to prevent the loss of precious time while EMTs knock at the front door.

If 9-1-1 is not used as the emergency number in your community, post your local emergency telephone number by all telephones and keep the number with you if you travel with a cell phone. Having to find a telephone directory to look up a number will consume critical time. **Box 1-3** describes other issues you may encounter with telephones.

In some remote locations, you may not be near a telephone. In these cases you may need to care for the victim for a longer time until the victim receives medical assistance. **Chapter 23** discusses common first aid situations in remote areas. In most other areas, however, your shouts for help will likely attract someone who can reach a telephone quickly to call 9-1-1.

Legal Concepts In First Aid

The United States is often said to be a litigious society because lawsuits are common. We hear so much in the media about people being sued that often we are afraid to act – even to help one

(continues on page 12)

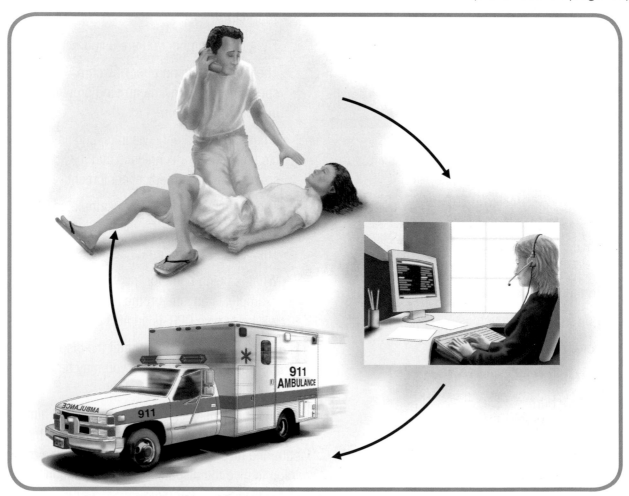

Figure 1-7 *Call 9-1-1 to get emergency help on its way.*

BOX 1-3: 9-1-1 AND TELEPHONE ISSUES

Internet telephone services, commonly called VoIP (voice over Internet) services, have become increasingly popular for computer users with broadband Internet service. In 2005, after incidents in which people were unable to call 9-1-1 on their computer phones, the FCC ruled that all VoIP telephone services must allow a connection to EMS through the 9-1-1 number. In late 2008, however, the FCC issued a consumer advisory warning that in some situations a 9-1-1 call over VoIP may still not be properly routed and urged anyone depending on VoIP telephone service to contact their provider to ensure reliability of this service. Many VoIP telephone users do not realize, in addition, that their telephone will work only as long as their computer and Internet connection are functioning. In a power outage, for example, a VoIP telephone connected to a computer without an independent power source may stop working, potentially leaving the user no way to call 9-1-1.

Similarly, many people do not realize that most cordless telephones also require electrical power – not just a charged battery in the handset. In a power failure, a wired land telephone should still work, being powered by the telephone line rather than the power circuit, but most cordless telephones will not, even if connected to a land telephone line. Cell phones are not affected by local power outages but may not have a strong signal in all locales.

By one method or another, it is important to ensure that you can always call 9-1-1 in an emergency, even when the power is off.

Note that cell phone users have been encouraged to put a personal contact in their phone directory under the name "ICE" or "In Case of Emergency" so that emergency responders can learn who to call if needed. As a first aider you would not check a victim's telephone or try to contact family members, but you may want to carry your own "in case of emergency" phone number.

 Learning **Checkpoint 3**

1. What number should you call to access EMS?

    a. 9-1-1 (if your community uses that number)

    b. The local emergency number (if not 9-1-1)

    c. Your employer's emergency number (when company policy)

    d. All of the above

2. Call 9-1-1 for –

    a. medical problems only.

    b. police and fire services only.

    c. medical problems and fires only.

    d. medical problems and all emergencies.

3. Who usually arrives first at the scene after you have called 9-1-1? _____ EMR → EMT _____

_____

4. List seven things you should be prepared to tell the EMS dispatcher when you call. _____

_____

(continued from page 10)

another – because we worry we might be sued if something goes wrong. Although legal problems very seldom arise in first aid situations, certain legal concepts are important when you interact with another person to give first aid. If you follow certain simple guidelines, you need not be concerned about being sued. If you give first aid as you are trained to do in this course and do your best, there is little chance of being found legally liable even if the victim does not recover.

To protect yourself, follow these general guidelines:

- Act only as you are trained to act.
- Get a victim's consent before giving first aid.
- Do not move a victim unnecessarily.
- Call for professional help.
- Keep giving care until help arrives.

Good Samaritan Laws

Most states have **Good Samaritan laws** designed to encourage people to help others in an emergency without having to worry about being sued. These laws vary somewhat from state to state, but in general they are designed to protect people who give first aid in an emergency.

These laws do not provide blanket protection, however, regardless of the person's actions. In general, first aiders are legally protected only:

- when acting in an emergency, voluntarily and without compensation.
- when acting as a reasonable, prudent person with the same training would act.
- when performing first aid techniques as trained.
- when not doing something outside their training.
- when not abandoning a victim after starting to give care.

Ask your instructor about the specific Good Samaritan laws in your area. Remember, however, that regardless of specific laws, first aiders who act with good intentions and as they have been trained will very rarely face any legal issues.

Must You Give First Aid?

In most places private citizens or bystanders at the scene of an emergency have no legal obligation to give first aid. Many people feel an ethical or moral obligation to help others in need, but this is different from a legal obligation.

Because laws do vary in different areas, however, ask your instructor about the law in your area.

There are three important exceptions to the principle that you are not legally required to give first aid. First, once you begin giving first aid in an emergency, you are obligated to continue giving care if you can and to remain with the victim. By beginning to give care you accept and take on an obligation to continue giving care in an emergency. Abandoning a victim in this situation could lead to the worsening of an injury or illness, disability or death.

The second exception is that some people are required to give first aid as a job responsibility. As a paid employee with this job requirement, you then are legally obligated. This is called a **duty to act**, and you may be held liable for failing to act or for acting inappropriately. Off the job, however, depending on your state's laws, you are usually not legally required to give first aid except in special cases.

The final exception is a parent or guardian who is responsible for a child, who has the duty to give the child adequate care. Federal and state laws against child abuse and neglect require parents and guardians to prevent harm and provide medical treatment (see **Chapter 21**).

Consent

Before you give first aid, you must have the victim's **consent**. This means the victim gives you permission to help him or her using first aid techniques. Touching another person without consent is a criminal action called battery. Consent may be either expressed or implied.

Expressed consent means the victim explicitly gives you permission to give first aid. To ask for consent, first tell the victim who you are and that you have had first aid training, and say what you want to do to help. The victim should understand that you are asking for consent, not stating what you plan to do regardless of what the victim wishes. A victim who is responsive (awake and alert) and able to communicate must give you expressed consent before you can give first aid. The victim may give consent by telling you it is okay or by nodding agreement. With an injured or ill child, a parent or guardian present must give expressed consent **(Figure 1-8)**.

If an adult is unresponsive, however, or a child's parent or guardian is not present and cannot be reached quickly enough for consent, then you have **implied consent** to give first aid in an emergency. In this case you can assume, unless there is some evidence to the contrary, that the person would, if able, consent to receiving care for a life-threatening condition. Similarly, if a person who initially refused consent becomes unresponsive, consent for care is now implied.

Refusing Consent

Most competent victims of a medical emergency will give consent for first aid when they understand the importance of this first aid. **Competent** means the person is able to understand what is happening and the implications of his or her decision about receiving first aid. A victim may not be competent because of intoxication, the influence of a drug, or altered mental status caused by a severe injury or a diabetic emergency.

Rarely, however, a competent victim may refuse your care when you seek consent. The person may have religious reasons, may be afraid, may not trust you or may have some other reason. A competent adult has the right to refuse medical care, even care that has already begun and you must not try to force care on this person. Refusal may be expressed through words, by shaking the head or signaling you to stop, or by

trying to push you away. If this happens, follow these guidelines:

- Make sure 9-1-1 has been called even though the victim may seem to refuse all care. The victim may accept treatment from a medical professional.

- Do not try to argue with the victim, especially about personal beliefs. Keep talking to the victim, who may change his or her mind. Explain that you respect his or her right to refuse care but ask the person to reconsider. Explain what may happen if the victim does not receive care.

- To protect yourself legally, make sure someone else at the scene sees or hears the victim's refusal to accept your care.

Scope of Care

As noted earlier, first aiders should perform first aid only as they have been trained. The set of first aid techniques one learns in a first aid course is called the **scope of care**. Acting outside your scope of care as a first aider, such as trying to do something you have heard about but have not been trained to do, may make you legally liable for the results of your actions.

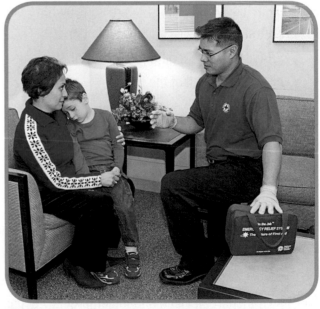

Figure 1-8 *A parent or guardian present at the scene must give consent for first aid for a child.*

Standard of Care

While scope of care refers to what you do, **standard of care** refers generally to how you perform first aid. Standard of care refers to what others with the same training would do in a similar situation. It is important to give first aid only as you are trained. Any other actions could result in the injury or illness becoming worse.

Negligence

Legally, you may be liable for the results of your actions if you do not follow accepted standards of care when providing first aid; this is called **negligence**. If you are negligent, an injured party may sue you to recover financial damages for the result of your actions. For you to be found guilty of negligence, three conditions must be met:

1. You had a duty to act (for example, first aid is your job responsibility).

2. You breached that duty (by not acting or by acting incorrectly).

3. Your actions or inaction caused injury or damages (including such things as physical injury or pain).

Examples of negligent actions could include moving a victim unnecessarily, doing something you have not been trained to do or failing to give first aid as you have been trained.

 Learning **Checkpoint 4**

1. True or False: The best thing to do in any emergency is to move the victim to your car and rush to an emergency department.

2. You have a duty to act when –

   a. you stop at the scene of an emergency.

   b. you have taken a first aid course.

   c. you have a first aid kit with you.

   d. your job requires you to give first aid when needed.

3. To which of the following victims do you have consent to give first aid? (Check all that apply.)

   ____ An unresponsive adult victim

   ____ A child without parent or guardian present

   ____ All victims, all of the time

   ____ A victim who nods when you ask if it is okay to give him or her first aid

   ____ A child whose parent or guardian gives consent for him or her

4. Check off things you should always do when giving first aid.

   ____ Move the victim.

   ____ Do what you have been trained to do.

   ____ Try any first aid technique you have read or heard about.

   ____ Ask for the victim's consent.

   ____ Stay with the victim until another trained person takes over.

   ____ Transport all victims to the emergency department in your vehicle.

Abandonment

Once you begin giving first aid in an emergency, do not stop until another trained person takes over. Stay with the victim until help arrives or someone with the same or a higher level of training takes over. If you leave the victim and the injury or illness becomes worse, this is called **abandonment**, a type of negligence. Note that abandonment is different from justified instances of stopping care, such as if you are exhausted and unable to continue or you are in imminent danger because of hazards at the scene.

Confidentiality

When giving first aid you may learn private information about the victim. That information should not be shared with anyone other than EMS professionals arriving at the scene to take over care of the victim. Although laws vary in terms of precise definitions regarding violation of privacy, **confidentiality** is the general principle that you should not give out any private information about a victim to anyone except for those caring for the victim.

Concluding Thoughts

How often have you heard people say something like "It can't happen to me?" No one ever expects to be injured seriously or experience a sudden crisis of illness, yet it happens to tens of millions of us every year. In fact, it is almost inevitable that eventually you or someone close to you will need first aid – and you can be the one who makes the difference. The following chapters will help you to be prepared.

Learning Outcomes

You should now be able to do the following:

1. List the four primary goals of first aid.
2. Explain why there is a need for first aid training.
3. Decide to help in an emergency.
4. Describe how to stay prepared for emergencies.
5. Describe the EMS system and the different types of EMS professionals.
6. Explain when to call 9-1-1 and what information to give the dispatcher.
7. Explain what first aiders need to understand about legal issues related to first aid.

Review Questions

1. The goals of first aid include –

   a. keeping the victim alive until he or she receives medical care.

   b. preventing the victim's condition from getting worse.

   c. ensuring the victim receives appropriate medical care.

   d. All of the above

2. If you are in a crowd of people when someone is suddenly injured, it is best to –

   a. wait to see if someone steps forward to help the victim.

   b. be confident and do not hesitate to offer your help.

   c. offer your cell phone to anyone who wants to call for help.

   d. stay nearby and wait to see if the victim asks for help.

3. Most nonfatal injuries occur in –
   a. workplaces.
   b. homes.
   c. public places.
   d. schools.

4. Your primary role in the EMS system is to –
   a. call 9-1-1 in an emergency.
   b. assist the EMS crew in caring for a victim.
   c. diagnose the victim's condition to determine which EMS personnel should come.
   d. advise the dispatcher on how many emergency responders to send.

5. Before calling 9-1-1, you should know –
   a. where you are.
   b. the telephone number you are calling from.
   c. whether the victim is responsive.
   d. All of the above

6. For which conditions should you call 9-1-1?
   a. Not breathing normally or difficulty breathing
   b. Poisoning, drug overdose
   c. Vomiting blood or having seizures
   d. All of the above

7. You are obligated to give first aid when –
   a. any person who is alone needs it.
   b. the victim is seriously injured.
   c. you have already begun voluntarily giving it.
   d. All of the above

8. You usually have automatic consent to give first aid to –
   a. all victims.
   b. all responsive victims.
   c. all unresponsive adults.
   d. all child victims.

9. If a responsive, competent adult refuses your first aid, what should you do?
   a. Give first aid anyway.
   b. Ask the person's spouse for consent to give first aid.
   c. Walk away.
   d. Call 9-1-1 and keep talking to the victim.

10. Standard of care refers to –
    a. what others with your training would do in a similar situation.
    b. the standard duty to act.
    c. having a written authorization to give first aid.
    d. guidelines published by the government.

Chapter 2 • Acting in an Emergency

Chapter Preview

- Preventing Disease Transmission
- Responding to Emergencies
- After an Emergency

You are driving home from work when you see a vehicle swerve off the road. It strikes a telephone pole, which breaks off, and a power line falls down on top of the vehicle. You pull to a stop some distance back. You can see the driver inside, and he is not moving. What should you do?

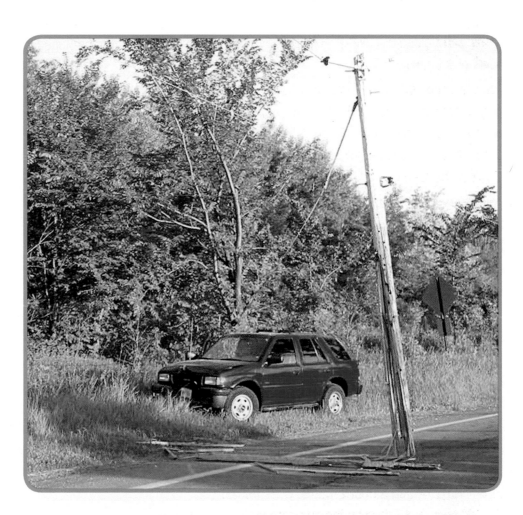

A medical emergency caused by injury or sudden illness can occur at any time in any place. Emergencies vary in many different ways. These may include:

- The nature of the injury or illness
- The severity of the injury or illness
- The presence of other injuries or factors affecting the victim's well-being
- The scene of the emergency (indoors, outdoors, potential hazards present, etc.)
- The victim (child, adult, elderly person, friend, stranger, etc.)

Because of these and other factors, no two emergency situations are identical. Yet certain key principles apply to all emergencies. In all emergencies involving injury or illness you should always follow the same basic steps outlined in this chapter.

Preventing Disease Transmission

In any emergency situation there is some risk of a first aider contracting an infectious disease from a victim who has a disease. That risk is very low, however, and taking steps to avoid being infected greatly reduces that risk.

How Are Infectious Diseases Transmitted?

The transmission of infectious disease occurs through a process involving four stages **(Figure 2-1)**:

1. The process begins with *someone or something having the infection.*

2. *The infectious pathogen (disease-causing bacteria, virus, fungus or parasite) leaves the infected person's body.* For example:

   - The person may bleed from a cut, and the pathogen is in that person's blood.
   - The person may sneeze out little droplets carrying the pathogen.

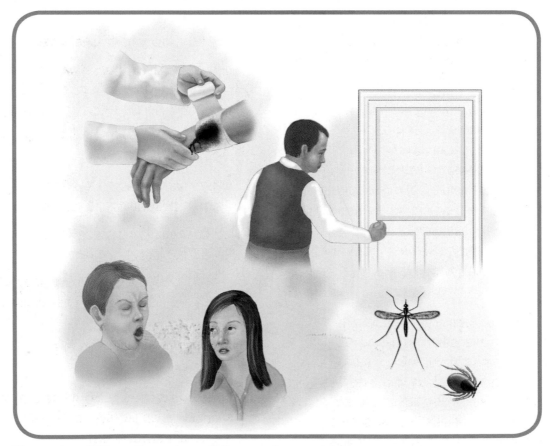

Figure 2-1 *Different modes of disease transmission.*

3. *The infectious pathogen reaches another person and enters his or her body.* This can happen in a number of ways:

   - The person may come into contact with the infected person's blood, other body fluid or infectious material in a way that allows the pathogen to enter his or her body through mucous membranes or non-intact skin (**bloodborne transmission**).

   - The person may inhale the pathogen in tiny droplets from the air (**airborne transmission**).

   - The person may be bitten by an insect, such as a tick or mosquito, carrying the pathogen (**vector transmission** of bloodborne pathogen).

   The transmission of a pathogen from one person to another is said to occur through direct or indirect contact:

   - **Direct contact** occurs from contact with an infected person or with fluids or substances from that person.

   - **Indirect contact** occurs from contact with contaminated objects, food or drink, droplets in the air, or vectors such as insects.

4. *The second person develops the infection.* Simply having the pathogen enter the body does not automatically mean a person will become ill. If vaccinated against the disease, the body will kill the pathogen before it can cause disease. A person's immune system may be able to kill some pathogens and thereby prevent illness. If it does not, a person may become infected. The process then starts all over again.

Bloodborne Diseases

Several serious diseases can be transmitted from one person to another through contact with the infected person's blood. These are called bloodborne diseases. Bacteria or viruses that cause such diseases, called pathogens, are also present in other body fluids, such as semen, vaginal secretions, and bloody saliva or vomit.

Body fluids such as nasal secretions, sweat, tears and urine do not normally transmit pathogens. Three serious bloodborne infections are HIV, hepatitis B and hepatitis C **(Table 2-1)**.

Protection Against Bloodborne Disease

Because these bloodborne diseases cannot be cured, they should be prevented. The best prevention is to avoid contact with all victims' blood and body fluids. You cannot know whether a victim (even a close friend) is infected, as often these diseases do not produce signs and symptoms. Even victims may not know that they are infected.

The Centers for Disease Control and Prevention (CDC) recommends taking **standard precautions** whenever you give first aid. The term **universal precautions** is also used to describe measures to prevent infection **(Box 2-1)**. Take these precautions for all victims, all the time, and always assume that blood and other body fluids may be infected. Follow these recommendations to avoid coming into contact with a victim's blood or body fluids:

- Use personal protective equipment.

- If you do not have medical examination gloves with you, put your hands in plastic bags or have the victim dress his or her own wound.

- Wash your hands with soap and water before and after giving first aid.

- Keep a barrier (such as gloves or a dry cloth) between body fluids and yourself.

- Cover any cuts or scrapes on your skin with protective clothing or gloves.

- Do not touch your mouth, nose or eyes when giving first aid (e.g., do not eat, drink or smoke).

- Do not touch objects soiled with blood or body fluids.

- Be careful to avoid being cut by anything sharp at the emergency scene, such as broken glass or torn metal.

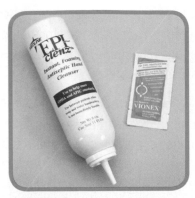

Figure 2-2 *Waterless antibacterial hand washing liquid and towelette.*

- Use absorbent material to soak up spilled blood or body fluids, and dispose of it appropriately. Clean the area with a commercial **disinfectant** or a freshly made 10% bleach solution.

- If you are exposed to a victim's blood or body fluid, wash immediately with soap and water and call your health care provider. At work, report the situation to your supervisor.

Hand Washing

Effective hand washing is essential for preventing disease transmission. Follow these guidelines (see Skill: "Hand washing"):

- Wash any exposed skin with soap and water as soon as possible after an exposure.

- While washing, be gentle with any scabs or sores.

- Wash all surfaces, including the backs of hands and wrists, between the fingers, and under fingernails.

- Wash hands immediately after removing gloves or other personal protective equipment.

- Before handling any potentially infectious materials, know where the nearest hand-washing facility is. You can use facilities such as restrooms, janitor closets and laboratory sinks, as long as soap is available.

- Do not use sinks in areas where food is prepared.

- Merely wetting the hands will not prevent infection.

- If antiseptic towelettes or antibacterial hand-washing liquid is used without water for the initial cleaning after an exposure, a thorough scrubbing with soap and water is still needed as soon as possible **(Figure 2-2)**.

Personal Protective Equipment

Personal protective equipment (PPE) is any equipment used to protect yourself from contact with blood or other body fluids. PPE includes gloves, barrier devices and other devices.

Gloves

Most important, keep **medical examination gloves** in your first aid kit and wear them in most first aid situations **(Figure 2-3)**. Gloves are a type of barrier; like other barriers, they separate you from potentially infectious materials (see Skill: "Putting on Gloves" and Skill: "Removing Contaminated Gloves"). Medical examination gloves suitable for protection from bloodborne pathogens are made of nitrile, vinyl, **latex**, or other waterproof materials **(Box 2-2)**. For added barrier protection, two pairs of gloves may be worn together in some situations.

When using gloves it is important to remember the following:

- **Check that your gloves are intact.** Check before you put them on and periodically afterward. If a hole or tear is present, replace the glove immediately with a new one.

- **Do not use petroleum-based hand lotions.** These lotions may cause latex gloves to disintegrate.

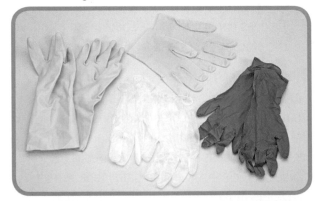

Figure 2-3 *Wear gloves to protect yourself from contact with blood or other body fluids.*

BOX 2-1: INFECTION CONTROL TERMINOLOGY

Because of changes in infection control terminology over the last two decades, there has been some confusion about the exact meanings and applications of the terms "universal precautions," "standard precautions" and "body substance isolation."

Universal precautions is the term Centers for Disease Control and Prevention (CDC) originally promoted in 1987 for actions to protect providers of first aid and health care from exposure to bloodborne pathogens. Universal precautions apply to all people's blood, semen, vaginal secretions and other body fluids containing visible blood or to any objects potentially contaminated with any of these. In its 1991 Bloodborne Pathogens Standard, the Occupational Safety and Health Administration (OSHA) required the use of universal precautions, which it defined as an approach to infection control*. According to the concept of Universal Precautions, all human blood and certain human body fluids are treated as if known to be infectious for HIV, HBV and other bloodborne pathogens." Many health care and first aid providers continue to use the term universal precautions, in part because this is the term used in federal and many state laws.

At the same time, many health care institutions were following principles of **body substance isolation (BSI)**, an infection control concept that originated in efforts to control all infections (not just bloodborne pathogens) that occur within health care facilities. BSI precautions assume that any body fluid or moist body tissue is potentially infectious.

In 1996, CDC published new guidelines called **standard precautions** intended primarily for infectious disease control within health care facilities. Standard precautions combine the major features of universal precautions and BSI precautions. Although some providers believe standard precautions have replaced universal precautions, CDC states: "Standard precautions were developed for use in hospitals and may not necessarily be indicated in other settings where universal precautions are used, such as child care settings and schools." (Source: http://www.cdc.gov/ncidod/hip/Blood/UNIVERSA.HTM)

Because standard precautions are more rigorous than universal precautions, this text will use the term "standard precautions". Recognize, however, that in many first aid situations universal precautions are appropriate.

*View the OSHA Standard, Bloodborne Pathogens (1910.1030) at http://www.osha.gov/pls/oshaweb/owadisp.show_documnet?p_table=STANDARDS&p_id=10051.

BOX 2-2: LATEX GLOVE ALLERGY

Medical examination gloves are often made of latex rubber, to which some people are allergic. Signs and symptoms of latex allergy may include skin rashes, hives, itching eyes or skin, flushing, watery or swollen eyes, runny nose or an asthmatic reaction. Use gloves made of vinyl or other material if you have any of these symptoms or if you work with patients who may have a latex allergy.

- **Remove contaminated gloves carefully**. Do not touch any part of the contaminated outside of the gloves.

- **Dispose of gloves properly**. After working with any material that may be infected by bloodborne pathogens, dispose of your gloves in a container clearly marked for biohazardous waste.

- **Handle sharp objects carefully**. Gloves protect against infectious substances but not against sharp objects, such as needles, that may also transmit infection.

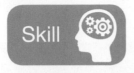 Skill Hand Washing

1 Remove any jewelry and your watch. Use a paper towel to turn on water and adjust the temperature to warm.

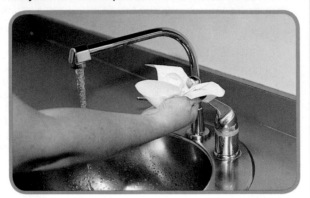

2 Wet your hands to above the wrists and lather up with soap. Keep your hands below your elbows throughout the hand washing process.

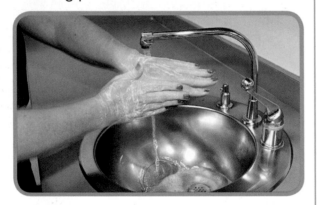

3 Wash all areas of your hands and wrists. Interlace fingers to scrub between them. If your hands were exposed to infectious material, scrub beneath fingernails with a nail brush or nail stick.

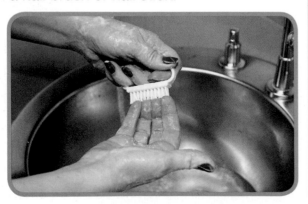

4 Rinse wrists and hands well. (Repeat soaping and washing if your hands were exposed to infectious material.)

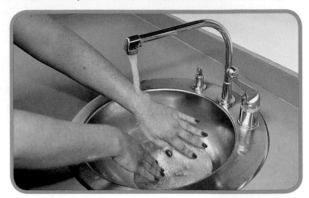

5 Dry hands thoroughly with paper towel and dispose of it properly. Use a new, dry paper towel to turn off the water faucet and open the door, and dispose of it properly.

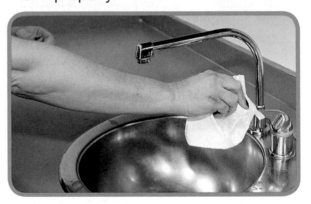

Table 2-1: **Bloodborne Diseases**

Disease	Prevalence	Modes of Transmission	Signs and Symptoms	Testing	Prevention
Acquired immunodeficiency syndrome (AIDS) Caused by human immunodeficiency virus (HIV). Eventually fatal.	More than 1 million HIV-positive people in the United States, one-fifth of whom are unaware of their infection.	Through infected person's body fluids, including: - Blood - Semen - Vaginal secretions - Breast milk - Other body fluids if blood is present Not by casual contact.	HIV often has no symptoms. AIDS symptoms may include: - Loss of appetite - Weight loss - Fever - Skin rashes - Swollen lymph nodes - Diarrhea - Fatigue - Night sweats - Inability to fight off infection	Blood test recommended after a potential exposure. Generally positive 2-8 weeks after exposure. Confirmation test recommended 3-6 months after an exposure.	No vaccine currently available. Antiretroviral treatment may be begun immediately following a known exposure. Safe first aid practices significantly reduce the risk of contracting HIV or other infectious diseases. - Regular hand washing - Use of barriers - Standard precautions
Hepatitis B (serum hepatitis) Caused by the hepatitis B virus (HBV). Major cause of liver damage, cirrhosis and liver cancer.	About 40,000 new infections yearly. Between 800,000 and 1.4 million chronic carriers. 3,000 people die of liver problems associated with HBV infection every year.	Transmitted by blood and materials contaminated with blood or body fluids. Blood and semen are the most infectious. - By injection (**needlestick** or puncture wound) - Through mucous membranes (blood contamination through eye or mouth) and non-intact skin - Through sexual activity - From infected mother to newborn at birth. Virus may survive for several days in dried body fluids on surfaces.	Often no symptoms. Symptoms usually appear gradually: - Loss of appetite - Nausea - Fatigue - Muscle or joint aches - Mild fever - Stomach pain - Occasional jaundice (yellow tint to whites of eyes or skin)	Blood test.	Use same precautions as with HIV. Vaccine is available and recommended for health care workers and professional rescuers. Employees at risk must be offered free vaccinations by employer. Vaccine also recommended for: - Those having unprotected sex with a partner with HBV or with multiple partners - Those having anal sex - Those using intravenous drugs - Those with hemophilia - Those who frequently work in countries where HBV is common - Those who live with someone with chronic HBV

SARAH FERNANDES

Table 2-1: **Bloodborne Disease** (continued)

Disease	Prevalence	Modes of Transmission	Signs and Symptoms	Testing	Prevention
Hepatitis C Caused by the hepatitis C virus (HCV). Causes liver disease; may result in eventual liver failure.	About 18,000 new infections every year. 2.7 to 3.9 million people in the United States have chronic HCV infection. 12,000 people die of liver problems associated with HCV infection every year.	Spread most often through drug injections with contaminated needles. May result from unclean tattoo or body piercing tools or from any item contaminated with blood. Spread through any direct contact with infectious blood.	Usually no symptoms. Occasionally one or more of the following symptoms: - Fatigue - Loss of appetite - Nausea - Anxiety - Weight loss - Alcohol intolerance - Abdominal pain - Loss of concentration - Jaundice	Blood test. Anyone testing positive should have follow-up test. Testing recommended for: - Health care workers exposed to HCV-positive blood - Anyone who has used intravenous recreational drugs - Anyone receiving a blood transfusion, organ transplant or kidney dialysis before 1992 - Anyone treated with a blood product prior to 1987 - Anyone with signs of liver disease	No vaccine available. Use same precautions as with HIV: - Follow barrier practices to prevent contact with blood. - Avoid recreational intravenous drug use. - Do not share toothbrushes, razors or other items that may be contaminated with blood. - Remember health risks associated with tattoos and body piercing if sanitary practices are not followed.

Source: Centers for Disease Control and Prevention, http://www.cdc.gov. Accessed March 1, 2011.

Barrier Devices

A **barrier device** is a pocket face mask or face shield used when giving rescue breaths during CPR. This device should be in the first aid kit and you should always use it for added protection. Because giving rescue breaths with a barrier device can greatly reduce the chance of an infectious disease being transmitted from or to a victim, the use of a barrier device is always recommended **(Figure 2-4)**. **Chapter 5** discusses uses of airway barrier devices more fully.

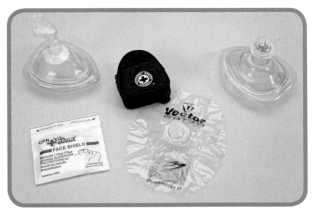

Figure 2-4 *A variety of barrier devices.*

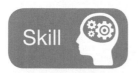
1 Pull glove onto one hand.

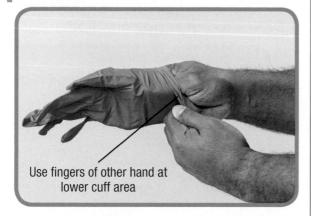

Use fingers of other hand at lower cuff area

2 Pull glove tight.

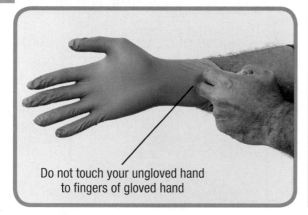

Do not touch your ungloved hand to fingers of gloved hand

3 Put on other glove.

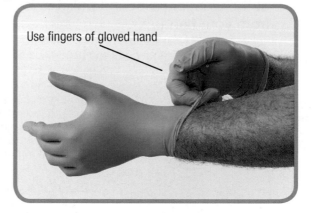

Use fingers of gloved hand

2 • Acting in an Emergency

Other PPE Devices

Other PPE devices include eye protection, masks and gowns or aprons. These are not required in most first aid situations, although OSHA requires such protections be available in some workplaces. In such cases, OSHA requires employees to be trained in the use of this PPE. Health care workers, for example, are required to wear masks and protective eyewear or face shields during procedures that are likely to generate droplets of blood or body fluids and gowns or aprons when blood or body fluid may be splashed.

Disposal and Disinfection of Supplies and Equipment

Preventing disease transmission also involves correct disposal or disinfection of used first aid supplies and equipment after caring for a victim.

First aid kits include many disposable supplies, such as dressings and bandages, that may become soiled by a victim's blood or other body fluids. These must be appropriately disposed of because such items may remain infectious for some time after use. Never reuse any equipment or supplies that are meant to be disposable. Other equipment, such as tweezers, require disinfection after use.

If EMS arrives to care for a victim of an emergency, they will usually manage the disposal of any soiled or infectious materials resulting from first aid care you have given. When professional rescuers are not involved, however, you need to ensure that soiled materials do not come into contact with other people. Many workplaces have a system in place for disposing of hazardous

(continues on page 27)

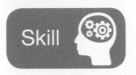

Skill **Removing Contaminated Gloves**

1 With one hand, grasp your other glove at the wrist or palm and pull it away from your hand.

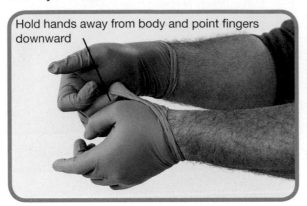

Hold hands away from body and point fingers downward

2 Pull the glove the rest of the way off.

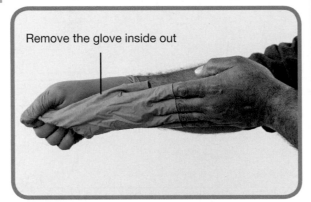

Remove the glove inside out

3 Holding the removed glove balled up in the palm of your gloved hand, insert two fingers under the cuff of the remaining glove.

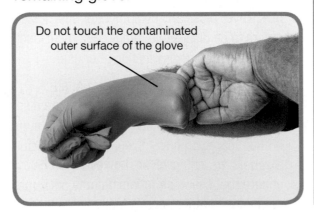

Do not touch the contaminated outer surface of the glove

4 Remove the glove by stretching it up and away from the hand and turning it inside out as you pull it off.

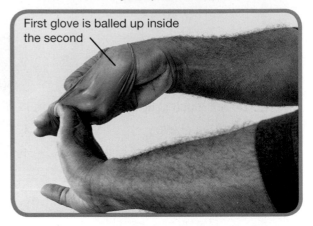

First glove is balled up inside the second

5 Dispose of gloves in a biohazard container and wash your hands.

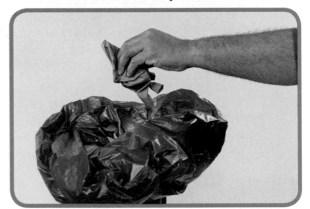

Learning Checkpoint 1

1. True or False: Bloodborne diseases are transmitted only through contact with an infected person's blood.

2. True or False: The risk of contracting a serious infectious disease by giving first aid is greatly reduced when you take precautions.

3. Standard precautions include:

   a. Treat all victims as if their body fluids are infected.

   b. Always wear gloves if blood may be present.

   c. Do not touch your mouth, nose or eyes when giving first aid.

   d. All of the above

4. Check off which of the following situations could lead to your getting an infectious disease.

   ____ a. Touching a bloody bandage in a trash can

   ____ b. Shaking hands with a person infected with HIV

   ____ c. Receiving a hepatitis B vaccination

   ____ d. Not wearing gloves and giving first aid if you have a cut on your finger

   ____ e. Being near a person with hepatitis C who is coughing

   ____ f. Contact with an unresponsive victim's urine

5. List at least three symptoms of a latex glove allergy.

(continued from page 25)

wastes; follow your company's policy. In the home, soiled supplies should be sealed inside a heavy plastic bag that is then sealed inside a second bag before being put in the trash. Make sure others do not come into contact with this trash. For contaminated sharps, such as needles used for insulin injections or lancets used to draw blood for glucose testing, special containers are required to prevent risks to those handling the trash. Talk with your health care provider about how to properly dispose of these objects.

To disinfect equipment or surfaces that are soiled by blood or other body fluids, use a commercial body fluid disposal kit or a 10% solution of household bleach in water. Wear gloves and clean the items or area thoroughly. If clothing or other fabrics are soiled, wash them by themselves in hot, soapy water for at least 25 minutes. Be sure to take a shower and wash well because your skin may have been contaminated through the clothing.

Responding To Emergencies

There are six basic actions to take in any emergency:

1. Recognize the emergency.

2. Check the scene.

3. Check the victim.

4. Call 9-1-1 (when appropriate).

5. Give first aid.

6. Have the victim seek medical attention (when appropriate).

Recognize the Emergency

You usually recognize an emergency when you see one. You see an injured or ill victim, or someone acting strangely. You may hear sounds of an emergency and realize that someone may be hurt. For example, you might look in the door of a co-worker's office and see a coffee cup overturned on the desk and the telephone receiver off the hook – and then see the man collapsed on the other side of the desk. You may see a crushed bicycle unattended alongside the road – and after checking further, see a child lying in the ditch. In situations like this the victim's life may depend on someone recognizing the signs that something is wrong and taking the time to investigate.

Check the Scene

Once you realize there is an emergency and someone is injured or ill, before going to the victim look to see if there may be other victims. You may need to call immediately for help for multiple victims. Look for any clues that may help you to determine what happened and what first aid may be needed. Also, look for bystanders who may be able to help give first aid or to go to a telephone to call 9-1-1.

When we see that someone needs our help, our first tendency is often to rush in. In many emergency situations, however, hazards may be present at the scene. For example, if you saw smoke coming out of a window of a house where you know an elderly man lives, your first thought might be to rush inside to rescue him. Consider, however, that you too might be overcome by smoke. Not only would you not have helped the original victim, but you would have become a second victim yourself for others to rescue and care for.

Therefore it is important, when you recognize that an emergency has occurred, to always check the scene before approaching a victim. Remember that you must be safe yourself if you are to help another. Look for any hazards such as the following:

- Smoke or flames
- Spilled gasoline or chemicals, fumes
- Downed electrical wires
- Risk of explosion or building collapse
- Roadside dangers or high-speed traffic

- Deep water or ice
- Potential for violence from someone present at the scene

If the scene is dangerous and you cannot safely approach the victim, *stay away and call for help*. Remember that help is usually only minutes away. The 9-1-1 dispatcher will send a crew with the appropriate training and equipment to safely reach and care for the victim. You may be able to monitor the scene from a safe distance and provide responding EMS personnel with critical information such as the location of the victim. **Box 2-3** describes some specific examples of hazardous situations.

Scene safety also includes protecting yourself from exposure to potentially infectious body fluids or other materials. As you approach a victim, for example, consider the need for using PPE as discussed earlier in this chapter.

Check the Victim

When you reach the victim, first check for life-threatening conditions requiring immediate first aid. These include being unresponsive, not breathing normally or severe bleeding. If the victim does not have a life-threatening condition, you then go on to look for lesser conditions requiring first aid. **Chapter 4** describes in detail both of these assessments. Unless the scene is dangerous or it is necessary to care for a life-threatening problem, do not move the victim. **Chapter 24** describes how to move a victim when necessary.

Call 9-1-1

Call 9-1-1 (or your local or company emergency number) immediately if you recognize a life-threatening injury or illness. Do not try to transport a victim to the emergency department yourself in such cases. In some exceptional circumstances you may give about two minutes of care before calling 9-1-1.

If the victim is responsive and may not be seriously injured or ill, go on to the next step to check the victim further before calling 9-1-1 – and then call 9-1-1 or a health care provider if needed.

BOX 2-3: HAZARDOUS SCENES

Traffic Collisions

Vehicle crash scenes can be extremely dangerous for rescuers because of the risks from passing vehicles, downed electrical wires, fire or explosion, vehicle instability, or other conditions. Rescuers have also been injured by unintentionally setting off an automatic airbag when attempting to reach a victim pinned inside a vehicle. For all of these reasons it is crucial to ensure that the scene is safe before approaching the vehicle. Do not try to stabilize the vehicle unless you have special training. Never try to remove a victim trapped inside a vehicle, but wait for professional rescuers. You may be able to provide some first aid through an open window or from the back seat.

Fire Scenes

Never enter a burning or smoky building unless you have special training and are functioning as a part of a fire department. Firefighters are highly trained and use special equipment that protects against fire and smoke. Do not let others enter or approach a fire scene. Make sure 9-1-1 has been called and then try to gather information for responding fire and EMS units, such as the possible number and location of victims, the cause of the fire, the presence of any explosives or chemicals and other relevant facts.

Electricity

Downed electrical lines at an emergency scene are a major hazard to both the victim and rescuers. Never try to move downed wires; instead, call 9-1-1 immediately. If downed wires are across a vehicle, do not touch the vehicle. If victims are in the vehicle, tell them to remain still and not exit the vehicle. Never attempt to remove a victim from a vehicle with a downed wire across it, no matter how seriously injured the victim may be. If downed wires are across a chain link fence, metal structure or body of water, do not approach the scene.

Water and Ice Hazards

Water and ice create several hazards. Never enter deep water to reach a victim unless you have been properly trained, and then do so only as a last resort. Instead, try to get a flotation device or rope to the victim (See **Chapter 24**). Fast-flowing water is a common hazard following natural disasters such as floods and hurricanes. Never enter moving water; instead, wait for trained rescue personnel. A fast-water rescue requires careful planning, proper equipment and training. Ice is also treacherous. Cold-water immersion is very serious and can quickly doom even the best swimmers. Ice rescue should be left for specially trained personnel who have the necessary safety equipment.

Natural Disasters

Natural disasters include such events as tornadoes, hurricanes, earthquakes, forest and range fires, and floods. Rescue efforts after a natural disaster are usually coordinated through a federal or state emergency management agency. If you find yourself in a natural disaster, make personal safety your highest priority. Natural disasters often involve more hazards than you might think, including electrical risks, hazardous materials and fast-moving water (See Appendices C, D, E and F).

Hazardous Materials

A hazardous material is any substance, liquid or solid, that is highly flammable, explosive, caustic, toxic, radioactive or otherwise dangerous. Hazardous materials are usually marked with warning placards **(Figure 2-5)**, but treat any unknown substance as a hazard until proven otherwise. Avoid any spilled liquid or powder as well as possible fumes. Especially dangerous is a vehicular collision involving a truck carrying hazardous materials. Stay well out of the area of a hazardous material spill and keep bystanders away. Call 9-1-1 and let trained hazmat professionals handle the emergency.

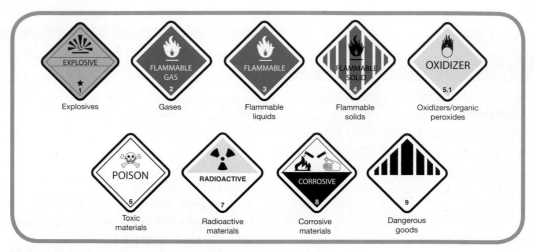

Figure 2-5 *A variety of hazardous materials placards.*

BOX 2-3: HAZARDOUS SCENES (continued)

Hazardous materials are not limited to industrial sites and transportation. There are many potential hazards in the home, including natural gas, gasoline, kerosene, pesticides and others. Many hazardous materials are odorless and not easily detected. Some hazardous materials, such as natural gas, are explosion hazards. A seemingly harmless action such as turning on a light switch or using a cell phone may create a spark and set off an explosion.

Unsafe Buildings/Structures

Buildings and other structures may be unsafe because of fire, an explosion, a natural disaster or deterioration. Never enter an unsafe building alone because of the risk of collapsing structures, hazardous materials, fire and so on. Call 9-1-1 and let properly trained and equipped professionals manage the rescue.

Wreckage

Wreckage from an automobile, aircraft or machinery is hazardous because of the presence of sharp pieces of metal, glass, fuel and moving parts. The wreckage may also be unstable. Stay away from the scene and call 9-1-1.

Suicide

If a person is threatening suicide and has a weapon, do not enter the scene – call 9-1-1 or law enforcement personnel. **Chapter 21** discusses behavioral emergencies such as suicidal or potentially violent victims.

Hostile Victim/Family

Occasionally a victim or family member may be hostile when you approach or offer first aid. Rage or hostility in a victim may be due to the injury or illness or to emotional factors. Many emergency victims are afraid of losing control, and their fear may become anger. Drug or alcohol abuse may also cause hostile behavior. If a victim seems hostile, first try to quietly explain who you are and that you are there to help. Often after the victim realizes that you are not a threat but are there to help, the hostility will dissipate. But if the victim refuses your care or threatens you, retreat from the scene and call 9-1-1. Never try to restrain, argue with or force care upon a victim. **Chapter 21** discusses how to deal with behavioral emergencies such as violent people.

Hostile family members also can be a problem, usually because they are fearful. Listen to what they have to say and act accordingly. If the situation remains hostile, retreat to a safe distance and wait for police officers and other EMS personnel. If at any time your personal safety appears threatened, leave the scene immediately.

Give First Aid

Give first aid once you have checked the victim and know his or her condition. Later chapters describe the first aid for the conditions you are likely to find. **Basic life support** is first aid given to a victim with a life-threatening problem involving breathing or circulation. Generally you provide basic life support to keep the victim alive until advanced help arrives. In most cases, however, the victim's condition is not life-threatening and your first aid consists of simple actions you can take to help the victim.

Note that first aiders do not administer medications to victims because of the risks of allergy or other complications. In some cases first aiders may help victims to take their own medications if needed.

Have the Victim Seek Medical Attention

As noted earlier, call 9-1-1 immediately for any emergency (life-threatening) condition. In many cases the injury or sudden illness is not an emergency and you do not need to call 9-1-1, but the victim still needs to see a health care provider. For example, a victim may have a serious cut on the arm that stops bleeding quickly when you give first aid. Because of the risk of infection, or because the cut may need stitches to heal well, the victim needs medical attention and should be transported to a hospital emergency department or his or her health care provider. Later chapters about specific injuries and problems describe when a victim needs to go to the emergency department or see a health care provider. When in doubt, call a health care provider to see if medical care may be needed.

After An Emergency

Arriving EMS professionals will take over the care of the victim **(Figure 2-6)**. Continue giving first aid until EMS personnel ask you to stop, as it may take a few minutes for emergency responders to prepare equipment and take over. Then you may still assist with crowd control, obtaining information from bystanders or assisting the emergency responders in other ways. Depending on the situation, you may have other follow-up activities. If the emergency

was traumatic or especially stressful, you may also need help coping with the effects of stress.

After giving first aid, be sure to wash your hands and clean the area well. If the emergency involved bleeding or contamination of the area with other body fluids, disinfect surfaces using a 10% bleach solution or other approved disinfectant. Dispose of all potentially contaminated materials appropriately. If you were in contact with any of the victim's body fluids, report this to the emergency responders so they can take appropriate action.

Follow-Up Activities

Arriving EMS professionals who take over the care of the victim will ask you questions about what happened, what you observed about the victim and what first aid you gave. Answer as fully as you can, because the details you provide may be important for the victim's medical care. Review the entire experience in your mind to make sure you have not forgotten to relay some important piece of information. For example, a victim who became unresponsive while you were giving him first aid may have experienced a poisoning, and anything the victim said or did when you first saw him may offer medical workers a clue about his condition.

Your descriptions to EMS personnel of what happened and what you did may be, in some situations, a form of legal documentation of actions. If you have any reason to think you may

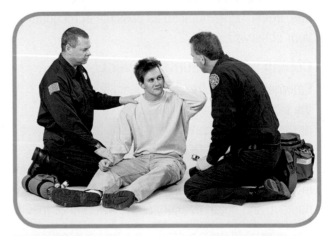

Figure 2-6 *EMS personnel with advanced training will take over care of an injured or ill victim after 9-1-1 is called.*

Learning Checkpoint 2

1. True or False: If you see someone injured in an emergency, the first thing to do is get to him or her quickly and check his or her condition.

2. When you encounter an injured victim, you should —

   a. give first aid until help arrives.

   b. help a victim only if the scene is safe.

   c. call 9-1-1 for life-threatening injuries.

   d. All of the above

3. Which of the following scenes are unsafe?

   ___ Spilled hazardous materials

   ___ Structure fires

   ___ Downed electrical wires

   ___ Hostile person with a weapon

be questioned in the future about your actions, it may be helpful to write down what happened and exactly what you did.

Some emergencies may be related to a crime, such as injuries resulting from an assault or abuse. In such cases the first responders to the scene will help ensure that possible evidence is not destroyed or altered, and law enforcement officials will arrive to preserve and investigate the scene. If you gave first aid to the victim of a crime, your descriptions of what you witnessed may become legal evidence. It is important to cooperate fully with police officers and, again, be as detailed as possible in recounting your observations.

Coping with a Traumatic Event

Emergencies are stressful, especially when the victim does not survive. Not even medical professionals can save every victim. Injuries, illness or circumstances are often beyond our control. Particularly stressful emergencies include those that involve multiple victims, children, victims of abuse or neglect, and death or injury of a co-worker or friend.

It is normal to have a strong emotional reaction during and immediately after a stressful emergency. Often this reaction diminishes with time, but in some cases the stress remains and problems may result. Stress can cause irritability when interacting with others, difficulty sleeping, problems concentrating, general anxiety or depression, and even physical symptoms. If you recognize that you are feeling or behaving differently after experiencing a traumatic emergency, you may need help coping.

- Talk to others: family members, co-workers, local emergency responders or your own health care provider (without breaching the confidentiality of the victim).

- Remind yourself that your reaction is normal, and that we all need help sometimes.

- Do not be afraid or reluctant to seek professional help. Students should ask at the student health center and workers should check with their human resources department about an employee assistance program or member assistance program. Your health care provider can also make a referral.

Concluding Thoughts

Emergency situations vary widely, but in all cases you respond to the emergency in the same basic way: Make sure the scene is safe, check the victim for life-threatening conditions and call 9-1-1, and give the appropriate first aid using standard precautions to minimize your exposure to infectious disease. These principles for acting in an emergency not only guide your response but also ensure your safety while you give the most effective care to someone in need.

Learning Outcomes

You should now be able to do the following:

1. Explain how bloodborne pathogens may be transmitted from an infected person to someone else.

2. List several common serious bloodborne diseases.

3. Describe standard precautions to take to prevent disease transmission when giving first aid.

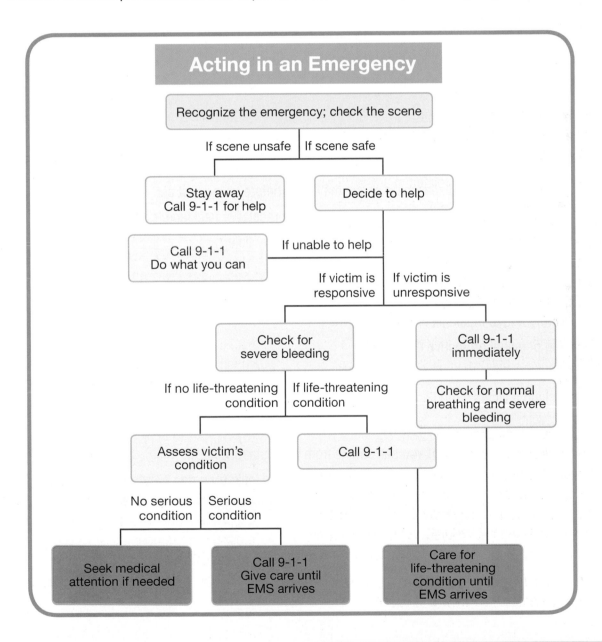

Review Questions

1. A bloodborne pathogen can easily enter your body through –

    a. any break in your skin.

    b. food cooked by someone else.

    c. the municipal water supply.

    d. any physical touching of the victim's skin.

2. Bloodborne pathogens may also be transmitted in –

    a. semen.

    b. vaginal secretions.

    c. bloody vomit.

    d. All of the above

3. HIV infection can be prevented when giving first aid by –

    a. avoiding all contact with known HIV-positive individuals.

    b. following standard precautions.

    c. getting vaccinated.

    d. wearing a face mask.

4. An effective way to avoid becoming infected when giving first aid is to –

    a. ask the victim what diseases he or she may have before giving first aid.

    b. check an unresponsive victim for a medical alert bracelet or necklace.

    c. use barriers to prevent contact with any blood or body fluid.

    d. never touch the victim.

5. Standard precautions include –

    a. wearing a face mask.

    b. using personal protective equipment.

    c. asking a victim about any communicable diseases before giving first aid.

    d. checking a victim's medical record after giving first aid.

6. If you believe someone may be inside a house where you see smoke coming from a window, you should –

    a. enter only the first floor if you see smoke from an upstairs window.

    b. take a deep breath and hold it while you run inside to look; try not to breathe once inside.

    c. search the house, staying low to the floor on hands and knees.

    d. not go inside but call 9-1-1 immediately.

7. You witness a low-speed car crash into a telephone pole. The driver has no obvious wounds and says he is okay. But he has not moved from behind the wheel and he looks pale and shaky. What should you do?

a. Call 9-1-1 and let the dispatcher decide what help may be needed.

b. Call 9-1-1 only if the driver first gives his consent for you to call.

c. Ask the driver to get into your vehicle so you can drive him to the nearest hospital.

d. Wait for a police car to stop; the officer will decide whether help is needed.

8. When you have given first aid to a victim, you should tell arriving EMS personnel –

a. what happened.

b. what you observed about the victim.

c. what first aid you gave.

d. All of the above

Chapter 3 • The Human Body

Chapter Preview

- Primary Areas of the Body
- Body Systems
- The Respiratory System
- The Cardiovascular System
- The Nervous System
- The Musculoskeletal System
- The Integumentary System
- The Gastrointestinal System
- The Lymphatic and Immune System
- The Endocrine System
- The Urinary System
- The Reproductive System

You are called to the storage area at the back of the warehouse where an employee has just been found lying on the floor. As you approach, you believe she may have fallen from the stepladder or a higher shelf, but you do not immediately see what is wrong.

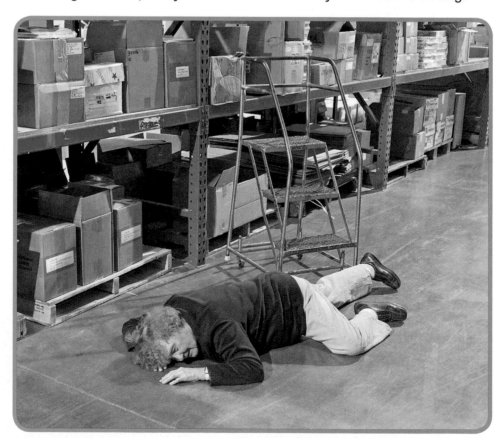

The human body is composed of many different organs and tissues, all working together to sustain life and allow for activity. In health, each organ performs its functions in concert with other body parts and organs. With injury or illness, however, one or more parts of the body are damaged or functioning less effectively. A minor injury may damage only a specific body part or function, but a serious injury or sudden illness can threaten body functions that are necessary for life. Understanding the human body will help you recognize the effects of injuries and illnesses and give effective first aid until the victim receives medical attention.

Primary Areas of the Body

A detailed understanding of medical language is not necessary for giving first aid and communicating with medical professionals, or when speaking with the 9-1-1 dispatcher. It is helpful, however, to understand the general areas of the body when describing an injury or the victim's signs and symptoms of illness. Following are key terms referring to major body areas **(Figure 3-1)**:

- *Extremities*. This refers to both the arms and the legs. Many first aid principles are the same for all the extremities, so this term is often used rather than saying "arms and legs."

- *Thorax*. This refers to the chest area enclosed by the ribs (including the back of the body). The thoracic cavity is the area inside the chest where the heart and lungs are located.

- *Abdomen*. This refers to the area immediately below the thoracic cavity. The stomach, intestines and other organs are located in the abdominal cavity. For the purposes of describing the location of injuries or signs and symptoms, the abdomen is often divided into quadrants based on the body's midline and an imaginary horizontal line through the umbilicus (navel) **(Figure 3-2)**. The **diaphragm**, the primary muscle used in breathing, is located between the thoracic cavity and the abdominal cavity.

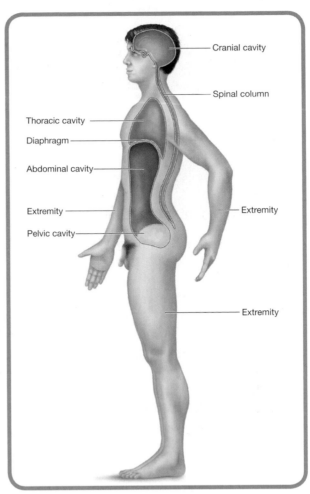

Figure 3-1 *Major areas of the body.*

- *Pelvis*. This refers generally to the area below the abdomen and specifically to the pelvic bones between the hip and the lower spine. The bladder and reproductive organs are located in the pelvic cavity.

- *Spine (spinal column)*. This **refers to the bones (vertebrae) of the back and neck extending from the base of the brain to the tailbone**, as well as to the **nerves, or spinal cord**, running through the vertebrae. *Spine* is generally used in first aid to refer to injuries to these bones or nerves rather than the less specific words *neck* or *back*.

With these terms you can generally describe the location of injuries and symptoms. Although health care professionals use a variety of directional and spatial terms to pinpoint exact locations in the body, first aiders can successfully communicate

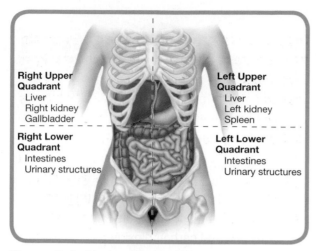

Figure 3-2 *Abdominal quadrants.*

locations with general words such as *above* or *below, left* and *right* and so on. Remember that *left* and *right* refer to the *victim's* left and right sides – not yours when facing the victim.

Body Systems

Life depends on the body carrying out a number of important functions, such as taking oxygen from the air and transporting it to all body cells, extracting nutrients from food, removing wastes, and managing the growth and repair of injured cells. An **organ** is a body part that accomplishes one or more specific functions. In most cases, several organs work together to achieve a larger body function. For example, the stomach and intestines accomplish much of the digestive process, but the gallbladder, pancreas and liver also play important roles. The combination of organs that work together to perform a major body function is called a **body system**. Following are brief descriptions of some of the primary functions of the different body systems. Each is described more fully later in this chapter along with its relevance to first aid.

- *Respiratory system.* Provides the oxygen needed by body cells and removes the waste product (carbon dioxide).

- *Cardiovascular system.* Moves the blood, which transports both oxygen and nutrients, throughout the body to supply cells and remove wastes.

- *Nervous system.* Controls all body functions and movement and allows for sensory perception and consciousness.

- *Musculoskeletal system.* Gives the body shape and strength and makes movement possible.

- *Integumentary system (skin and related structures).* Protects the body from the environment and germs and helps regulate body temperature.

- *Gastrointestinal system.* Extracts nutrients from food to meet the body's needs for energy and eliminates solid wastes.

- *Immune system.* Helps fight disease.

- *Endocrine system.* Produces hormones that help regulate many body functions.

- *Urinary system.* Removes liquid wastes from the body and helps maintain the body's water balance.

- *Reproductive system.* Makes human reproduction possible.

Although we sometimes talk about each system as if it were separate from others, body systems are closely interrelated and work together to perform many functions. For example, blood is part of the cardiovascular system, which pumps it to all areas of the body. Blood carries oxygen from the lungs (respiratory system) to the body cells, all of which need a continuous supply of oxygen to stay alive. Nerve sensors (nervous system) detect the amount of oxygen and carbon dioxide in the blood and speed up or slow down the heartbeat and breathing rate to control the oxygen level. If body temperature drops, muscles of the extremities (musculoskeletal system) may start shivering to produce heat, which is carried by the blood to vital organs. The kidneys (urinary system) filter the blood to remove waste products, which leave the body through the urine. These are just a few examples of the many complex ways body systems work together.

As you learn about different kinds of first aid throughout this text, remember that different parts of the body are often closely related. This will help you understand what is happening in the body during periods of injury and illness so you can provide first aid most effectively. For example, in someone with asthma, inhaling a substance such as smoke may cause muscles in the airway to spasm and swell, making breathing difficult. As oxygen levels in the blood reaching the brain drop, the person feels dizzy. Changes then occur in the respiratory, cardiovascular and nervous systems. In this case, understanding how a breathing problem can affect a victim's mental status (responsiveness) can help you focus on correcting the cause.

As you will learn in later chapters, life-threatening injuries and illnesses most often affect the respiratory, circulatory and nervous systems. Problems affecting these systems may impair the essential delivery of oxygen to body tissues, leading to death. First aiders, therefore, must first assess a victim for problems related to breathing and circulation and then assess problems related to other body systems.

The Respiratory System

The primary organs of the respiratory system are the structures of the airway and the lungs **(Figure 3-3)**. The **airway** is the path air takes from the nose and mouth to the lungs. Air entering the nose or mouth passes through the **pharynx** (throat) to the **trachea** (windpipe). The trachea branches into the left and right **bronchi** (singular: bronchus), the passageways into the lungs. The bronchi branch into smaller tubular passages in the lungs and eventually end in the **alveoli**, the tiny air sacs where oxygen and carbon dioxide pass into and out of small blood vessels called capillaries.

Because the pharynx also leads to the **esophagus**, the tube that carries food to the stomach, another structure, called the **epiglottis**, is very important for breathing. The epiglottis is a tissue flap that prevents solids and liquids from entering the trachea and blocking the airway or reaching the lungs. The epiglottis directs food and drink to pass from the throat to the esophagus and stomach.

Breathing depends on muscular movements that are under the control of the nervous system. When

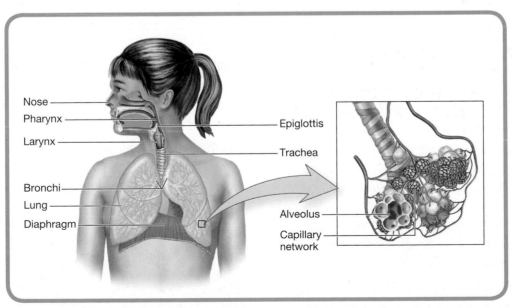

Figure 3-3 *The respiratory system.*

Nose
Pharynx
Larynx
Bronchi
Lung
Diaphragm
Epiglottis
Trachea
Alveolus
Capillary network

Table 3-1: Normal Reference Values for Breathing Rate

	Breaths per minute
Adult	12-20
Child	15-30
Infant	25-50

the **diaphragm** (the large muscle below the lungs) contracts, the thoracic cavity and lungs expand, pulling air into the lungs from which oxygen can move into the blood. When the diaphragm relaxes, the size of the thoracic cavity is reduced and air carrying out carbon dioxide flows back out of the lungs. **Table 3-1** provides some normal reference values for breathing.

The main function of the respiratory system is to allow oxygen to enter the blood from air that is breathed in (inhaled) and to remove carbon dioxide, a waste product of respiration, from the blood into air that is breathed out (exhaled). This is called **external respiration**. **Internal respiration** is the process of oxygen and carbon dioxide moving into and out of the blood within internal body tissues.

Emergencies Related to the Respiratory System

Respiration is one of the most vital functions in the body, and many different injuries and illnesses can affect it. Any factor that impedes the flow of air into and out of the lungs can affect respiration and become life-threatening. An **airway obstruction** is a physical blockage of the airway that prevents the flow of air. For example, a person who is eating may have a piece of food lodged in the pharynx, a condition called **choking**. In an unconscious person lying on his or her back, the tongue may block the opening into the pharynx. An injury to the head or neck may also cause the soft tissues of the upper airway to swell and obstruct the airway. All of these are life-threatening situations.

Another potential problem with the airway is a failure of the epiglottis to prevent substances from entering the trachea. The swallowing reflex normally prevents this, but in an unconscious person this reflex may not be functioning. This can result in liquids or solids entering the trachea and lungs. For example, an unconscious person lying on his or her back may vomit, and the vomit may flow back down the throat and into the trachea and lungs, impeding respiration and possibly causing a severe lung infection. This is one reason why an unresponsive victim is never given anything to drink – the fluid may flow into the lungs.

Chest injuries may also affect respiration. A broken rib may puncture a lung, making breathing ineffective. A penetrating injury into the lungs from the outside, such as that caused by a bullet or sharp object, may alter the lung pressures needed for inhaling and keep the lungs from filling with air.

Because breathing is controlled by the brain, other factors that affect the nervous system may also cause respiratory emergencies. A poisoning or drug overdose, for example, may severely depress nervous system functions, slowing breathing to the point where the body is not getting enough oxygen. An electric shock may interrupt the normal nervous system control of respiration and cause breathing to stop.

Finally, some illnesses also cause breathing difficulties. Asthma is a common condition, especially in children, in which airway tissues swell and make it hard for the person to breathe. Chronic lung diseases, more common in the elderly and in smokers, may reduce lung functioning so much that the person struggles to catch a breath.

If the body is not receiving enough oxygen, other organs will begin to fail. The heart will soon stop and brain cells will begin to die within minutes. In **Chapter 5** you will learn how to recognize breathing emergencies and the appropriate first aid to give victims depending on the cause.

The Cardiovascular System

The cardiovascular system consists of the heart, blood and blood vessels **(Figure 3-4)**. The primary functions of the cardiovascular system are to transport oxygen and nutrients in the blood to all parts of the body and to remove carbon dioxide and other wastes from tissues. Other functions include transporting hormones that regulate other body functions, helping regulate body temperature, transporting cells and substances that fight infection, and helping maintain the body's fluid balance.

The heart has four chambers: the left and right atria and the left and right ventricles. The **ventricles** pump the blood through two loops, or cycles, in the body. First, blood is pumped to the lungs to pick up oxygen and release carbon dioxide. The blood returns to the heart, which pumps it to all areas of the body, releasing oxygen for use by body cells and picking up carbon dioxide for removal. The term **cardiac** refers to the heart. The heart is also part of the body's muscular system, as the heart is composed of a unique kind of muscle (**myocardium**) that contracts to make the pumping action. This pumping action, called **contraction**, is controlled by electrical signals that are in turn controlled by the nervous system.

The blood flows from the heart to body areas through an extensive network of **arteries** **(Figure 3-5)**. With the heartbeat, pulsing **blood pressure** changes occur in the arteries that can be felt in certain body locations as the **pulse**. Arteries progressively branch into smaller vessels that eventually reach **capillaries**, which are very small blood vessels with thin walls where oxygen and carbon dioxide are exchanged with body cells. From the capillaries the blood drains back to the heart through an equally extensive system of **veins**. Blood flows more evenly through veins, which do not have a pulse. Arteries are generally deeper in the body than veins and are therefore more protected and less likely to be damaged by injuries.

The heart rate, which can be measured as the pulse, is affected by many factors. With exercise, fever, or emotional excitement, the heart rate increases to meet the body's greater need for oxygen. Various

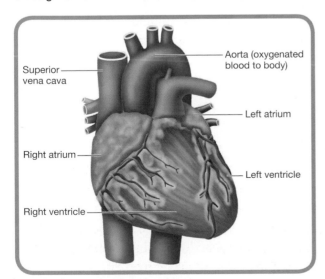

Figure 3-4 *The heart.*

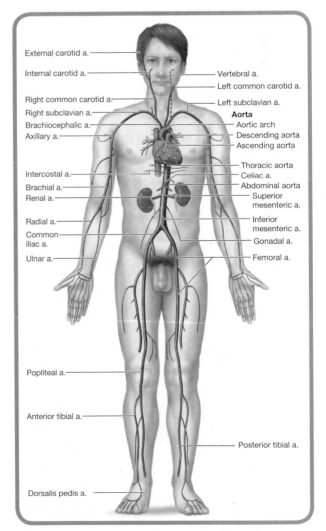

Figure 3-5 *Major arteries of the body.*

injuries and illnesses may either increase or decrease the heart rate. **Table 3-2** provides some normal reference values for heart rate.

Emergencies Related to the Cardiovascular System

As with the respiratory system, the cardiovascular system's functions are vital for life, health and well-being. The most vital function is carrying oxygen to the body's tissues. As noted earlier, cells begin to die in vital organs such as the brain after only a few minutes without oxygen. Any injury or illness that affects respiration, therefore, also diminishes the ability of the cardiovascular system to deliver oxygen to the body.

Blood vessel problems may also affect cardiovascular functioning. Bleeding, which often occurs with injuries, may be so severe that not

Table 3-2: **Normal Reference Values for Heart Rate**	
	Beats per minute
Adult	60-100
Child	60-150
Infant	120-150

enough blood is left in circulation to adequately provide the oxygen the body needs.

Arterial bleeding is most severe because the blood may spurt out under pressure, leading within minutes to the life-threatening condition called **shock**. Shock occurs when vital body organs are not receiving enough oxygen (see **Chapter 9**).

 ## Learning Checkpoint 1

1. Name two organs inside the thoracic cavity.

   _____

2. Which of the following is a function of the respiratory system?

   a. Inhaling and exhaling

   b. Moving oxygen into the blood

   c. Moving carbon dioxide out of body tissues

   d. All of the above

3. At what structure is an airway obstruction most likely to occur?

   _____

4. The heart pumps blood to all body tissues through which blood vessels?

   a. Arteries

   b. Veins

   c. Capillaries

   d. All of the above

5. Check off which cardiac problems can affect tissue oxygenation.

   ___ Cardiac arrest   ___ Diabetes

   ___ Kidney failure   ___ Myocardial infarction

   ___ Asthma   ___ Tetanus infection

   ___ Dysrhythmia

Bleeding from veins is generally slower but can still be serious or life-threatening if it continues. Capillary bleeding is generally minor and usually stops by itself as the blood clots. **Chapter 8** describes the first aid techniques to control bleeding.

Stroke is another type of blood vessel problem involving arteries in the brain. A blood clot or bleeding in the brain may reduce circulation to a part of the brain, causing mental and physical impairments. **Chapter 16** describes the first aid for stroke.

Problems involving the heart can also affect tissue oxygenation. Some conditions, such as congestive heart failure, reduce the heart's ability to pump to effectively meet the body's needs. If the heart muscle itself does not receive enough oxygenated blood because of blocked cardiac arteries, part of the heart muscle may die. This is called a heart attack, or **myocardial infarction**. The heart may also stop (**cardiac arrest**), in which case the person needs CPR, as described in **Chapter 5**. Dysrhythmia, or an abnormal heartbeat, is another type of heart problem that may reduce the heart's pumping effectiveness.

The Nervous System

The nervous system has three general sets of functions:

1. Sensory receptors in the skin, eyes, ears, nose and mouth, as well as throughout the body, gather information about the internal and external environment and send this information to the brain.

2. The brain integrates and analyzes information, both consciously and automatically, for immediate and future uses.

3. Nerve signals from the brain lead to movements and other actions throughout the body to accomplish specific tasks or to maintain **homeostasis**, a balanced state within the body necessary for effective functioning.

The nervous system controls the actions of most other body systems. For example, when nervous system receptors detect a low level of oxygen in the blood, the brain directs the muscles of breathing to speed up the respiratory rate and the heart to beat faster to ensure that the body gets enough oxygen.

The brain controls the nervous system (**Figure 3-6**). Specific areas in the brain control different functions, such as controlling heart rate, storing memories, creating visual images and directing muscle movements. The brain connects directly with the spinal cord, the pathway to and from nerves throughout the body. The brain and spinal cord form the **central nervous system**. After

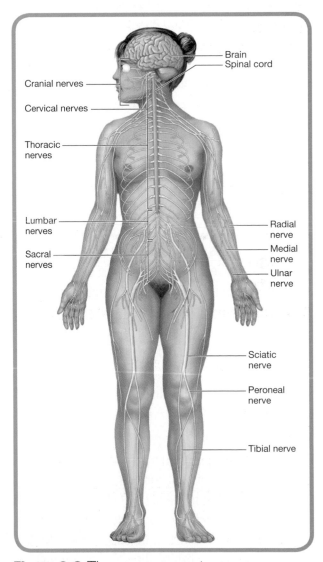

Figure 3-6 *The nervous system.*

leaving the skull the spinal cord is encased inside vertebrae, the bones of the spine **(Figure 3-7)**. Nerves project out from the spinal cord between the vertebrae of the neck and back and extend throughout the body. Generally, nerves exiting the spinal cord nearer the top control movement and other functions higher in the body, and nerves from the spinal cord nearer the bottom control functions lower in the body.

Emergencies Related to the Nervous System

Injury or illness affecting the nervous system can have general or very specific effects on the body. Head and spinal injuries can have serious or life-threatening effects. An injury to a part of the brain, or a disease process such as a stroke that damages a particular brain area, may destroy or impair the function of that brain tissue. If the respiratory center in the brain is damaged, the person may stop breathing. If a muscle control center is damaged, a part of the body may be paralyzed. Head injuries may also cause bleeding or swelling of the brain. Because the brain is tightly encased in the skull, bleeding or swelling puts pressure on the brain and may cause more widespread effects.

Brain functions can also be more generally affected by injury or illness. **Altered mental status** is a phrase used to describe changes in a person's responsiveness, such as becoming confused, disoriented, lethargic or comatose. Altered mental status may result from such things as head injuries; any injury causing reduced oxygenation; and sudden illness such as stroke, seizure, diabetic emergencies, severe infection, high fever, poisoning or drug overdose. **Chapter 16** describes the first aid for such emergencies.

Damage to the spinal cord may occur at any level between the base of the skull and the lower back. Significant damage to the cord, such as complete severing caused by a neck or back fracture, often results in a complete loss of function in body areas controlled by nerves exiting the spine below that level. A lower back injury may result in a loss of

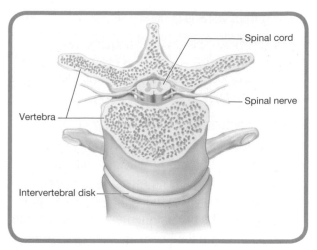

Figure 3-7 *The spinal cord.*

feeling in the legs and inability to move the legs (**paralysis**). A similar injury to the spinal cord in the neck area may result in paralysis and loss of feeling in the entire body below the neck. The neck is a particularly vulnerable area because any trauma to the head, such as the head being snapped forward in a vehicle crash or striking a hard object after diving in shallow water, may injure neck vertebrae and the spinal cord. **Chapter 12** describes how to assess an injured victim for a possible head or spine injury and how to protect the spinal cord from additional injury caused by movement.

In addition to head and spinal injuries, injuries elsewhere in the body, as well as some illnesses, also affect the nervous system. Pain will result from damage to nerve fibers in many areas of the body and therefore pain is always assessed as a symptom that may reveal something about a victim's injury or illness. The pain caused by injured nerves in a cut finger is obvious, but pain within the body is not always so clear-cut. A crushing pain in the chest that extends into the left arm may be caused by a heart attack. Abdominal pain that begins in the area of the umbilicus (navel) and then settles into the lower abdomen on the right side may be a sign of appendicitis. Although pain is not always present with serious conditions, pain should be taken seriously whenever it occurs. The level of pain, however, should not be taken as an indicator of the severity of an injury or illness.

The Musculoskeletal System

The musculoskeletal system combines two closely related body systems and is composed of bones, muscles and the structures that join them (ligaments and tendons). The bones of the body have several functions **(Figure 3-8)**:

- The skeleton provides shape and support for the body as a whole.

- Groups of bones protect vital internal organs (e.g., the ribs protect the heart and lungs, the skull protects the brain, the vertebrae protect the spinal cord).

- Bone marrow inside certain bones produces blood cells.

- Bones store calcium for use by the rest of the body when needed.

- Bones act as levers to allow movement at joints when muscles act on them.

Skeletal muscles attach to bones to create body movements **(Figure 3-9)**. Another function is to produce body heat through movement or shivering.

The phrase *musculoskeletal* usually refers to skeletal (voluntary) muscles, but the body also has other kinds of muscle tissue with special functions (called involuntary muscle tissue). As noted earlier, the heart's muscle tissue provides its beating force. The esophagus is a muscular tube with special movements that aid in swallowing and moving food to the stomach. Muscle tissue throughout the gastrointestinal system keeps the products of digestion moving through the digestive tract. The diaphragm is a thin muscle below the lungs that does the primary work of breathing. Muscle tissue inside blood vessels helps keep blood moving through the body. All muscle activity is controlled by the nervous system.

Tendons are fibrous tissues that connect muscles to bones. **Ligaments** are tough bands of tissue that join bones together at joints.

Emergencies Related to the Musculoskeletal System

Musculoskeletal injuries include fractures, dislocations, sprains and strains. A **fracture** is a broken bone. Although fractures can be serious

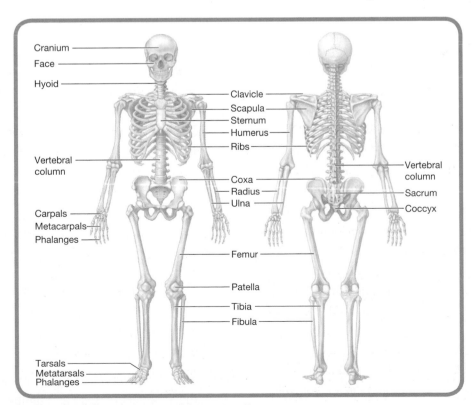

Figure 3-8 *Major bones of the body.*

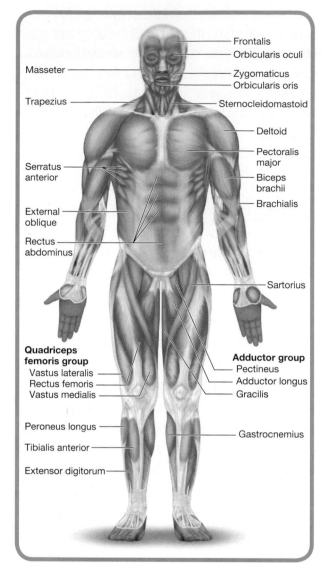

Figure 3-9 *Major muscles of the body.*

injuries, particularly when nearby organs or blood vessels are damaged by the broken bone ends, most fractures are not life-threatening. Dislocations and sprains are both joint injuries. In a **dislocation**, one or more bones move out of their normal position in a joint, preventing the joint from functioning as usual. Finger and shoulder dislocations are among the most common dislocations. A **sprain** is damage to ligaments and other structures in a joint; the ankle and wrist are commonly sprained by forces on these joints. A **strain** is a tearing of muscle or tendon tissue usually caused by overexertion of the muscle. All of these injuries require first aid, as you will learn in **Chapter 14**.

Musculoskeletal injuries are often associated with other injuries. Vertebral fractures are likely to injure the spinal cord and cause nervous system damage. Fractures of the **femur**, the long bone in the thigh, often cause much soft tissue damage and bleeding. A fracture of the pelvis may damage the bladder or other organs in the pelvic cavity. A skull fracture may cause brain damage.

The musculoskeletal system is also affected by illnesses, although most of these do not occur suddenly and therefore seldom require first aid. Arthritis (chronic joint inflammation causing pain and restricted motion), muscular dystrophy (disorders of progressive degeneration of muscles) and osteoarthritis (weakening of bones, usually with aging) are all common musculoskeletal system diseases.

The Integumentary System

The integumentary system consists of the skin, nails, hair and accessory structures such as sweat and oil glands **(Figure 3-10)**. The primary function of the skin is to protect the body from the external environment (temperature extremes, pathogens and other substances). Other functions include:

- *Regulating body temperature.* When the body is hot, blood vessels in the skin widen to bring heat to the surface to dissipate; sweating also helps cool the skin. When the body is cold, blood vessels constrict to conserve heat and muscle movements occur such as shivering and "goose bumps" (tiny muscle reactions in the hair follicles).

- *Preventing water loss from the body.* The skin acts as a barrier to prevent water loss.

- *Waste removal.* Through sweating, the skin removes some body wastes.

- *Vitamin production.* Skin cells produce vitamin D.

- *Sensation.* Nerve sensors in the skin react to touch, pressure, pain and temperature.

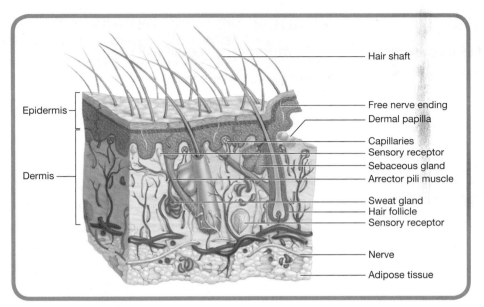

Figure 3-10 *Anatomy of the skin.*

Labels: Hair shaft, Free nerve ending, Dermal papilla, Capillaries, Sensory receptor, Sebaceous gland, Arrector pili muscle, Sweat gland, Hair follicle, Sensory receptor, Nerve, Adipose tissue, Epidermis, Dermis

Emergencies Related to the Integumentary System

Because skin is the organ most exposed to the environment, it is frequently damaged by traumatic injuries. Cuts and scrapes are common causes of bleeding. The blood vessels in the skin are relatively small, and bleeding from the skin seldom involves as much blood loss as from deeper blood vessels. Any openings in the skin, however, may allow pathogens into the body. As described in **Chapter 2**, **pathogens** are germs capable of causing disease, including bloodborne pathogens that can cause serious illnesses. Take precautions if you will be exposed to a victim's body fluids.

Exposure to temperature extremes can damage the skin. Skin exposed to freezing temperatures may get **frostbite**, in which tissue freezes and dies. Very high temperatures and many chemicals cause skin **burns**, which destroy tissue and may allow loss of body heat and body fluid (See **Chapter 11**). Because sunburn damages skin in a way that makes skin cancer more likely later on, precautions should be taken to protect the skin from sun exposure.

Although skin functions help regulate body temperature, when a person is exposed to cold or heat, regulatory mechanisms may not be able to keep the body at its normal temperature. The skin of a victim of hypothermia (whole body cooling) often looks pale and cool. In heatstroke, a life-threatening condition in which the body becomes overheated, sweating stops and the skin is flushed and very hot to the touch. **Chapter 20** describes the first aid for heat and cold emergencies.

The skin often reveals important information about the condition of the body. For example, when blood oxygen levels are low, the skin may look bluish, especially at the lips, under the nails and around mucous membranes. This skin color is called cyanosis. The skin of a victim in shock is often cool, clammy or sweating and pale or bluish. Sweating and pale skin are also signs of a possible heart attack. Many sudden illnesses also cause sweating and skin color changes (flushed or pale). In dark-skinned individuals, the skin color generally becomes ashen rather than pale.

Because skin condition is a sensitive indicator of circulatory status, the skin can also help you monitor the effects of some first aid techniques. For example, when a victim's fractured arm or leg is splinted, the skin of the fingers or toes is periodically checked to ensure that circulation to the extremity has not been cut off.

Learning Checkpoint 2

1. Check off injuries and illnesses that may cause altered mental status.

___ Head injuries   ___ Stroke

___ Seizure   ___ Diabetic emergencies

___ High fever   ___ Poisoning

___ Drug overdose   ___ Severe infection

2. A spinal injury may result in –

a. myocardial infarction.

b. lung infection.

c. paralysis.

d. All of the above

3. Define a dislocation.

_____

4. Why might a fractured femur be life-threatening?

a. Loss of calcium stored in the bone

b. Severe bleeding

c. Injury to soft tissues of the leg

d. All of the above

5. In what situation can even a small skin cut be very serious?

_____

The Gastrointestinal System

The primary function of the gastrointestinal system is to digest food and extract nutrients to meet the body's needs for energy and specific dietary substances. Food and fluids pass through the esophagus to the stomach and then to the small and large intestines, where nutrients are absorbed into the blood to be transported to body cells **(Figure 3-11)**. Wastes are eliminated through the anus.

Accessory organs of digestion include the pancreas and liver, which produce substances that aid in digestion, and the gallbladder, which stores bile made by the liver. The liver has several other important functions.

Emergencies Related to the Gastrointestinal System

Because the abdominal cavity is not protected by bones, gastrointestinal organs can be easily injured by traumatic forces. In a closed abdominal injury the skin is not broken, but pain or tenderness along with a swollen or rigid abdomen may suggest an internal injury. In an open abdominal wound, internal organs may be exposed to the outside, raising the risk of infection. **Chapter 13** describes first aid for abdominal injuries.

The gastrointestinal system may also be involved in a number of sudden illnesses and conditions. An ingested poison is absorbed in the same manner as nutrients from food and once in the blood can affect the entire body.

Various illnesses can cause vomiting or diarrhea. If either continues for a prolonged period, the victim may become dehydrated, a serious condition in which the body loses needed water. Infants, especially, can lose significant amounts of body fluid from diarrhea, which quickly becomes a medical emergency. Vomiting blood is likely a sign of serious illness.

The liver too is affected by many illnesses as well as by chronic alcohol use. As noted in **Chapter 2**, hepatitis is a bloodborne disease that frequently causes liver damage. Because the liver is a vital organ whose functions are necessary for life, it is critical to take appropriate precautions to prevent the transmission of hepatitis in first aid situations.

The Lymphatic and Immune Systems

The lymphatic system consists of the lymph nodes and lymphatic vessels located throughout the body, along with other organs **(Figure 3-12)**.

The lymphatic system helps the body to absorb fats and maintain a fluid balance, but its primary function is to help defend against disease as part of the immune system. Lymphocytes, a type of white blood cell, help fight infection. Other organs and the cells of the immune system work together with the lymphatic system to provide defense mechanisms against pathogens and foreign substances that enter the body.

Emergencies Related to the Immune System

Although many illnesses and other health problems may result from problems in the immune system, seldom do these occur suddenly and require first aid or immediate treatment. A wound that is not properly cared for, however, may develop an infection if the body's immune system does not eliminate pathogens that may enter the body through the wound. As described in **Chapter 2**, HIV, an infection attacking the immune system and causing AIDS, may also enter the first aid provider's body as a result of exposure to an

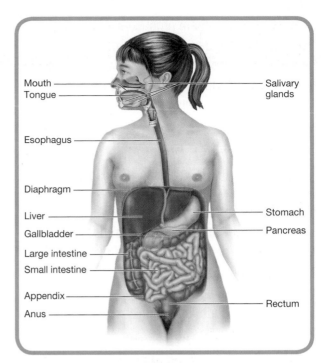

Figure 3-11 *The gastrointestinal system.*

infected victim's body fluids. Taking precautions against infection is necessary in all emergencies.

The related concept of **immunity** is also important in first aid. A **vaccine** is a form of preventive care that bolsters the body's immune system to prevent the vaccinated person from becoming infected by a specific pathogen. A vaccine is available for hepatitis B, for example, which health care workers and professional rescuers often receive because of the risk of acquiring this bloodborne infection when caring for victims of injury. Tetanus vaccine similarly gives protection against wounds being infected by the deadly tetanus bacterium, which is commonly present in the environment.

The Endocrine System

The endocrine system includes a series of glands in various body areas that produce hormones. **Hormones** are chemical messengers that are carried in the blood and affect the functioning of organs throughout the body. More than two dozen hormones are produced in the body, each with specific functions and effects. For example, the thyroid gland produces hormones that regulate growth and development. The gonads (testes in men, ovaries in women) produce steroid hormones that stimulate the development of male and female sex characteristics and allow reproductive functions. The pancreas secretes a hormone called **insulin** that helps regulate blood sugar levels.

Emergencies Related to the Endocrine System

All hormones affect a person's health and the over- or underproduction of each can cause disease. Most of these problems develop more slowly, however and are seldom issues for first aid – with one major exception. **Diabetes** is a metabolic disorder affecting over 16 million people in the United States. Diabetics either do not produce enough insulin or have developed

resistance to the effects of insulin. A person with diabetes may suddenly become very ill because of very high or very low blood sugar levels related to this insulin problem. Without treatment or first aid, a diabetic crisis can quickly progress to a medical emergency (see **Chapter 16**).

The Urinary System

The urinary system removes dissolved metabolic wastes from the body through the urine and helps the body maintain fluid and electrolyte balances. Metabolic wastes result from cellular functions within the body. The blood transports these wastes to the **kidneys**, which filter them out and produce urine **(Figure 3-13)**. Urine is transported to the **bladder**, which stores urine until it is passed to the outside.

Emergencies Related to the Urinary System

Traumatic injury may damage the bladder or kidneys, possibly resulting in blood in the urine. Blood in the urine is always a sign of a problem requiring medical attention.

Many medical problems affecting the urinary system do not develop suddenly and therefore are usually not first aid issues.

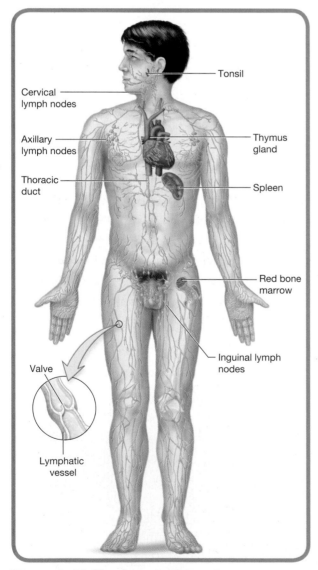

Figure 3-12 *The lymphatic system.*

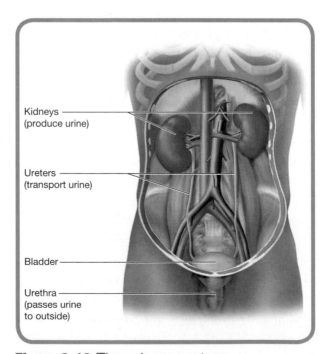

Figure 3-13 *The urinary system.*

Learning Checkpoint 3

1. What is important about vomiting?

   a. It can lead to dehydration.

   b. It may be a sign of serious illness.

   c. Vomiting blood often indicates a serious illness.

   d. All of the above

2. Name a vaccination *all* people should have periodically throughout their lives.

3. Diabetes involves a problem in the body with which hormone?

   a. Insulin

   b. Bile

   c. Steroids

   d. Any of the above

4. Blood present in the urine always means –

   a. a sexually transmitted disease is present.

   b. the person has a yeast infection.

   c. the person should seek medical attention.

   d. the person needs to restore electrolyte balance.

Because frequency and amount of urine passed depends in part on how much water is present in the body, changes in urination may indicate the presence of a health problem. A long period without urination in an infant, for example, may be a sign of dehydration, a medical emergency.

The Reproductive System

Unlike other body systems that are identical or similar in males and females, the reproductive system involves different organs in males and females. The reproductive system in males produces sperm, the male reproductive cell, and transports the sperm for delivery into the female vagina. In females the system produces eggs, the female reproductive cells, and supports and nurtures in the uterus an egg fertilized by sperm as it develops into a fetus; other functions relate to childbirth and lactation (producing milk for breastfeeding infant). The term **genitals** refers to the male and female sex organs (penis and testicles in males; the labia, clitoris and vagina in females).

Emergencies Related to the Reproductive System

Abdominal injuries may damage the genitals or reproductive organs, and such wounds may require special first aid (see **Chapter 10**). Because our culture views the genitals as a very private body area, care for these injuries should include concern for the victim's privacy and be performed with sensitivity.

In rare situations a pregnant woman may develop complications. Occasionally childbirth may occur without the pregnant woman being attended by a doctor, midwife or other person trained in childbirth. In such cases a first aider may need to assist the pregnant woman. Childbirth is usually a normal, natural process that takes place without problems or complications. Sometimes, however, a medical emergency may occur. **Chapter 22** describes first aid in pregnancy and childbirth.

Concluding Thoughts

When you encounter a victim in need of first aid, the nature of the problem may be obvious or it may be difficult to judge. A simple cut that is bleeding, for example, does not require knowledge of the cardiovascular system before you can give first aid. With many injuries and illnesses, however, understanding what is going on in the body will help you assess the problem and remember what first aid to give. Understanding how a breathing problem can cause altered mental status, for example, or how a person with diabetes may experience a sudden emergency, can help you to know what actions to take. The general principles described in this chapter will become more meaningful as you learn about specific injuries and illnesses throughout the rest of this text.

Learning Outcomes

You should now be able to do the following:

1. Describe the primary areas of the body.

2. List the 10 body systems and explain a key function of each.

3. For each body system, describe at least one injury or illness that affects the functioning of that system.

Review Questions

1. The main function of the respiratory system is to —

   a. filter the blood.

   b. transport nutrients to body tissues.

   c. protect the body from pathogens.

   d. provide oxygen for body tissues.

2. A problem in one body system —

   a. can also affect the functioning of other body systems.

   b. affects only that system.

   c. affects only that system plus the nervous system.

   d. affects every system in the body.

3. A person who is choking is said to have —

   a. altered mental status.

   b. an airway obstruction.

   c. a dysrhythmia.

   d. a metabolic disorder.

4. What life-threatening problem occurs when vital organs are not receiving enough oxygen?

   a. Diabetes

   b. Hypothermia

   c. Shock

   d. Seizures

5. Inside the vertebrae is the –

   a. central nervous system.

   b. spinal cord.

   c. spinal ligament.

   d. peripheral nervous system.

6. Heart attack may cause –

   a. crushing pain in the chest.

   b. severe bleeding.

   c. seizures.

   d. airway obstruction.

7. The functions of the musculoskeletal system include –

   a. protecting internal organs.

   b. producing lymph.

   c. circulating blood.

   d. regulating hormones.

8. Skin changes may help you determine when a victim has –

   a. hypothermia.

   b. heatstroke.

   c. sudden illness.

   d. All of the above

9. A sign of an internal abdominal injury is –

   a. sweating.

   b. seizures.

   c. a swollen or rigid abdomen.

   d. All of the above

10. A person with diabetes may have an emergency caused by –

    a. very high blood sugar levels.

    b. very low blood sugar levels.

    c. either very high or very low blood sugar levels.

    d. a fluid balance problem.

Chapter 4 • Assessing the Victim

Chapter Preview

- The Initial Assessment
- The Recovery Position
- The Secondary Assessment
- Monitor the Victim

Late in the afternoon you stop by your supervisor's office to drop off a report. When you knock on the door it swings open. You look inside and see him slumped over his desk. You call his name as you approach, but he doesn't respond, so you tap him on the shoulder and shout, "Are you okay?" He still does not respond. What do you do now?

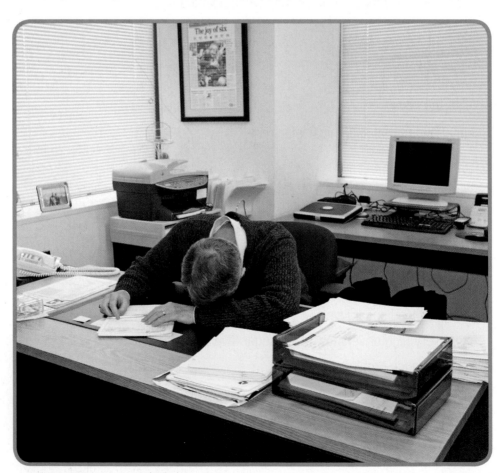

As described in **Chapter 2**, after you recognize the emergency and check the scene for safety, you then check the victim to see what problems may need emergency care or first aid. This check, called an **assessment**, has two primary steps:

1. In the **initial assessment**, check for immediate life-threatening conditions. Check for responsiveness, normal breathing and severe bleeding. Give immediate care for any life-threatening condition found.

2. In the **secondary assessment**, get the victim's history (find out what happened and what may have contributed to the emergency) and perform a physical examination of a responsive victim to check for any injuries or other signs of sudden illness.

Then while giving first aid for any injuries you find and while waiting for help to arrive, continue with a third step:

3. Monitor the victim for any changes.

Always perform these steps in this order. If you find a life-threatening problem, such as the absence of normal breathing, the victim needs immediate help. This victim could die if you first spend time looking for broken bones or asking bystanders what happened. **Always remember to conduct the initial assessment first.**

The Initial Assessment

In the initial assessment you check the victim for life-threatening conditions. Even as you come up to the victim, be looking immediately for responsiveness, normal breathing and severe bleeding. The entire initial assessment should take just a few seconds.

Because of the risk of aggravating a spine injury, do not move the victim to perform this assessment except when absolutely necessary for two circumstances:

1. The patient faces an immediate danger if not moved, because

   • fire is present or likely to occur.

   • explosives are present or there is a danger of explosion (e.g., a natural gas leak).

   • the patient cannot be protected from other hazards at the scene.

   • you are unable to gain access to other patients who need lifesaving care.

   • you cannot make the scene safe (e.g., a structure about to collapse).

2. You cannot give lifesaving care because of the patient's location or position (e.g., a victim who needs CPR is slumped in a chair or lying on a bed).

Check for Responsiveness

As you approach, you may notice immediately whether the victim is responsive. Responsive means a person is conscious and awake. A victim who is speaking, coughing, crying or moving is responsive. Even if the victim cannot talk because of an injury, he or she may be able to move and thereby signal responsiveness. A victim who cannot talk or move may be paralyzed but may still be able to respond through purposeful eye movements or other signs. This is why we say *responsive* rather than *conscious*: we cannot always know whether a person is conscious or unconscious, but we do know whether that person responds to us.

Just knowing the victim is responsive is not enough, however. Any victim who can talk is obviously responsive and is able to breathe — but the victim may have severe bleeding, a life-threatening condition. A victim who is awake and moving is responsive, but if this person is not speaking, crying or coughing, the victim may be unable to breathe because of an obstructed airway (choking) or other breathing problem. Therefore, even with a responsive victim, you must still continue to check for normal breathing and severe bleeding.

If the victim is not speaking, making other sounds or moving, tap the person on the shoulder and shout, "Are you okay?" **(Figure 4-1)**. Be careful not to move the victim in any way when assessing responsiveness. Do not shake the victim's shoulder or touch the head or neck, because the victim may have a spinal injury that any movement could worsen. If the victim still does not respond to your touch and voice, this is a life-threatening emergency and you must act quickly. If someone else is present, have that person call 9-1-1 immediately while you continue to check the unresponsive victim.

Unresponsiveness may be a sign of an urgent, life-threatening problem (such as not breathing) or it may result from a less urgent problem, but you cannot know that. Regardless of its cause and regardless of whether other life-threatening problems are present, *unresponsiveness in itself is considered an emergency.* For example, if the victim is on his or her back, the tongue may move back in the throat and block the airway, preventing breathing.

The degree of a victim's responsiveness is frequently assessed using the AVPU scale (Box 4-1). This scale is useful for noting changes in a victim's responsiveness during the time you are providing care and for communicating this information to arriving EMS professionals.

Check for Normal Breathing

At the same time you are checking for responsiveness, look for normal breathing. An unresponsive victim who is only gasping is not breathing normally and needs basic life support. If the victim can speak or cough, then he or she is breathing.

BOX 4-1: THE AVPU SCALE

A = **Alert**. The victim is aware of the time and where he or she is.

V = Responds to **Verbal** stimuli. The victim is not clearly oriented to time and place but responds when spoken to.

P = Responds to **Painful** stimuli. The victim does not respond when spoken to but moves or responds to pain, as when pinched between the neck and shoulder.

U = **Unresponsive** to all stimuli. The victim's eyes are closed and there is no movement or other response to painful stimuli.

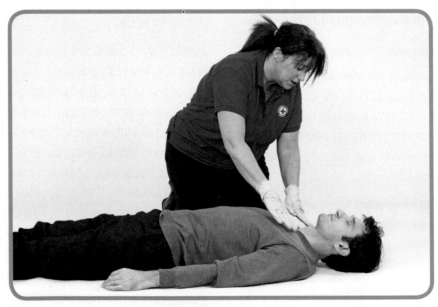

Figure 4-1 *Check the victim for responsiveness by tapping the shoulder and shouting, "Are you okay?"*

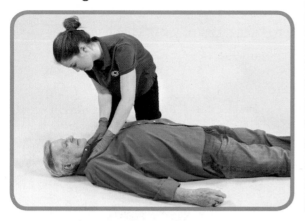
1 Check for responsiveness and normal breathing.

2 If the victim is unresponsive, call 9-1-1. If the victim is unresponsive and not breathing, also call for an AED and provide basic life support.

3 If the victim is breathing, check for severe bleeding and other threats to life.

4 Care for any life-threatening conditions before continuing to check the victim and provide other care.

If you find an unresponsive person in a position other than lying on his or her back, do not immediately roll the victim onto his or her back to begin providing care. Moving a victim unnecessarily may cause additional injury, especially if the victim may have a spinal injury. If the victim is seen to be breathing normally, leave him or her in the position found while continuing your assessment.

Remember, if an unresponsive victim is not breathing normally, you must immediately start CPR as described in **Chapter 5**.

Check for Severe Bleeding

After ensuring that the victim is breathing normally, check for severe bleeding. If the victim is bleeding profusely, vital organs are not receiving enough oxygen to sustain life.

Check for severe bleeding by quickly looking over the victim's body for obvious blood. Check for blood-saturated clothing or blood pooled under the body. Control any severe bleeding with direct pressure (see **Chapter 8**).

This step completes the initial assessment (see Skill: "Initial Assessment"). As described in the following chapters on basic life support, if the initial assessment reveals a life-threatening condition, you immediately begin to provide care for it. Only if it is clear that the victim is breathing normally and not bleeding severely do you move on to the secondary assessment to check for additional injuries or signs of a sudden illness requiring care. An unresponsive victim should be positioned on his or her side in the recovery position following the initial assessment.

BOX 4-2: HELMET REMOVAL

Helmets are worn by people in a variety of activities: bicycle riders, motorcycle riders, athletes playing sports such as football and construction site workers. If an injured victim is wearing a helmet, it should be removed only if absolutely necessary to care for a life-threatening condition, because removal involves the risk of moving the victim's head or neck and possibly worsening a spinal or head injury. Leave the helmet in place for arriving EMS professionals, unless a full-face helmet absolutely must be removed to perform CPR. With many sports helmets, the face guard can be removed so that the helmet can be left on while CPR is given.

The Recovery Position

An unresponsive victim who is breathing normally and who is not suspected of having a spinal injury, should be put in the **recovery position**. This position is used for several reasons:

- It helps keep the airway open.

- It allows fluids to drain from the mouth so that the victim does not choke on blood, vomit or other fluids.

- It prevents the victim from inhaling stomach contents if the victim vomits.

If possible, unless this could worsen the victim's injury, put the victim on his or her left side. Because of anatomical differences in the body, the left side has more benefits for protecting the victim. On the left side, vomiting is delayed, the movement of poison into the small intestine is slower and in a pregnant woman there is less pressure on the vena cava, the large vein that returns blood to the heart. The modified HAINES (High Arm IN Endangered Spine) position is recommended because it reduces movement of the neck in case of potential spinal injury (see Skill: "HAINES Recovery Position").

For an unresponsive, breathing infant, hold the infant face down over your arm with his or her head slightly lower than the body **(Figure 4-2)**.

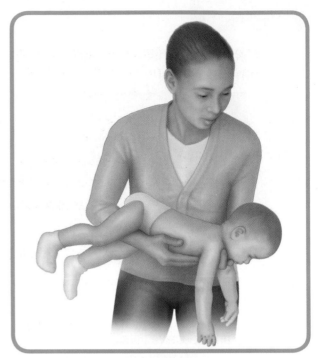

Figure 4-2 *Infant recovery position.*

Support the head and neck with your hand and keep the nose and mouth clear.

Once the victim is in the recovery position, continue to monitor breathing while waiting for advanced help to arrive and observe the victim for bleeding, medical alert bracelets or insignia and any deformities that may indicate a serious injury. Give this information to responding EMS professionals.

Learning Checkpoint 1

1. You first encounter a victim lying quietly on the floor. Number the following actions in the correct order.

    _____ a. Look around his body for a pool of blood.

    _____ b. Check to see if victim responds to your voice or touch.

    _____ c. Look for normal breathing.

2. Describe when you should not immediately proceed to the secondary assessment from the initial assessment.

    _____

3. True or False: If you hear a victim coughing, you can assume he or she is breathing.

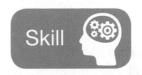
1 Extend the victim's arm that is farther from you above the victim's head.

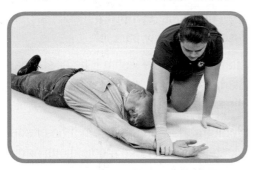

2 Position the victim's other arm across the chest.

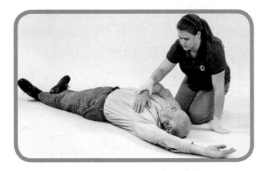

3 Bend the victim's nearer leg at the knee.

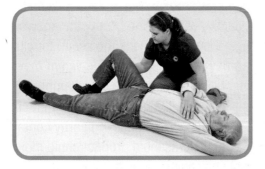

4 Put your forearm under the victim's shoulder with your hand around the back of the neck to support the head and neck.

5 Carefully roll the victim away from you by pushing on the victim's flexed knee and lifting with your forearm while your hand stabilizes the head and neck. The victim's head is now supported on the raised arm.

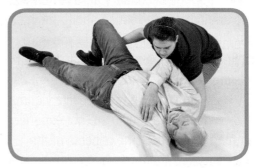

6 While continuing to support the head and neck, position the victim's hand palm-down with fingers under the armpit of the raised arm, with forearm flat on the surface at 90 degrees to the body.

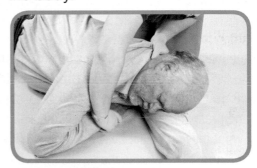

7 Bend both legs so the victim's position is stabilized.

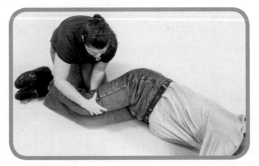

8 With victim now in position, check the airway and open the mouth to allow drainage.

4 • Assessing the Victim

The Secondary Assessment

Remember that the secondary assessment is performed only for victims without life-threatening conditions. Do not interrupt care for a serious problem in order to carry out a secondary assessment. But if the victim's condition seems stable and no threats to life require your attention, then the secondary assessment can provide additional information about the injury or illness. That information may help you care for the victim and may be of value to arriving EMS professionals. The secondary assessment can usually be performed with responsive victims of injury or sudden illness who are not experiencing a breathing problem. Some aspects of the secondary assessment may be performed with unresponsive victims.

The secondary assessment has two primary parts: the history and the physical examination. In both parts, focus your attention primarily on the injured area, taking into account the cause and nature of the injury (often called the "mechanism of injury").

Get the Victim's History

After the initial assessment, get the victim's **history** to try to find out more about what happened and the victim's condition. Talk to a responsive victim. With an unresponsive victim, ask bystanders about what they know or saw. With a potentially serious injury, try to assess the forces involved. For example, a victim who fell from a height or was struck in the head by a heavy object is at greater risk of having a spinal injury and you must be careful not to move this victim during your assessment or when giving first aid.

When taking the history of a responsive victim of sudden illness, ask fully about the victim's situation to learn possible causes. For example, in a case of poisoning the victim may not immediately associate present symptoms with something ingested an hour or more ago. Or a victim could be experiencing the effects of carbon monoxide breathed inside a building, even though you encountered the victim outside.

Use the **SAMPLE** format to ensure that you cover the victim's full history:

S = **Signs and symptoms**. What can you observe about the victim (**signs**)? Ask the victim how he or she feels (**symptoms**) and ask for a description of any pain felt.

A = **Allergies**. Ask the victim if he or she has any allergies to foods, medicines, insect stings or other substances. Look for a medical alert ID.

M = **Medications**. Ask the victim if he or she is taking any prescribed medications or over-the-counter products, including vitamins, supplements and herbal remedies.

P = **Previous problems**. Ask the victim if he or she has had anything like this before or if he or she has any other illnesses. Again, a medical alert ID may indicate the victim has a condition such as diabetes or epilepsy.

L = **Last food or drink**. Ask the victim what he or she last ate and when.

E = **Events**. Ask the victim what happened and try to identify the events that led to the current situation. When did the victim first begin to experience the problem?

If the victim is unresponsive, ask family members or bystanders whether they know the answers to these questions. Also check the scene for clues to what may have happened. The victim may have just taken a medication, for example or you may see something like a syringe that could indicate possible drug abuse. A nearby container of a poisonous household product could indicate a possible poisoning. Consider the environment: a very cold or hot environment may produce a temperature-related emergency or contribute to sudden illness. Finally, consider the victim's age. A younger person who slips on ice and falls may have only a bruise, whereas an elderly woman who falls is more likely to have broken her hip.

The information from the SAMPLE history may help you to give the right first aid. When help arrives, give the information you gathered to the EMS professionals. It will help them to provide the appropriate medical care.

Physical Examination

The secondary assessment of an injured or ill victim who is responsive also includes a **physical examination**. With this examination you may find other injuries that need first aid or additional clues to the victim's condition. Remember that you do not stop giving first aid for a serious condition just to perform or complete this examination. Instead, keep the victim still and calm and wait for EMS professionals.

Remember that an unresponsive victim without a possible spinal injury should be kept in the recovery position until EMS professionals arrive. Continue to monitor the victim's breathing and observe the victim for bleeding and other signs of serious injury.

Allow a responsive victim to remain in the position he or she finds most comfortable while conducting the physical examination. The victim does not need to be moved to lie on his or her back as shown in the illustrations.

Ask a responsive victim for consent to do a physical examination, as with any other first aid, and describe what you are about to do before touching the victim. Keep away from any body area the victim tells you is very painful. Watch for a victim's facial expression or stiffening of a body part, which may reveal pain or tenderness the victim does not tell you about.

Focus on the area the victim knows is injured. You do not need to touch every body area, for example, if the victim has an injured arm and the nature of the injury does not suggest other body areas may be injured.

The physical examination of a responsive adult includes examining the victim from head to toe looking for anything out of the ordinary **(Box 4-3)**. You begin at the head because injuries here are more likely to be serious than injuries in the

BOX 4-3: SIGNS AND SYMPTOMS OF INJURY AND ILLNESS

The victim may tell you about:
- Pain, tenderness
- Dizziness, feeling faint
- Nausea
- Tingling or abnormal sensation, no sensation
- Thirst
- Hot, cold

You may see:
- Painful expression, guarding against movement
- Bleeding, wound, bruise, swelling
- Abnormal skin color
- Deformity, inability to move part
- Unusual chest movement
- Vomit, incontinence

You may feel:
- Damp skin
- Hot or cold skin
- Swelling
- Deformity

You may hear:
- Noisy breathing
- Groaning, sounds of pain
- Stress in victim's voice
- Sucking chest wound

You may smell:
- Odor of a drug used
- Odor of poisonous or hazardous substance
- Fruity smelling breath (diabetic emergency)

extremities or lower in the body. As a general rule, look for the following signs and symptoms of injury or illness throughout the body, comparing one side of the body to the other:

- Pain when an area moves or is touched

- Bleeding or other wounds

- An area that is swollen or deformed

- Skin color (flushed, pale or ashen), temperature (hot or cold), moisture (dry, sweating or clammy)

- Abnormal sensation or inability to move the area

While performing the examination, watch for changes in the victim's condition. For example, the victim may at first be fully responsive and alert, but as you continue to check different body areas, the victim may become disoriented or dizzy, suggested changing mental status. The victim's breathing may change or stop. Call 9-1-1 if the victim's condition becomes more serious and the call was not made earlier.

You may have to remove some of the victim's clothing to examine an injured body area. Remove clothing or shoes only when necessary, such as to apply pressure on a wound to control bleeding, because moving the body part could cause additional injury. Protect the victim's privacy and prevent exposure to the cold. Follow these guidelines for removing clothing:

- Carefully roll or fold up a sleeve to expose an arm.

- To remove a jacket or shirt when an arm is injured, remove the uninjured arm from its sleeve first and then carefully work the jacket or shirt around the body and down off the injured arm while supporting it.

- Gently pull up a pants leg to expose the calf or knee. With scissors, carefully cut along the seam to expose the thigh.

- Support the victim's ankle when removing a shoe. Leave long boots on.

- If you cannot easily slide off a tight sock, lift it gently with your fingers and cut it open with scissors.

The acronym **DOTS** is often used as a reminder of what to look for in the physical examination of an injured victim:

D = Deformities

O = Open injuries

T = Tenderness (pain)

S = Swelling

Check the Head and Neck

Do not move the head or neck during the examination. Gently feel the skull for bleeding, bumps or depressions. Check the ears and nose for blood or a clear fluid. Check the pupils of both eyes, which should be of equal size and should respond to light when you cover and uncover the eyes with your hand. Check the victim's breathing for ease and regularity, and note any unusual breath odor. Check the mouth for burned areas. Check the neck for a medical alert necklace, deformity or swelling, bleeding, and pain. Observe the skin of the head and neck for color, temperature and moisture.

Check the Torso

Check the chest and sides, feeling for deformity, wounds or tender areas. Look for blood in any area. Ask the victim to take a deep breath, and feel and look for easy, symmetrical expansion of the chest with breathing or for signs of pain on breathing. Gently feel along the collarbones and shoulders for deformity, swelling or pain.

If you suspect a problem in the abdominal or pelvic areas, gently check the abdomen for rigidity, pain or bleeding and gently feel both sides of the hips and pelvis to check for pain or deformity.

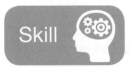

If you find any problems in any body area, do not let the victim move. Wait for help.

1 Being careful not to move the victim's head or neck, check the head.

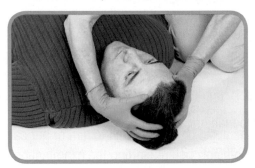

2 Check neck area for medical alert necklace, deformity or swelling, and pain. Do not move the neck.

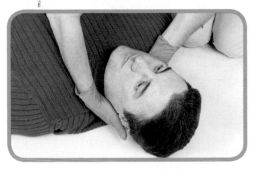

3 Check skin appearance, temperature and moisture.

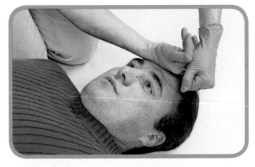

4 Check chest. Ask victim to breathe deeply.

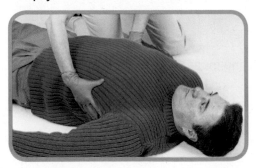

5 Check abdomen.

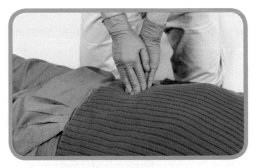

6 Check pelvis and hips.

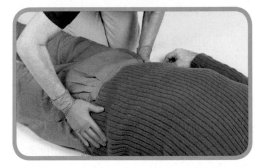

7 Check upper extremities. Look for medical alert bracelet.

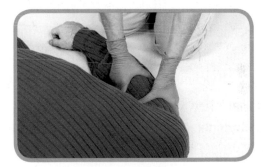

8 Check lower extremities.

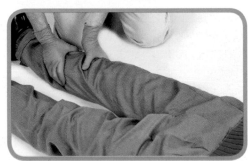

4 • Assessing the Victim

Check the Extremities

Check the arms for bleeding, deformity and pain. Ask the victim to bend his or her elbows, wrists and fingers. Look for a medical alert bracelet. Touch the fingers and ask if the sensation feels normal to the victim. Check the skin color and temperature of the hand to detect impaired circulation. Ask the victim to shrug the shoulders.

Check the legs for bleeding, deformity and pain. Unless you suspect a back, abdominal or pelvic injury, ask the victim to point and wiggle the toes. Check the skin temperature and color of the feet. Touch the feet and ask if the sensation feels normal to the victim.

If you find anything unusual in the extremities, compare that extremity with the opposite side and note differences (see Skill: "Physical Examination").

Examining a Child or Infant

The assessment of a child or infant is similar to that of an adult, taking into account physical differences and the child's different language skills and emotional state. Use simple questions to gather the history, such as, "Where does it hurt?" Talk with the child's parents or guardians, if possible, and involve them in the physical examination **(Figure 4-4)**. Allow a parent or guardian holding an infant or young child to continue to hold the victim during the examination. With a young child it is often better to perform the physical examination from toe to head rather than from the head first, to allow the child to get used to you. Because a child is more likely to become upset or anxious, talk to him or her calmly and soothingly before starting the examination and look for signs of anything unusual before touching the child. A child who is upset often reacts with physical changes that may mask or confuse the signs of injury.

Monitor The Victim

Give first aid for injuries or illness you discover in your assessment, as described in the following chapters. With very minor conditions the victim

Learning Checkpoint 2

1. When is the secondary assessment performed?

    a. Immediately before giving CPR when needed

    b. In all victims, right after the initial assessment

    c. After checking for responsiveness

    d. After determining that there are no life-threatening conditions

2. Write what each letter in the SAMPLE history stands for

    S = _____

    A = _____

    M = _____

    P = _____

    L = _____

    E = _____

3. Describe what signs and symptoms of injury you are looking for as you examine each part of a victim's body.

    _____

    _____

may need no more than your first aid. In other situations the victim may need to see a health care provider or go to the emergency department. With all life-threatening or serious conditions, you should have called 9-1-1 and will now be awaiting the arrival of help.

While waiting, monitor the victim to make sure his or her condition does not worsen. With an unresponsive victim or a victim with a serious injury, repeat your assessment of breathing at least every 5 minutes.

Concluding Thoughts

You can see why a victim of injury or sudden illness is assessed in two stages: If the initial assessment reveals a life-threatening problem, then you must provide basic life support immediately without going on to the history and physical examination. Chapter 5 is the first of three chapters describing basic life support for life-threatening problems. Remember: A breathing problem is an immediate threat to life, requiring action within seconds because body tissues will begin to die within minutes.

Learning Outcomes

You should now be able to do the following:

1. Explain how to check the victim's responsiveness and normal breathing.

2. Demonstrate how to move a victim into the recovery position and explain when this is done.

3. Explain the importance of each element in the SAMPLE history.

4. Demonstrate how to perform a physical examination of a responsive victim without a life-threatening problem.

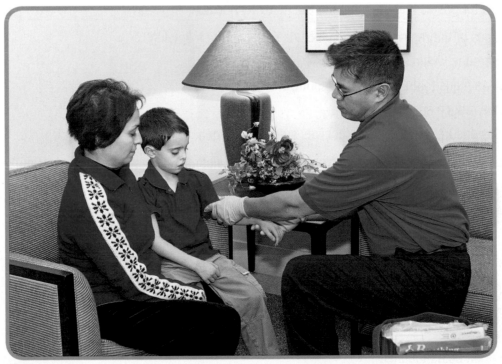

Figure 4-4 *Involve the child's parent or guardian in the history and physical examination.*

Review Questions

1. The initial assessment checks the victim for –
   a. bone fractures.
   b. severe bleeding.
   c. severe allergies.
   d. spinal injuries.

2. Assess an adult or child victim for responsiveness by –
   a. tapping the shoulder and shouting, "Are you okay?"
   b. pinching the cheek between thumb and forefinger.
   c. checking for pupil reactions to light.
   d. checking skin for normal color and temperature.

3. If a victim can talk to you, you can be sure he or she –
   a. does not have a life-threatening condition.
   b. does not have a spinal injury.
   c. is breathing.
   d. All of the above

4. At what point do you begin providing care for a victim who is not breathing normally?
   a. Immediately.
   b. As soon as the 9-1-1 dispatcher tells you to.
   c. As soon as you complete the secondary assessment.
   d Right after positioning the victim in the recovery position.

5. Advantages of the recovery position include which of the following?
   a. It lowers the victim's blood pressure.
   b. It allows fluids to drain from the mouth.
   c. It helps reduce shock.
   d. It helps ensure that the brain receives sufficient oxygen.

6. When gathering a SAMPLE history from a suddenly ill victim, which should you ask about?
   a. Allergies and medications taken
   b. Age and weight
   c. Favorite foods
   d. Most recent annual physical examination

7. During the physical examination, what are you looking for?
   a. Bleeding or wounds
   b. A swollen area
   c. Pain upon being touched
   d. All of the above

Chapter 5 • Cardiovascular Emergencies and Cardiopulmonary Resuscitation (CPR)

Chapter Preview

- Overview of Basic Life Support
- Cardiovascular Illness and Emergencies
- Respiratory Emergencies

- Cardiac Chain of Survival
- Call First/Call Fast
- CPR

You are walking past your neighbor's house when you hear a scream for help. You knock on the door and offer to help. Your neighbor lets you in, and you find her husband unresponsive on the floor. "He just collapsed," she tells you. You send her to call 9-1-1 and quickly check to see whether he is breathing normally. He is not breathing. How do you handle this situation?

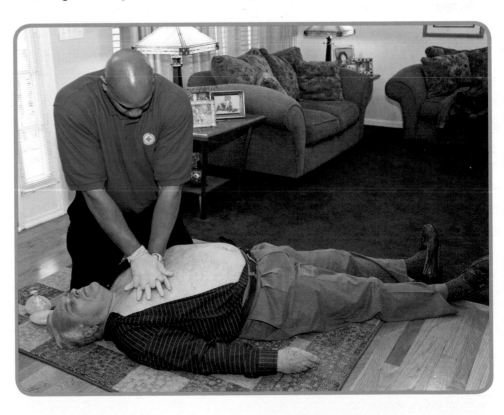

Cardiac and respiratory emergencies are among the most serious threats to life. Basic life support is needed for a victim whose heartbeat or breathing has stopped. If the victim's heart has stopped beating normally, chest compressions are needed to circulate blood to vital organs. Rescue breaths are also given to oxygenate the blood.

Chest compressions combined with rescue breaths is called **cardiopulmonary resuscitation (CPR)** The chapter discusses cardiac and respiratory emergencies and the basic life support care given to victims with these threats to life.

Overview of Basic Life Support

Basic life support (BLS) refers to first aid given if the victim's breathing or heart stops. Many things can cause breathing or the heart to stop. Whenever either breathing or the heart stops, the other also stops very soon. BLS is often needed for victims of:

- Heart attack

- Drowning

- Choking

- Other injuries or conditions that affect breathing or the heart

Basic life support consists of several first aid skills, often called **resuscitation**.

A victim who is not breathing normally needs CPR to circulate oxygenated blood in the body to keep vital organs alive and to move oxygen into the body. A victim whose heart is in a condition called ventricular fibrillation, which is common after heart attacks and other situations, needs an electric shock given by an automated external defibrillator (AED) to restore a more normal heart rhythm. A victim who is choking also needs first aid to clear the airway to allow either natural breathing or rescue breaths.

This chapter focuses on cardiovascular and respiratory emergencies and the use of CPR. The additional skills for using an AED and giving choking care are described in the following two chapters.

Differences Among Adults, Children and Infants

Because of size and other differences, there are some distinctions in how BLS skills are used with adults, children and infants. These differences result from anatomical and physiological differences in the human body at different ages. The standard age groups for BLS are defined in the following way. Remember these age categories in reference to CPR and the use of an AED:

- An *infant* is up to 1 year of age.

- A *child* for purposes of CPR and choking care is 1 year up to the onset of adolescence or puberty (as determined by the occurrence of secondary sex characteristics, such as the presence of armpit hair in boys or breast development in girls); for AED only, a child means ages 1 to 8.

- An *adult* for all BLS skills except for AED means at or past puberty; for AED only, adult means older than 8.

Cardiovascular Illness and Emergencies

CPR is most commonly needed by victims in cardiac arrest as a result of a heart attack.

Learning Checkpoint 1

1. Basic life support helps keep a victim alive when _____ or _____ stops.

2. For purposes of using an AED a child is defined as someone between the ages of _____ and _____.

Because a heart attack is usually caused by cardiovascular disease, preventing cardiovascular illnesses by maintaining a healthy lifestyle is the most effective way to prevent heart attacks and other cardiovascular emergencies such as stroke.

The term *cardiovascular illness* refers to several different diseases involving the heart and blood vessels (Figure 5-1). Cardiovascular disease becomes more common as a person ages, but as Figure 5-2 shows, these diseases are surprisingly common even in young adults. The three most common cardiovascular diseases are:

- Heart disease, such as **coronary heart disease** (blockage of vessels supplying heart muscle with blood, often leading to heart attack)

- **Stroke** (sudden impairment of blood circulation in a part of the brain)

- **Hypertension** (high blood pressure, a very common condition that can lead to both heart attack and stroke)

Heart disease remains the most common cause of death in Americans, resulting in about 616,000 deaths a year.[1] More than 17 million people in the United States have coronary heart disease and about 785,000 first-time heart attacks occur each year, plus another 470,000 repeat heart attacks.[2]

Stroke has been and remains the number three cause of death overall. About 795,000 people a year have a stroke, resulting in about 136,000 deaths.[3] More than 5 million people are living with the effects of stroke, which often include severe disability. Stroke is discussed in **Chapter 16**.

[1]*National Safety Council [NSC]. (2011). Injury Facts®, 2011 Edition. Itasca, IL: Author.*

[2]*Centers for Disease Control and Prevention. http://www. cdc.gov/heartdisease/facts.htm Accessed March 29, 2011.*

[3]*American Heart Association, http://circ.ahajournals.org/ cgi/reprint/CIR.0b013e3182009701 Accessed March 29, 2011.*

CVD Prevalence, United States	
CVD	81,100,000
Hypertension	74,500,000
CHD	17,600,000
Acute Myocardial Infarction (AMI)	8,500,000
Angina Pectoris	10,200,000
Stroke	6,400,000
Heart Failure	5,800,000
Congenital Heart Defects	1,000,000
Atrial Fibrillation	2,200,000
Peripheral Arterial Disease	8,000,000

Data from National Institutes of Health at http://www.nhlbi.nih.gov/ resources/docs/2009_ChartBook.pdf Accessed March 4, 2011.

Figure 5-1 *Percentage breakdown of deaths from cardiovascular disease.*

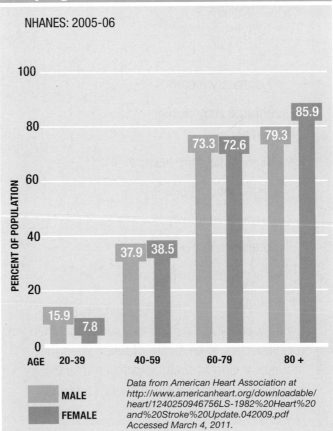

Prevalence of cardiovascular diseases in Americans 20 and older by age and sex.

NHANES: 2005-06

Data from American Heart Association at http://www.americanheart.org/downloadable/ heart/1240250946756LS-1982%20Heart%20 and%20Stroke%20Update.042009.pdf Accessed March 4, 2011.

Figure 5-2

Almost one-third of all people in the United States have high blood pressure – more than 76 million people. Although this disease directly results in more than 57,000 deaths a year,[4] hypertension contributes as a risk factor to many more deaths caused by heart attack, stroke or other diseases.

Taken together, these three cardiovascular diseases along with the others shown in **Figure 5-1** constitute the number one health problem in the United States today. Yet many of the risk factors leading to these diseases can be prevented.

Cardiovascular Risk Factors

A risk factor is anything that makes it more likely that a person will develop a particular disease. Some risk factors are beyond our control, but others are lifestyle factors that a person can avoid or change. Following are the known risk factors for cardiovascular disease:

Risk factors that cannot be changed

- Increasing age
- Gender
- Race
- Hereditary factors

Preventable risk factors

- Smoking
- High cholesterol levels
- High blood pressure
- Physical inactivity
- Obesity and overweight
- Uncontrolled diabetes
- Stress

Even though some risk factors cannot be changed, it is important to be aware of them when they increase your risk of cardiovascular disease. In general, the risks of these diseases rise with increasing age. As shown in **Fig. 5-2**, at some ages men are more likely to have cardiovascular disease than women, while at other ages the prevalence is higher in women; neither gender should feel immune to heart attacks and other problems. African-Americans generally have a higher prevalence of high blood pressure than Caucasians and therefore have a greater risk for cardiovascular disease. Hereditary factors such as a family history of heart disease also can increase one's risk.

If you know your risk for cardiovascular disease is high because of risk factors beyond your control, it is all the more important to focus on those risk factors you can control. Risk factors often have an additive effect: the more risk factors you have, the higher your danger overall for developing disease.

Prevention of cardiovascular disease, therefore, involves eliminating risk factors by living a healthy lifestyle. In general, this means:

- Not using tobacco
- Eating healthy foods to prevent overweight, to help lower cholesterol levels and blood pressure, and to help prevent diabetes
- Maintaining low cholesterol levels, with medication when appropriate
- Controlling high blood pressure with diet, exercise, weight control and medication if needed
- Getting sufficient regular exercise to help prevent overweight, high blood pressure, diabetes and stress
- Preventing or managing stress

You should notice how these risk factors are interrelated. For example, inactivity puts one at risk for being overweight and weight control helps prevent hypertension as well as helping one manage stress. Eating well also helps prevent overweight and helps to control blood pressure. These interrelated risk factors are sometimes referred to as a *constellation* of factors. To maintain

[4]*American Heart Association, http://circ.ahajournals.org/cgi/reprint/CIR.0b013e3182009701 Accessed March 29, 2011.*

good cardiovascular health, we should focus not on one or two factors but on a whole constellation of healthy choices that together result in a healthy lifestyle.

Maintaining Cardiovascular Health

Cardiovascular health can be attained and maintained with a lifestyle that includes good diet, exercise, weight and blood pressure control, and stress management.

All of these factors involve behavioral habits that typically begin in childhood, although they may also develop later in life. Adults who understand that they need to eat healthily and get exercise, for example, may have difficulty doing so if they have habitually behaved otherwise. The following sections, therefore, focus on establishing good habits early in childhood as well as developing them later in life when needed.

In recent years more media attention has been given to the cardiovascular health of children. The problems of childhood obesity, high cholesterol levels, poor diet and lack of exercise are now recognized. Although few children actually experience heart disease other than rare congenital problems, from a very early age they form habits that often stay with them for life.

Smoking

Smoking and other uses of tobacco contribute to poor cardiovascular health. Smokers have a risk for cardiovascular disease that is two to four times higher than nonsmokers. Children learn about smoking at a very early age by observing adults. About 90% of adults who use tobacco began before age 18, starting at the average age of 13.[5] Do not smoke around children, both because of the risks of secondhand smoke and because you as an adult caregiver are a role model and would be implicitly teaching children it is okay to smoke. Support the efforts of schools and other organizations to teach children that all tobacco use is unhealthy.

Most adults who smoke know that it is an unhealthy habit yet still have difficulty quitting.

More than 45 million Americans still smoke (23% of men, 21% of women).[6] Many smoking cessation programs have been developed and have proved effective when one is motivated to stop. For information, contact the American Cancer Society, American Lung Association or American Heart Association. The U.S. Surgeon General has stated that a program for quitting smoking is most effective if it includes these five steps:

1. Get ready.

2. Get support.

3. Learn new skills and behaviors.

4. Get medication and use it correctly.

5. Be prepared for relapse or difficult situations.

Admittedly, it is not easy to quit smoking, as nicotine is a highly addictive substance. But a commitment to quitting along with a realistic attitude and plan has led to millions of adults successfully breaking the habit. Your cardiovascular health and risk for cancer begin to improve the day you quit.

Diet

Good nutrition affects a child's health in the present and influences habits that will affect cardiovascular health later on. Children's food preferences are influenced by many factors, such as what the family eats at home, what they see other children eat at childcare or at school, and what television commercials "teach" them to eat. You cannot counteract all of these influences, of course, but encouraging good eating habits is the responsibility of all adult caregivers.

Most current nutritional research continues to support what we have known for some time: High-fat and high-sugar foods are unhealthy and eating a variety of foods with an emphasis on

[5]Illinois Department of Public Health, http://www.idph.state. il.us/public/hb/hbsmoke.htm Accessed March 1, 2011.

[6]American Heart Association, http://www.americanheart. org/presenter.jhtml?identifier=4559 Accessed March 1, 2011.

fruits, vegetables and whole grains and cereals is healthy and promotes a normal weight. In 2010 a federal government panel reviewed previous dietary recommendations and issued the revised guidelines for adults and children older than 2 listed in **Box 5-1**. In addition, certain dietary changes are recommended for specific population groups, such as older adults, pregnant women, overweight adults and others. Talk to your health care provider about changes that may be important for you.

In almost all instances, healthy alternatives to unhealthy foods and snacks are available that taste just as good. Choose low-fat frozen yogurt or frozen fruit bars rather than ice cream, skim or low-fat milk rather than whole milk, whole wheat bread, rather than white bread and so on. This will help you set the stage for a lifetime of cardiovascular health.

Cholesterol

Cholesterol is a fatty substance the body needs to carry out important functions. Cholesterol is taken into the body from the diet, especially from foods high in animal fats, and is manufactured in the liver. Hereditary factors also affect your cholesterol level. Because of these factors outside your control, you cannot assume you have a low blood cholesterol level just because you eat well.

High blood cholesterol levels are very common in the United States. About 102 million people, or 45% of the population, have borderline-high or high levels of low-density lipoprotein (LDL), the *bad* type of cholesterol.[7] This is due in part to a generally poor diet and lack of exercise. Cholesterol affects cardiovascular health because it is deposited in the arteries along with other substances as **plaque (Figure 5-3)**. A buildup of plaque leads to the condition called **atherosclerosis**, a narrowing and "hardening" of the arteries. Atherosclerosis in coronary arteries can cause a heart attack and in arteries in the brain can cause a stroke.

[7]*American Heart Association. http://www.americanheart. org/presenter.jhtml?identifier=4506 Accessed March 1, 2011.*

Because high blood cholesterol levels are a risk factor for cardiovascular disease, adults need regular testing. Increasingly pediatricians are testing children as well. Only a blood test can determine your cholesterol level.

If you are found to have high blood levels of LDL, you can take several steps to control this risk factor:

- Avoid high-cholesterol foods such as animal fats.

- Maintain a healthy weight (cholesterol levels rise in overweight people).

- Get more exercise (cholesterol levels generally rise with inactivity). Make it your goal to get 30 to 60 minutes of exercise on most or all days of the week.

- Talk with your health care provider about whether a cholesterol-lowering medication is appropriate for you. If you do take a medication, do so consistently. For a variety of reasons, less than half of people prescribed these medications are still taking them a year later even though they still need them – perhaps because they feel fine. Remember that usually you can't feel the results of plaque building up in your arteries and threatening your health.

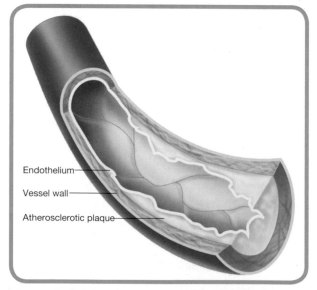

Endothelium

Vessel wall

Atherosclerotic plaque

Figure 5-3 *High blood cholesterol levels contribute to buildup of plaque inside arteries.*

Exercise

It has become a cliché but is nonetheless true: Most children and adults do not get enough exercise. Almost 40% of the population reports no leisure-time physical activity at all, with many more not engaging in any activity regularly. Television, computer games and the Internet have contributed to children becoming more sedentary than decades ago. Adults often say they are too busy with work and family responsibilities to engage in activities that provide exercise.

Exercise is good not only for the muscles but for the heart, lungs and blood vessels. Like diet, exercise helps both adults and children be healthier now while building a foundation for future cardiovascular health and a longer, healthier, happier life. **Box 5-2** provides the 2008 federal recommendations for physical activity for different groups of people.

Both children and adults get more exercise if it is fun. Almost all age-appropriate sports and energetic activities that children enjoy are good forms of cardiovascular exercise. Adults can choose from a full range of exercise programs developed for use at home or at a fitness center. Even brisk walking counts.

BOX 5-1: DIETARY GUIDELINES FOR AMERICANS, 2010 KEY RECOMMENDATIONS

Balancing Calories to Manage Weight

- Prevent and/or reduce overweight and obesity through improved eating and physical activity behaviors.

- Control total calorie intake to manage body weight. For people who are overweight or obese, this will mean consuming fewer calories from foods and beverages.

- Increase physical activity and reduce time spent in sedentary behaviors.

- Maintain appropriate calorie balance during each stage of life – childhood, adolescence, adulthood, pregnancy and breastfeeding, and older age.

Foods and Food Components to Reduce

- Reduce daily sodium intake to less than 2,300 milligrams (mg) and further reduce intake to 1,500 mg among persons 51 and older and those of any age who are African-American or have hypertension, diabetes or chronic kidney disease. The 1,500-mg recommendation applies to about half of the U.S. population, including children and the majority of adults.

- Consume less than 10 percent of calories from saturated fatty acids by replacing them with monounsaturated and polyunsaturated fatty acids.

- Consume less than 300 mg per day of dietary cholesterol.

- Keep trans fatty acid consumption as low as possible by limiting foods that contain synthetic sources of trans fats, such as partially hydrogenated oils, and by limiting other solid fats.

- Reduce the intake of calories from solid fats and added sugars.

- Limit the consumption of foods that contain refined grains, especially refined grain foods that contain solid fats, added sugars and sodium.

- If alcohol is consumed, it should be consumed in moderation – up to one drink per day for women and two drinks per day for men – and only by adults of legal drinking age.

(continues)

BOX 5-1: DIETARY GUIDELINES FOR AMERICANS, 2010 KEY RECOMMENDATIONS (continued)

Foods and Nutrients to Increase

Individuals should meet the following recommendations as part of a healthy eating pattern while staying within their calorie needs.

- Increase vegetable and fruit intake.

- Eat a variety of vegetables, especially dark-green and red and orange vegetables and beans and peas.

- Consume at least half of all grains as whole grains. Increase whole-grain intake by replacing refined grains with whole grains.

- Increase intake of fat-free or low-fat milk and milk products, such as milk, yogurt, cheese or fortified soy beverages.

- Choose a variety of protein foods, which include seafood, lean meat and poultry, eggs, beans and peas, soy products, and unsalted nuts and seeds.

- Increase the amount and variety of seafood consumed by choosing seafood in place of some meat and poultry.

- Replace protein foods that are higher in solid fats with choices that are lower in solid fats and calories and/or are sources of oils.

- Use oils to replace solid fats where possible.

- Choose foods that provide more potassium, dietary fiber, calcium and vitamin D, which are nutrients of concern in American diets. These foods include vegetables, fruits, whole grains, and milk and milk products.

Building Healthy Eating Patterns

- Select an eating pattern that meets nutrient needs over time at an appropriate calorie level.

- Account for all foods and beverages consumed and assess how they fit within a total healthy eating pattern.

- Follow food safety recommendations when preparing and eating foods to reduce the risk of foodborne illnesses.

Source: US Department of Agriculture, http://www.health.gov/dietaryguidelines/dga2010/DietaryGuidelines2010.pdf Accessed March 1, 2011.

Adults who are presently out of shape, especially those older than 50 who have become sedentary, should talk to their health care provider before beginning an exercise program. Often it is best to begin slowly and gradually increase your workouts to a comfortable yet effective level.

As with other lifestyle changes, it is important to have a realistic attitude when beginning an exercise or fitness program. People often join a fitness club or purchase exercise equipment for home use, begin strenuously and soon quit. A long-term commitment is needed, developing a plan that realistically fits your lifestyle and personal interests.

Make physical activity a routine part of the day, not a special requirement at certain times.

Everyone needs to think of physical activity as being as "normal" in their life as eating or sleeping, not something special to be done just when you feel like it or to meet a specific weight goal. It is important to help children to develop this attitude, too.

Weight Control

Almost 30% of adults in the United States are obese by current standards and another 35% are overweight.[8] Overweight and obesity contribute to many other diseases in addition to cardiovascular disease.

[8]WebMD www.webmd.com/diet/news/20100210/percentage-of-overweight-obese-americans-swells Accessed March 1, 2011.

(continues on page 77)

BOX 5-2: 2008 PHYSICAL ACTIVITY GUIDELINES FOR AMERICANS

Key Guidelines for Children and Adolescents

- Children and adolescents should do 60 minutes (1 hour) or more of physical activity daily.

  - **Aerobic**: Most of the 60 or more minutes a day should be either moderate- or vigorous-intensity aerobic physical activity and should include vigorous-intensity physical activity at least 3 days a week.

  - **Muscle-strengthening**: As part of their 60 or more minutes of daily physical activity, children and adolescents should include muscle-strengthening physical activity at least 3 days of the week.

  - **Bone-strengthening**: As part of their 60 or more minutes of daily physical activity, children and adolescents should include bone-strengthening physical activity at least 3 days of the week.

- It is important to encourage young people to participate in physical activities that are appropriate for their age, that are enjoyable and that offer variety.

Key Guidelines for Adults

- All adults should avoid inactivity. Some physical activity is better than none and adults who participate in any amount of physical activity gain some health benefits.

- For substantial health benefits, adults should do at least 150 minutes (2 hours and 30 minutes) a week of moderate-intensity or 75 minutes (1 hour and 15 minutes) a week of vigorous-intensity aerobic physical activity or an equivalent combination of moderate- and vigorous intensity aerobic activity. Aerobic activity should be performed in episodes of at least 10 minutes and, preferably, should be spread throughout the week.

- For additional and more extensive health benefits, adults should increase their aerobic physical activity to 300 minutes (5 hours) a week of moderate intensity or 150 minutes a week of vigorous intensity aerobic physical activity or an equivalent combination of moderate- and vigorous-intensity activity. Additional health benefits are gained by engaging in physical activity beyond this amount.

- Adults should also do muscle-strengthening activities that are moderate or high intensity and involve all major muscle groups on 2 or more days a week, as these activities provide additional health benefits.

Key Guidelines for Older Adults

The Key Guidelines for Adults also apply to older adults. In addition, the following Guidelines are just for older adults:

- When older adults cannot do 150 minutes of moderate-intensity aerobic activity a week because of chronic conditions, they should be as physically active as their abilities and conditions allow.

- Older adults should do exercises that maintain or improve balance if they are at risk of falling.

- Older adults should determine their level of effort for physical activity relative to their level of fitness.

- Older adults with chronic conditions should understand whether and how their conditions affect their ability to do regular physical activity safely.

(continued)

5 • Cardiovascular Emergencies and CPR

BOX 5-2: 2008 PHYSICAL ACTIVITY GUIDELINES FOR AMERICANS (continued)

Key Guidelines for Safe Physical Activity

To do physical activity safely and reduce the risk of injuries and other adverse events, people should:

- Understand the risks yet be confident that physical activity is safe for almost everyone.

- Choose to do types of physical activity that are appropriate for their current fitness level and health goals, because some activities are safer than others.

- Increase physical activity gradually over time whenever more activity is necessary to meet guidelines or health goals. Inactive people should "start low and go slow" by gradually increasing how often and how long activities are done.

- Protect themselves by using appropriate gear and sports equipment, looking for safe environments, following rules and policies and making sensible choices about when, where and how to be active.

- Be under the care of a health care provider if they have chronic conditions or symptoms. People with chronic conditions and symptoms should consult their health care provider about the types and amounts of activity appropriate for them.

Key Guidelines for Women During Pregnancy and the Postpartum Period

- Healthy women who are not already highly active or doing vigorous-intensity activity should get at least 150 minutes of moderate-intensity aerobic activity a week during pregnancy and the postpartum period. Preferably, this activity should be spread throughout the week.

- Pregnant women who habitually engage in vigorous-intensity aerobic activity or who are highly active can continue physical activity during pregnancy and the postpartum period, provided that they remain healthy and discuss with their health care provider how and when activity should be adjusted over time.

Key Guidelines for Adults With Disabilities

- Adults with disabilities, who are able to, should get at least 150 minutes a week of moderate-intensity or 75 minutes a week of vigorous-intensity aerobic activity or an equivalent combination of moderate- and vigorous-intensity aerobic activity. Aerobic activity should be performed in episodes of at least 10 minutes and, preferably, should be spread throughout the week.

- Adults with disabilities, who are able to, should also do muscle-strengthening activities of moderate or high intensity that involve all major muscle groups on 2 or more days a week, as these activities provide additional health benefits.

- When adults with disabilities are not able to meet the Guidelines, they should engage in regular physical activity according to their abilities and should avoid inactivity.

- Adults with disabilities should consult their health care provider about the amounts and types of physical activity that are appropriate for their abilities.

Key Messages for People With Chronic Medical Conditions

- Adults with chronic conditions obtain important health benefits from regular physical activity.

- When adults with chronic conditions do activity according to their abilities, physical activity is safe.

- Adults with chronic conditions should be under the care of a health care provider. People with chronic conditions and symptoms should consult their health care provider about the types and amounts of activity appropriate for them.

Source: U.S. Department of Health and Human Services, http://www.health.gov/paguidelines/guidelines/summary.aspx Accessed March 4, 2011.

(continued from page 74)

Overweight and obesity are categorized in relation to a person's **body mass index (BMI)**, a measure of weight in relation to a person's height. The higher the BMI number, the greater the percentage of fat in a person's body. Overweight is defined as a BMI of 25 to 30, and obesity is a BMI of 30 or higher. The chart in **Figure 5-4** provides an approximate BMI for adults based on height and weight.

The habits that lead to overweight start early in life. Prevention is a better approach than having to lose weight later on and keep it off. The earlier recommendations for diet and exercise, while promoting good health generally, are also the keys to preventing a weight problem from developing.

The cornerstones of all effective weight-loss programs combine a healthy diet with adequate physical activity, as detailed in the previous section.

Many different programs have been developed, including a large number of programs that involve fad diets or dietary supplements that promise to burn off the fat. Research shows, however, that controlling caloric intake and getting exercise are the only factors that result in successfully losing weight and keeping it off. Like other major lifestyle changes, such as quitting smoking, weight control requires commitment, a realistic attitude and plan and time and effort. An excellent starting point is talking with your health care provider to learn what kind of program will work best for you.

High Blood Pressure

As noted earlier, more than 74 million people in the United States have high blood pressure – and in many this condition is not controlled. Hypertension is often called the "silent killer" because in most

Body Mass Index (BMI) Table

	NORMAL						OVERWEIGHT					OBESE									
BMI	19	20	21	22	23	24	25	26	27	28	29	30	31	32	33	34	35	36	37	38	39
HEIGHT (inches)	BODY WEIGHT (pounds)																				
58	91	96	100	105	110	115	119	124	129	134	138	143	148	153	158	162	167	172	177	181	186
59	94	99	104	109	114	119	124	128	133	138	143	148	153	158	163	168	173	178	183	188	193
60	97	102	107	112	118	123	128	133	138	143	148	153	158	163	168	174	179	184	189	194	199
61	100	106	111	116	122	127	132	137	143	148	153	158	164	169	174	180	185	190	195	201	205
62	104	109	115	120	126	131	136	142	147	153	158	164	169	175	180	186	191	196	202	207	213
63	107	113	118	124	130	135	141	146	152	158	163	169	175	180	186	191	197	203	208	214	220
64	110	116	122	128	134	140	145	151	157	163	169	174	180	186	192	197	204	209	215	221	227
65	114	120	126	132	138	144	150	156	162	168	174	180	186	192	198	204	210	216	222	228	234
66	118	124	130	136	142	148	155	161	167	173	179	186	192	198	204	210	216	223	229	235	241
67	121	127	134	140	146	153	159	166	172	178	185	191	198	204	211	217	223	230	236	242	249
68	125	131	138	144	151	158	164	171	177	184	190	197	203	210	216	223	230	236	243	249	256
69	128	135	142	149	155	162	169	176	182	189	196	203	209	216	223	230	236	243	250	257	283
70	132	139	146	153	160	167	174	181	188	195	202	209	216	222	229	236	243	250	257	264	271
71	136	143	150	157	165	172	179	186	193	200	208	215	222	229	236	243	250	257	265	272	279
72	140	147	154	162	169	177	184	191	199	206	213	221	228	235	242	250	258	265	272	279	287
73	144	151	159	166	174	182	189	197	204	212	219	227	235	242	250	257	265	272	280	288	295
74	148	155	163	171	179	186	194	202	210	218	225	233	241	249	256	264	272	280	287	295	303
75	152	160	168	176	184	192	200	208	216	224	232	240	248	256	264	272	279	287	295	303	311
76	156	164	172	180	189	197	205	213	221	230	238	246	254	263	271	279	287	295	304	312	320

Source: National Institutes of Health, http://www.nhlbi.nih.gov/guidelines/obesity/bmi_tbl.htm, accessed February 24, 2011.

Figure 5-4 *Body mass index.*

people it causes no symptoms and the person can be completely unaware of having it. Yet hypertension is linked to high death rates caused by heart attack, stroke or other diseases.

Although in some cases hypertension is caused by an underlying condition that may be treated, in the great majority of cases it exists without a specific known cause that can be addressed. Hypertension is diagnosed by regular blood pressure tests. The current standards classify different levels of hypertension according to seriousness. Prehypertension is a systolic blood pressure of 120 to 139, stage 1 hypertension is 140 to 159 and stage 2 hypertension is 160+. By these standards, even those in the prehypertension category are at some risk and should take steps to control their blood pressure. Because blood pressure generally rises with age, it is now estimated that by age 55, more than half of all adults have more than a 50% chance of being hypertensive – a percentage that rises to more than 70% by age 75.[9]

Recommendations for controlling blood pressure involve both lifestyle changes and medications. For people with prehypertension, lifestyle changes alone are generally sufficient:

- Maintain a normal weight.
- Get more physical activity.
- Reduce salt intake.

Many individuals with stage 1 or 2 hypertension will also need medication to lower their blood pressure. The risks of hypertension are among the reasons that everyone should have periodic physical examinations by a health care provider, who will give appropriate recommendations for controlling high blood pressure.

Stress

Stress is an emotional or mental state that is generally considered a risk factor for cardiovascular disease. Long-term, frequent stress is thought to have various negative effects on a person's physical health, although it is difficult for research studies to study the exact effects of stress because of issues of quantifying and measuring stress and separating this factor from other risk factors. Nonetheless, there is some evidence that excessive stress lowers the body's immune functions and has other negative effects, and that stress reduction in some cases has a positive benefit. Interestingly, some of the other healthy lifestyle decisions described previously, such as exercise and a good diet, also help control or reduce stress. People who frequently feel stressed, however, would benefit from talking to their health care provider about programs for stress reduction.

Respiratory Emergencies

Any illness or injury that causes a victim to stop breathing, or to breathe so ineffectively that the body is not receiving enough oxygen, is a respiratory emergency. The two primary types of breathing emergencies are respiratory arrest and respiratory distress.

All body tissues need a continual supply of oxygen to function and to maintain life. As described in **Chapter 3**, the respiratory system, working primarily with the cardiovascular system, provides this needed oxygen. In the lungs, oxygen moves out of the air into the blood, which is then circulated throughout the body. Carbon dioxide, a waste product of cellular metabolism, is also picked up from the tissues by the blood and eliminated in the lungs. The functioning of the respiratory and cardiovascular systems also depends on the muscles of breathing and nervous system control of breathing and the heart. A problem in any of these areas can result in a respiratory emergency. For example:

- A physical obstruction in the airway, such as food blocking the pharynx or immersion in water, can make it impossible for air to reach the lungs.
- An injury to the chest can penetrate the lungs and hinder the movement of air into and out of the lungs with breathing.

[9]*Centers for Disease Control and Prevention, http://www. cdc.gov/bloodpressure/facts.htm Accessed March 1, 2011.*

- Breathing in carbon monoxide from a faulty furnace or smoke from a fire can reduce the availability of oxygen in the lungs and cause less oxygen to be present in the blood for body tissues.

- A heart problem can result in insufficient blood being circulated in the body, reducing the amount of oxygen available for tissues.

- An electric shock can disrupt the nervous system's control of either breathing or the heartbeat, thereby disrupting the flow of oxygen to the body.

- A drug overdose or poisoning can depress nervous system control of breathing such that insufficient oxygen reaches body tissues.

These are just a few of the many ways in which respiratory emergencies may occur. Regardless of the cause, body cells begin to die soon after losing their oxygen supply. Brain cells are very susceptible to low levels of oxygen and begin to die as soon as four minutes after oxygen is cut off. Within six minutes brain damage is likely **(Figure 5-5)**. Death is likely soon after.

Respiratory Arrest and Respiratory Distress

Respiratory arrest means that breathing has completely stopped. Again, this condition may result from many different causes. You do not need to know the exact cause, however, because the BLS steps for respiratory arrest are the same in all cases.

With **respiratory distress**, on the other hand, the victim is still breathing, but the breathing is difficult and may become so ineffective that the victim's blood-oxygen content drops to a life-threatening level. Respiratory distress may occur with different illnesses and injuries. Someone with asthma, for example, may experience great difficulty breathing when tissues of the airway swell and make it difficult to move air into and out of the lungs. A severe allergic reaction may cause a similar problem.

The first aid for victims of respiratory distress is somewhat different because the victim is still

breathing. In this case care focuses on easing the breathing crisis and addresses the cause of the problem if possible. Conditions causing respiratory distress are described in **Chapter 16**. Note, however, that respiratory distress can progress to respiratory arrest, in which case the victim needs CPR as described in this chapter.

Prevention of Respiratory Arrest

Respiratory arrest can be prevented by preventing its common causes, including drowning and sudden infant death syndrome (SIDS), as well as all general injury prevention measures. The prevention of choking, a common cause of respiratory arrest, is described in **Chapter 7**. Because breathing stops when the heart stops, preventing cardiac arrest also prevents respiratory arrest.

Preventing Drowning

About 3,400 people die each year from drowning in the United States.[10] More than a fifth of these drownings are children younger than 14. For every child who dies from drowning, another four receive emergency department care for a near-drowning,[11]

[11]*Centers for Disease Control and Prevention, http://www. cdc.gov/HomeandRecreationalSafety/Water-Safety/ waterinjuries-factsheet.html Accessed March 1, 2011.*

[10]*National Safety Council. (2011). Injury Facts®, 2011 Edition. Itasca, IL: Author.*

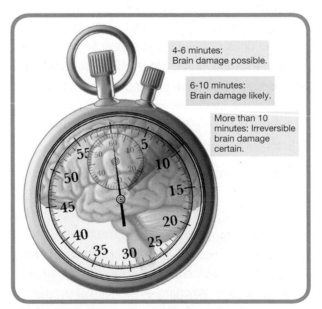

4-6 minutes: Brain damage possible.

6-10 minutes: Brain damage likely.

More than 10 minutes: Irreversible brain damage certain.

Figure 5-5 *Without oxygen, vital organs soon begin to die.*

and many of these have permanent disabilities from brain damage caused by lack of oxygen during submersion or related factors.

Although drowning is the second leading cause of injury-related death for children 1 to 14 years old[11], most parents say they do not worry about their child drowning. This overconfidence and lack of concern is likely a significant factor in the poor supervision of children around water. Among children, the huge majority of drownings occur with an adult "supervising" but distracted by other factors.

The prevention of drowning is based on understanding the primary risk factors:

- Most infant victims drown in bathtubs, buckets or toilets. An infant should never be left unsupervised near water, even to a depth of an inch or two, for even a moment.

- Most victims one to four years old drown in residential swimming pools with one or both parents at home at the time – with the child usually out of sight for less than 5 minutes. Never leave a young child alone in or near the water, even if the child has had beginning swimming lessons or promises to stay out of the water in your absence. All children should be supervised by an adult who maintains continuous visual contact and does not engage in distracting activities such as talking on the telephone or reading. Pools should have protective barriers with effective locks. Parents should never trust floating toys, rafts or inner tubes to keep their children afloat.

- Up to half of drowning deaths in the age group with the most drownings, adolescents and adults, are associated with alcohol use during water recreational activities.[11] Alcohol influences balance, coordination and judgment, which are key factors in situations that lead to drowning. Prevention is simple: do not drink and go into or near the water. Swim with a buddy, never dive into shallow or unknown water, and wear a life jacket during water sports.

- About 72% of the 709 annual deaths during boating activities result from drowning. Most victims are not wearing life jackets and in about 20% of cases alcohol is involved.[11] Following safe boating guidelines can help prevent most of these drowning deaths.

Preventing SIDS

Sudden infant death syndrome (SIDS), sometimes also called crib death, is the sudden death of an infant younger than one of unexplained causes. It occurs most commonly between 2 and 4 months of age and is the most common cause of infant death after 1 month of age. More than 2,200 infants die of SIDS in the United States every year[12], a number that has dropped in recent years with efforts to educate parents and caregivers. Current research suggests that SIDS may result from certain congenital differences that make some infants more susceptible, but evidence also indicates that preventive efforts can prevent SIDS from occurring in most cases. It has also been estimated that as many as 900 of the deaths that are attributed to SIDS may have resulted from simple suffocation[13] because these infants are found in suffocating environments and positions, often lying on the stomach with nose and mouth covered by soft bedding.

To reduce the risk of SIDS and suffocation:

- Always place infants on their backs to sleep. This step alone can lower the risk of SIDS by more than 50%.

- Use a firm, flat crib mattress that meets safety standards.

- Remove pillows, comforters, toys and other soft objects from the crib.

- Do not cover the infant's head during sleep.

[12]*National Sudden and Unexpected Infant/Child Death & Pregnancy Loss Resource Center, http://www.sidscenter.org/Statistics.html Accessed March 1, 2011.*

[13]*Virginia Department of Health, http://www.vahealth.org/Injury/data/factsheets/Infant_Child%20Suffocation%20Fact%20Sheet.pdf Accessed March 1, 2011.*

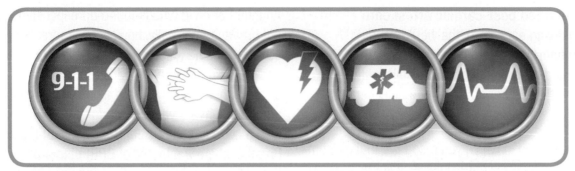

Figure 5-6 *Cardiac Chain of Survival.*

- If a blanket must be used, use a thin blanket, tuck it under the edges of the mattress, and keep it at chest level and below to reduce the likelihood of the infant pulling it over his or her face.

- Avoid smoking. When a woman smokes during pregnancy, the infant is three times more likely to have SIDS, and an infant exposed to passive smoke has a much higher than normal risk.

- Avoid overheating during sleep; dress the infant in light sleep clothing and keep the room at a temperature that is comfortable for an adult.

- Do not have the infant sleep in a bed shared with siblings or parents. Experts recommend having the infant's crib beside the bed when parents wish to be close and to facilitate breastfeeding.

- Give an infant between 1 and 12 months of age a clean, dry pacifier at bedtime.

Cardiac Chain of Survival

Any victim whose breathing or heart stops needs CPR. Cardiac arrest and respiratory arrest victims both need CPR. **Cardiac arrest** refers to a sudden stop in the beating of the heart. **Respiratory arrest** refers to a cessation of breathing, in which case cardiac arrest will also soon occur.

To recognize the urgent need for quick actions to save the lives of cardiac arrest victims, the

Citizen CPR Foundation created the concept of the **Cardiac Chain of Survival (Figure 5-6)**. This chain has five crucial links:

1. **Immediate recognition of cardiac arrest and activation of the emergency response system**. *Recognize that a victim whose heart has stopped needs help immediately!* It is also important that you recognize the signs and symptoms of a potential life-threatening condition such as a heart attack or a stroke in a responsive person (see **Chapter 16**). Do not wait until a person becomes unresponsive to start the chain of events needed to keep him or her alive. Call 9-1-1 and get help on the way. The victim needs early access to advanced medical care.

2. **Early CPR with an emphasis on chest compressions**. For an unresponsive victim who is not breathing normally, start CPR immediately. This helps keep the brain and other vital organs supplied with oxygen until an AED arrives.

3. **Rapid defibrillation**. An AED, now present in many public and work places, can help get the heart beating normally again after a cardiac arrest. Send someone right away to get the AED.

4. **Effective advanced life support**. The sooner the victim is treated by emergency care professionals, the better the chance for survival. You can help make sure the victim reaches this link in the chain by acting immediately with the earlier links.

5. **Integrated post-cardiac arrest care.**
Following early care, the victim needs
continued, integrated medical care by a team
of medical professionals, typically within a
hospital or other advanced medical center.

Call First/Call Fast

In any situation in which you recognize that a victim
of injury or illness is unresponsive, if someone else
is present at the scene, have that person call 9-1-1
immediately. Shout for anyone who may hear you
and have them call 9-1-1 and go for an AED.

When you are alone, however, you need to decide
whether to call immediately or to first begin
to provide care for the victim. The rule that lay
rescuers should follow depends on the victim's
age. An adult who is found unresponsive and not
breathing normally is more likely to be the victim
of a heart attack and therefore needs defibrillation
urgently. For an adult, therefore, if you are alone
with the victim, call 9-1-1 immediately and then
return to provide CPR. **Remember: Call first**.

An infant or child who is found unresponsive and
not breathing normally, however, is more likely to
be experiencing an airway or breathing problem
and less likely to need defibrillation. For an infant
or child, therefore, if you are alone with the victim
and no one hears your shouts for help, you should
give 5 cycles of chest compressions and rescue
breaths (about 2 minutes of CPR) before pausing
to call 9-1-1 and then continuing to provide CPR.
Remember: Start CPR first but call fast.

CPR

CPR is used for all unresponsive victims who are
not breathing normally. Remember that airway and
respiratory problems can cause breathing to stop,
followed by cardiac arrest. Cardiac arrest is also
commonly caused by:

- Heart attack or other heart disease
- Drowning
- Suffocation
- Stroke

(continues on page 83)

Learning Checkpoint 2

1. CPR stands for –

   a. cardiac position for recovery.

   b. cardiopulmonary resuscitation.

   c. chest pump rescue.

   d. None of the above

2. Put a check mark next to risk factors for cardiovascular disease.

   _____ Smoking   _____ High cholesterol levels

   _____ Regular aspirin use   _____ Inactivity

   _____ High blood pressure   _____ Family history of heart disease

   _____ Growing older   _____ Working full-time

3. The first crucial link in the Cardiac Chain of Survival is _____

4. *Call first* (before starting CPR) for which of these victims? (Check all that apply.)

   _____ Unresponsive adult not breathing normally

   _____ Unresponsive infant not breathing normally

   _____ Unresponsive child not breathing normally

(continued from page 82)

- Allergic reaction
- Diabetic emergency
- Prolonged seizures
- Drug overdose
- Electric shock
- Certain injuries

You do not need to know the cause of cardiac or respiratory arrest, however, before starting CPR. The technique for CPR is the same regardless of cause.

CPR helps keep the victim alive by circulating some oxygenated blood to vital organs. Compressions on the **sternum** (breastbone) increase pressure inside the chest, resulting in movement of some oxygen-carrying blood to the brain and other tissues. Rescue breaths move oxygen into the lungs, where it is picked up by the blood. The circulation of blood resulting from CPR is not nearly as strong as the circulation from a heartbeat, but it can help keep brain and other tissues alive until a normal heart rhythm is restored. Often an electric shock from an AED (see **Chapter 6**) or other medical procedures called **advanced cardiac life support (ACLS)** are needed to restore a heartbeat – and CPR can keep the victim viable until then. In some instances, the heart may start again spontaneously with CPR.

CPR has been clearly demonstrated to save lives in many circumstances. With the most common cause of cardiac arrest, a heart attack, CPR and defibrillation within 3 to 5 minutes after the victim collapses can save more than 50% of victims. Given that sudden cardiac arrest occurs in almost 900 people with heart disease *every day*, with 95% dying before reaching a hospital, you can see that CPR followed by AED can save many thousands of lives every year.[14] The exact number of lives saved is unknown because no agency collects all national data on CPR use in all circumstances. Remember that CPR is only one step in the cardiac chain of survival, however. In most cases CPR serves only

[14]*Heart Rhythm Foundation http://www.heartrhythm foundation.org/facts/scd.asp Accessed March 1, 2011.*

to keep the victim alive until an AED and/or EMS professionals arrive at the scene.

Chest Compressions in CPR

The general technique of CPR involves alternating chest compressions and rescue breaths. After determining the victim is unresponsive and not breathing normally, start CPR with chest compressions followed by rescue breaths. For a victim of any age, these are the general steps of CPR:

1. Bare the chest and find the correct hand position on the lower half of the breastbone in the middle of the chest in adults and children **(Figure 5-7)**. In infants, the position is just below the nipple line. For adults, place the heel of one hand in the correct position; then put the second hand on top of the first and interlock fingers. For children, depending on their size and your strength, use both hands or the heel of one hand. For infants, use two fingers.

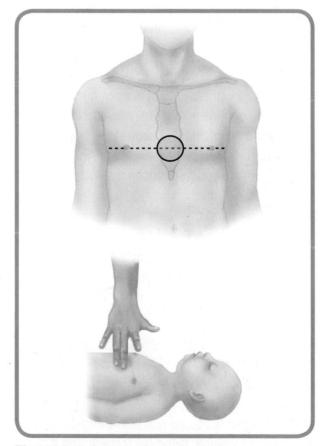

Figure 5-7 *Proper placement for compressions.*

2. Compress the chest hard and fast at a rate of at least 100 compressions per minute. Compressions in an adult should be at least 2 inches deep. In an infant or child, compressions should be at least ⅓ the depth of the chest (about 1½ inches in an infant or about 2 inches in a child). Between compressions let the chest return to its normal height by taking your weight off your hands, but do not remove your hands (or fingers for infants) from the chest.

3. Alternate 30 chest compressions and 2 rescue breaths for all victims. For all victims, give each breath over 1 second.

Rescue Breaths in CPR

Giving rescue breaths is the technique of blowing air into a non-breathing victim's lungs to oxygenate the blood. Rescue breaths are given along with chest compressions, which help circulate the oxygenated blood to vital organs, keeping the victim alive until the victim is resuscitated or EMS personnel arrive to give advanced care.

Rescue breaths are given with the first aider's own air unless special equipment is available. The air around us contains about 21% oxygen and the breath we exhale contains about 16% oxygen – still enough oxygen to increase the oxygen level in the victim's blood to maintain life. When a first aider blows air into the victim's mouth or nose, this air moves into the lungs in a manner similar to natural breathing. The chest rises as the lungs expand and oxygen moves into the blood in the small vessels within the lungs. After each breath the chest is allowed to fall and the air is "exhaled" out, then the next breath is given.

Rescue breaths are given along with chest compressions to any victim who is not breathing normally. An unresponsive victim who is occasionally gasping is not breathing and needs CPR. Also have someone call 9-1-1 immediately. If an AED is available, send someone to get it (see **Chapter 6**).

Techniques for Giving Rescue Breaths

After beginning CPR with 30 chest compressions, open the victim's airway to give two rescue breaths. This is done by tilting the head back and lifting the chin as shown in **Figure 5-8**. This is called the head tilt–chin lift. This position moves the tongue away from the opening into the throat to allow air to pass through the airway. Then you can give the rescue breaths.

Use a barrier device if you have one, to protect against disease transmission, but do not delay giving rescue breaths to get one. Even without a barrier device the risk of contracting an infectious disease from rescue breathing is very low.

The basic technique is to blow air slowly into the victim while watching the chest rise to make sure your air is going into the lungs. Do not try to rush the air in or blow too forcefully. Do not take a big breath in order to exhale more air into the victim; just take a normal breath. Give each breath over 1 second. If the breath does not go in – if you feel resistance or do not see the victim's chest rise – then try again to open the airway. If your breath still does not go in, then the victim has an airway obstruction and needs care for choking (see **Chapter 7**). If your initial breath does go in, give a second breath over 1 second and then resume chest compressions.

Remember these key points:

- Do not blow harder than is needed to make the victim's chest rise.

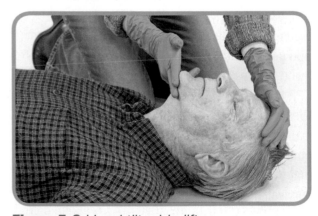

Figure 5-8 *Head tilt–chin lift.*

- After each breath remember to let the air escape and the chest fall.

- Blowing in too forcefully or for too long is ineffective and may put air in the stomach, which may cause vomiting.

Mouth to Barrier

Barrier devices are always recommended for giving rescue breaths and should be kept in the first aid kit **(Figure 5-9)**. The two most common types of barrier devices are pocket masks and face shields. Both types of devices offer protection from the victim's saliva and other fluids, as well as from the victim's exhaled air when equipped with a one-way valve. With either device, keep the victim's head positioned to maintain an open airway as you deliver rescue breaths through the device.

A pocket mask is positioned on the victim's face over both the mouth and nose. A one-way valve in the mouthpiece lets your air flow into the victim but directs the victim's exhaled air out another way so that it does not reach you directly during rescue breathing. With a face mask, as with any barrier device, make sure it is well sealed to the victim's face and watch the victim's chest rise to confirm that your air is going into the victim.

A face shield is also positioned over the victim's mouth as a protective barrier. The victim's nose is pinched closed when giving a rescue breath to prevent the air from coming out the nose instead of entering the lungs.

Mouth to Mouth

If you do not have a barrier device, pinch the victim's nose shut and seal your mouth over the victim's mouth. Blow into the victim's mouth, watching the chest rise to confirm that the air is going in.

Mouth to Nose

If the victim's mouth cannot be opened or is injured, or if you cannot get a good seal with your mouth over the victim's mouth, you can give rescue breaths through the nose. Hold the victim's mouth closed, seal your mouth over the nose to blow in and then allow the mouth to open to let the air escape.

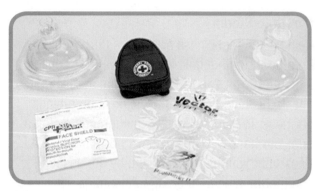

(a)

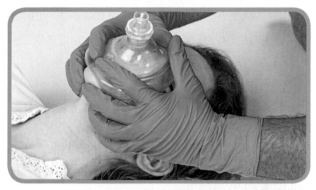

(b)

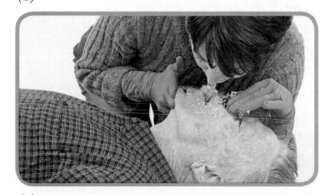

(c)

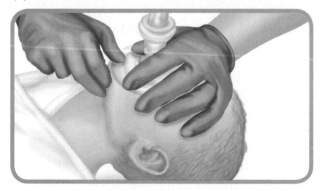

(d)

Figure 5-9 *(a) Barrier devices. (b) Position pocket mask over mouth and nose. (c) Position face shield over mouth and pinch nose. (d) Mask used with an infant.*

Mouth to Stoma

Because of past illness or injury, some people breathe through a hole in their lower neck called a stoma (**Figure 5-10**). In the initial assessment, check this hole to see if the victim is breathing normally. To give rescue breaths through a stoma, cup your hand over the victim's nose and mouth to prevent your air from leaving by the nose and mouth instead of going to the lungs. Then seal your mouth over the stoma and give rescue breaths as usual. Or you can use a round pediatric face mask if you have one.

Mouth to Nose and Mouth

Because of their smaller size, infants and very small children are generally given rescue breaths through both their mouth and nose. Seal your mouth over both the nose and mouth and give gentle breaths as usual, watching to see the chest rise with each breath.

Rescue Breaths for Infants

Rescue breathing for infants is similar to that for adults and children, with these differences:

- Gently tilt the head back to open the airway and check breathing – do not overextend the neck.

- If no barrier device is available, cover both mouth and nose with your mouth to give breaths. (Use the mouth or nose only if you cannot cover both.)

Special Circumstances for Rescue Breaths

In some circumstances you may have to adjust how you give rescue breaths, including a victim vomiting, a victim wearing dentures and a victim with facial injuries.

Vomiting

In some cases, the air provided with rescue breaths may move into the stomach rather than the lungs. If the airway is not sufficiently open, if rescue breaths are given too quickly or if you continue to blow in air even after the lungs have expanded and the chest has risen, air may be forced into the stomach. In this situation, not only is the victim possibly not receiving enough air in the lungs to oxygenate the blood, but the air in the stomach makes vomiting more likely. Vomiting presents two problems. First, if an unresponsive victim vomits during BLS care, you have to roll the victim onto his or her side to drain the victim's mouth and then wipe the mouth clean before continuing. The time required to do this takes time away from the chest compressions of CPR, which are essential for moving oxygenated blood to vital organs. Second, when the victim vomits there is a risk of aspiration, which is the movement of vomit or other fluids or solids into the lungs, which can cause a serious infection and other problems. For these reasons, when giving rescue breaths be sure to:

- Open the airway first.

- Watch the chest rise as you give breaths.

- Blow slowly and steadily rather than too quickly.

- Stop each breath when the chest rises rather than continuing to blow.

- Let the chest fall between breaths.

Dentures

A victim's dentures are usually left in place during rescue breathing. If they are loose and make it difficult to give breaths, or may fall back in the mouth and block the airway, remove dentures before giving rescue breaths.

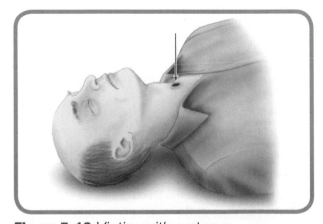

Figure 5-10 *Victim with a stoma.*

$\frac{60}{5} = 12$

Facial Injuries

If the victim's mouth cannot be opened or is injured or if you cannot get a good seal with your mouth over the victim's mouth, you can give rescue breathing through the nose. Hold the victim's mouth closed, seal your mouth over the nose to blow in and then allow the mouth to open to let the air escape.

Note: A victim with injuries may have blood in the mouth, which needs to be drained before giving rescue breathing. If suction equipment is available and you are trained in its use, you may suction either blood or vomit from the victim's mouth (see **Appendix A**).

BOX 5-3: PROBLEMS WITH CPR TECHNIQUE

It is well known that CPR saves lives and that CPR training is needed to effectively use this procedure. CPR is taught in the classroom using manikins, of course, and thus the skill is typically learned in ideal circumstances rather than real-life situations, which may be very different. It is often difficult to evaluate the effectiveness of CPR given in the field because of the many variables that determine victim outcome.

Studies have shown two key problems in the chest compression technique of many rescuers. Often compressions are not delivered steadily and constantly at all times during the resuscitation efforts. Equally important, compressions are often too shallow, resulting in ineffective blood flow.

Studies have also shown that only good-quality CPR improves the victim's chances of survival. The quality depends mostly on giving chest compressions at the correct rate and depth.

This research clearly indicates the importance of performing CPR as learned – especially the depth and rate of chest compressions. Understanding the importance of these factors should help first aiders remember to focus on their technique in order to provide the quality CPR the victim needs to survive.

 Learning **Checkpoint 3**

1. Rescue breaths are needed to –

    a. get oxygen into the victim's blood.

    b. circulate the blood to vital organs.

    c. open the victim's airway.

    d. All of the above

2. True or False: Blow as hard as you can into the victim's mouth during rescue breathing.

3. What is the best way to confirm that your breaths are going into the victim's lungs?

    a. Listen at the victim's mouth for escaping air.

    b. Place one hand on the victim's abdomen to feel movement.

    c. Watch the victim's chest rise and fall.

    d. None of the above

4. When giving rescue breaths, give each breath over _____ second(s).

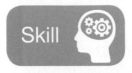

Skill — CPR for Adults, Children and Infants (1 Rescuer)

1 Determine that the victim is unresponsive and not breathing normally. Have someone call 9-1-1 or call yourself if alone, and get an AED.

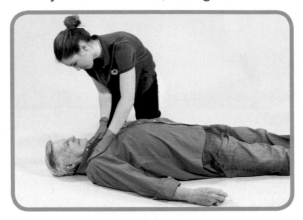

2 Expose the chest. Put your hand on the lower half of the breastbone in the middle of the chest for chest compressions. For an adult, put your second hand on top of the first and interlock the fingers. For a child, use 1 or both hands. For an infant, put 2 middle fingers of 1 hand just below the nipple line.

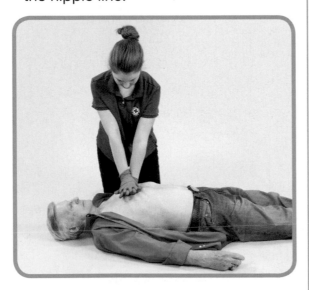

3 Give 30 chest compressions hard and fast at least 2 inches deep in an adult and at least ⅓ the depth of the chest in an infant (about 1½ inches) or child (about 2 inches) at a rate of at least 100 per minute. Count aloud for a steady fast rate: "One, two, three…" Then give 2 breaths.

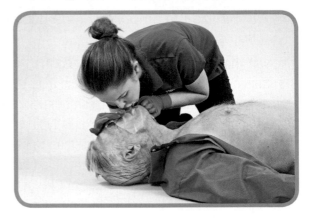

4 Open the airway and give 2 rescue breaths, each lasting 1 second, to cause a visible chest rise. (If the first breath does not go in, reposition the victim's head and try again; if the second breath does not go in, give choking care (see **Chapter 7**).

5 Continue cycles of 30 compressions and 2 breaths.

6 Continue CPR until:
- The victim wakes up.
- An AED is brought to the scene and is ready to use.
- Personnel with more training arrive and take over.

7 a. If the victim starts breathing normally but is unresponsive, put the victim in the recovery position and monitor breathing.

   b. When an AED arrives, start the AED sequence.

ALERT
Chest Compressions

- Be careful with your hand position for chest compressions. Keep fingers off the chest (except the 2 fingers for an infant).
- Do not give compressions over the bottom tip of the breastbone.
- When compressing, keep your elbows straight and keep your hands in contact with the chest at all times.
- Remember to compress the chest hard and fast, but let the chest recoil completely between compressions.
- Minimize the amount of time used giving rescue breaths between sets of compressions.
- Performing chest compressions only is called Hands-Only CPR. It can be used by any bystander to treat adult victims of out-of-hospital cardiac arrest.

 Learning Checkpoint 4

1. When is it appropriate to start CPR?

    a. As soon as you determine the victim is unresponsive.

    b. As soon as you determine the victim is not breathing normally.

    c. As soon as you determine the victim is both unresponsive and not breathing normally.

    d. Only when you have called 9-1-1 and the dispatcher tells you to start CPR.

2. Describe how to find the site for chest compressions in an adult or child victim.

    _____

    _____

3. Chest compressions in an adult should be at least _____ inches deep. In an infant or child, compress to a depth of at least _____ of the chest depth.

4. What is the correct ratio of chest compressions to breaths in single-rescuer CPR?

    a. 15 to 1

    b. 15 to 2

    c. 30 to 1

    d. 30 to 2

5. If you are performing CPR on an adult victim when an AED is brought to the scene and is ready to use, what action should you take?

    a. Use the AED as soon as it is ready.

    b. Continue CPR for at least 15 cycles before using the AED.

    c. Use the AED only if you can feel the victim's heart quivering in his or her chest.

    d. Use the AED only if the victim showed signs and symptoms of having a heart attack; otherwise, do not use it but continue CPR.

Technique of CPR for Adults and Children

See the "Skill: CPR for Adults, Children and Infants" for the steps for combining chest compressions with rescue breaths in CPR for adults and children.

Compression-Only CPR

An unresponsive victim who is not breathing normally needs both rescue breaths and chest compressions to move oxygenated blood to vital organs. However, if for any reason you cannot or will not give rescue breaths, you should still give the victim chest compressions. This gives the victim a better chance for survival than doing nothing.

Concluding Thoughts

Remember to check for normal breathing in any unresponsive victim. If an unresponsive victim is gasping or is not breathing, give CPR beginning with chest compressions. Remember also that, as important as CPR is for sustaining life, in many cases of cardiac arrest the victim also needs defibrillation to restore a normal heartbeat. The use of an AED, the final step for lay rescuers in basic life support, is described in **Chapter 6**.

Learning Outcomes

You should now be able to do the following:

1. List the risk factors for cardiovascular disease.

2. Explain general principles for maintaining cardiovascular health and preventing cardiovascular disease and respiratory arrest.

3. Describe the age categories for adults, children and infants related to differences in basic life support skills.

4. List the steps in the Cardiac Chain of Survival.

5. Describe when to call 9-1-1 before starting CPR and when to give 2 minutes of CPR before calling 9-1-1.

6. Demonstrate the procedure for giving CPR.

Review Questions

1. Preventable risk factors for cardiovascular disease include –
   a. smoking.
   b. high cholesterol levels.
   c. inactivity.
   d. All of the above

2. For the purposes of CPR, when does an infant become a child?
   a. At 6 months
   b. At 1 year
   c. At 15 pounds
   d. At 25 pounds

3. Call 9-1-1 first before beginning CPR for –
   a. an unresponsive adult who is not breathing normally.
   b. an unresponsive child or infant who is not breathing normally.
   c. a responsive adult.
   d. a responsive child or infant.

4. The correct hand position for chest compressions in adults is –

    a. on the top of the breastbone below the neck.

    b. on the lower end of the breastbone just above the abdomen.

    c. on the lower half of the breastbone in the middle of the chest.

    d. three finger-widths above where the ribs join.

5. How long should it take to deliver one rescue breath?

    a. ½ second

    b. 1 second

    c. 1½ seconds

    d. 2 seconds

6. Why should a barrier device be used with rescue breaths?

    a. To help get more air into the victim

    b. To prevent vomiting

    c. To protect against infectious disease

    d. To prevent air from entering the esophagus

7. Vomiting during rescue breaths may result from –

    a. blowing in too forcefully.

    b. blowing in for too long.

    c. blowing in too fast.

    d. All of the above

8. The correct ratio of chest compressions to breaths in single-rescuer CPR is –

    a. 5 to 2.

    b. 10 to 2.

    c. 15 to 2.

    d. 30 to 2.

9. If a victim begins breathing normally after you have given CPR but remains unresponsive, what do you do?

    a. Put the victim in the recovery position.

    b. Continue chest compressions and rescue breaths.

    c. Continue giving only chest compressions.

    d. Give rescue breaths only.

10. When should you send someone to bring an AED to the scene when you encounter an unresponsive adult?

    a. As soon as you see the victim is unresponsive

    b. As soon as the 9-1-1 dispatcher tells you to

    c. After 1 minute of CPR

    d. It depends on the cause of the victim's condition

Chapter 6 • Automated External Defibrillators (AED)

Chapter Preview

- Public Access to Defibrillation
- The Heart's Electrical System
- How AEDs Work
- Using an AED

- Special Considerations
- Potential AED Problems
- AED Maintenance

You are called to the scene where a man is lying unresponsive on the floor. Someone has already called 9-1-1. You know where an AED is located in the building, and you send someone for it as you check the victim for normal breathing. The victim is not breathing, and you begin CPR starting with chest compressions. About one minute later the other person returns with an AED and first aid kit. What series of actions should you now take?

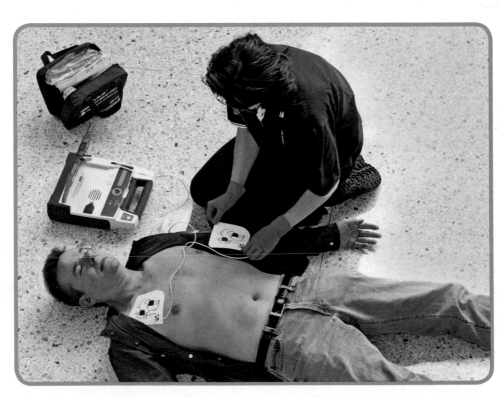

Not every victim who receives BLS needs an automated external defibrillator (AED), but many do. In many cases of cardiac arrest, the victim's heart has an abnormal rhythm that does not circulate the blood and this rhythm can often be corrected with the AED. Remember the Cardiac Chain of Survival: an AED should be used with any unresponsive victim who is not breathing. The early use of an AED for a heart attack victim doubles the chances for survival, and the American Heart Association estimates that the widespread availability and use of AEDs could save the lives of many thousands of people every year in the United States.[1]

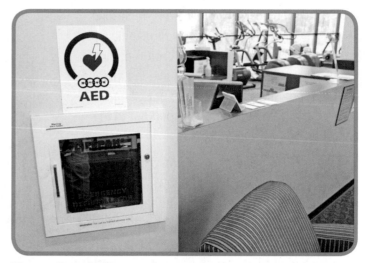

Figure 6-1 *AEDs are increasingly common in public places.*

Public Access to Defibrillation

To give a victim of cardiac arrest the best chance for resuscitation, CPR and **defibrillation** must begin as soon as possible. Ideally an AED should reach the victim within minutes. All ambulances and many other emergency responders such as police officers carry AEDs and reach the scene quickly after 9-1-1 is called, but the availability of AEDs in public places where people may experience heart attacks helps to ensure that a unit is present when needed by a trained first aider or first responder. Public access to defibrillation (PAD) programs have worked to make AEDs available in workplaces, public gathering places and other facilities for use by trained rescuers and first aiders. Increasingly visible are signs in public places indicating where AEDs are located **(Figure 6-1)**. Many states have laws requiring AEDs to be present in various public places.

In many areas a health care provider oversees the placement and use of the AED, as well as AED training. For professional rescuers, this is called medical direction. Your course instructor will inform you how to meet any legal requirements in your area for using an AED. The Food and Drug Administration (FDA) approves nonprescription AEDs for home use, and AED units that do not

[1]*American Heart Association. http://circ.ahajournals.org/cgi/reprint/CIRCULATIONAHA.106.172289v1 Accessed March 4, 2011.*

require specific training are present in homes and other settings. These devices have been demonstrated to be safe for use by lay people who follow the instructions printed on the device and the device's voice prompts during use. AED training will always offer benefits, but AEDs are generally simple and safe to use.

The Heart's Electrical System

The heart pumps blood to the lungs to pick up oxygen and then pumps oxygenated blood to all parts of the body. The heart consists of four chambers: the left atrium, the right atrium, and the left and right ventricles. The ventricles, the lower chambers of the heart, do most of the pumping. The heart's electrical system keeps the four chambers of the heart synchronized and working together. The sinoatrial and atrioventricular (AV) nodes help organize and control the rhythmic electrical impulses that keep the heart beating properly **(Figure 6-2)**.

With a heart attack or other heart problems, this rhythmic electrical control may be disrupted, causing an abnormal heart rhythm such as ventricular fibrillation.

Ventricular Fibrillation

Ventricular fibrillation (V-fib) is an abnormal heart rhythm that commonly occurs with heart attacks and stops circulation of the blood.

Although we say a victim in V-fib is in cardiac arrest, the heart is not actually completely still but is beating abnormally. **Fibrillation** means the ventricles of the heart are quivering instead of beating rhythmically. Blood is not filling the ventricles and is not being pumped out to the lungs or body as usual.

Heart attack is the most common cause of cardiac arrest, and ventricular fibrillation is a common dysrthymia that may result from heart attack, electrocution, hypothermia, trauma and other causes. Studies show that in approximately half the cases of cardiac arrest, the victim's heart is in fibrillation and therefore would benefit from a shock delivered by the AED.

How AEDs Work

The AED automatically checks the victim's heart rhythm and advises whether the victim needs a shock. The pads placed on the victim's chest are connected by cables to the main unit, which contain wires through which an electrical current passes.

The pads monitor the heart's electrical activity and the unit determines whether an abnormal rhythm is present for which a shock is needed. If the victim's heart is in V-fib, the machine will advise giving an electric shock to return the heart

to a normal rhythm. This is called defibrillation or stopping the fibrillation of the heart **(Figure 6-3)**.

The AED's **electrodes**, or pads, are placed on the victim's chest (or, with some AED models, on the front and back of the chest of a small child). When the unit delivers a shock, electricity travels through the cables to the pads, then through the body to the heart, and "jolts" the heart's electrical system in an attempt to restore a normal heartbeat. Because electrical current passes through the pads, it is important to position them correctly on the body and to avoid water, metal and any other substance that conducts electricity.

AEDs are simple to use, but they must be used right away. With every minute that goes by before defibrillation begins, the victim's chances for survival drop by about 10%.

The AED Unit

AEDs are complex inside despite their ease of use. They contain a battery and are portable.

Some models have a screen that tells you what to do; all models give directions in a clear voice. AED

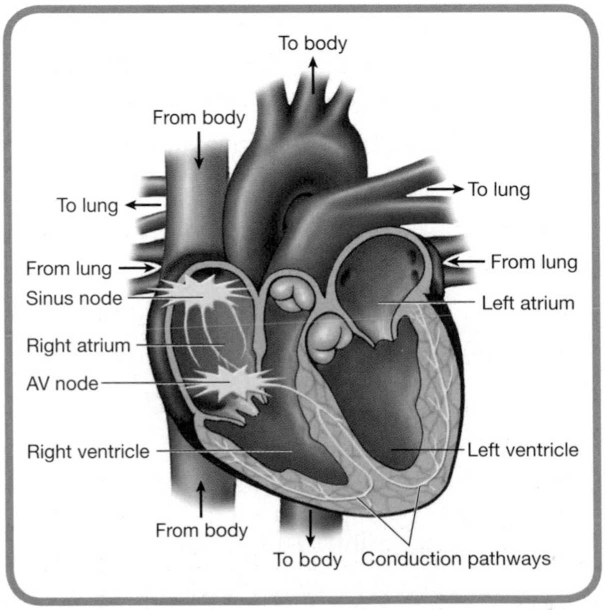

Figure 6-2 *The heart's electrical system.*

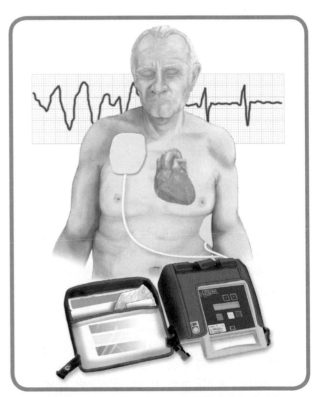

Figure 6-3 *An AED gives a shock to the heart.*

Learning Checkpoint 1

1. True or False: An AED works by giving a shock to a fibrillating heart to restore it to a normal rhythm.

2. True or False: It is very risky to use an AED because the unit cannot tell whether the victim's heart is beating normally or not.

3. About what proportion of cardiac arrest victims are in fibrillation and require a shock?

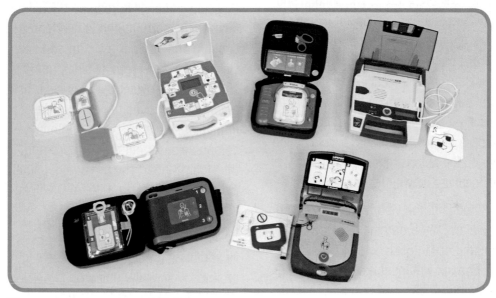

Figure 6-4 *A variety of AEDs.*

models vary somewhat in other features, but all work in the same basic way **(Figure 6-4)**.

Using an AED

In any situation in which a victim suddenly collapses or is found unresponsive, be thinking about the possibility of cardiac arrest even as you approach. If someone else is present and you know an AED is available nearby, send that person to call 9-1-1 and get the AED. It is better to have it right away and not use it than to need it and have to wait for it.

Determine the Need for AED

As always, with any unresponsive victim, send someone to call 9-1-1 and to get an AED. If the victim is not breathing normally, you will need to use the AED.

Start CPR

Remember BLS and the Cardiac Chain of Survival. Give CPR until the AED arrives at the scene and is ready to use. If you arrive at the victim with an AED, check the victim for normal breathing, and then use the AED immediately on an adult victim before starting CPR. If another rescuer is present, one should begin CPR while the other sets up the device. Continue CPR until the unit is ready to analyze the victim's heart rhythm, and then stop and follow the unit's instructions.

For a child found unresponsive and not breathing normally (not observed to have collapsed suddenly), give 5 cycles of CPR (about 2 minutes) before using the AED. This is different from the protocol for adults, because in most cases the child's heart is not in V-fib.

Attach the AED to Victim

Be sure the victim is not in water or in contact with metal. Water or metal conduct electricity that may pose a risk to you or others. Place the AED near the victim's shoulder next to the rescuer who will operate it. Turn it on and attach the pads (electrodes) to the victim's chest. Most AED units have a diagram on the pads or the unit itself to remind you where to position the pads **(Figure 6-5)**. Typically, the first pad is placed on the right side below the collar bone and to the right of the breastbone. The second pad is placed below and to the left of the left nipple and above the lower rib margin. On an infant or small child, the AED unit may indicate to position the pads on the front and back of the chest instead. If you have only adult pads, use them on the infant or child because this is their only hope; position the pads on the front and back of the chest if they would be too close together on the anterior chest and possibly cause an electrical arc between them.

Attach the AED pads to the victim only if the victim is unresponsive and not breathing. Expose the victim's chest and dry the skin with a towel or dry clothing (heart attack victims are often sweating). If the victim has heavy chest hair, quickly shave the pad areas. If a razor is not available, use scissors or trauma shears (which should be kept with the AED) to trim the hair and allow skin contact with the pads. Remove the backing from the pads and apply the pads firmly on the victim's chest. If required with your AED model, plug the pad cables into the main unit.

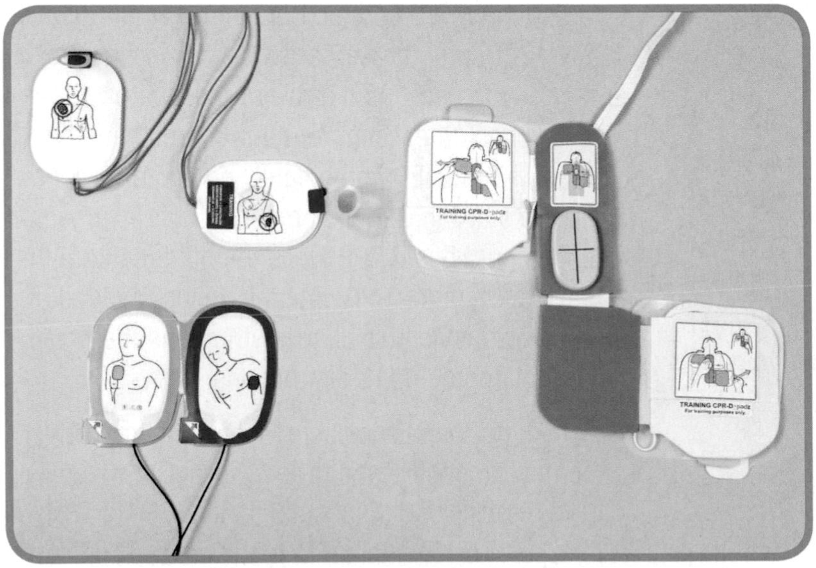

Analyze and Shock

With the pads in place and the AED unit on, most AED models then automatically analyze the victim's heart rhythm. Do not move or touch the victim while it is analyzing. After it analyzes the heart rhythm, the unit will advise you whether to give a shock or to resume CPR. If a shock is advised, be sure no one is touching the victim. Look up and down the victim and say, "Everybody clear!" Once everyone is clear, administer the shock (when advised) or stay clear as the AED automatically gives the shock. After the shock, immediately resume CPR, beginning with chest compressions, until the AED prompts to analyze the victim's heart rhythm again, usually after about 2 minutes. Then the AED will advise another shock if needed or prompt you to continue CPR (with the pads left in place).

Note that different AEDs may use slightly different prompts. Follow the unit's voice and visual prompts through this process. Some units are programmed to administer the shock automatically rather than prompt the user to push the "shock" button; in this case always follow the unit's prompts.

If the victim recovers (moves and is breathing normally), put an unresponsive breathing victim in the recovery position and continue to monitor his or her breathing. Keep the AED pads in place as some victims may return to V-fib and require defibrillation again.

The AED may also say no shock is indicated. This means the victim's heart will not benefit from defibrillation. If this is so, immediately continue CPR (see Skill: "Using an AED").

Figure 6-5 *AED pads usually include diagrams showing correct pad placement.*

Special Considerations

Some situations involve special considerations in the use of the AED.

Children

AEDs are now designed and recommended to be used for both children and infants. Follow the adult guidelines for children older than age 8.

Although sudden cardiac arrest in younger children is much rarer, it can occur from causes such as:

- Sudden infant death syndrome
- Poisoning
- Drowning
- A heart problem

In most cases, however, cardiac arrest in a child is not caused by a heart problem and the child's heart is not in V-fib. Therefore, give a child or infant 2 minutes of CPR before using the AED, unless the child or infant was witnessed to collapse suddenly. If the child does not recover, then use the AED as usual. This is different from the protocol for adults, in whom cardiac arrest is more likely to be the result of heart attack and on whom the AED should be used immediately.

Most AED units can be used with children and infants, using different pads specially designed for children and infants **(Figure 6-6)**. It is important to use only approved pediatric AED electrode pads, which are smaller than those for adults and produce lower-energy shocks on a child younger than 8. Usually the pads have a distinctive appearance to prevent confusing adult and pediatric pads, such as pink connectors and teddybear emblems. If pediatric pads are not available, however, using adult pads is better than not using the AED at all. Pediatric pads should not be used for an adult, however, because the lower energy is insufficient to affect the heart rhythm.

Be sure to follow the device's instructions for pad placement on a small child. For example,

the AED shown on the right in **Figure 6-6** uses pad placement on the front and back of the child's chest. Testing has demonstrated that with small children it can be difficult to position both the pads on the front of the chest and studies have shown placement on the front and back also delivers an effective shock (see **Box 6-1**).

BOX 6-1: CHANGING AED TECHNOLOGY

AEDs were first designed for use on adults and older children and, therefore, originally had pads that came in one size only and were placed in the typical manner on the upper right and lower left chest, as described earlier. When research showed the benefit of lower-energy shocks for pediatric victims, newer units were developed that used separate pediatric pads, sometimes placed on the front and back of the chest. AED technology continues to evolve, with some units able to determine characteristics of the victim and adjust the shock level automatically. Other new units now use the same pads for all victims, regardless of size and weight, but have a separate switch on the unit to use for pediatric victims. With such advances, separate pediatric pads may eventually become obsolete.

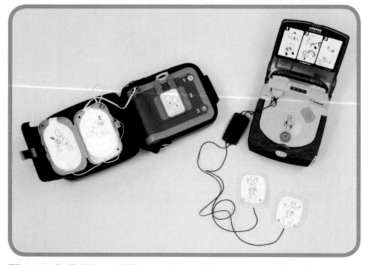

Figure 6-6 *The AED on the right has pediatric pads and the one on the left uses a key to reduce the amount of joules (electrical charge) to the adult pads so they can be used for infants and children.*

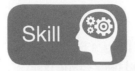 Skill **Using an AED**

1 Position the victim away from water and metal. Place the unit by the victim's shoulder and turn it on.

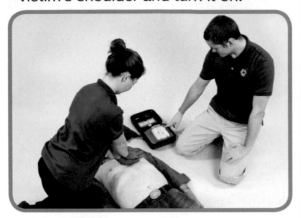

2 Expose the victim's chest and quickly dry or shave the pad placement area if necessary.

3 Apply pads to the victim's chest as shown on pads. If needed, plug the cables into the unit.

Use adult pads for a victim 8 or older. For an infant or child younger than 8, use a unit with pediatric pads if available, applied as directed by the unit; if pediatric pads are unavailable, use adult pads.

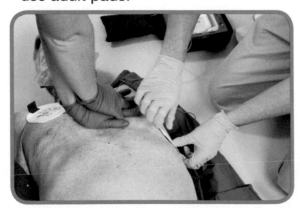

4 Stand clear during rhythm analysis.

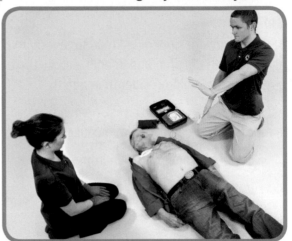

5 Follow prompts from the AED unit to do one of three things: (1) press the "shock" button, (2) stay clear while the AED automatically delivers a shock or (3) do not shock but immediately give CPR with the pads remaining in place, starting with chest compressions.

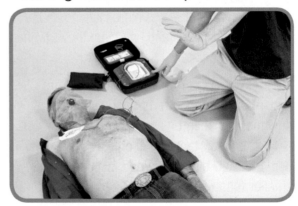

6 Follow the AED's prompts to analyze the rhythm again after 5 cycles of CPR (about 2 minutes).

7 Continue steps 5 and 6 until the victim wakes up or more advanced help arrives and takes over.

8 If the victim begins breathing normally but is unresponsive, put the victim in the recovery position (with pads remaining in place) and continue to monitor breathing and pulse.

ALERT

- Move the victim away from metal or standing water before using the AED.
- Remove any medication pads with a gloved hand and dry the victim's chest well before attaching the electrodes.
- Avoid any flammable materials, including oxygen flowing through a mask. Do not use alcohol to wipe the victim's skin.
- Do not use the AED when in motion in a vehicle or boat.
- Do not use a cell phone or two-way radio within 6 feet of an AED.
- Remember not to touch the victim while the AED is analyzing the rhythm or administering a shock.

 Learning **Checkpoint 2**

1. Which statement is true about the pads (electrodes) of an AED?

   a. The AED has two pads that must be correctly positioned.

   b. The AED has four pads that must be correctly positioned.

   c. The AED has two pads, but only one needs to be put on the victim's chest (the other is a spare).

   d. The pads are used only if a heart rhythm is not detected when the machine is placed in the center of the victim's chest.

2. If the AED unit advises you to give a shock, what do you do next?

   a. Continue CPR while asking someone else to push the "shock" button.

   b. Place a wet towel over the victim's chest and push the "shock" button.

   c. Make sure everyone is clear of the victim and then push the "shock" button.

   d. Wait about one minute for the unit to confirm analysis of a shockable rhythm.

3. What do you do immediately after the AED administers a shock?

_____

Traumatic Injury

Cardiac arrest in a severely injured victim is usually caused by the traumatic injury, not by a heart rhythm problem such as V-fib. In such cases your local medical direction may specify not to use the AED. However, if the injury seems minor, the victim's cardiac arrest may respond to defibrillation. You should attach the pads and follow the prompts from the AED. When in doubt, use the AED.

Internal Pacemaker or Defibrillator

When you expose the victim's chest to apply the AED pads, you may see a bulge or lump beneath the victim's skin from an implanted **pacemaker** or defibrillator, often on the upper left side of the chest **(Figure 6-7)**. Do not place a pad directly over this area, but instead place it at least 1 or more inches away. If the victim's chest or body is jerking, there may be an implanted defibrillator that is giving shocks; wait until jerking has ended before applying the pads.

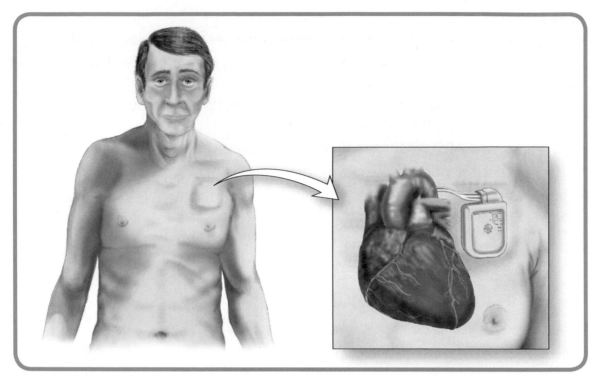

Figure 6-7 *Vary AED pad placement if the victim has an implanted device.*

Hypothermia

Detecting breathing in a victim of hypothermia (low body temperature) can be difficult. Handle a hypothermic victim very carefully because jarring may cause cardiac arrest. Follow your local guidelines for AED use if you find no signs of breathing. Typically, if the AED finds a shockable rhythm and advises shocks, no more than one shock is given, and then CPR and rewarming is performed until help arrives.

Medication Patches

If the victim has a medication patch or paste on the chest, remove it with a gloved hand and wipe the chest before applying the AED pads **(Figure 6-8)**.

Potential AED Problems

An AED must be maintained regularly and the battery kept charged. With regular maintenance, an AED should not have any problems during use.

The AED may also prompt you to avoid problems. If you get a low-battery prompt, change the battery before continuing. Another prompt may advise you to avoid moving the victim if the AED detects motion.

AED Maintenance

AEDs require regular maintenance. Check the manufacturer's manual for periodic scheduled maintenance and testing of the unit.

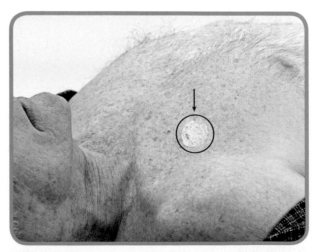

Figure 6-8 *Remove medication patches prior to AED use.*

AED INSPECTION CHECKLIST

Date: _____ Location: _____ AED Model: _____

Inspected by:_____ Signed:_____

Criteria	ok/no	Corrective action/remarks
AED unit		
Verify correctly placed	_____	_____
Clean, clear of objects	_____	_____
No cracks or damage to case	_____	_____
Cables/connectors present and not expired	_____	_____
Fully charged battery in place	_____	_____
Charged spare battery present	_____	_____
Check status/service light indicator	_____	_____
Check absence of service alarm	_____	_____
Power on, self-test	_____	_____
Supplies		
Two sealed sets of electrode pads	_____	_____
Verify expiration date on pad packages	_____	_____
Razor	_____	_____
Medical examination gloves	_____	_____
Hand towels	_____	_____
Scissors or trauma shears	_____	_____
Pocket mask or face shield	_____	_____

Figure 6-9 *Example of an AED inspection checklist.*

 Learning Checkpoint 3

1. Name at least one situation in which a young child may experience sudden cardiac arrest and could benefit from the use of a pediatric AED.

   _____

2. Describe where to put the AED pads if you see that a victim has an implanted pacemaker or defibrillator.

   _____

3. What should you do with the AED pads if the victim has a medication patch on his or her chest?

   _____

Table 6-1: Summary of Basic Life Support

Step	Infant (younger than 1 year)	Child (1 year through Puberty, except 1-8 for AED)	Adult
1. Check for respon-siveness and normal breathing.	Stimulate to check response. Observe whether breathing normally.	Tap shoulder and shout "Are you OK?" while observing for normal breathing (only gasps are not normal).	
2. If unresponsive, have someone call for help.	Send someone to call 9-1-1. If alone, give 2 min-utes of care before calling 9-1-1 (and getting AED).	Send someone to call 9-1-1. If alone, unless the child has a known heart problem, give 2 minutes of care before calling 9-1-1 (and getting AED).	Send someone to call 9-1-1. If alone, call 9-1-1 and get an AED immediate-ly (give 2 minutes of care first for drowning victim).
3. If unresponsive and not breathing normally, give CPR, starting with chest compressions.	For compressions use 2 fingers just below the nip-ple line. Compress chest to ⅓ the depth of chest (about 1½ inches).	For compressions use one or two hands in the center of the chest between nipples. Compress chest to ⅓ the depth of chest (about 2 inches).	For compressions use both hands, one on top of other, in the center of the chest between nipples. Compress chest at least 2 inches.
3a. Chest compressions in CPR.	Chest compressions at a rate of at least 100 per minute.		
3b. Ratio of compressions and breaths.	Cycles of 30 compressions and 2 breaths.		
4. Give 2 breaths.	Use barrier device or cover mouth, nose or stoma. Each breath lasts 1 second.		
4a. If breaths do not go in, reposition head and try again.	Each breath lasts 1 second.		
4b. If breaths still do not go in, continue with chest compressions.	Continue with chest compressions. Check the mouth for an object each time breaths are given and remove it if seen.		
5. Use AED as soon as available.	Use pediatric electrode pads if available. If not available, use adult pads.		Use adult AED electrode pads.
6. If victim recovers normal breathing, put in recovery position.	Hold infant and monitor breathing.	Lay on side in HAINES recovery position and monitor breathing.	

A daily inspection of the unit helps ensure that the AED is always ready for use and all needed supplies are present. Professional rescuers usually inspect the unit at the beginning of their shift. Most facilities with an AED use a daily checklist form **(Figure 6-9)**. A checklist should always be adapted for the specific AED model, including the manufacturer's daily maintenance guidelines. In addition, many units come with a simulator device used to check that the AED is correctly analyzing rhythms and delivering shocks; this may be part of the daily inspection routine.

Concluding Thoughts

Remember that an AED is needed for most victims who are in cardiac arrest – CPR alone is often not enough. Always call or send someone for an AED for a victim who is unresponsive and not breathing normally.

Learning Outcomes

You should now be able to do the following:

1. Explain how AEDs work to correct an abnormal heart rhythm.

2. Describe when an AED should be used and the basic steps for use.

3. Demonstrate how to use an AED with an adult or child victim.

4. List special considerations to be aware of when using an AED with certain types of victims or in certain situations.

Review Questions

1. What is occurring during ventricular fibrillation?

   a. The ventricles of the heart have stopped moving.

   b. The ventricles of the heart are contracting too slowly.

   c. The ventricles of the heart are quivering rather than pumping.

   d. The ventricles of the heart are contracting with opposing rhythms.

2. An AED administers a shock to the victim –

   a. whenever you turn it on.

   b. automatically about 15 seconds after the unit is turned on.

   c. when you push the "shock" button after being prompted to do so.

   d. about 3 seconds after the pads are applied to the victim.

3. What should you do before using an AED?

   a. Ensure that the victim is not breathing.

   b. Administer CPR until the AED is ready to use.

   c. Place it next to the victim and turn it on.

   d. All of the above

4. The AED pads should be positioned where on the victim?

   a. Where the diagram on the unit indicates placement.

   b. Below the nipples on both sides of the chest.

   c. In both armpits.

   d. One on the chest and the other on the abdomen.

5. While the AED is analyzing the victim's heart rhythm –

   a. continue CPR.

   b. do not touch the victim.

   c. push the "shock" button.

   d. push down on the pads to hold them in place.

6. If the AED indicates no shock is needed, you should then –

   a. wait 20 seconds and try again.

   b. give CPR starting with chest compressions.

   c. give a lower-power shock.

   d. take the pads off and reposition them.

7. An AED may be used with a child 1 to 8 years old, ideally with –

   a. special pediatric pads.

   b. the voltage knob turned to a lower setting.

   c. the pads on the legs to lower the voltage through the heart.

   d. petroleum jelly between the skin and the pads.

8. When using an AED with a victim of hypothermia –

   a. briskly rub the victim's chest to warm up the skin below the pads.

   b. handle the victim very carefully.

   c. put oil on the pads to provide better conductivity.

   d. wait until you have fully warmed the body before applying the pads.

Chapter 7 • Airway Obstructions

Chapter Preview

- Choking Emergencies
- Preventing Choking
- Airway Obstruction

You are having a cup of tea in the lunch room when you see a man at the next table suddenly bring his hands up to his throat. He looks frantic and his mouth is open, but he is not speaking. The others at his table are looking at him but no one has moved to help – they do not seem to know what to do. You approach the man, who you think may be choking. What should you say and do?

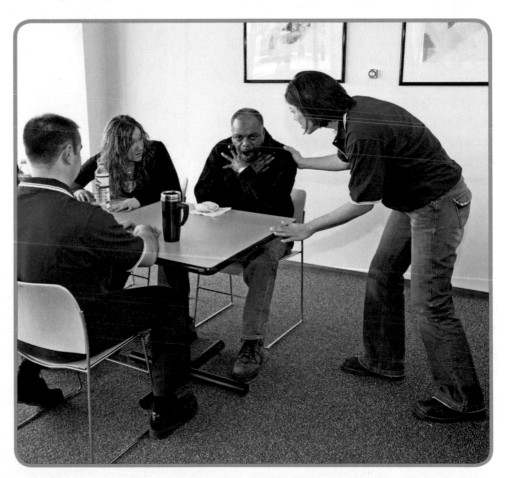

As described in **Chapter 5**, the inability to breathe is a life-threatening emergency, and body cells not receiving oxygen begin to die within minutes. The inability to breathe because of an airway obstruction is commonly called choking. Choking is a common cause of respiratory arrest (the stopping of breathing). Because time is so critical in these emergencies, it is important to be prepared to give immediate care to responsive and unresponsive choking victims.

Choking Emergencies

With airway obstructions, the victim cannot breathe because the airway is blocked by a foreign object, an anatomical structure such as the tongue, or fluid or vomit. These emergencies require immediate care to clear the obstruction and enable the victim to breathe **(Figure 7-1)**.

Preventing Choking

Choking is common in both adults and children. About 4,600 people die from choking each year in the United States. Although people often think of choking as a problem primarily for infants and young children, in fact the age group that experiences choking most frequently is adults 65 and older, who are more than twice as likely to die from choking as younger adults. Perhaps because most parents and caretakers know about the choking risk for younger children, fewer children – about 140 children younger than 4 – die each year from choking. Yet virtually all of these cases of choking could have been prevented.[1]

In adults, choking often results from trying to swallow large pieces of food that have not been chewed sufficiently, either from eating too quickly or from eating while engaged in other activities. Choking is more common in people under the influence of alcohol or drugs. Choking is also more

likely in those wearing dentures, apparently because of a diminished sensation for how well food has been chewed before attempting to swallow.

Choking is a serious threat to infants and children up to 3 to 4 years of age and a significant cause of death. An infant or young child may put any small object in his or her mouth, and nonfood items account for most choking deaths in young children. Coins, balloons, small balls and toy parts are the most common causes of choking in young children.[2] In older children, the most common items choked on are food, candy and gum.[3] Follow these guidelines to prevent choking in infants and children:

- Do not leave any small objects within reach of an infant (such as buttons, beads, coins, etc.). Ensure that small parts cannot break off toys or other items around the infant or young child.

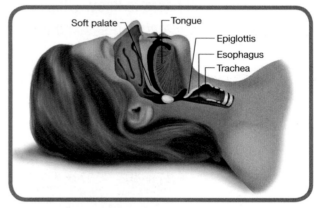

(a)

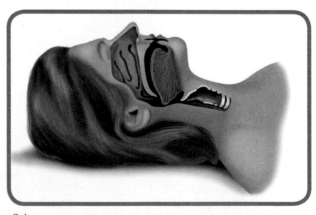

(b)

Figure 7-1 *(a) Food lodged in the airway, obstructing breathing. (b) The tongue blocking the airway in an unresponsive victim.*

[1]*National Safety Council. (2011). Injury Facts®, 2011 Edition. Itasca, IL: Author.*

[2]*Safe Kids USA, http://www.safekids.org/our-work/ research/fact-sheets/choking-and-suffocation- prevention-fact-sheet.html Accessed March 1, 2011.*

[3]*Healthline, http://www.healthline.com/galecontent/ choking-1 Accessed March 1, 2011.*

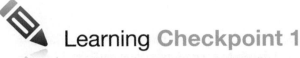

Learning Checkpoint 1

1. List at least four situations in which choking is a risk for an adult.

_____

_____

_____

_____

2. Put a check mark next to food items that should not be given to a child younger than 3.

_____ Popcorn   _____ Grapes

_____ Jell-O   _____ Corn kernels

_____ Marshmallows   _____ Soft bread slices

_____ Spaghetti   _____ Gum

- Feed infants only soft foods that do not require chewing.

- Have children sit in a high chair or at a table to eat. Never let a child move around while eating.

- Teach children not to eat too fast or to talk or laugh while eating.

- Cut up foods a child could choke on, such as hot dogs, into small pieces.

- Do not give children younger than 3 certain foods, including:
  - Peanuts
  - Popcorn
  - Grapes
  - Chunks of raw vegetables (such as baby carrots) or fruits
  - Marshmallows
  - Gum

- Supervise young children while they eat and be prepared to care for a child who chokes.

Airway Obstruction

A victim is choking when the airway is obstructed either partially or fully. A victim can choke on:

- Food or other foreign bodies in the mouth

- The tongue (in an unresponsive victim lying on his or her back)

- Teeth or other body tissues resulting from injury

- Vomit

A complete **airway obstruction** means the victim is getting no air at all and, consequently, no oxygen is entering the blood. This victim will soon become unresponsive and not long after breathing stops, the heart will stop, too. Choking care is urgently needed.

A partial obstruction means something is partly blocking the airway but the victim is still getting some air into the lungs around the obstructing object. The victim may be getting enough air to cough out the obstructing object – or breathing may be very difficult and the victim might be unable to cough strongly enough to expel the object.

Assessing Choking

Most cases of choking in adults occur while eating. Most cases of choking in infants and children occur while eating or playing. Often, therefore, someone is present and recognizes the choking event while the victim is still responsive. Choking may be either mild or severe. With a mild obstruction the victim is usually coughing forcefully in an attempt to expel the object. The victim is getting some air and may be making wheezing or high-pitched sounds with breaths, along with coughing. Do not interrupt the person's coughing or attempts to expel the object, and do not pound the person on the back in an effort to help.

With severe choking, however, the victim is getting very little air or none at all. The person may look frantic and be clutching at the throat (Figure 7-2). You may notice a pale or bluish coloring (cyanosis) around the mouth and nail beds. A victim who is coughing very weakly and silently, or not coughing at all, is unlikely to expel the obstructing object. The victim cannot speak. Simply ask the victim if he or she is choking. If the victim cannot answer but indicates that he or she is choking, ask for permission to help and begin choking care for a responsive victim.

An unresponsive victim who may be choking receives the same initial assessment as any unresponsive victim as described in **Chapter 4**. If the victim is not breathing normally, start CPR with 30 chest compressions. If your first breath does not go into the victim after opening the airway, try again to open the airway and attempt a second breath. If it still does not go in, then assume the victim has an obstructed airway.

Care for Choking Adults and Children

Choking care depends on whether the victim is responsive or unresponsive and whether, in an unresponsive victim, the obstruction is mild or severe:

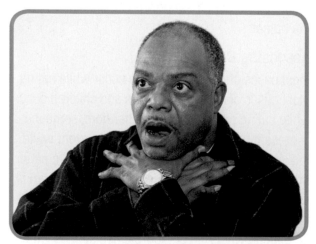

Figure 7-2 *The universal sign of a responsive victim who is choking.*

- For a **responsive choking victim who is coughing**, encourage the victim to continue coughing to clear the object. Stay with the victim and call 9-1-1 if the object is not immediately expelled.

- For a **responsive choking victim who cannot speak or cough forcefully**, give abdominal thrusts as described in the Skill: "Choking Care for Responsive Adult or Child."

- For **an unresponsive choking victim who is not breathing normally and who may be choking**, immediately call (or have someone call) 9-1-1 and begin CPR.

With a responsive victim, after quickly asking for consent, telling the victim what you intend to do and having someone else call 9-1-1, stand behind the victim and reach around to the abdomen. Place one leg forward between the victim's legs to help you brace in case the victim becomes unresponsive and falls. Keep your head slightly to the side in case the victim's head snaps back during the abdominal thrusts.

Make a fist with one hand and place the thumb side of the fist against the victim's abdomen just above the navel. Grasp the fist with your other hand and thrust inward and upward into the victim's abdomen with quick thrusts. The pressure of each thrust serves to force air from the lungs up the trachea to expel the object. Pause only briefly after each abdominal thrust to see if the victim is able to breathe or cough; if not, continue with additional thrusts.

If you are giving abdominal thrusts to a child or someone much shorter than you, kneel behind the victim. If the victim is much taller than you, ask the victim to kneel or sit because it is important that your thrusts are upward as well as inward, which is impossible if you have to reach up to the victim's abdomen.

Note that because abdominal thrusts may sometimes cause internal injury, a victim who is

(continues on page 110)

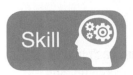

Choking Care for Responsive Adult or Child

1 Stand behind an adult victim with one leg forward between the victim's legs. Keep your head slightly to one side. For a child, move down to the child's level or kneel behind the child. Reach around the abdomen.

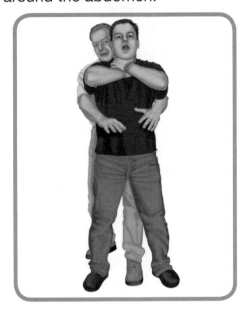

2 Locate the person's navel with a finger from one hand. Make a fist with the other hand and place the thumb side of the fist against the person's abdomen just above the navel.

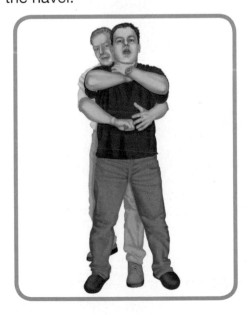

3 Grasp your fist with your other hand and thrust inward and upward into the victim's abdomen with quick thrusts. Continue abdominal thrusts until the victim expels the object or becomes unresponsive.

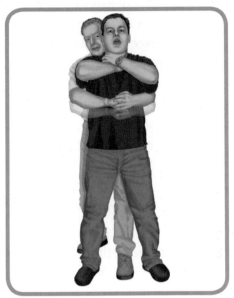

4 For a responsive pregnant victim, or any victim you cannot get your arms around or cannot effectively give abdominal thrusts to, give chest thrusts in the middle of the breastbone from behind the victim. Avoid squeezing the ribs with your arms.

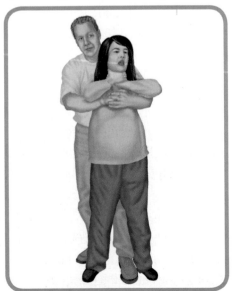

(continued from page 108)

given abdominal thrusts is recommended to be examined by a health care provider.

When a severe airway obstruction is not cleared, the victim will become unresponsive within minutes. You may have found the victim in an unresponsive condition, or the victim may become unresponsive while you are giving abdominal thrusts if the object is not expelled. In the latter case, quickly and carefully lower the victim and lay him or her on his or her back on the floor. Make sure 9-1-1 has been called. Begin the CPR sequence as usual with 30 chest compressions delivered hard and fast. Then, when you open the victim's mouth to give a rescue breath, look first for an object in the mouth. If you see an object in the victim's mouth, remove it. If the object is expelled, give 2 rescue breaths as usual and continue CPR unless the victim recovers and is breathing normally.

If the obstruction remains, the chest compressions of CPR may expel the foreign object. While giving CPR, each time you open the victim's mouth to give breaths, check first to see if an object is visible; if so, remove it.

Care for Choking Infants

If a responsive choking infant can cry or cough, watch carefully to see if the object comes out. If the infant is responsive but cannot cry or cough, have someone call 9-1-1 and assume the airway is obstructed. Give alternating back blows (slaps) and chest thrusts in an attempt to expel the object. Support the infant in one hand against your thigh as you sit or stand, keeping the infant's head lower than the body. To prevent spinal injury, be sure to support the infant's head and neck during these maneuvers. The detailed steps for back blows (slaps) and chest thrusts are described in the Skill: "Choking Care for Responsive Infant."

If an infant to whom you were giving responsive choking care then becomes unresponsive, be sure 9-1-1 has been called and start CPR with chest compressions. As with an adult or child, the chest compressions may cause the object to be expelled.

Check for an object in the mouth each time you open the airway before you give a breath, and remove any object you see. Never do a finger sweep of the mouth if you do not see an object, because this could force an object deeper into the throat.

When you encounter an unresponsive infant, first check for normal breathing as usual. If the infant is not breathing normally, begin CPR with chest compressions. If your first breath does not go in after opening the airway and the infant's chest does not rise, try again after repositioning the infant's head to open the airway. If the second breath does not go in, assume that the infant has an airway obstruction and continue CPR, checking the mouth for an object each time you open it to give a rescue breath.

Self-Treating Choking

If you are choking when alone, give yourself abdominal thrusts to try to expel the object. You may try using your hands, or leaning over and pushing your abdomen against the back of a chair or other firm object **(Figure 7-3)**.

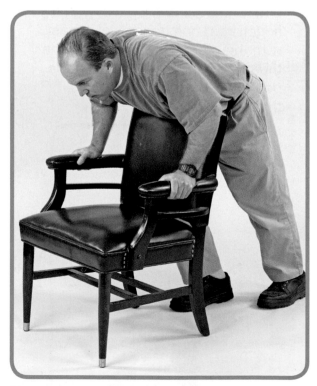

Figure 7-3 *Abdominal self-thrusts.*

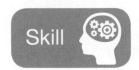
Choking Care for Unresponsive Adult, Child or Infant

1 If the victim is unresponsive and not breathing normally, start CPR with 30 chest compressions at least 2 inches deep in an adult and at least ⅓ the depth of the chest in a child (about 2 inches) or infant (about 1½ inches) at a rate of at least 100 per minute. Count aloud for a steady fast rate: "One, two, three, . . ."

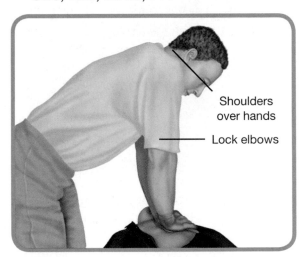

Shoulders over hands

Lock elbows

2 Open the airway with the head tilt–chin lift.

3 Give 2 rescue breaths, each lasting 1 second. If the first breath does not go in and the chest does not rise, position the victim's head again to open the airway and try again.

4 If breaths still do not go in, continue CPR with chest compressions, in a ratio of 30 compressions and 2 breaths.

5 Look inside the mouth before giving breaths after each cycle of compressions and remove any object you see. Then give 2 breaths.

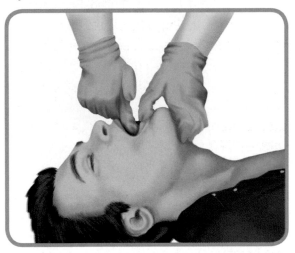

6 Continue CPR until:
- The victim recovers and is breathing normally.
- Professional help arrives and takes over.

7 • Airway Obstructions

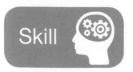

Skill — Choking Care for Responsive Infant

1 Support the infant face-down by holding the head in one hand, with the torso on your forearm against your thigh. Give up to 5 back blows (slaps) between the shoulder blades with the heel of your hand.

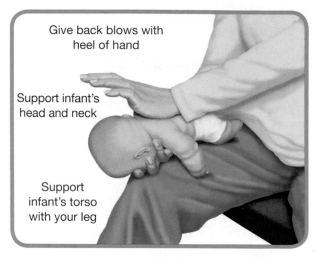

Give back blows with heel of hand

Support infant's head and neck

Support infant's torso with your leg

2 Check for an expelled object. If not present, continue with next step.

3 With your other hand on the back of the infant's head, roll the infant face-up, supporting the back of the infant's head with your hand.

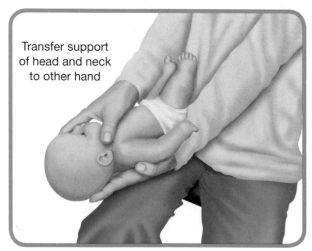

Transfer support of head and neck to other hand

4 Give up to 5 chest thrusts with two fingers on sternum just below the nipple line, about 1 per second. Each thrust should be 1½ inches deep. Check mouth for expelled object.

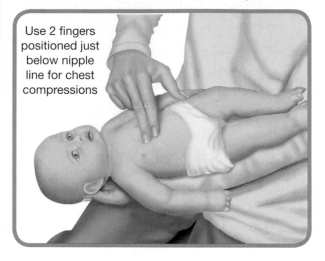

Use 2 fingers positioned just below nipple line for chest compressions

5 Continue cycles of 5 back blows (slaps), 5 chest thrusts and checking the mouth. If alone, call 9-1-1 after 1 minute. Continue until the object is expelled or the infant becomes unresponsive. If the infant becomes unresponsive, give CPR. Look inside the mouth before giving breaths after each cycle of compressions and remove any object you see.

Learning Checkpoint 2

1. For a responsive adult victim who is choking and cannot cough, you should –

   a. start CPR immediately.

   b. alternate back blows and chest thrusts.

   c. give abdominal thrusts.

   d. wait until the victim becomes unresponsive.

2. True or False: A choking victim who is coughing forcefully is still able to breathe and may be able to cough out the foreign body.

3. True or False: A choking victim who is unable to breathe will soon become unresponsive.

4. For a responsive choking infant –

   a. support the head as you position the infant.

   b. alternate back blows (slaps) and chest thrusts.

   c. check the infant's mouth for an expelled object.

   d. All of the above

5. Explain why CPR is given to a choking victim who becomes unresponsive.

   _____

   _____

   _____

   _____

Concluding Thoughts

You have now learned the basic life support skills of CPR, AED use and care for choking victims. **Chapter 8** continues with another important skill: bleeding control. Severe bleeding is another life-threatening condition.

Learning Outcomes

You should now be able to do the following:

1. List ways to prevent choking.

2. Demonstrate choking care for a responsive adult, child and infant.

3. Demonstrate choking care for an unresponsive adult, child and infant.

Review Questions

1. What increases the risk of choking in an adult?

   a. Taking high blood pressure medication

   b. Overcooking foods

   c. Having gum disease

   d. Drinking alcohol with meals

2. A victim with a severe airway obstruction –

    a. cannot speak or cough forcefully.

    b. cannot speak but can cough forcefully.

    c. can speak and cough weakly.

    d. can speak but only in short sentences.

3. To give abdominal thrusts to a responsive choking adult, what hand position is used?

    a. Both hands together on the bottom edge of the breastbone

    b. Both hands together just above the navel

    c. One hand at the navel and one hand at the "V" where the lower ribs meet

    d. One hand on the bottom rib at each side

4. What is important when giving choking first aid to a responsive infant?

    a. Alternate series of back blows (slaps) and chest thrusts.

    b. Keep the infant's head raised above the body.

    c. Give CPR in the usual way.

    d. Perform a more gentle version of the adult responsive choking technique.

Chapter 8 • Controlling Bleeding

Chapter Preview

- Effects of Blood Loss
- External Bleeding
- Internal Bleeding

You receive a call that a worker in the shipping department is injured. You grab the first aid kit and arrive at the scene within a minute. The injured man is holding a bloody rag wrapped around his hand. He says he was using a box cutter, which slipped and made a gash in his palm. He unwraps the rag to show you, and you see a deep laceration that is still bleeding. What are the important steps you should take?

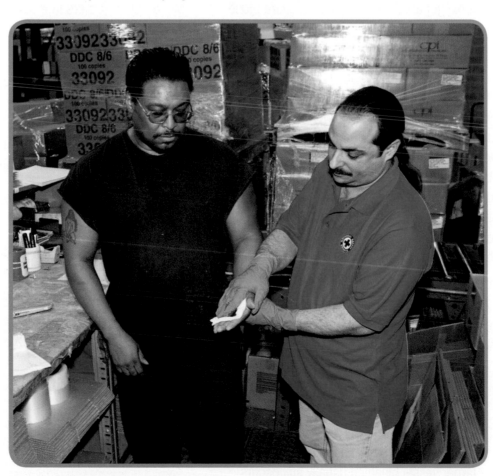

Blood carries oxygen from the lungs to all parts of the body. Many kinds of injuries damage blood vessels and cause external or internal bleeding. Bleeding may be minor or life-threatening. Severe loss of blood can threaten the ability of the cardiovascular system to get the needed oxygen to vital organs. Severe bleeding, therefore, can be as great a threat to life as respiratory or cardiac arrest. This is why the victim is examined for severe bleeding in the initial assessment. Fortunately, most external bleeding is not that severe and can be controlled with first aid techniques.

Effects of Blood Loss

As you learned in **Chapter 3**, the cardiovascular system has several important functions. Of all these, none is more important than transporting oxygen to the body. Without oxygen, vital tissues begin to die within minutes. Although the other functions of blood are also essential for life, the lack of oxygenation resulting from severe blood loss is the most serious first aid issue.

Fortunately, the body can compensate for a small blood loss without ill effects **(Figure 8-1)**. This is why it is possible for a healthy person to donate blood periodically without problems. A larger blood loss, however, can have serious effects, potentially leading to death. **Table 8-1** shows the amount of blood loss that causes shock and the loss that becomes lethal if not immediately corrected. Note that in infants and children, severe bleeding becomes critical more quickly than in adults because the same amount of blood lost represents a higher percentage of the body's blood volume.

When a blood vessel is damaged and blood escapes, the body attempts to control the bleeding through three processes:

- **Vascular spasm** is a mechanism in which the damaged blood vessel constricts to slow the bleeding and to allow clotting to occur. With an injured small vessel, this constriction may be sufficient to stop the bleeding, but with a larger vessel bleeding usually still occurs.

- **Platelets** in the blood then stick to each other and to the walls of the injured vessel to form a **platelet plug**, which may reduce or stop minor bleeding.

- **Clotting** (coagulation) is the process in which **fibrin** produced from blood proteins clumps together with platelets and other blood cells in a fibrin web to seal the leak in the vessel **(Figure 8-2)**. These three mechanisms working together may be able to stop or reduce bleeding after an injury. In a more serious injury, however, these mechanisms may not be sufficient to stop the bleeding, or bleeding may continue long enough that the victim shows the effects of reduced blood volume. Controlling bleeding is therefore an important first aid action.

Bleeding occurs when blood from injured vessels escapes the body through a wound (external bleeding) or gathers in a body space or cavity (internal bleeding). Although many of the signs and symptoms of each are different, as is the first aid given, both external and internal bleeding can be life-threatening when severe and uncontrolled.

External Bleeding

External bleeding typically occurs when skin and other underlying tissues are damaged by trauma,

Table 8-1: **Lethal Blood Loss**

Hemorrhage	Percent of Total Blood Volume Lost	Effects
Class I	Less than 15%	Generally well tolerated
Class II	15% to 30%	Shock occurs; victim needs rapid transport
Class III	30% to 40%	Severe shock occurs; victim needs immediate transfusion
Class IV	More than 40%	Rapidly fatal

Note: A 15% volume loss in a 150-lb. person is about 750 mL. A 30% loss is about 1.5 liters and a 40% loss is about 2 liters.

Blood loss after an injury may occur quickly with severe bleeding, but usually the body passes through a series of stages as blood volume drops:

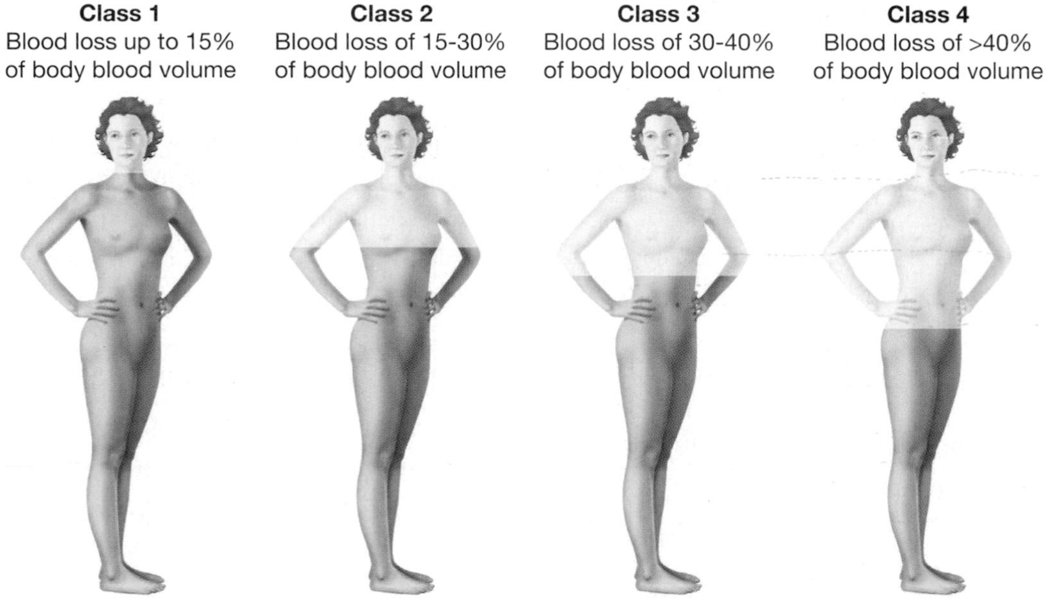

Class 1	**Class 2**	**Class 3**	**Class 4**
Blood loss up to 15% of body blood volume	Blood loss of 15-30% of body blood volume	Blood loss of 30-40% of body blood volume	Blood loss of >40% of body blood volume

With a loss of up to 15% of blood volume, the body can compensate for the loss of volume by constricting (shrinking) blood vessels to maintain blood pressure and can continue to transport oxygen to organs. The victim remains alert, and blood pressure and pulse are close to normal.

With a loss of 15% to 30% of blood volume, constricting blood vessels maintain blood flow to vital organs such as the brain and heart while reducing blood flow to other body areas. The skin looks pale or ashen, cool and dry. Heart and respiratory rates increase in an attempt to compensate. The victim may feel restless and confused.

With a loss of 30% to 40% of blood volume, the body can no longer compensate. Blood pressure falls and the victim experiences shock, a serious condition in which vital organs are not receiving enough oxygenated blood. The victim is confused or anxious. Without medical treatment soon, vital organs will fail and the victim will die.

With a loss of more than 40% of blood volume, blood pressure falls further and vital organs begin to fail. The victim becomes lethargic, stuporous and eventually unresponsive. Death occurs when the brain and other vital organs fail from lack of oxygen.

Figure 8-1 *Effects of Blood Loss.*

and blood from cut or torn blood vessels flows out through the wound. The rate at which bleeding occurs depends on the size and type of the vessel(s) damaged. Larger blood vessels are usually deeper in the body and more protected, and therefore most superficial wounds damage only smaller blood vessels **(Figure 8-3)**. This is not true in all body areas, however, and a wound where a major vessel is close to the skin surface may result in very heavy bleeding, such as at the wrist or neck.

Types of External Bleeding

There are three types of blood vessels: **arteries**, which carry blood from the heart to body tissues; **veins,** which carry blood back to the heart from body tissues; and **capillaries**, which are tiny vessels between the arteries and veins where oxygen and nutrients in the blood pass into tissues, and carbon dioxide and wastes move into the blood for removal. Therefore there are three types of external bleeding **(Figure 8-4):**

- **Bleeding from injured arteries** is more likely with deep injuries and is generally more serious. The blood is bright red and may spurt from the wound; blood loss can be very rapid. This bleeding needs to be controlled immediately.

- **Bleeding from injured veins** is generally slower and steady but can still be serious. The blood is darker red and flows steadily rather than spurting. This bleeding is usually easier to control.

- **Bleeding from capillaries** oozes from shallow cuts or scrapes and often stops soon by itself. The wound still needs attention to prevent infection.

Controlling External Bleeding

For minor bleeding that stops by itself, clean and dress the wound as described in **Chapter 10**. The bleeding should stop by itself or with light pressure on the dressing, such as the pressure provided by an adhesive bandage around a cut finger.

For more serious bleeding, first aid is needed immediately to stop the bleeding.

Applying direct pressure on the wound is sufficient to stop the bleeding in most cases (see Skill: "Controlling Bleeding"). Direct pressure on the wound controls bleeding by squeezing shut the

bleeding vessel at the point where it is damaged. Press directly on the wound with a sterile dressing and your gloved hand. If gloves are not available, you can improvise with any impermeable substance as a barrier to prevent contact between the victim's blood and your skin. This pressure stops the blood from flowing out. When the blood stops flowing, the natural body processes involved in clotting have a chance to function more effectively because platelets and fibrin are not "washed out" of the damaged area by the flow of blood. This is why sometimes pressure is needed only for a short time – the body's natural processes control the bleeding

(continues on page 120)

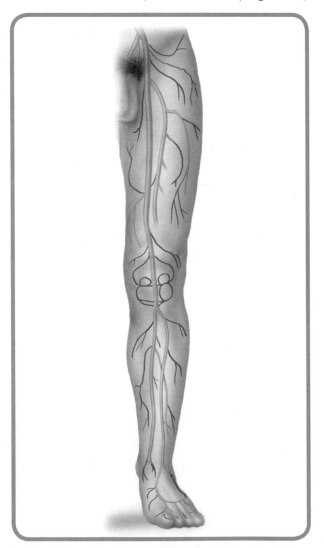

Figure 8-3 *Arteries of the leg. Note that the larger arteries are deeper within the leg and the arteries nearer the skin surface are generally much smaller and will bleed less.*

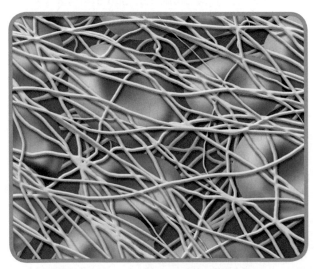

Figure 8-2 *View of blood clot showing blood cells in a web of fibrin.*

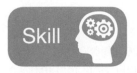

Skill — Controlling Bleeding

1 Put on gloves.

Improvise a barrier if no barrier is available.

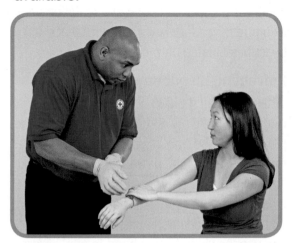

2 Place a sterile dressing or clean cloth on the wound.

3 Apply firm direct pressure with your hand for about 5 minutes.

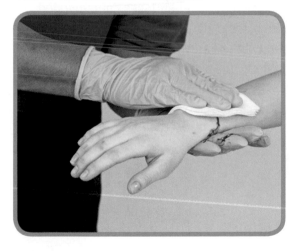

4 Reevaluate the bleeding: if it continues, put another dressing or cloth pad on top of the first and keep applying pressure.

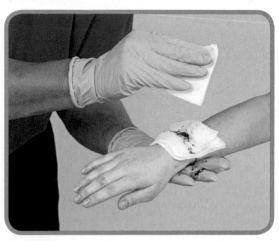

5 If needed, apply a pressure bandage to keep pressure on the wound, wrapping from the end of the extremity toward the center of the body.

The pressure is sufficient if the bandage is snug but you can slip a finger under it.

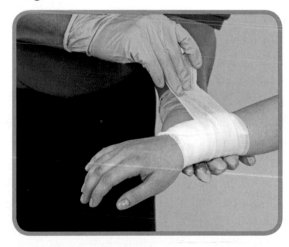

6 If appropriate, treat the victim for shock (see **Chapter 9**) and call 9-1-1.

ALERT

- Do not put pressure on an object in a wound.
- Do not put pressure on the scalp if the skull may be injured.
- Tourniquets should only be used as an extreme last resort by rescuers trained in their use, because of the high risk of complications (see **Chapter 23**).

(continued from page 118)

once they have the opportunity to work. With more severe vessel damage, however, pressure may have to be maintained for some time before clotting is successful. Releasing the pressure on the wound too soon would allow the normal blood pressure to break through the "dam" made of platelets, fibrin and other cells. This is also the reason why you should add more dressings on top of blood-soaked bandages when bleeding continues, rather than removing the first dressings – because removing them would release pressure and remove blood that is clotting.

Direct pressure should not be put on certain wounds, such as skull fractures or objects impaled in the wound, because the pressure may cause additional damage. In such cases pressure is applied around the wound or object, as described in **Chapter 10**.

Call 9-1-1 for any severe bleeding or bleeding that does not stop quickly. The victim should seek medical attention for any significant wound (see **Chapter 10**). Do not remove the dressing or bandage; the wound will be cleaned later by medical personnel.

Pressure Bandages

To control severe bleeding as quickly as possible, apply direct pressure with your gloved hand on a sterile dressing (or clean cloth) placed on the wound. If needed, you may apply a **pressure bandage** over a wound in an extremity to maintain this pressure so you can give other first aid as needed. Use a roller bandage wrapped around the limb to completely cover the wound and to maintain sufficient pressure to keep bleeding from starting again (see Skill: "Applying a Pressure Bandage").

Whenever you apply a bandage around an extremity, be sure that it is not so tight that it cuts off circulation to the limb. As a general rule, the pressure is sufficient if the bandage is snug but a finger can be slipped under it. Periodically check the victim's fingers or toes for signs of good circulation: normal skin color, warmth and sensation (not tingling or numbness). If you find

signs that circulation is reduced, loosen the bandage and apply it less tightly. Note that injuries often cause swelling that may increase after you apply the bandage, making the bandage tighter and possibly cutting off circulation. Therefore continue to check for signs of circulation until the victim receives medical attention. **Chapter 10** describes bandaging more fully.

Preventing Bloodborne Infection

When giving first aid to control bleeding, remember to follow standard precautions to prevent disease transmission. If you do not have medical examination gloves with you, put your hand in a plastic bag or use a barrier such as plastic wrap between your hand and the wound. If nothing is available to use as a barrier, you can use the victim's own hand to apply pressure on the wound.

After providing care for bleeding, remember also not to touch your face or other parts of your body until you have thoroughly washed your hands. Because objects or surfaces contaminated with blood can remain infectious for some time afterward, be sure to dispose of soiled supplies properly and disinfect all contaminated items. **Chapter 2** describes guidelines for preventing bloodborne disease transmission.

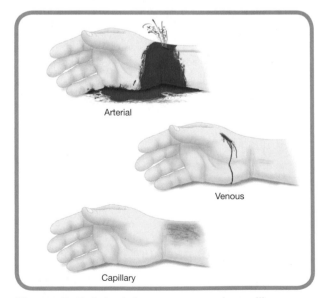

Figure 8-4 *Arterial, venous and capillary bleeding.*

Skill 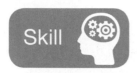 Applying a Pressure Bandage

1 Place a sterile dressing or clean cloth on wound. Start wrapping an elastic or self-adhering roller bandage below the wound dressing, wrapping from the end of the extremity toward the center of the body.

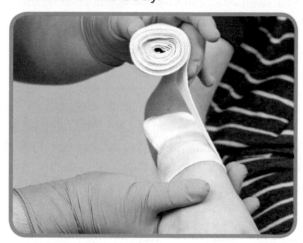

2 Make several circular turns, then overlap turns by about ½ of previous turn.

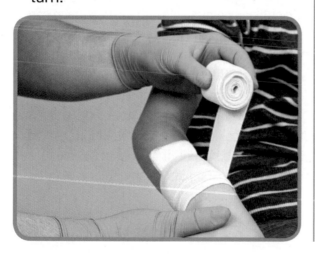

3 Work up the limb to cover the dressing completely. The pressure is sufficient if the bandage is snug but a finger can be slipped under it.

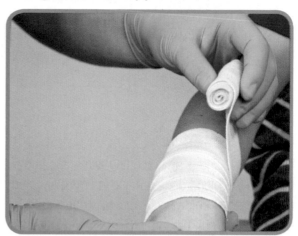

4 Fix or tie the end of the bandage in place.

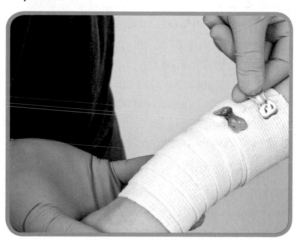

Learning Checkpoint 1

1. True or False: Arterial bleeding is the most serious because blood loss can be very rapid.

2. True or False: The first thing to do with any bleeding wound is wash it and apply antibiotic ointment.

3. Describe the skin characteristics of a victim who has been bleeding severely.

_____

4. If you do not have medical examination gloves with you, what other materials or objects can be used as a barrier between your hand and the wound when applying direct pressure?

_____

Internal Bleeding

Internal bleeding is any bleeding within the body in which the blood does not escape from an open wound. Internal bleeding is typically caused by a blunt impact on the body. The body may be impacted by a large force, such as being struck by a car, or a smaller force that leaves only a bruise. A serious injury can cause organs deep within the body to bleed severely. This bleeding, although unseen, can be life-threatening. A closed wound resulting from a minor injury may involve only minor local bleeding in the skin and other superficial tissue, appearing as a bruise (also called a contusion). Internal bleeding may also occur in the absence of trauma, such as with a bleeding ulcer.

Because you cannot see internal bleeding, it is important to consider the mechanism of injury when you assess the victim. With any injury involving a fall or a moving vehicle, even a bicycle, consider the possibility of internal bleeding. The victim may complain of pain. With internal bleeding the victim may experience shock – which may cause cool, clammy skin that is pale or bluish or ashen – thirst, and possible confusion or lightheadedness. In some cases the victim may vomit or cough up blood, or blood may be present in urine or stool (bloody or black). With bleeding into the abdominal cavity, the victim's abdomen may be tender, swollen, bruised or hard.

Minor bleeding just below the skin surface can be reduced to some extent with a cold pack or ice and wrapping an injured extremity (see First Aid: "Simple Bruises"). Deeper internal bleeding cannot be controlled by first aid. Call 9-1-1 immediately if you suspect internal bleeding, and treat for shock (see **Chapter 9**). Be prepared to give basic life support if the victim's condition worsens (see First Aid: "Internal Bleeding").

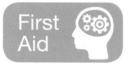

Simple Bruises
Signs, Symptoms and Care

When You See

- **Bruising**
- **Signs of pain**

Do This First

1 Check for signs and symptoms of a fracture or sprain (see **Chapter 14**) and give appropriate first aid.

2 Place a plastic bag with an ice-water mix on the injured area to reduce swelling and lessen pain; put a wet barrier such as a cloth between the plastic bag and the skin. A cold pack also can be used. Apply the cold for 20 minutes (or 10 minutes if it produces discomfort), then remove it for 30 minutes. Repeat the process for 24 to 48 hours or until the victim receives medical help.

3 With an arm or leg, wrap the area with an elastic roller bandage. Keep the part raised to help reduce swelling.

Additional Care

- Seek medical attention if you suspect a more serious injury such as a fracture or sprain.

Internal Bleeding
Signs, Symptoms and Care

When You See

- **Abdomen is tender, swollen, bruised or hard**
- **Blood vomited or coughed up or present in urine or stool (bloody, black or tarry)**
- **Cool, clammy skin; may be pale, bluish or ashen in color**
- **Thirst**
- **Possible confusion or lightheadedness**

Do This First

1 Have the victim lie on his or her back.

2 Call 9-1-1.

3 Be alert for vomiting. Put a victim who vomits or becomes unresponsive in the recovery position.

4 Keep the victim from becoming chilled or overheated.

5 If the victim becomes unresponsive, monitor breathing and be ready to give basic life support (BLS) as needed.

Additional Care

- Calm and reassure the victim.
- Treat for shock (see **Chapter 9**).

ALERT

- Do not give the victim anything to drink even if he or she is thirsty.

Learning Checkpoint 2

1. True or False: Internal bleeding is seldom life-threatening because there is no loss of blood from the body.

2. Put a check mark next to the signs and symptoms of internal bleeding.

   ___✓ Cool, clammy skin   ___✓ Confusion or lightheadedness

   ___✓ Vomiting or coughing up blood   ___✓ Blood in urine or stool

   ___✓ Tender, swollen or hard abdomen   ___✓ Bruise

3. First aid for serious internal bleeding includes –

   a. calling 9-1-1.

   b. positioning the victim lying down.

   c. keeping the victim from becoming chilled or overheated.

   d. All of the above

Concluding Thoughts

Many people are frightened of, or upset by, bleeding. Fortunately, in most cases the body's own mechanisms make it easy to control external bleeding with direct pressure. Because serious bleeding can be life-threatening, however, always call 9-1-1. In **Chapter 9**, you will learn more about caring for a victim who is in shock as a result of serious bleeding.

Learning Outcomes

You should now be able to do the following:

1. Explain the effects of blood loss and the body's mechanisms to control bleeding.

2. Describe the different types of external bleeding.

3. Demonstrate the steps for controlling external bleeding.

4. Demonstrate the steps for applying a pressure bandage.

5. List the steps for caring for a bruise.

6. List the signs and symptoms of internal bleeding and describe the first aid to give.

Review Questions

1. The body attempts to slow or stop bleeding from a damaged blood vessel by –

   a. skeletal muscle contraction.

   b. blood clotting.

   c. producing more red blood cells.

   d. stopping the heartbeat.

2. Which type of bleeding is usually most serious?

    a. Arterial bleeding

    b. Venous bleeding

    c. Capillary bleeding

    d. All bleeding is equally serious.

3. To prevent bloodborne disease transmission, apply pressure on a bleeding wound with –

    a. your gloved hand.

    b. any impermeable substance.

    c. the victim's hand.

    d. Any of the above

4. What do you do if blood soaks through the pressure bandage?

    a. Ignore the blood but maintain the pressure.

    b. Put a new bandage on top of the first and maintain pressure.

    c. Replace the bloody bandage with a new bandage and maintain pressure.

    d. Apply a tourniquet on top of the bandage.

5. A pressure bandage is applied –

    a. around the extremity from the joint above the wound to the joint below the wound, to apply equal pressure to the whole area.

    b. above the wound to cut off the blood flow.

    c. on the wound to control bleeding.

    d. both above and below the wound to control blood flow and bleeding.

6. Which is a sign or symptom that a pressure bandage is too tight on the arm?

    a. Red color under the fingernails

    b. Hot fingers

    c. Cold fingers

    d. Extreme thirst

7. Internal bleeding into the abdomen may result in the abdomen feeling –

    a. hard.

    b. hot.

    c. pulsing.

    d. soft and squishy.

8. Severe internal bleeding may cause –

    a. the victim to feel thirsty.

    b. the victim's skin to be cool and clammy.

    c. the victim to be confused.

    d. All of the above

Chapter 9 • Shock

Chapter Preview

- Shock
- Anaphylaxis

Seated at a nearby table at a local Mexican restaurant are a woman, her two daughters and her daughter's friend. They are sharing a variety of dishes and having a good time – until the friend abruptly puts down her fork and leans back in her seat, looking ill. You notice her face seems puffy around the mouth and she is obviously having trouble breathing. The mother and two daughters are asking her if she is okay but don't seem to know what to do. With your first aid training, you recognize the situation as a possible food allergy. What should you do?

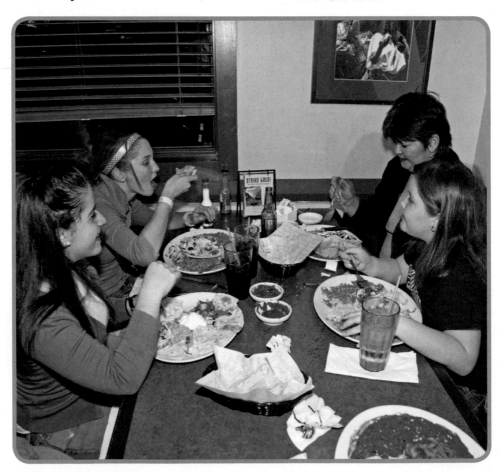

126 | Shock

Shock is a dangerous condition in which not enough oxygen-rich blood reaches vital organs in the body. The brain, heart and other organs need a continuous supply of oxygen. Anything that happens to or in the body that significantly reduces blood flow can cause shock. Severe bleeding is a common cause of shock in first aid situations.

Shock is a life-threatening emergency. It may develop quickly or gradually. Always call 9-1-1 for a victim in shock.

Shock

For enough blood to reach the body's vital organs and keep them well oxygenated, three general conditions must be met:

1. The heart must be efficiently pumping blood.

2. Blood volume in the body must be sufficient to fill blood vessels so the pumping action circulates blood to vital organs.

3. Blood vessels throughout the body must be intact and functioning normally. A loss of blood through injured blood vessels may reduce the blood volume to the point where not enough blood is circulated to vital organs. Certain conditions may also dilate blood vessels to the extent that there is not enough blood volume to fill blood vessels.

Normally the body easily meets these conditions. The heart rate varies as needed to pump more or less blood throughout the body. The body controls blood volume by moving fluid into or out of the blood as needed. Blood vessels constrict or dilate in different conditions to ensure that enough blood is circulated to vital organs at all times. In a healthy person these mechanisms work automatically to supply the constant supply of oxygen that the brain, heart and other vital organs need.

In cases of injury or illness, however, one or more of these necessary conditions may be disrupted. Disruption of the heart, the blood volume and the blood vessels may reduce the blood flow to vital organs, causing shock **(Figure 9-1)**.

Causes of Shock

Shock may develop in a victim in many different situations. Following are descriptions of the primary types of shock. You do not need to know which exact type a victim has, as long as you recognize the problem and give appropriate first aid. **Box 9-1** lists the specific types of injuries and conditions that may lead to shock.

- **Hypovolemic shock** occurs when blood volume drops. Severe bleeding, either external or internal, is a common cause of shock when not enough blood is left circulating in the body to bring required oxygen to vital organs (this is called **hemorrhagic shock**). Other conditions may also lower blood volume. Severe burns result

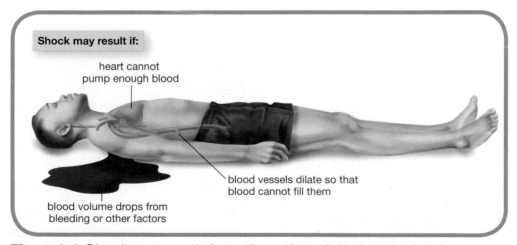

Shock may result if:

heart cannot pump enough blood

blood vessels dilate so that blood cannot fill them

blood volume drops from bleeding or other factors

Figure 9-1 *Shock may result from disruption of the heart, blood volume and blood vessels.*

BOX 9-1: INJURIES AND CONDITIONS THAT MAY CAUSE SHOCK

- Severe bleeding
- Severe burns
- Heart failure
- Heart attack
- Head or spinal injuries
- Severe allergic reactions

- Dehydration (common with heatstroke or severe vomiting or diarrhea)
- Electrocution
- Serious infections
- Extreme emotional reactions (temporary, less dangerous form of shock)

in a loss of fluid from the blood. Severe vomiting or diarrhea and other causes of dehydration may also result in the body moving fluid from the blood to meet other body needs, causing shock. Infants and young children are especially vulnerable to hypovolemic shock caused by persistent vomiting or diarrhea.

- **Cardiogenic shock** occurs when any condition causes the heart function to be reduced to the point that blood is not circulating sufficiently. Heart attack is a common cause. An abnormal heartbeat, such as ventricular fibrillation, is another cause of inadequate circulation. As described in the chapters on basic life support, CPR and an AED are used to restore a normal heartbeat and keep blood moving to vital organs, thereby helping to prevent the occurrence of shock.

- **Neurogenic shock** occurs when a problem related to the nervous system's control of blood vessels allows vessels to dilate excessively. If blood vessels throughout the body expand too much, the volume of blood is not sufficient to fill blood vessels and not enough blood can be pumped to vital organs. Certain spinal cord injuries may cause neurogenic shock. A similar condition may result from extreme fear or similar emotions

that cause fainting when blood vessels temporarily dilate because of the nervous system reaction.

- **Anaphylactic shock** is an extreme allergic reaction, typically to an insect sting, a particular food, medication and some other substance. Anaphylaxis produces shock because part of the allergic reaction causes the dilation of blood vessels and the movement of fluid out of the blood through capillary walls. Because anaphylaxis causes other signs and symptoms and requires different first aid treatment, it is discussed separately later in this chapter.

First Aid for Shock

A victim in shock has various signs and symptoms depending on the cause and severity. Note, however, that the victim's signs and symptoms are not always correlated with the severity of the shock; therefore all cases of shock should be treated as severe. A victim with any serious injury should be assumed to be at risk of shock, even if you do not see all the signs and symptoms. Remember that internal bleeding can be life-threatening even though you cannot see it or know for certain whether it is occurring.

Shock generally occurs in stages that may progress either gradually or so quickly that the victim is in full shock very soon after the injury. In the first stage, compensatory shock, early signs include feelings of anxiety, restlessness and fear, along with increased breathing and heart rates. In the second stage, decompensatory shock, mental status continues to deteriorate, leading to confusion, disorientation and sleepiness. Breathing becomes rapid and shallow, and the heartbeat becomes rapid (but the pulse weak because of decreased blood volume). The skin becomes pale or ashen and cool as blood is shunted from the extremities to vital organs. Nausea and thirst occur as blood is shunted from the digestive system. As oxygen levels drop in body tissues, the lips and nail beds may look bluish. The victim ultimately becomes unresponsive. Without medical treatment, the third stage, irreversible shock, leads to respiratory and cardiac arrest. Once it develops, shock cannot be reversed without professional medical care, so it is important to recognize situations in which shock is likely or is beginning to occur and to give care to minimize it.

Not all victims experience all symptoms of shock or have them in the same order. But a victim who has several of these signs and symptoms after a serious injury is probably beginning to experience shock. It is crucial to call 9-1-1 immediately because once it begins, shock will continue to develop unless medical treatment begins. EMS professionals often refer to the "golden hour" – the period of time from when a shock-producing traumatic injury occurs until the victim is receiving emergency medical treatment in a hospital. A victim reaching medical care later has a much lower chance of survival. Calling 9-1-1 immediately is necessary to start the emergency response process so the victim can receive help before shock leads to death.

After EMS is called, first aid for shock is directed at helping minimize or delay the onset; first aid at the scene cannot reverse shock. If the victim is bleeding, it is essential to control the bleeding immediately to prevent further blood loss. Then, position the victim lying on his or her back with legs raised such that the feet are 6 to 12 inches above the ground, unless the victim may have a spinal injury or head injury or may have had a

stroke. This is often called the *shock position*. Put a victim who is having breathing difficulty into the position of easiest breathing, typically a reclining position partly sitting up. Ensure that the airway is open. Help the victim to maintain normal body temperature, if necessary, by covering him or her with a blanket or coat, but avoid overheating. Outdoors in cold weather, also put a blanket or coat under the victim unless the victim may have a spinal injury (see First Aid: "Shock").

Blood loss in infants or children may quickly lead to shock, and young children and infants are also more susceptible to shock caused by dehydration resulting from repeated vomiting or diarrhea. Call 9-1-1 for any infant or child with persistent vomiting or diarrhea; do not wait for the signs of shock to develop.

Early shock may be less obvious in children because a child's body is generally more efficient at compensating initially for the blood volume decrease. By the time the classic signs of shock occur, the child's blood volume is usually already very low. As shock progresses, the child's condition declines very rapidly. An infant or child in shock may become limp and unresponsive, with eyes partially open or closed and the skin pale, bluish and ashen. Call 9-1-1 immediately. Treatment is the same as for adults, but because the child's decline is rapid, you should be prepared to give basic life support as needed.

Anaphylaxis

As described earlier, **anaphylaxis**, also called anaphylactic shock, involves a severe allergic reaction. In addition to the circulatory problems of shock, the victim's airway may swell, making breathing difficult or impossible. The breathing problem is usually the immediate life-threatening emergency. Always call 9-1-1 for an anaphylaxis emergency.

Causes of Anaphylaxis

The immune system has several mechanisms that protect the body from foreign substances that enter the body. When the individual is allergic

Learning Checkpoint 1

1. True or False: Because a shock victim is thirsty and may be dehydrated, offer clear fluids to drink.

2. True or False: A spinal injury can cause shock.

3. Which of these actions should you take first for a victim in shock because of external bleeding?

   a. Stop the bleeding.

   b. Raise the legs.

   c. Loosen tight clothing.

   d. Cover the victim with a blanket.

4. A shock victim is likely to have which signs and symptoms?

   a. Vomiting; diarrhea; red, blotchy face

   b. Nausea, thirst or clammy skin

   c. Incontinence, hives or swollen legs

   d. Headache, painful abdomen or coughing

5. What is the most important action to take for all shock victims?

   Call 9-1-1

to the substance (called an **allergen**), such as pollen that is inhaled or a food that is ingested, the normal action of the immune system results in a physiological response that includes various signs and symptoms, depending on the type and strength of the allergy. Typical mild allergic reactions include nasal congestion; watery eyes; and itching, blotchy skin.

Anaphylaxis, or anaphylactic shock, is a more extreme allergic reaction in some people that causes severe signs and symptoms that can rapidly become life-threatening. The most common causes of anaphylaxis are:

- Certain drugs (such as penicillins and sulfa)

- Certain foods (such as peanuts, shellfish and eggs)

- Insect stings and bites (such as bees or wasps)

The signs and symptoms of anaphylactic shock may begin within minutes, even seconds, of the victim's contact with the allergen. As a general rule,

the more quickly the reaction occurs, the more serious it is likely to be. Anaphylaxis is frightening and demands immediate action because you cannot know if the reaction will continue to worsen and become fatal without medical care. Even if the victim has had what feels like a similar reaction in the past, he or she cannot know for certain that it will not be worse this time.

Prevention of Anaphylaxis

Prevention of anaphylaxis resulting from an allergic reaction depends on avoiding the specific allergen.

Food allergies are the most common cause of anaphylaxis and death resulting from anaphylaxis.[1] Unfortunately, most reactions occur in people without a history of reaction because allergic reactions develop from repeated exposures to the particular allergen, making prevention difficult. Health care professionals

(continues on page 132)

[1]*National Institute of Allergy and Infectious Diseases http://www.niaid.nih.gov/topics/foodAllergy/understanding/Pages/anaphylaxis.aspx Accessed March 1, 2011.*

First Aid — Shock
Signs, Symptoms and Care

When You See

- **Anxiety, confusion, agitation and restlessness**
- **Dizziness, lightheadedness**
- **Cool, clammy or sweating skin; pale, bluish and ashen in color**
- **Rapid, shallow breathing**
- **Thirst**
- **Nausea or vomiting**
- **Changing responsiveness**

Do This First

1 Check for responsiveness, normal breathing and severe bleeding and care first for life-threatening injuries.

2 Call 9-1-1 and be ready to give basic life support if needed.

3 a. Position a responsive victim with trauma on his or her back using a blanket or coat as a pad. If there is no evidence of trauma, raise the legs such that the feet are 6-12 inches above the ground.

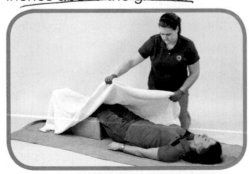

b. Put a breathing, unresponsive victim (if no suspected spinal injury) in the recovery position.

4 Loosen any tight clothing.

5 Be alert for the possibility of vomiting; if vomiting occurs, turn the victim's head to drain the mouth.

6 Maintain the victim's normal body temperature. If necessary, maintain the victim's body heat with a blanket or coat over the victim.

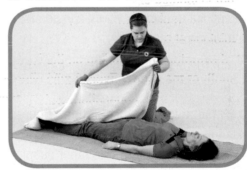

Additional Care

- Stay with the victim and offer reassurance and comfort.
- Keep bystanders from crowding around the victim.

ALERT

- Do not let a shock victim eat, drink or smoke.
- Note that sweating in a shock victim is not necessarily a sign of being too warm. If in doubt, it is better to maintain a shock victim's body temperature by keeping the victim warm.

(continued from page 130)

are trained to watch for the early effects of an anaphylactic reaction, however, and to provide early treatment. Following are preventive actions for people with known medication allergies:

- Maintain a complete history of medication reactions and share this with health care providers.

- Wear a medical alert ID in case you cannot communicate about an allergy in an emergency.

- For people allergic to nonprescription medications, read product labels carefully – many products may include a number of unexpected ingredients.

Food allergies occur in about 4% of adults and 6% of children younger than 3. Peanut and nut allergies are the most common; other common foods causing allergies include milk, eggs, wheat, soy, fish and shellfish.[2] About 150 to 200 people die every year in the United States from food-induced anaphylaxis[3] – mostly adolescents and young adults. Prevention depends on avoiding foods known to cause a reaction, which can be more difficult than it may seem:

- Check food product labels for alternate names of foods.

- In restaurants and other settings where exact ingredients cannot be known, do not trust what wait staff or other people may say. Avoid foods that may contain hidden ingredients, such as sauces that may have been prepared using equipment contaminated by an allergenic food.

- Educate a child's caretakers, teachers and friends' parents about an allergy and its dangers to prevent the child from eating something shared by another child.

About 3% of adults and 1% of children have an allergic reaction to the venom of stinging insects, including honeybees, hornets, wasps, yellow jackets and fire ants. About 40 deaths every year

in the United States are attributed to anaphylactic reactions to such stings.[4] Again, prevention is based on avoiding stinging insects whenever possible. When outdoors, these actions help you to avoid attracting or provoking stinging insects:

- Stay away from insect nesting areas. Check around the home for insect nests to destroy.

- Do not wear bright colors or sweet-smelling perfumes or colognes.

- Wear clothing that covers arms and legs; wear shoes to prevent stings caused by stepping on insects.

- Do not swat at or try to wave insects away.

- When getting into a car, if the windows were left open, check for insects that may have flown in.

- Be cautious when near areas where insects gather, such as around flowering plants and garbage cans.

- If stung, do not pull out the stinger with your fingers because the attached venom sac may eject more venom when squeezed; instead, scrape it off with something similar in size and rigidity to a credit card **(Figure 9-2)**. **Chapter 19** provides additional information about bites and stings.

Immunotherapy, often called *allergy shots*, is also available to lessen a person's reaction to insect venoms. Injections, usually given over three years, gradually desensitize the body, eventually preventing allergic reactions in most people undergoing therapy. People with severe insect allergies should see their health care provider for information about immunotherapy.

[2]*The Food Allergy and Anaphylaxis Network http://www. foodallergy.org/downloads/FoodAllergyFactsandStatistics. pdf Accessed March 1, 2011.*

[3]*American Academy of Allergy Asthma & Immunology, http://www.aaaai.org/media/statistics/allergy-statistics. asp#foodallergy Accessed March 1, 2011.*

[4]*American Academy of Allergy Asthma & Immunology, http://www.aaaai.org/media/statistics/allergy-statistics. asp#insectstingallergy Accessed March 29, 2011.*

As described in the following section, emergency medication is also available for people at risk for severe allergic reactions. Although this medication cannot prevent the exposure to the allergen, it can stop the progress of an allergic reaction and prevent the victim from experiencing anaphylaxis.

First Aid for Anaphylaxis

If the victim knows he or she has the allergy and knows about the exposure, the victim may be able to tell you about the allergy when the reaction begins. Following the guidelines for the SAMPLE history in **Chapter 4**, ask all victims about allergies and the things they ate or drank most recently. For example, a victim who is severely allergic to bee stings and who has just been stung, may say he or she needs medication immediately to prevent anaphylaxis. Or, someone who is allergic to nuts may feel the start of the reaction and wonder if there were nuts in something he or she just ate. In many cases, however, the person may not know about the allergy and may not have had an allergic reaction before. Therefore you cannot depend on having this information but should suspect an allergic reaction based on the situation and the victim's signs and symptoms.

The early signs and symptoms of anaphylaxis include skin flushing, itching or burning, and rash; sneezing and watery eyes and nose; coughing or a feeling of a tickle or lump in the throat that does not go away; and gastrointestinal upset.

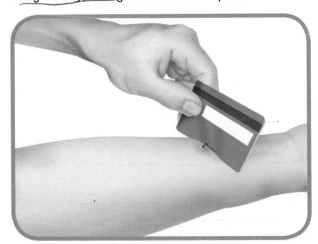

Figure 9-2 *Use a rigid piece of plastic to scrape away a stinger.*

As symptoms worsen, the victim becomes anxious and may have the feeling that the throat is closing and the chest is becoming tight. Other signs include fast breathing, coughing, wheezing and hoarseness, and altered mental status. The victim may have severe headache, a feeling of weakness or fainting, and pale or ashen skin or cyanosis (bluish color of lips and nail beds), along with other shock signs and symptoms.

First aid begins with making sure 9-1-1 is called; medical care is urgently needed because first aid usually cannot stop or reverse anaphylactic shock. Help the victim into a position for easiest breathing and offer reassurance. Be prepared to give basic life support if needed. If the victim becomes unresponsive, put him or her in the recovery position and continue to monitor breathing.

Some people who know they have a severe allergy carry an emergency epinephrine auto-injector such as an **EpiPen**, EpiPen Jr. (for children), Anakit and Twinject **(Figure 9-3)**. This medication usually will stop the anaphylactic reaction temporarily. Ask a victim about this and

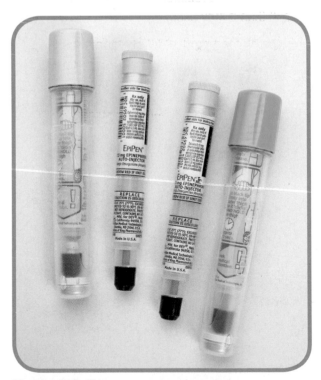

Figure 9-3 *Emergency epinephrine auto-injectors.*

help him or her to open and use the auto-injector as needed. If the victim cannot use his or her prescribed epinephrine auto-injector, you may administer it yourself if permitted by state law. The EpiPen is removed from its case and the safety release cap removed. The tip is then jabbed into the outer part of the thigh muscle and held there for 10 seconds while the medication is injected.

The effects of the emergency epinephrine will last 15 to 20 minutes, during which time you should stay with the victim until EMS professionals arrive and take over care. You may observe the victim experiencing the side effects of epinephrine: fast heartbeat, breathing difficulty, nausea and vomiting, dizziness or nervousness and headache (see First Aid: "Anaphylaxis").

Learning Checkpoint 2

1. True or False: Ask a victim having an anaphylactic reaction about any allergies and medication for allergies.

   ✓

2. True or False: A bee sting can cause a severe allergic reaction.

3. The major risk for a victim in anaphylaxis is —

   a. swelling around the eyes.

   b. heart attack.

   c. internal bleeding.

   ✓ d. breathing problems.

4. How should a victim in anaphylaxis be positioned if he or she is having trouble breathing?

   _____ recovery position. _____

First Aid

Anaphylaxis
Signs, Symptoms and Care

When You See

- **Difficulty breathing, wheezing**
- **Complaints of tightness in throat or chest**
- **Swelling of the face and neck, or puffy eyes**
- **Anxiety or agitation**
- **Nausea or vomiting**
- **Changing levels of responsiveness**

Do This First

1 Call 9-1-1.

2 Help a responsive victim use his or her emergency epinephrine auto-injector, such as an EpiPen, Ana-Kit or or TwinJect. If the victim cannot use his or her prescribed auto-injector, you may administer it yourself if permitted by state law.

   a. Take the auto-injector out of its case and remove the safety cap.

   b. To administer the medication, the victim jabs the pen tip into the outer thigh and holds it there for 10 seconds while the medication is injected.

   c. The medication should provide relief for 15-20 minutes.

3 Monitor the victim's breathing and be ready to give CPR if needed.

4 Help a responsive victim sit up in a position of easiest breathing. Put an unresponsive victim who is breathing in the recovery position.

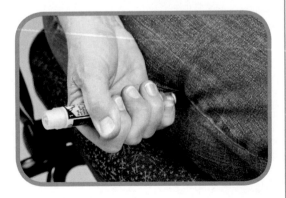

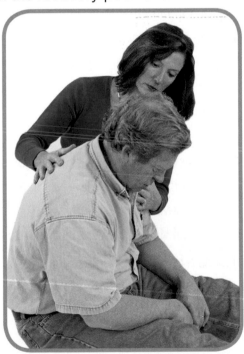

Additional Care

- Stay with the victim and offer reassurance and comfort.

Concluding Thoughts

Most commonly, shock is caused by heavy blood loss, so the most important thing to do for a victim who is bleeding is to control the bleeding as quickly as possible. Call 9-1-1 because shock is a serious threat to life. In most cases the first aid for a victim in shock is primarily supportive, but a victim with severe allergies may carry an emergency epinephrine auto-injector that can be used to treat anaphylactic shock caused by an allergic reaction.

Learning Outcomes

You should now be able to do the following:

1. Explain what happens inside the body with severe blood loss.

2. List common causes of shock.

3. Describe first aid steps for a victim in shock.

4. Describe ways to prevent exposure to known allergens.

5. Describe the first aid for anaphylaxis.

6. Demonstrate how to use an emergency epinephrine auto-injector (if training pens are available).

Review Questions

1. Which is fundamental to the definition of shock?

   a. Not enough oxygen reaching vital organs

   b. Too much waste building up in the urine

   c. The heartbeat stopping

   d. An abdominal injury

2. When should you call 9-1-1?

   a. Call only if the shock victim becomes unresponsive.

   b. Call only for blood loss of more than 30% of blood volume.

   c. Call for all victims in shock.

   d. Call for all victims who had any bleeding.

3. Which is a possible cause of shock?

   a. Bleeding

   b. Spinal cord injury

   c. Severe burn

   d. All of the above

4. Which is a part of first aid for shock?

   a. Giving the victim water to drink to replace lost fluids

   b. Raising the victim's legs

   c. Keeping the victim moving to prevent his or her becoming unresponsive

   d. Applying ice to the injury

5. Signs and symptoms of shock include –

   a. confusion.

   b. rapid, shallow breathing.

   c. pale, bluish and ashen skin.

   d. All of the above

6. Shock in a child is similar to shock in an adult except –

   a. a child's condition may decline more rapidly.

   b. early shock is more dramatically obvious in a child.

   c. a greater blood loss is required in a child to produce shock.

   d. a child's skin does not become pale with shock.

7. Anaphylaxis is commonly caused by a severe allergic reaction to –

   a. campfire smoke.

   b. insect stings.

   c. poison ivy.

   d. animal fur.

8. How soon may a severe allergic reaction occur following exposure?

   a. Within seconds or minutes

   b. Within about 30 minutes

   c. Within 1 to 2 hours

   d. Within 6 to 12 hours

9. If a person who has just been stung by a bee says he is allergic to bee stings, you should –

   a. call 9-1-1 immediately.

   b. wait for the development of signs and symptoms, then call 9-1-1.

   c. send someone to the nearest drugstore to buy an EpiPen.

   d. use the shock position and see if that reverses the problem.

10. First aid for a victim experiencing anaphylaxis includes –

   a. cooling the victim's body with ice packs.

   b. giving the victim an aspirin as quickly as possible.

   c. positioning the victim for easiest breathing.

   d. using pressure points on arms and legs.

Chapter 10 • Wounds and Soft Tissue Injuries

Chapter Preview

- Types of Open Wounds
- Cleaning Wounds
- Wound Infection
- Dressing and Bandaging Wounds
- When to Seek Medical Attention for a Wound
- Special Wounds

Your co-worker has cut his arm while trying to repair some office equipment. It is not bleeding heavily, but the wound seems dirty. You get the first aid kit and put on gloves, then take him to a nearby sink. How should you wash the wound? What other first aid should you give?

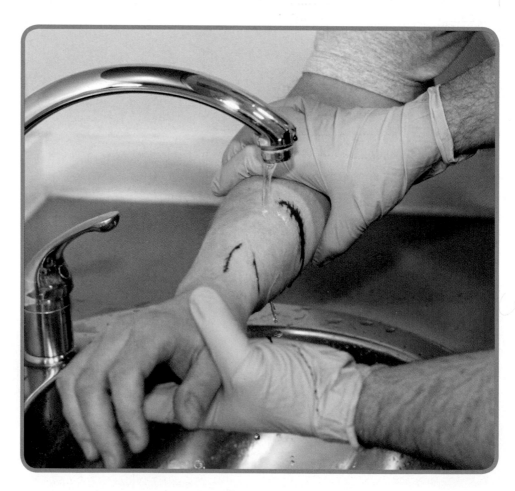

A wound is an injury to the skin and sometimes other deeper soft tissues. In an **open wound** the skin is torn or cut open, often leading to bleeding. Different types of wounds require different specific first aid, but all wounds have a risk for becoming infected by pathogens that may enter the body through the break in the skin. In addition to controlling bleeding (see **Chapter 8**), first aiders should also know how to care for different kinds of wounds and how to apply dressings and bandages.

Wound care involves cleaning and dressing a wound to prevent infection, and protecting the wound so healing can occur. Remember: *Do not waste time cleaning a wound that is severely bleeding. Controlling bleeding is always the priority.* Health care personnel will clean the wound as needed.

This chapter describes first aid for open wounds. Care of internal bleeding caused by **closed injuries** is described in **Chapter 8**. The care of musculoskeletal injuries, another type of closed injury, is described in **Chapter 14**.

Types of Open Wounds

Different mechanisms of injury cause different types of damage to soft tissues. The main types of open wounds are abrasions, lacerations, punctures, avulsions and amputations. The type and amount of bleeding caused by an injury depend on the type of wound, its location and its depth. Different types of wounds also have different implications for first aid.

- **Abrasions** occur when the top layers of skin are scraped off **(Figure 10-1)**. Skinned elbows or knees, for example, are common in children. Abrasions are often painful but are not serious injuries because underlying tissues are not usually injured. Bleeding is usually limited to capillary bleeding that typically stops soon by itself. Foreign material may be present in the wound, which can cause infection.

- **Lacerations** or cuts, frequently penetrate the skin and may also damage underlying tissue **(Figure 10-2)**. Lacerations are either smooth cuts with straight edges (called incisions), such as those caused by knives or other sharp objects, or jagged cuts with rough edges. Depending on the depth and location of the cut, lacerations may cause heavier bleeding. A laceration through a major artery may cause life-threatening bleeding.

- **Punctures** occur when sharp objects penetrate the skin and possibly deeper tissues **(Figure 10-3)**. The wound may penetrate through the body part, as with a gunshot wound, causing both entrance and exit wounds. Puncture wounds are more likely to trap foreign material in the body, increasing the risk for infection.

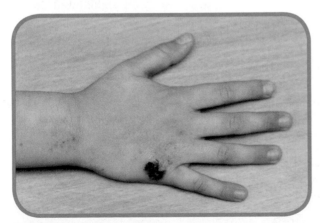

Figure 10-1 *Abrasion.*

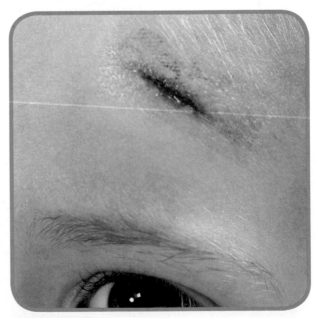

Figure 10-2 *Laceration.*

- An <u>avulsion</u> is an area of skin or other soft tissue <u>torn</u> partially from the body, like a flap **(Figure 10-4)**. Any area of skin or a whole soft tissue structure, like the ear, may be avulsed.

- An **amputation** is the complete <u>cutting</u> or tearing off of all or <u>part of an extremity</u>: a finger or toe, hand or foot, arm or leg. This wound is often called <u>a traumatic</u> amputation to distinguish it from an amputation performed surgically. Depending on the nature of the wound and the time that passes before the victim reaches the hospital, the amputated part may be reattached.

- **Burns** are damage caused to skin and other tissue by <u>heat</u>, <u>chemicals or electricity</u>. Because of the significant differences among first aid approaches for burns, burn care is covered in detail in **Chapter 11**.

First aid care for open wounds varies depending on their location on the body. Wounds to certain body areas require special first aid measures as described later in this chapter.

Cleaning Wounds

When a <u>wound is bleeding heavily, the first</u> aid priority is to control the <u>bleeding</u> (see **Chapter 8**). Do not delay or interrupt efforts to stop bleeding in order to clean the wound. Health care professionals who treat the victim later will clean the wound. Even after you have stopped the bleeding with direct pressure or other means, do not remove the dressing from the wound

to clean it. Removing the dressing may disturb clotted blood and start the wound bleeding again.

Unless the wound is very large, deep or bleeding seriously, or the victim has other injuries needing attention, the first step in minor wound care is to clean the wound to help prevent infection. Wash your hands first and wear gloves if available. You may need to expose the wound first by removing clothing, taking care to avoid contact with the wound. Then, gently wash a shallow wound or abrasion with large amounts of warm or room-temperature water with or without soap to remove dirt. Irrigate a deeper wound under large amounts of running water to remove foreign matter **(Figure 10-5)**. Do not merely soak the wound in water; instead, actively run water over it. Washing out a wound under running water is called **irrigation**. Then carefully pat the wound dry. Apply antibiotic ointment only to an abrasion or superficial wound and only if the victim is not allergic to the antibiotic. Apply a sterile dressing and bandage to protect and keep the dressing in place (see First Aid: "Wound Care").

Wound Infection

Infection is an invasion of the body by a pathogen that may potentially cause disease. Because a wound lacks the protection offered by intact skin and allows pathogens into body tissues and/or the blood, infection may occur with any open wound. Some pathogens cause local tissue damage, while others spread throughout the body and may become life-threatening. The bloodborne diseases described in **Chapter 2** may be transmitted from

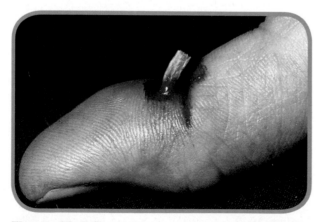

Figure 10-3 *Puncture.*

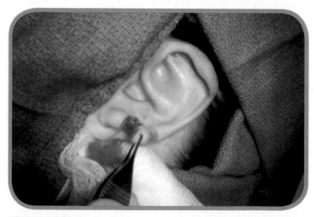

Figure 10-4 *Avulsion.*

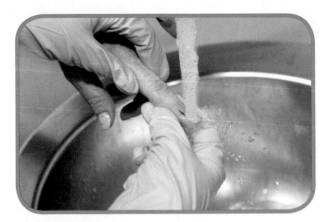

Figure 10-5 *Irrigate a shallow wound with running water to help clean it.*

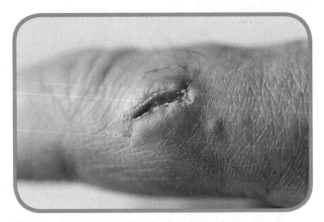

Figure 10-6 *An infected wound.*

one person to another through an open wound, but many other pathogens are also present in the environment. Pathogens may be transmitted into a wound by the object that caused the wound, by any substance that comes into contact with the wound or even by pathogens in the air. Because infection is an ever-present threat, wound care includes steps to prevent infection.

Although infection is a risk with all open wounds, some types of wounds are at greater risk, including wounds resulting from bites (even human bites); puncture wounds; wounds contaminated with dirt or other substances; and wounds with jagged, uneven edges that are not easily cleaned.

As noted earlier, to help healing and prevent infection, **antibiotic** ointment may be used on abrasions or shallow wounds in a person who is not allergic to the antibiotic, after the wound is cleaned. Antibiotic ointment should not be used on other types of open wounds because the ointment may seal the wound and block the drainage that is part of the normal healing process. If you see signs of infection occurring in a wound, do not just apply an antibiotic ointment and hope it will kill the pathogen. See a health care provider before the infection becomes worse **(Box 10-1)**.

Any wound can become infected **(Figure 10-6)**, in which case medical attention is needed. The signs and symptoms of an infection are:

- Wound area is red, swollen and warm.

- Pain
- Pus
- Fever
- Red streaks or trails on the skin near the wound are a sign the infection is spreading – see a health care provider immediately.

Dressing and Bandaging Wounds
Dressings

Dressings are placed on wounds to help stop bleeding, prevent infection and protect the wound while it is healing.

Types of Dressings

First aid kits should include sealed sterile dressings in many sizes **(Figure 10-7)**. Common types of dressings include:

- Gauze squares of various sizes
- Roller gauze
- Nonstick pad dressings
- Adhesive strips such as Band-Aids and other dressings combined with a bandage
- Bulky dressings, also called **trauma dressings** (for large wounds or to stabilize an object impaled in a wound)
- **Occlusive dressings** (which create an airtight seal over certain types of wounds)

(continues on page 143)

First Aid ⚙️🧠 Wound Care
Signs, Symptoms and Care

When You See

- **A shallow, open wound**

Do This First

1 Wash your hands and put on gloves if available.

2 Gently wash shallow wounds and abrasions with large amounts of warm or room-temperature water with or without soap to remove dirt.

3 Irrigate a deeper wound under large amounts of running water to remove foreign matter.

4 Do not use alcohol, hydrogen peroxide or iodine on the wound.

5 Pat the area dry.

6 Apply antibiotic ointment only to an abrasion or superficial wound, and only if the victim is not allergic to the antibiotic.

7 Cover the wound with a sterile dressing and bandage (or adhesive bandage with nonstick pad).

Additional Care

- Change the dressing daily or if it becomes wet. (If a dressing sticks to the wound, soak it in water first.)
- Seek medical attention for the following:
  - If the person's tetanus vaccination is out of date
  - The wound may be infected
  - A deep or puncture wound
  - An impaled object
  - A wound that may require stitches (cuts on the face or hands when the edges do not close together, gaping wounds, and cuts longer than 1 inch)

ALERT

- Do not try to clean a major wound after controlling bleeding – it may start bleeding again. Health care personnel will clean the wound as needed.
- Do not put antibiotic ointment on a puncture wound or deep wound; use only on abrasions and shallow wounds.
- Do not use alcohol, hydrogen peroxide or iodine on the wound. Such substances may not kill pathogens or may damage healthy body tissue.
- Avoid breathing or blowing on the wound, as this may transmit pathogens.
- Do not attempt to remove clothing stuck to a wound; cut around the clothing and leave it in place for health care providers to manage.
- Do not scrub a wound, as this can cause further tissue damage.

BOX 10-1: TETANUS

Tetanus, also called lockjaw because a stiff neck and jaw is an early symptom, is an infection caused by common bacteria. Tetanus bacteria are found in soil, on skin surfaces and elsewhere in the environment, including the home and other indoor locations. The bacteria enter the body through a wound, multiply and produce a powerful toxin that acts on the nervous system, causing death in up to 15% of cases.[1]

The number of cases of tetanus in the United States has fallen dramatically since immunization became common in the late 1940s. Tetanus immunization is included in routine childhood vaccinations, but adults need a tetanus booster at least every 10 years. A tetanus booster may be recommended before 10 years in a victim with a significant wound. Tetanus infection is more common following puncture wounds or deep lacerations but can occur also with abrasions or any break in the skin, including burns, dental infections and animal bites. It is important, therefore, for adults to maintain their immunization status with periodic boosters. In addition, medical attention should be sought for any deep or puncture wound. A tetanus shot must be given within 72 hours of receiving a wound to be effective.[2]

[1]*WebMD, http://emedicine.medscape.com/article/786414-overview*

[2]*Mayo Clinic, http://www.mayoclinic.com/health/tetanus/DS00227/DSECTION=prevention Accessed March 1, 2011.*

(continued from page 141)

In some situations it may be necessary to improvise a dressing. If a sterile dressing is not available, use a clean cloth as a dressing; non-fluffy cloth works best because it is less likely to stick to the wound. Look for a clean towel, handkerchief or other material. Avoid using cotton balls or cotton cloth if possible because cotton fibers tend to stick to wounds. To improvise bulky dressings, use sanitary pads if available, which, although not sterile, are generally individually wrapped and very clean. Bulky dressings can also be made of towels, baby diapers or many layers of gauze. A ring dressing can be used around an area on which direct pressure should not be used **(Box 10-2)**.

Guidelines for Using Dressings

After washing and drying the wound, apply the dressing this way:

1. Wash hands and wear gloves.

2. Choose a dressing larger than the wound. Do not touch the part of the dressing that will contact the wound.

3. Carefully lay the dressing on the wound (do not slide it on from the side). Cover the entire wound **(Figure 10-8)**.

4. If blood seeps through, do not remove the dressing; instead, add more dressings on top of it.

5. Apply a bandage to hold the dressing in place.

When a dressing is later removed – to clean the wound or change a soiled dressing, for example

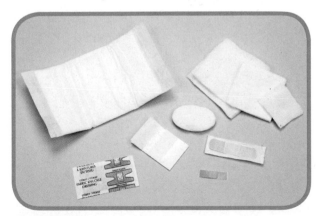

Figure 10-7 *A variety of dressings.*

– do not tug on a dressing that sticks to the wound. Soak it in warm water to release the dressing.

Bandages

Bandages are used for covering a dressing, keeping the dressing on a wound and maintaining pressure to control bleeding. Because only dressings touch the wound itself, bandages need to be clean but not necessarily sterile. As described in **Chapter 14**, bandages are also used to support or immobilize an injury to bones, joints or muscles and to reduce swelling.

Types of Bandages

Different types of bandages are available for different uses **(Figure 10-9)**. The following are common types of bandages:

- Adhesive compresses or strips for small wounds that combine a dressing with an adhesive bandage

- Adhesive tape rolls (cloth, plastic or paper)

- Tubular bandages for fingers or toes

- Elastic bandages

- Self-adhering bandages

- Gauze roller bandages

- Triangular bandages (or folded square cloths)

- Any cloth or other material improvised to meet the purposes of bandaging

Guidelines for Bandaging

Follow these guidelines for bandaging:

1. To put pressure on a wound to stop bleeding or to prevent the swelling of an injury, apply the bandage firmly but not so tightly that it cuts off circulation. The pressure is sufficient if the bandage is snug but you can slip a finger under it. Never put a circular bandage around the neck. With a bandage around a limb, check the fingers or toes for color, warmth and sensation (normal touch, not tingling) to make sure circulation is not cut off. If there are signs of reduced circulation, unwrap the bandage and reapply it less tightly.

2. Do not cover fingers or toes unless they are injured. Keep them exposed so they can be checked for adequate circulation.

3. Because swelling continues after many injuries, keep checking the tightness of the bandage. Swelling may make a loose bandage tight enough to cut off circulation.

4. With a bandaged wound, be sure the bandage is secure enough that the dressing will not move and expose the wound to possible contamination.

5. With elastic and roller bandages, anchor the first end and tie, tape, pin or clip the ending section in place. Loose ends could get caught on something and pull the bandage loose or disrupt the wound.

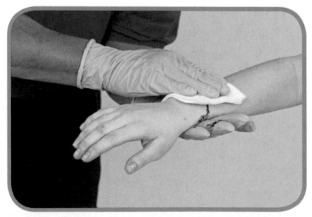

Figure 10-8 *Cover the wound with a sterile dressing.*

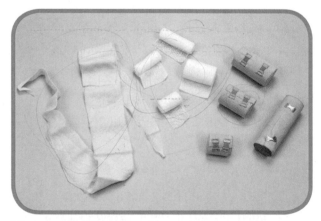

Figure 10-9 *Types of bandages.*

BOX 10-2: RING PAD

Direct pressure should not be used over the entire surface of certain types of wounds. For example, pressure should not be put on a skull fracture (see **Chapter 12**), a fractured bone protruding from a wound (see **Chapter 14**) or an object impaled in a wound. Cover the open wound with a sterile dressing as usual but do not apply direct pressure on the wound. In these cases bleeding is controlled around the object or fracture. A dressing made into a pad in a ring shape is appropriate for controlling bleeding and dressing such wounds.

Make a ring pad from a long strip of gauze or other material. First make a circular wrap the right size to surround the area. With the remainder of

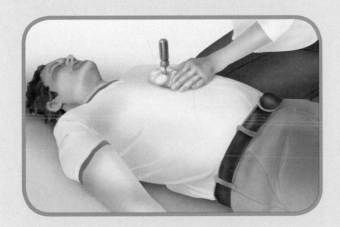

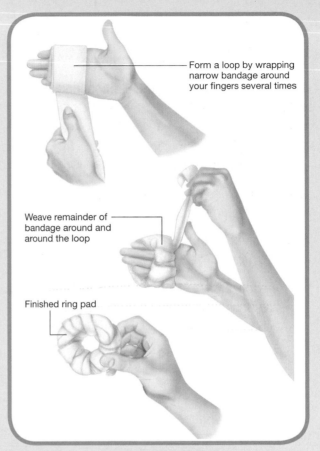

Form a loop by wrapping narrow bandage around your fingers several times

Weave remainder of bandage around and around the loop

Finished ring pad

the strip or an additional strip, wrap around the circular wrap to give the ring more bulk. Then position the ring around the wound and apply indirect pressure as needed.

6. Use an elastic roller bandage to make a pressure bandage around a limb to control bleeding and protect the wound (see **Chapter 8**).

7. An elastic roller bandage is used to support a joint and prevent swelling. At the wrist or ankle a figure-eight wrap is used (see **Chapter 14**).

8. Wrap a bandage from the bottom of the limb upward toward the heart to avoid cutting off circulation.

9. Avoid bending a joint once it has been bandaged because movement may loosen the dressing or cut off circulation.

When to Seek Medical Attention for a Wound

Remember: Call 9-1-1 for severe bleeding. In addition, the victim should see a health care provider as soon as possible in the following cases:

- Bleeding that is not easily controlled

- Any deep or large wound (e.g., wounds into muscle or bone)

- Significant wounds on the face

- Signs and symptoms that the wound is infected

- Any bite from an animal or human

- Foreign object or material embedded in the wound

- Puncture wounds

- The victim is unsure about tetanus vaccination

- Any wound you are unsure about

- Wounds that may require stitches **(Figure 10-10)**:

  – Cuts on the face or hands when the edges do not close together

  – Gaping wounds

  – Cuts longer than 1 inch

Special Wounds

In addition to the general guidelines for all wounds, certain types of wounds require special first aid considerations. These include puncture wounds, impaled objects, amputations and injuries to the genitals, head or face.

Injury Prevention

Wounds may occur anywhere in the body as a result of any kind of trauma. Prevention focuses on injury prevention in general, as described throughout this text. Following are guidelines for preventing certain special kinds of wounds:

- Many traumatic amputations result from industrial emergencies and the use of power tools in the home. Always follow OSHA guidelines in the work setting to prevent injury and, when using power tools at home, follow the specific guidelines provided by the tool's manufacturer. Never disassemble safeguards built into tools or equipment.

- Wearing the appropriate helmet at work or during sports and recreational activities can prevent skull injuries and injuries to the face and ears.

- Eye injuries frequently result from small objects or particles being unexpectedly propelled into the eye. Eye shields should be worn whenever one is working with power equipment.

- The American Dental Association recommends wearing a mouthguard during any activity that can result in a blow to the face or mouth. Ask your dentist about having a custom mouthguard made to provide a safe, comfortable fit.

- To avoid breaking a tooth, do not chew ice, hard candy or popcorn kernels.

- To prevent injuries to the genitals, males engaging in contact sports should wear an athletic cup; females should wear a pelvic shield or groin pad or protector.

(continues on page 148)

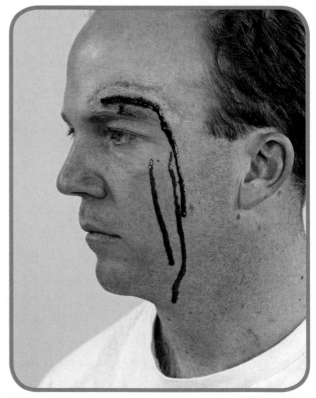

Figure 10-10 *A large, open wound may require stitches.*

Learning Checkpoint 1

1. Check off the actions that are included in wound care:

   ✓ Irrigate minor wounds with running water.

   _____ Pour rubbing alcohol on any wound.

   _____ Wash major wounds to help stop the bleeding.

   ✓ Cover any wound with a sterile dressing and bandage.

   _____ Let a scab form before washing a minor wound.

   ✓ See a health care provider for a deep wound or puncture wound.

   _____ Blow on a minor wound to cool the area and relieve pain.

2. If you are changing a wound dressing a day after the injury and the dressing sticks to the wound, what should you do?

   _____

3. True or (False): Puncture wounds have little risk for infection.

4. True or False: You don't need to bother putting on gloves to dress a minor wound if you know the victim well.

5. For what type(s) of wound(s) is an antibiotic ointment appropriate?

   _____Abrasion_____

6. Check off which signs and symptoms may indicate a wound is infected:

_____ Headache	_____ Cool, clammy skin
✓ Warmth in the area	_____ A scab forms that looks dark brown
✓ Red, swollen area	✓ Nausea and vomiting
✓ Fever	✓ Pus drains from the wound

7. Which of these victims need to seek medical attention? (Check all that apply.)

   ✓ Jose has a deep laceration from a piece of equipment, but you managed to stop the bleeding in 15 minutes.

   ✓ Rebecca had lunch in a nearby park and was bitten by a squirrel she was feeding, but the bleeding was minor and stopped almost immediately.

   _____ Carl scraped his knee when he fell off his bicycle on the way to work, but the abrasion washed out clean and you have applied an antibiotic ointment.

   ✓ Kim got a bad gash on her cheek when a bottle broke in the supply room, but she had already stopped the bleeding by the time you saw her.

8. True or False: To control bleeding, make a pressure bandage as tight as you can get it.

9. You have put a pressure bandage around a victim's arm to control bleeding from a laceration. A few minutes later she says her fingers are tingling. You feel her hand, and her fingers are cold. What should you do?

   _____untied_____

10. When applying a bandage over a dressing, the bandage should

    a. hold down only the corners of the dressing so the wound can breathe.

    b. be soaked first in cold water.

    ✓ c. cover the entire dressing.

    d. be loose enough so it can be slid to one side to change the dressing.

(continued from page 146)

- To prevent stretching and potentially tearing ligaments and other supportive breast tissues, women should wear a sports bra during exercise or sport activities.

Puncture Wounds

Puncture wounds may involve deeper injuries you cannot see. If the puncturing object may have penetrated the body, check also for an exit wound. In general, puncture wounds carry a greater risk of infection than other types of wounds because often they bleed less, and therefore germs may not be flushed out. In addition to routine wound care, follow these steps:

1. Irrigate the wound with large amounts of warm or room-temperature water with or without soap to remove foreign matter.

2. Gently press on wound edges to promote bleeding.

3. Dry the area. Do not put any medication inside or over the puncture wound.

4. Cover the wound with a sterile dressing and bandage.

5. Seek medical attention.

Impaled Objects

Removing an object from a wound could cause more injury and bleeding, because often the object is sealing the wound or damaged blood vessels. Leave it in place and dress the wound around it **(Figure 10-11)**. Use bulky dressings (trauma dressings) to stabilize the object and keep it from moving. If there is blood or sweat on the skin, adhesive tape may not stick well enough to hold bulky dressings in place; use a roller bandage or strips of cloth to tie the bandage in place around the impaled object. Follow these guidelines:

1. Control bleeding by applying direct pressure around the edges of the object.

2. Dress the wound around the object.

3. Stabilize the object in place with large dressings or folded cloths.

4. Support the object while bandaging the dressings in place.

5. Keep the victim still and seek medical attention.

An impaled object in the eye or the cheek is a unique circumstance requiring special care, as described in the later sections on eye and cheek injuries.

Avulsions and Amputations

An avulsion is a piece of skin or other soft tissue torn partially from the body, like a flap. Try to move the skin or tissue back into its normal position unless the wound is contaminated, and then control bleeding and provide wound care.

If the avulsed tissue is completely separated from the body, care for it the same as you would for an amputated part.

In an amputation, a part has been severed from the body. Control the bleeding and care for the victim and the wound first, then recover and care for the amputated part. Bleeding can usually be controlled with the same measures as for other wounds, using bulky dressings. Follow these steps to care for the severed body part, which surgeons may be able to reattach to the victim:

1. Wrap the severed part in a dry, sterile dressing or clean cloth. Do not wash it.

2. Place the part in a plastic bag or container and seal it.

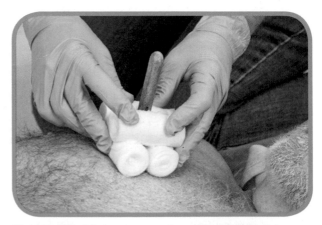

Figure 10-11 *Leave an impaled object in place and use bulky dressings to keep it from moving.*

3. Place the sealed bag in another bag or container with ice. Do not let the part touch water or ice directly, and do not surround it with ice **(Figure 10-12)**.

4. Make sure the severed part is given to emergency personnel or taken with the victim to the emergency department.

Genital Injuries

Injuries to the genitals are rare because of their protected location. Injuries may occur from blunt trauma, an impact that creates a wound or sexual abuse. Provide privacy for a victim when giving first aid for a wound in the genital area. Follow these guidelines:

- Use direct pressure with a sterile dressing or sanitary pad to control external bleeding. Then use a large triangular bandage applied like a diaper to secure the dressings in place **(Figure 10-13)**.

- For injured testicles, provide support with a towel wrapped between the legs like a diaper. For a closed injury caused by blunt trauma, a cold pack may help reduce pain.

- For vaginal bleeding, have the woman press a sanitary pad or clean folded towel to the area to control the bleeding.

- Call 9-1-1 for severe or continuing bleeding, significant pain or swelling, or the possibility of sexual abuse.

- In the case of rape or sexual abuse, preserve evidence for law enforcement personnel by following the guidelines in **Chapter 21**.

Head and Face Wounds

Wounds to the head or face may require special first aid. The following sections provide guidelines for these special injuries. Skull injuries, such as fractures, are described in **Chapter 12**.

With any significant injury to the head, the victim may also have a neck or spinal injury. If you suspect a spinal injury, be careful not to move the victim's head while giving first aid for head and face wounds.

Scalp Wound Without Suspected Skull Fracture

If signs and symptoms of a skull fracture are not present and the wound is restricted to the scalp, apply a dressing and use direct pressure as usual to control bleeding. Then apply a roller bandage, or a triangular bandage folded into a cravat, around the head to secure the dressing. Never wrap a bandage around the neck because of the risk of impeding breathing if the injury causes swelling (see First Aid: "Scalp Wound Without Suspected Skull Fracture").

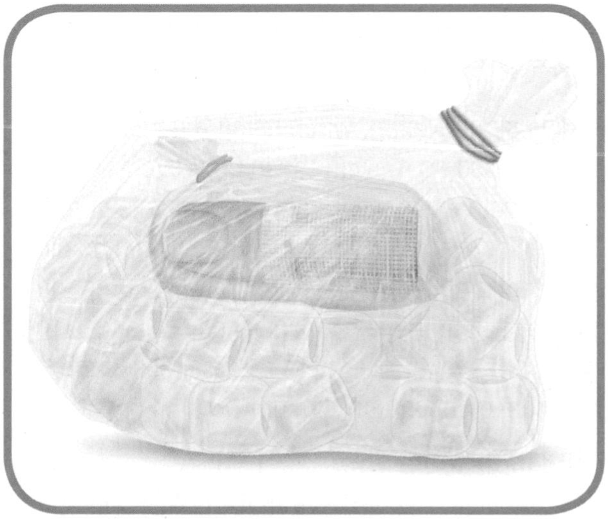

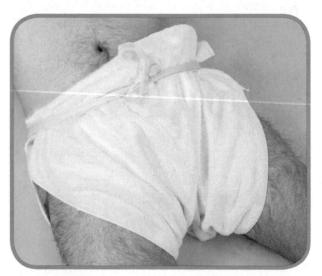

Figure 10-12 *Keep amputated part cold but not directly touching ice.*

Figure 10-13 *Apply a triangular bandage like a diaper to secure dressings in the genital area.*

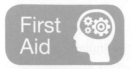

First Aid — Scalp Wound Without Suspected Skull Fracture
Signs, Symptoms and Care

When You See

- **Bleeding from the head**
- **No sign of skull fracture**

Do This First

1 Replace any skin flaps and cover the wound with a sterile dressing.

2 Use direct pressure to control bleeding.

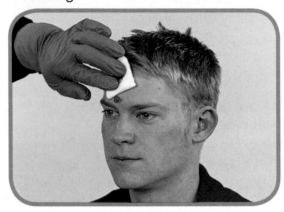

3 Put a roller or triangle bandage around the victim's head to secure the dressing.

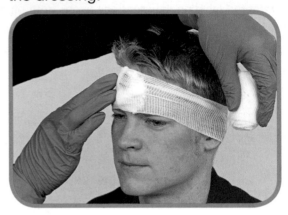

Additional Care

- Position the victim with head and shoulders slightly raised to help control bleeding.
- Seek medical attention if the victim later experiences nausea and vomiting, persistent headache, drowsiness or disorientation, stumbling or lack of coordination, or problems with speech or vision.

Eye Injuries

Eye injuries are serious because vision may be affected. Eye injuries include blows to the eye, impaled objects in the eye, dirt or small particles in the eye, and chemicals or other substances splashed into the eye. When caring for any eye injury, avoid putting pressure directly on the eyeball because this tissue is easily injured.

With most eye injuries, movement of the eye will continue to worsen the injury. Bandaging or otherwise covering an injured eye discourages the victim from moving it. Because the eyes move together, the unaffected eye must also be covered; otherwise the victim, when using the unaffected eye, will also be moving the injured eye. Having both eyes covered or bandaged is often frightening, especially to an injured victim. Explain what you are doing and why before covering the good eye. To minimize anxiety, keep talking to the victim or have another person offer reassurance with conversation and touch.

For a blow to the eye:

1. If the eye is bleeding or leaking fluid, call 9-1-1 or get the victim to the emergency department immediately.

2. Put a cold pack over the eye, with a barrier such as cloth between the cold pack and the eye, for up to 15 minutes to ease pain and reduce swelling, but do not put pressure on the eye. If the victim is wearing a contact lens, do not try to remove it **(Figure 10-14)**.

3. Have victim lie still. Cover the uninjured eye.

4. Seek medical attention if pain persists or vision is affected in any way.

For a large object embedded in the eye:

1. Do not remove the object. Stabilize it in place with dressings or bulky cloth. Be careful not to put any pressure on the eye from the object. With a large impaled object or one that may move, use a paper cup or something similar to stabilize the object and keep it from moving in the eye **(Figure 10-15)**.

2. Cover both eyes, because movement of the uninjured one causes movement of the injured one.

3. Call 9-1-1 or get the victim to the emergency department immediately.

For dirt or a small particle in the eye:

If the victim complains of something small caught in the eye, do not let the victim rub the eye with his or her hands, which could cause scratching of the eye or other soft tissue. The body's natural way to remove small particles from the eye is to wash it out with

tears and blinking. Wait a minute to see if the victim's tears flush out the object. If not, try these methods:

1. Gently pull the upper eyelid out and down over the lower eyelid. This allows the lower lashes to catch a particle caught under the upper eyelid.

2. If the particle remains, gently flush the eye with water from a medicine dropper or water glass. Have the victim tilt the head so that the affected eye is lower than the other; this prevents water from flowing into the unaffected eye. Flush from the corner nearer the nose. Ask the victim to hold the eyelids open with his or her fingers, if needed, and to look in all directions and blink during the flushing.

3. If the particle remains and is visible, carefully try to brush it out gently with a wet, sterile dressing. Lift the upper eyelid and swab its underside if you see the particle **(Figure 10-16)**.

4. If the particle remains or the victim has any vision problems or pain, cover the eye with a sterile dressing and seek medical attention. Also cover the uninjured eye to prevent movement of the injured one.

For a chemical or substance splashed in the eye:

1. Flush the victim's eye with large amounts of running water until EMS arrives. Use a specialized solution if available.

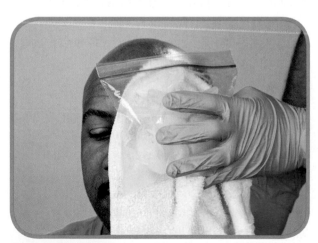

Figure 10-14 *For a blow to the eye, hold a cold pack on the eye.*

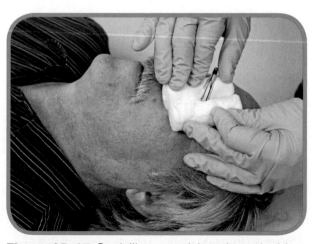

Figure 10-15 *Stabilize an object impaled in the eyeball.*

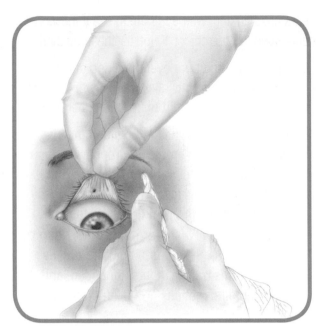

Figure 10-16 *Carefully remove a particle from the eyelid.*

2. Have a victim wearing contact lenses remove them.

3. Tilt the victim's head so water does not run into the other eye (see **Chapter 11**).

4. Call 9-1-1.

Ear Injuries

With bleeding from the external ear, control the bleeding with direct pressure and dress the wound.

Remember that bleeding or clear fluid (cerebrospinal fluid) from within the ear can be a sign of a serious head injury. Do not use direct pressure to try to stop fluid from coming out the ear. Give care as described in **Chapter 12**.

If the victim complains of a foreign object in the ear, do not try to remove it with any tool or object. Never insert tweezers, a pin or cotton swab into the ear in an attempt to remove an object. The object may be pushed further into the ear, or the tool may damage the eardrum or other tissues. Leave the object in place and seek medical attention. Only if the foreign object is clearly visible and easily grasped with your fingers is it safe to remove an object, but do not remove an impaled object. Occasionally an insect may crawl into the ear when a person is sleeping.

If you see or know that an insect is in the ear, gently pour lukewarm water into the ear to try to float it out. If it does not come out, seek medical attention.

For bleeding from within the ear, follow the guidelines in First Aid: "Ear Injuries."

Nose Injuries

Injury to the nose can cause heavy bleeding. Nosebleeds can also be caused by pressure changes or a child picking at the nose. Nosebleeds can usually be controlled, usually within a few minutes, by positioning the victim leaning slightly forward and pinching the nostrils closed until bleeding stops. For an unresponsive victim or a victim who cannot sit leaning forward, position the victim on one side with the head turned to allow drainage from the nose and mouth while you pinch the nostrils closed. Do not try to pack the nostrils with a dressing in an effort to control the bleeding.

Bleeding that runs from the back of the nose down the throat is more serious and needs immediate medical attention. Do not tilt the victim's head backward but keep the victim positioned to allow blood to drain out the mouth so that the airway is not threatened (see First Aid: "Nosebleed").

Small children often put small objects in their noses. If a foreign object is clearly visible and easily grasped with tweezers, you may safely remove it, but do not remove an impaled object. Do not push tweezers or your finger into the nostril to try to remove an object because of the risk of pushing it in deeper. Do not have a child try to blow an object out, because it may be sucked in deeper instead.

Cheek Injuries

A wound on the outside of the cheek is cared for by following the general guidelines for wounds. If an object is impaled in a wound in the cheek, check inside the mouth to see if the object has penetrated through. If you can see both sides of the object and can remove it safely, do so. *This is the one exception to the rule about not removing an impaled object from a wound.* The object

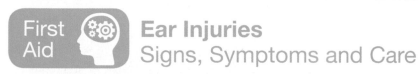
When You See

- **Bleeding or fluid from inside the ear**
- **Signs of pain**
- **Possible deafness**

Do This First

1 Clear fluid or watery blood from the ear could mean a skull fracture. Call 9-1-1.

2 Help victim to sit up, tilting the affected ear lower to let blood or other fluid drain.

3 Cover the ear with a loose, sterile dressing, but do not apply pressure.

4 Seek medical attention immediately if 9-1-1 was not called.

Additional Care

- Keep the ear covered to reduce the risk of infection.

ALERT

- Do not plug the ear closed to try to stop bleeding.

---

may pose a risk to the airway if it protrudes into the mouth or later falls into the mouth. Gently pull the object out, in the direction from which it penetrated the cheek, taking care with a sharp object not to cut the cheek further. Then place a dressing inside the mouth between the cheek wound and the teeth; watch that this dressing does not come out of position and block the airway. Apply another dressing to the outside of the wound, applying pressure as needed to control bleeding. For an unresponsive victim, roll the victim's body as a unit to position the head so that blood and other fluid will run out of the mouth (as described in **Chapter 12**).

Teeth and Mouth Injuries

Injuries to the mouth may cause bleeding anywhere in the mouth and may knock out a tooth. Bleeding is controlled with direct pressure on a dressing over the wound. A tooth that has been knocked out can usually be replanted if the tooth is properly cared for. The priority of first aid

for the mouth is always to ensure that the airway is open and that blood can drain from the mouth until bleeding is controlled.

A tooth that has been knocked out requires care if it is to be successfully reimplanted because delicate tissues attached to the tooth may quickly die. Do not try to put the tooth back in the socket. The tooth should not be allowed to dry out; immerse it in milk or water.

If a tooth is knocked loose enough that there is a risk it may fall out, make a pad from rolled gauze and have the victim bite down on it to keep the tooth in place until the victim reaches the dentist. If a tooth is broken, rinse the victim's mouth with saline or tap water and then apply a cold pack to reduce swelling and pain; see a dentist as soon as possible.

For a knocked-out tooth:

1. Have the victim sit with head tilted forward to let blood drain out.

(continues on page 155)

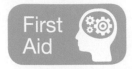

First Aid

Nosebleed
Signs, Symptoms and Care

When You See

- **Blood coming from either or both nostrils**
- **Blood possibly running from back of nose down into the mouth or throat**

Do This First

1 Have the victim sit and tilt head slightly forward with mouth open. Carefully remove any object you see protruding from the nose, but do not probe inside the nose.

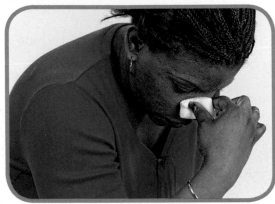

2 Have the victim pinch the nostrils together, just below the bridge of the nose, for 10 minutes. Ask victim to breathe through the mouth and not speak, swallow, cough or sniff.

3 If victim is gasping or choking on blood in the throat, call 9-1-1.

4 Place a cold compress on the bridge of the nose.

5 After 10 minutes, release the pressure slowly. Pinch the nostrils again for another 10 minutes if bleeding continues.

Additional Care

- Place a cold compress on the bridge of the nose.
- Seek medical attention if:
  - bleeding continues after two attempts to control it.
  - you suspect the nose is broken.
  - there is a foreign object in the nose.
  - the victim has high blood pressure.
- Have the person rest for a few hours and avoid rubbing or blowing the nose.

ALERT

- Do not tilt the victim's head backward.
- Do not have the victim lie down.

Blisters
Signs, Symptoms and Care

When You See

- **A raised, fluid-filled blister, often surrounded by red skin**

Do This First

1 Wash the blister and surrounding area with soap and water. Rinse and gently pat dry.

2 Cover the blister with an adhesive bandage big enough that the gauze pad covers the entire blister. Bandages with an adhesive strip on all four sides are best because they keep the area cleaner if the blister breaks. For a larger blister, use a donut-shaped dressing to surround the blister and prevent pressure on it.

Additional Care

- Prevent continued friction in the area

ALERT

- Never deliberately break a blister. This could lead to infection.

(continued from page 153)

2. Rinse the wound with saline solution or tap water.

3. Control the bleeding by having the victim bite down for 20 to 30 minutes on a gauze pad or cotton ball placed over the tooth socket **(Figure 10-17)**.

4. Save the tooth. Pick it up by the crown and place it in a container of milk (or clean water if milk is not available). Do not clean or scrub the tooth.

5. Have the victim see a dentist immediately.

For other bleeding in the mouth:

1. Have the victim sit with head tilted forward to let blood drain out.

2. **For a wound penetrating the lip**: Put a rolled dressing between the lip and the gum. Hold a second dressing against the outside lip.

3. **For a bleeding tongue**: Put a dressing on the wound and apply pressure.

4. Do not repeatedly rinse the mouth (this may prevent clotting).

5. Do not let victim swallow blood, which may cause vomiting.

6. When the bleeding stops, tell the victim not to drink anything warm for several hours.

7. Seek medical attention if bleeding is severe or does not stop.

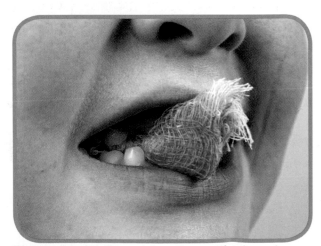

Figure 10-17 *Stop bleeding with dressing over tooth socket.*

Learning Checkpoint 2

1. Name one circumstance in which you might want to promote bleeding.

   _____

2. True or False: The first thing to do when you see an impaled object in a wound is to pull it out so you can put direct pressure on the wound to stop the bleeding.

3. True or False: An amputated part should be kept cold but not put in direct contact with ice.

4. With an eye injury, why would you cover the uninjured eye, too?

   _____

5. Describe three ways you can try to remove a small particle from the eye.

   _____

6. True or False: For bleeding from within the ear, roll a piece of gauze into a plug and try to seal the ear with it.

7. A nosebleed victim should first try to stop the bleeding by pinching the nostrils closed for _____ minutes. During this time, list two or three things the victim should not do.

   _____

8. True or False: A knocked-out tooth can be reimplanted if it is kept in milk (or clean water if milk is not available) and the victim reaches a dentist soon.

9. True or False: Repeatedly rinsing the mouth with cool water is the best way to stop bleeding in the mouth.

Blisters

Blisters usually occur because of friction on the skin, as when a shoe rubs the back of the ankle or heel. They can be painful and may become infected after breaking. Burns may cause a different kind of blister (see **Chapter 11**).

Blisters can usually be prevented by protecting the feet with socks or with tape where socks rub. A small blister can be protected with an adhesive bandage. Try to prevent it from breaking open, which can lead to infection. For a larger blister, cut a hole in several layers of gauze or moleskin and position this dressing over the blister with the blister itself protected within the hole (see First Aid: "Blisters").

If a blister breaks, wash the area and care for it as you would care for a wound (see **Chapter 10**).

Splinters

You can remove a splinter in the skin by coaxing it out with a sterile needle and then grasping the end with tweezers or your fingers. Cleanse the area with soap and water.

Crush Injuries

A crush injury is caused when strong pressure is exerted against the body. Depending on the force involved, a crushing injury can result in muscle, bone, nerve and tissue damage, shock, and internal and/or external bleeding.

Provide care for the injuries you find and call 9-1-1.

Concluding Thoughts

Wounds are among the most common injuries requiring first aid. In most cases the care is simple and straightforward: Clean the wound, apply a dressing and cover and secure the dressing with an appropriate bandage. Particular kinds of wounds and injuries in certain areas of the body require additional specific care. Following these guidelines will, in most cases, prevent infection of the wound and lead to effective healing.

Learning Outcomes

You should now be able to do the following:

1. Describe how to clean a wound.

2. Describe the signs and symptoms of an infected wound and what to do about it.

3. List standard guidelines for using dressings and bandages.

4. Explain how to determine when a wound needs medical attention.

5. Describe first aid for punctures, wounds with impaled objects, avulsions and amputations and for injuries of the genitals, scalp and specific facial areas.

Review Questions

1. What is the first priority for a severely bleeding wound?

   a. Seeking medical attention

   b. Controlling the bleeding

   c. Preventing infection

   d. Irrigating the wound

2. Infection is more likely in which kind of wound?

   a. Puncture

   b. Laceration

   c. Abrasion

   d. Avulsion

3. What is the best way to clean a wound?

   a. Soak in alcohol

   b. Apply iodine

   c. Irrigate with water

   d. Apply a cool, moist compress

4. Antibiotic ointment may be used on what kinds of wounds?

   a. Abrasions

   b. Punctures

   c. Deep burns

   d. Open abdominal wounds

5. A pressure bandage to control bleeding –

   a. should be applied directly over the wound.

   b. should be as tight as you can get it to stop the bleeding.

   c. should be made with an elastic roller bandage.

   d. All of the above

6. Signs of good circulation in a limb below a pressure bandage include –

    a. cool skin.

    b. normal skin color.

    c. tingling sensations.

    d. ability to move fingers or toes.

7. What wounds should be seen by a health care provider?

    a. Wounds through the skin into muscle tissue

    b. Human bite wounds

    c. Wounds that may require stitches

    d. All of the above

8. How would you best care for a traumatically amputated finger?

    a. Wash it under running water and put it in a glass or jar of ice water.

    b. Wrap it in a dressing, place it inside a plastic bag and put the bag on ice.

    c. Keep it dry and at body temperature (held against victim's body).

    d. Put it in a plastic bag and place the bag in the freezer until help arrives.

9. For a nonbleeding but painful blow to the eye –

    a. flush constantly with warm, running water for up to 30 minutes.

    b. have victim sit in a dark room with both eyes covered for 30 minutes.

    c. put a cold pack over the eye for up to 15 minutes.

    d. give the victim aspirin or ibuprofen.

10. Care for a nosebleed includes –

    a. having the victim "blow" the nose into a handkerchief to clear out blood.

    b. pinching the nostrils closed up to 10 minutes.

    c. packing the nose with sterile gauze.

    d. having the victim tilt head back while sucking on ice chips.

Chapter 11 • Burns

Chapter Preview

- What Happens With a Burn?
- Prevention of Fires and Burns
- Heat Burns
- First Aid for Heat Burns

- Smoke Inhalation
- Chemical Burns
- Electrical Burns and Shocks

While visiting your aunt at her home, you join her in the kitchen as she cooks pasta for dinner. On the stove front burner is a large pot of boiling water. She is telling you about something that happened earlier that day and is not paying close attention to her cooking. Before you can react to stop her, you see her reach across the boiling water for the kettle on the back burner. She yelps as the steam burns her forearm, and jerks her arm back. What should you do immediately? What additional care should you give for this burn?

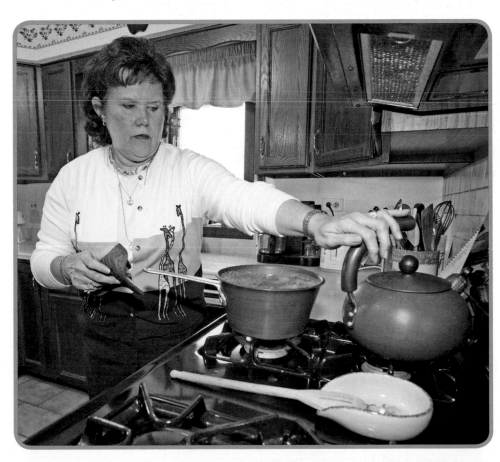

Fires and burns are a major cause of death and injury. There are about 3,200 deaths a year in the United States caused by fires and burns and about 416,000 burn injuries leading to emergency department visits.[1] Fires and burns may occur in almost any setting, but the great majority occur in the home and experts believe that most fires and burns can be prevented. Even with preventive steps, however, it is essential to know what to do when fire occurs and how to treat burn victims.

Burns of the skin or deeper tissues may be caused by the sun, heat, chemicals or electricity. Mild heat burns and sunburn may need only simple first aid, but severe burns can be a medical emergency.

What Happens With a Burn?

A burn is an injury to the skin and potentially deeper structures caused by heat, electricity or chemicals. Burns can cause severe adverse effects in the body because the skin has several important functions:

- *Protection.* The skin protects the body against the entry of **pathogens** that can cause infection, as well as other harmful substances. Specialized cells also have an immune function.

[1]*National Safety Council. (2011). Injury Facts®, 2011 Edition. Itasca, IL: Author.*

- *Fluid retention.* The skin prevents the loss of fluids and other important substances such as electrolytes.

- *Temperature regulation.* The skin has a major role in controlling the body's temperature, preventing heat loss in cold environments and promoting heat loss in hot environments.

- *Sensation.* The skin contains sensory and other nerves and blood vessels.

Although a minor burn such as a sunburn may damage only the **epidermis**, the outer layer of skin, more severe burns damage the **dermis**, or middle layer, which contains nerves and blood vessels, or the deepest layer of subcutaneous tissue, through which larger blood vessels and nerves pass **(Figure 11-1)**.

Burns that extend into the dermis expose tissues to the outside environment and carry a high risk of infection from pathogens present almost everywhere. The more extensive and deeper a burn, the more likely infection becomes because pathogens may enter more easily and medical treatment becomes more difficult.

Burns extending into the dermis or deeper also cause fluid loss. Injured capillaries in the dermis leak fluid; this is the cause of watery blisters

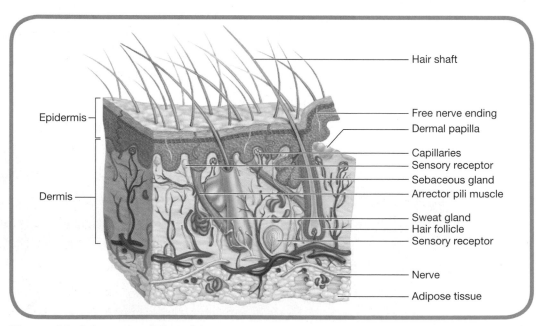

Epidermis

Dermis

Hair shaft
Free nerve ending
Dermal papilla
Capillaries
Sensory receptor
Sebaceous gland
Arrector pili muscle
Sweat gland
Hair follicle
Sensory receptor
Nerve
Adipose tissue

Figure 11-1 *Layers of the skin.*

in second-degree burns. Deeper burns cause fluid loss from larger blood vessels. Significant fluid loss from severe burns can cause shock, a further threat to the burn victim that can be life-threatening (see **Chapter 9**).

To function well, the human body must maintain a fairly consistent internal temperature. Because the skin helps regulate this function, a severe burn can cause a loss of body heat, further stressing vital organs. Therefore a victim with extensive severe burns should not be cooled with water over much of the body because of the increased risk of **hypothermia**, which would further threaten the victim's condition.

Because the skin is rich in sensory nerves, burns can be very painful due to damage to these nerves. With burns entirely through the skin, however, the victim may not feel pain because the nerve endings are completely destroyed. In such cases there are often less severely burned areas around the pain-free areas that do cause significant pain. Pain is therefore present in most burns but is not an indication of the burn's severity.

Finally, burns may damage body tissues other than just the skin. A full-thickness burn that penetrates all the way through the skin may damage muscle and fat tissue beneath as well as underlying organs, resulting in additional trauma to the body and increasing the urgency for medical treatment. Victims with burns caused by fires may also have respiratory damage caused by inhaling smoke, fumes or hot air. Respiratory tract tissues may swell, causing breathing difficulty.

Prevention of Fires and Burns
Common Causes of Burns
The huge majority of all deaths by fire and burns occur in the home. Following are some sobering facts and statistics about fires in the home:[2]

- In 2008, U.S. fire departments responded to an estimated 1,451,500 fires.

[2]*National Fire Protection Association. http://www.nfpa.org/ assets/files/PDF/FireOverview.pdf Accessed March 1, 2011.*

- On average, a fire department responded to a fire every 22 seconds.
- Fire claimed nine lives every day.
- Cooking is the leading cause of home fires and home fire injuries.
- Smoking has been the leading cause of home fire deaths for decades.
- Almost all U.S. homes have at least one smoke alarm, but 63% of home fire deaths resulted from fires in homes without working smoke alarms.
- Children younger than 5 and older adults face the highest risk of home fire death, but young adults face a higher risk of home fire injury.

The following are the most common causes of fires leading to injury or death:

- Smoking
- Heating
- Cooking
- Playing with fire
- Electrical wiring
- Open flames
- Appliances or other equipment

Preventing Burns
Preventing burns involves both preventing fires and preventing burns from hot water and other sources of heat such as stoves.

Preventing Fires
Follow these guidelines to prevent a fire in the home and other settings **(Figure 11-2)**:

- Make your home and workplace safe:
  - Make sure enough smoke detectors are installed and change batteries twice a year when you change your clocks for daylight-saving time.
  - Do not allow smoking, or ensure that it is done safely and materials are safely extinguished. Never allow smoking in bed.

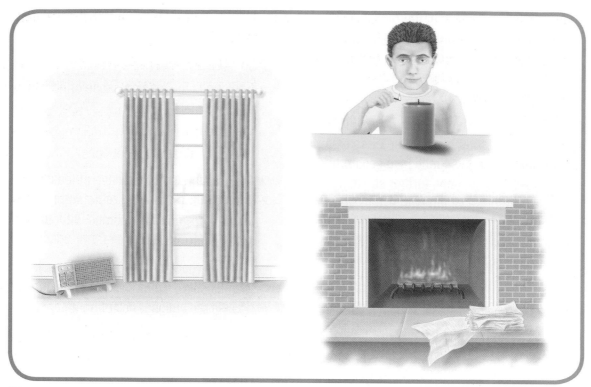

Figure 11-2 *Inspect all rooms for fire hazards and keep children away from flames and sources of heat.*

- Keep curtains and other flammable objects away from fireplaces and stoves; use fireplace screens.
- Have chimneys regularly inspected and cleaned to prevent chimney fires.
- Never store gasoline or other highly flammable liquids indoors.

• Prevent fires in the kitchen:

- Keep a fire extinguisher in the kitchen and know how to use it.
- Tie back long hair or loose clothing when cooking or working around flames.
- If food catches on fire in a microwave or toaster oven, leave the food there and turn off the appliance; keep other objects away until the flames go out.

• Prevent fires caused by electricity:

- Keep power cords safely out of the way and away from children.

- Check appliance cords for damaged areas or fraying.
- Do not overload electrical outlets or use multiple extension cords.
- Unplug appliances and extension cords when not in use.

• Keep children from playing with fire:

- Store matches, lighters, candles and other ignition sources away from children.
- Teach young children that matches, candles and lighters are only for adult use, and model safe behavior when using them yourself.
- Accept that "child-resistant" lighters are not childproof but can be used even by toddlers to start fires.
- Understand that children who know that fire is "bad" are likely to play with matches or lighters in their bedrooms or elsewhere where they think they will not be caught.

– Any child may play with fire because of peer pressure or simple curiosity. Teach all children the dangers of fire, and keep matches and ignition sources away from them. Remember that more than 50,000 structure fires every year are set by children.[3]

- Protect children from burns caused by fire:

  – Purchase only flame-resistant pajamas and bedding.

  – Plan escape routes and teach children where to go if a fire breaks out.

  – Teach children to "stop, drop and roll" if their clothing catches on fire.

If a Fire Occurs

Because a fire may occur even when you try to prevent it, know what to do if one should break out:

- Evacuate everyone first. Do not delay evacuation while you call 9-1-1 or use a fire extinguisher. Follow the rehearsed evacuation route.

- Do not use an elevator.

- Feel doors before opening them, and do not open a door that is hot.

- If the air is smoky, stay near the floor where there is more oxygen.

- Do not throw water on an electrical or grease (cooking) fire.

- If you cannot escape a building on fire, stuff clothing or rags in door cracks and vents; call 9-1-1 and give the dispatcher your exact location.

Preventing Heat Burns

After house fires, the most common cause of serious burns to children and the elderly is scalding from hot gases and liquids. Follow these

[3]*National Fire Protection Association, http://www.nfpa. org/categoryList.asp?categoryID=281&URL=Safety%20 Information/For%20consumers/Arson%20&%20 juvenile%20fire%20setting/Children%20playing%20 with%20fire Accessed March 1, 2011.*

guidelines to prevent burns from anything that may be hot:

- Do not use steam vaporizers; if you do, keep them away from areas children can reach.

- Keep hot irons, curling irons, toasters and similar appliances away from children. Never leave a child alone in a room with a hot object.

- Do not use space heaters on the floor or anywhere children can reach them. Install heat guards around radiators and heaters. Move a child's bed away from radiators or other heat sources.

- Keep children away from barbecue grills, which stay hot for a long time after use.

- Keep children away from campfires, which may contain hot or burning coals many hours after the fire was "put out." Never leave children unsupervised near a fire or use flammable liquids to start a campfire. Keep tents and other gear well away.

- Never let children use fireworks.

- In the bathroom:

  – Prevent scalding burns by turning down the temperature of the water heater to 120°F or lower. If you cannot do this (as in an apartment building with shared hot water), purchase an anti-scald device from a children's store or hardware store.

  – Check the temperature of bath water with your wrist. Stir the water with your hand to prevent hot spots.

  – Supervise children in the bathtub.

- In the kitchen:

  – When cooking, use the back burners on the stove and keep pot handles turned toward the back of the stove.

  – Do not store food near the stove because children may attempt to reach it on their own.

- Do not hold an infant when cooking or drinking a hot liquid.

- Do not open the oven door with a child nearby.

- Check the temperature of microwaved baby food or a baby bottle before feeding it to an infant.

- Do not let young children use a microwave oven by themselves.

- Keep high chairs away from the stove and counters where hot foods or electrical cords may be present.

Preventing Heat Burns in the Elderly

The elderly are less likely to hear, see or feel fire and burn threats and are less able to escape a fire. In addition to the guidelines described previously, take these preventive actions in a home with an elderly family member:

- Ensure that all exits are kept clear.

- Keep eyeglasses, a telephone and needed walking aids next to the bed.

- Wear short sleeves or tight garments when cooking and use oven mitts for protection.

- Avoid cooking when sleepy or when taking medications that cause drowsiness.

- Do not let anyone smoke near a device that supplies oxygen.

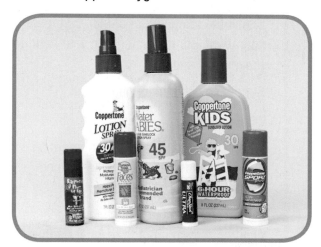

Figure 11-3 *Protect against sunburn with frequent use of sunscreen.*

- Use a timer to remind you to turn off electric heating pads and blankets.

- Be aware of the special risks of hot objects such as cooking materials and utensils.

- Understand the limitations imposed by any physical impairments or cognitive deficits.

- Contact an organization such as the American Burn Association (http://www.ameriburn.org) for additional safety tips on preventing burns among the elderly.

Preventing Sunburn

Sunburns cause pain and damage the skin. Because repeated sunburns can cause skin cancer later in life, steps should always be taken to prevent sunburns.

- Keep infants younger than 12 months out of direct sunlight as much as possible. Sun-blocking clothing and shade are recommended for infants younger than 6 months old, although sunscreen can safely be used on small areas of skin. Protect an infant's eyes from sunlight as well.

- For everyday outdoors activities, the American Cancer Society recommends applying sunscreen or sunblock with a sun protection factor (SPF) of at least 15 on all exposed areas of skin 20 minutes before sun exposure and at least every 2 hours while in the sun **(Figure 11-3)**. Use a higher SPF for prolonged sun exposure.

- Wear a wide-brimmed hat and protective clothing, and keep infants and young children covered with light clothing, hats and sunglasses.

- Limit sun exposure between 10 a.m. and 4 p.m.

- Be aware that reflective surfaces such as water and snow increase the risk of burning.

- Use sunscreen even on cloudy, hazy or foggy days, because sunburn may still occur.

- Use a lip balm with at least 15 SPF when in direct sun for an extended time.

Heat Burns

Heat burns may be caused by flames or contact with steam or any hot object. The severity of a burn depends on the amount of damage to the skin and other tissues under the skin.

Put Out the Fire!

If the victim's clothing is on fire, use a blanket or water to put out any flames, or have the victim roll on the ground. Even when the fire is out, the skin will keep burning if it is still hot, so cool the burn area with water immediately, except with very severe burns. Also, remove the victim's clothing and jewelry, if it is possible to do so without further injuring the victim, because they may still be hot and continue to burn the victim.

Assessing a Burn

Assess burns to determine the appropriate first aid to give and decide whether to call 9-1-1 or transport the victim to medical care. Assessment involves consideration of several factors:

- What type of burn(s) does the victim have (first-, second- or third-degree)?

- How extensive is the burn (how much body area)?

- What specific body areas are burned?

- Are special circumstances present (the victim's age and health status)?

Because these variables can be complex, there is no one simple rule for determining when to call 9-1-1 or seek medical care. Whenever any burn may be serious, call 9-1-1 and let medical professionals guide your decision.

Classification of Burns

Burns are classified according to their depth into or through the skin:

- **First-degree burns** (also called **superficial burns**) damage only the skin's outer layer, the epidermis, like a typical sunburn. The skin is red, typically dry and painful. These minor burns usually heal well by themselves but may require medical attention if they cover an extensive area.

- **Second-degree burns** (also called **partial-thickness burns**) damage the skin's deeper layer, the dermis. The skin is red, may look mottled and is very painful. Blisters are often present and may be weeping clear fluid. Scarring may be present after healing. Depending on size and other factors, second-degree burns may require medical attention.

- **Third-degree burns** (also called **full-thickness burns**) damage the skin all the way through the subcutaneous layer and may burn muscle or other tissues. The skin is charred or blackened or may look white and leathery. Pain is not present where the skin has burned through but is likely in adjacent areas. These burns are medical emergencies. Often a victim with serious burns has a mix of different burn classifications. One area may have a third-degree burn, for example, while nearby areas have first- or second-degree burns. Follow the first aid guidelines for the most severely burned area first.

Assessing Burn Size and Severity

In addition to burn depth, the size of the burned area is an important part of the assessment. This is usually calculated as a percentage of body surface area. A common method used by medical professionals to estimate the body surface area of a burn is the **rule of nines**. In this system the adult body is divided into a number of areas with percentages based on increments of 9%. As shown in **Figure 11-4**, the percentages are different for a small child.

- Each arm is 9% (front or back alone is 4.5%).

- Each leg is 18% (front or back alone is 9%).

- The front of the torso is 18% (9% for abdomen and 9% for chest).

- The back of the torso is 18% (9% for lower back and buttocks, 9% for upper back).

- The head is 9% (face or back of head alone is 4.5%).

- The genital region is 1%.

In some cases the percentage of body surface area burned influences the decision to call EMS and determines some aspects of advanced medical care. Any third-degree burn larger than a 50-cent piece or second-degree burn over more than 10% of the body in an adult (5% in a child or older adult) is an emergency. Seek medical attention also for a first-degree burn over more than 50% of the body.

Also important is the location of the burn on the body. Second- or third-degree burns on the face, genitals or hands or feet are considered emergencies and require immediate medical care. Circumferential burns that wrap around an extremity or a finger or toe should also receive immediate medical attention. Burns around the nose and mouth may affect breathing and are medical emergencies.

Finally, consider the victim's age and health. A burn in a child younger than five or an adult older than 55 is more serious than in a younger

adult. Many chronic health disorders also make burns more serious. When in doubt whether a victim needs immediate emergency treatment, call 9-1-1 (**Box 11-1**).

First Aid for Heat Burns

First aid for heat burns is based on four general principles of burn care:

1. Stop the burning and cool the area.

2. Protect the burned area from additional trauma and pathogens.

3. Provide supportive care.

4. Ensure medical attention.

The specific first aid varies somewhat depending on the severity of the burn.

Care for First-Degree Burns

First-degree burns include most cases of sunburn and minor burns caused by heat or scalding. The skin is pink or red and remains unbroken, but some swelling may occur. Although first-degree burns may seem minor, they still cause pain and damage the skin. The first goal, as with all burns, is to stop the burning by removing the heat source and cooling the area with cold running water; do not use ice, which can cause further damage. Be sure to use running water so that the water stays

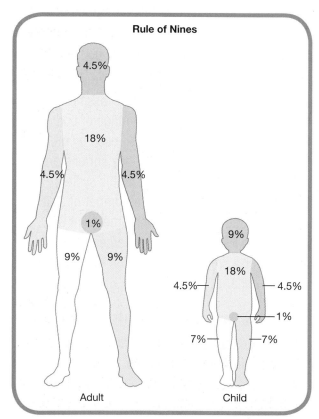

Rule of Nines

4.5%

18%

4.5%   4.5%

1%

9%   9%

9%   9%

9%

18%

4.5%   4.5%

1%

7%   7%

Adult   Child

Figure 11-4 *The rule of nines for calculating body surface area burned. These numbers represent one half (front or back) of the body.*

BOX 11-1: WHEN TO CALL 9-1-1 FOR A BURN

- The victim has a third-degree burn.

- The victim has a second-degree burn that is large (over 10% of body area in adult or 5% of body area in a child, older adult or someone with chronic illness) or that affects the head, genitals, or hands or feet.

- The victim is having trouble breathing.

- The victim may have inhaled smoke or fumes.

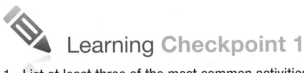

Learning Checkpoint 1

1. List at least three of the most common activities during which fires occur.

   _____

2. Describe at least three things you can do to help prevent fires from occurring in the kitchen.

   _____

3. True or False: If a fire breaks out in a building where you and others are present, the first thing you should do is call 9-1-1.

4. Name four factors that affect how serious a burn may be.

   _____

cold – a wet cloth put on a burn, for example, might absorb the burn's heat and no longer be cold. Because swelling may occur, jewelry and constrictive clothing should be removed from the area. Thereafter, protect the burned skin from contact with objects that may rub or put pressure on it. Do not apply ointment or other oily or greasy substances on the burn, although aloe vera gel may provide some comfort (see First Aid: "First-Degree Burns").

Care for Second-Degree Burns

A second-degree burn is deeper than a first-degree burn, involving the dermis and causing more damage to capillaries and nerve endings. The skin is red and swollen, often blotchy in appearance, and has blisters that may leak a clear fluid. If blisters break, pathogens may enter the skin and cause infection; first aid, therefore, includes protecting the skin. Pain is more severe than with a first-degree burn.

A small second-degree burn (smaller than your palm) may be treated at home, but a larger burn requires immediate medical attention. If larger than 10% of the body surface area (or 5% in a child, older adult or person with chronic illness), the burn should be treated as an emergency and 9-1-1 called. Stop the burning immediately and cool the area with cold running water. Remove jewelry and constricting clothing from the area.

While waiting for medical care, keep the burn covered with a dry, loose, nonstick dressing. As with all burns, do not apply ointment or other substances to the burn (see First Aid: "Second-Degree Burns").

Care for Third-Degree Burns

Third-degree burns are usually emergencies and when large may be life-threatening. Third-degree burns penetrate all the way through the skin and may damage underlying tissues. Infection is likely. It is important to act immediately to stop the burning and cool the burn, although a very large burn area (over 20% of body surface area) should not be immersed in water because of the risk of causing hypothermia. The victim may rapidly develop the signs of shock, a life-threatening condition requiring treatment in addition to the burn first aid. Call 9-1-1.

Stop the burning immediately and cool the area with cold running water. Remove jewelry and constricting clothing from the area. Cover the burn with a dry, loose, nonstick dressing. As with all burns, do not apply ointment or other substances to the burn. While waiting for emergency personnel, treat the victim for shock by having the victim lie down, elevating the legs and maintaining normal body temperature. Monitor the victim's breathing and give basic life support (BLS) if needed (see First Aid: "Third-Degree Burns").

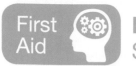

First-Degree Burns
Signs, Symptoms and Care

When You See

- **Skin is red, dry and painful**
- **May be some swelling**
- **Skin not broken**

Do This First

1 Stop the burning by removing the heat source.

2 Immediately cool the burn with cold running tap water until area is free from pain even after removal from water.

3 Remove clothing and jewelry or any other constricting item before the area swells.

4 Protect the burn from friction or pressure.

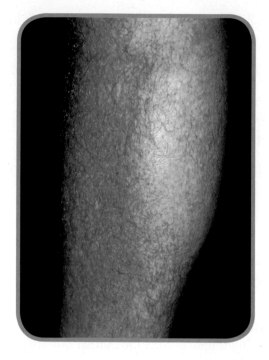

Additional Care

- Aloe vera gel can be used on the skin for comfort.

ALERT

- Do not put butter on a burn.
- Do not use ice on a burn because even though it may relieve pain, the cold may cause additional damage to the skin. Ice-cold water should not be used.

Smoke Inhalation

Any victim who was in the vicinity of a fire could have airway or lung injuries from inhaling smoke or other fumes resulting from fires. Even hot air can cause such injuries. This can be a medical emergency. The lining of the airway may swell and make breathing difficult. The small sacs in the lungs where oxygen enters the lungs, the alveoli, may be damaged and affect the ability of the body to receive enough oxygen through normal breathing. A victim of smoke inhalation may also have carbon monoxide poisoning (see **Chapter 17**).

The signs and symptoms of smoke inhalation include coughing, wheezing or hoarseness; burns or blackening around the mouth or nose; coughing up a sooty substance; and difficulty breathing. Note that symptoms from smoke inhalation may not become obvious for up to 48 hours after exposure.

Care for Smoke Inhalation

First, get the victim to fresh air or fresh air to the victim. A victim who can safely be moved should be assisted outdoors or to an area of fresh air. If the victim cannot be moved, ventilate the area by any means available to remove smoke and fumes. Call 9-1-1 immediately, even if the victim is not

(continues on page 171)

Second-Degree Burns
Signs, Symptoms and Care

When You See

- **Skin is swollen and red, may be blotchy or streaked**
- **Blisters that may be weeping clear fluid**
- **Signs of significant pain**

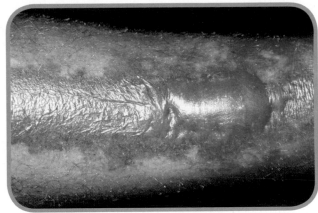

Do This First

1 Stop the burning by removing the heat source.

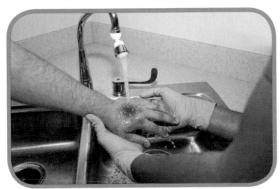

2 Immediately cool the burn with cold running tap water until area is free from pain even after removal from water.

3 For large burns, call 9-1-1.

4 Remove clothing and jewelry from the area before the area swells.

5 Put a nonstick dressing over the burn to protect the area, but keep it loose and do not tape it to the skin.

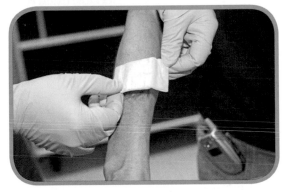

Additional Care

- For burns on the face, genitals, hands or feet, seek medical attention.

ALERT

- Do not break skin blisters; this could cause an infection.
- Be gentle when covering the area.

First Aid

Third-Degree Burns
Signs, Symptoms and Care

When You See

- **Skin damage; charred skin; or white, leathery skin**
- **May have signs and symptoms of shock (clammy, pale or ashen skin; nausea and vomiting; fast breathing)**

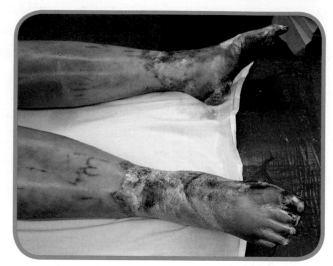

Do This First

1 Stop the burning by removing the heat source.

2 Immediately cool the burn with cold running tap water until area is free from pain even after removal from water. (Do not put ice on a burn, which would cause tissue injury.)

3 Remove clothing and jewelry before the area swells.

4 Call 9-1-1.

5 Treat for shock: have the victim lie down, elevate the legs if no trauma and maintain normal body temperature.

6 Carefully cover the burn with a nonstick dressing; keep it loose and do not tape it to the skin. Do not apply a cream or ointment.

Additional Care

- Watch the victim's breathing and be ready to give basic life support (BLS) if needed.

ALERT

- Do not attempt to cool the burn with cold water if it is larger than 20% of the body (e.g., one whole leg or torso from neck to waist), or 10% for child, because of the risk of hypothermia and shock.
- Do not touch the burn or put anything on it.
- Do not give the victim anything to drink.

Learning **Checkpoint 2**

1. True or False: For a victim with a second-degree burn, you should break skin blisters and cover the area with a burn ointment to promote faster healing.

2. For a victim with a third-degree burn, you should cool only a _____ area with water because of the risk of shock or hypothermia.

3. As you are leaving work, you see a man working on his car in the parking lot. He suddenly screams and backs away, his clothing on fire. What do you do? List in correct order the first four actions you should take.

(continued from page 168)

experiencing signs and symptoms, because injury may have occurred even though the effects are not yet showing. While waiting for medical care, help the victim into a position for easiest breathing (often semireclining), and keep him or her calm. If the victim becomes unresponsive, position him or her in the recovery position and monitor breathing. Be prepared to give basic life support if needed (see First Aid: "Smoke Inhalation").

Chemical Burns

Many strong chemicals found in workplaces and the home can burn skin on contact. Sometimes the burn develops slowly and in some cases the victim may not be aware of the burn for up to 24 hours. Acids and alkalis, liquids and solids can all cause serious chemical burns **(Figure 11-5)**.

Preventing Chemical Burns

- Read directions before using any household products. Heed warnings on products and keep all products in their original containers. Do not mix different products.

- Protect hands with heavy rubber gloves and cover other exposed areas of the body.

- Ensure adequate ventilation when using products with dangerous fumes.

Care for Chemical Burns

In most cases you can see the substance on the victim's skin, and the victim feels a burning or stinging sensation. Because the chemical reaction can continue as long as the substance is on the skin, you must remove it immediately. In a work setting,

check material safety data sheets (MSDS) for the care of a burn caused by the specific chemical. For a dry chemical, brush it off with a gloved hand, cloth, piece of cardboard or paper, spare article of clothing, or any other item available. Be careful not to get the chemical on your own skin or to spread it to other areas of the victim's skin. Wear gloves if available. Then, flush the area with water as soon as possible. Remove any clothing and jewelry from the burned area. For a liquid spilled on the victim's skin, start flushing with water immediately.

Call 9-1-1 for any chemical burn and keep flushing the burned area with water until medical care arrives (see First Aid: "Chemical Burns"). Remember that a chemical may give off fumes even if you cannot smell them; therefore, the victim should be moved (if safe) to fresh air. Even a dry chemical may give off fumes once it is in contact with water. Note: Do not try to neutralize an acid by applying an alkaline substance, or vice versa, because of the risk of further damage caused by the chemical reaction.

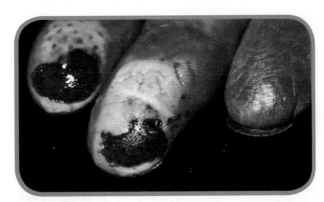

Figure 11-5 *A chemical burn.*

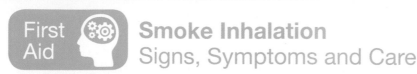

First Aid

Smoke Inhalation
Signs, Symptoms and Care

When You See

- **Smoke visible in area**
- **Coughing, wheezing or hoarse voice**
- **Possible burned area on face or chest**
- **Difficulty breathing**

Do This First

1 Get the victim to fresh air or fresh air to the victim.

2 Call 9-1-1.

3 Help the victim into a position for easiest breathing.

Additional Care

- Put an unresponsive victim in the recovery position.
- Be ready to give BLS if needed.

Learning Checkpoint 3

1. A co-worker has splashed an unknown liquid in her eye and is holding her hand over the eye. What should you do first?

   a. Have her keep holding the eye closed so her tears will wash out the chemical.

   b. Call 9-1-1 and wait for health care personnel to take care of her eye.

   c. Immediately flush the eye with running water.

   d. Mix baking soda with water and pour it into her eye.

2. Describe the first action to take if a victim has a dry chemical on the skin.

   _____

3. True or False: If a person who was in a smoky area near a fire does not have any signs and symptoms within an hour, that person does not need medical care.

Electrical Burns and Shocks

An electrical burn or shock occurs whenever any part of the body comes in contact with electricity. Typical electrical injuries occur from faulty appliances or power cords, or when an appliance comes into contact with water. Water easily conducts electricity to anyone who touches the water. Many deaths caused by electricity occur when an appliance such as a hair dryer or radio falls into bathwater.

Preventing Electrical Shocks and Burns

Electricity may cause life-threatening shocks as well as electrical burns. Follow these guidelines to stay safe **(Figure 11-6)**:

- Use outlet caps to block unused electrical outlets.
- Do not use a night light that looks like a toy in a young child's bedroom; it can cause an electrical burn if the child tries to play with it.

Chemical Burns
Signs, Symptoms and Care

When You See

- **A chemical on the victim's skin or clothing**
- **Complaints of pain or a burning sensation**
- **A spilled substance on or around an unresponsive victim**
- **A smell of fumes in the air**

Do This First

1 Send someone to check the MSDS for the chemical involved.

2 Move the victim away from fumes or ventilate the area.

3 With a gloved hand or piece of cloth, brush off any dry chemical but do not contaminate skin that has not been in contact with the chemical.

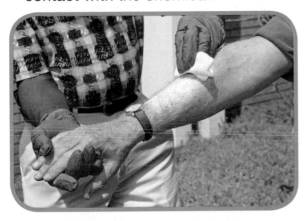

4 Flush the entire area as quickly as possible with large amounts of running water. Flush until EMS personnel arrive to give definitive care or until a toxic-specific solution is available.

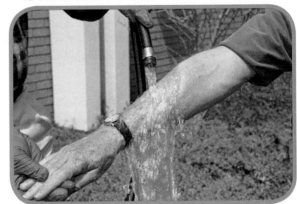

5 Remove clothing and jewelry from the burn area while flushing with water.

6 Call 9-1-1 for any chemical burn.

ALERT

Chemical in the Eyes

- For a chemical splashed into the eye, flush immediately with running water and continue until EMS personnel arrive. Have the victim remove contact lenses.
- Tilt the victim's head so the water runs away from the face and not into the other eye.

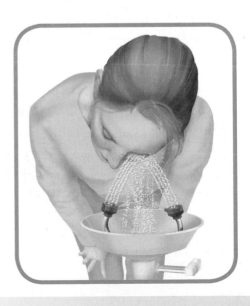

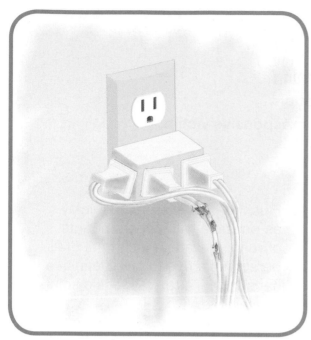

Figure 11-6 *Overloaded outlets or extension cords pose a risk of fire or electrical shocks.*

- Never use electrical appliances near water or when your hands are wet.

- Inspect electric cords for broken or frayed insulation.

- Be careful not to touch the wire prongs when inserting or removing electrical plugs from a receptacle. Pull the plug itself out, not the cord.

- Install a **ground fault circuit interrupter (GFCI)** in outlets in bathrooms and kitchens; this device automatically turns off electricity when appliances become wet.

- Outdoors, keep everyone away from downed power lines and do not let children play near electrical poles or fly kites near electrical wires.

Preventing Lightning Strikes

Each year, an estimated 700 people in the United States are struck by lightning, causing significant injuries and about 70 deaths.[4] If you are caught outdoors in a thunderstorm, follow these guidelines:

[4]*National Weather Service, http://www.lightningsafety. noaa.gov/medical.htm Accessed March 1, 2011.*

- Know that lightning is a risk even if the storm seems far off. Seek shelter if you hear thunder within 30 seconds of seeing a lightning strike. Lightning has been known to "jump" miles away from a storm cloud.

- Get out of water immediately or off a boat.

- Try not to be the tallest object around. Crouch near the ground or get beneath a group of trees – but not a tall, isolated tree. Avoid high ground and open spaces.

- Stay away from metal fences and power lines. Do not take shelter near metal objects.

- A closed motor vehicle is safer than being caught in the open. Keep the doors and windows completely shut.

- If you are caught in the open, crouch or squat down (but do not lie down) with your feet together. A group of people should stay about 15 feet away from each other.

- Indoors, stay away from doors and windows and do not use electrical appliances or devices. Also keep away from telephone lines and plumbing fixtures.

Care for Electrical Burns

Two possible injuries may occur from electricity:

- External burns caused by the heat of electricity

- Electrical injuries caused by electricity flowing through the body

High-voltage electricity flowing through the body can cause significant injuries to many different tissues. Heart damage may cause heart rhythm irregularities that threaten the victim's circulation or cause the heart to stop **(Box 11-2)**.

As with all types of burns, the urgent first step is to stop the burning. If the victim is still in contact with a source of electricity, ensure that the power is disconnected or turned off immediately. Do not touch a victim still in contact with electricity because of the risk of receiving a shock or burn yourself.

External burns resulting from heat or flames caused by electricity are cared for in the same manner as heat burns. Electrical injuries may cause only minor external burns where the electricity entered and left the body; these are called entrance and exit wounds **(Figure 11-7)**.

Internal damage caused by an electric shock is seldom as obvious as an external burn. Signs and symptoms may include seizures or changing levels of responsiveness. Call 9-1-1 and monitor the victim's breathing while waiting for medical assistance. Be prepared to give basic life support if needed (see First Aid: "Electrical Burns").

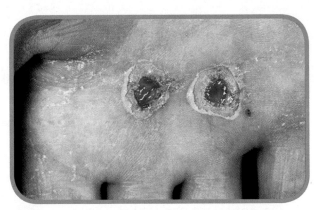

Figure 11-7 *An electrical burn.*

Learning Checkpoint 4

1. True or False: The first thing to do for an unresponsive victim in contact with an electrical wire is to pour water over the area of contact.

2. What is the safest way to stop the electricity when someone is shocked by an electrical appliance? How should you not try to stop it?

_____

3. Driving home from work, you are stopped behind a car that has struck a telephone pole. You get out to help the driver and see a power line dangling from the pole, in contact with the roof of the car. Your first action should be to –

   a. use your cell phone to call 9-1-1.

   b. look for a stick or piece of wood to push the wire away from the car.

   c. try to pull the victim out the car window.

   d. give any needed first aid by leaning in the car window.

BOX 11-2: HIGH-VOLTAGE SHOCKS

High Power Lines

If a power line is down, do not approach a victim in contact with the line. Call 9-1-1 immediately. Do not try to move the wire away using any object. Wait for emergency workers to arrive, and keep others away from the scene.

Lightning Strikes

Lightning strikes often cause serious injury. In addition to burns, the electrical shock may affect the heart and brain and cause temporary blindness or deafness, unresponsiveness or seizures, bleeding, bone fractures, or cardiac arrest. Call 9-1-1 immediately and give basic life support, treating the most serious injuries first.

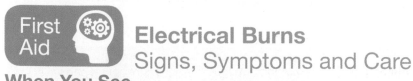

Electrical Burns
Signs, Symptoms and Care

When You See

- **A source of electricity near the victim: bare wires, power cords, an electrical device**
- **Burned area of skin, or possibly both entrance and exit wounds**
- **Changing levels of responsiveness**

Do This First

1 Do not touch the victim until you know the area is safe. Unplug or turn off the power.

2 Call 9-1-1.

3 For an unresponsive victim, give BLS.

4 Care for the burn (stop the burning, cool the area, remove clothing and jewelry, and cover the burn with a sterile dressing).

5 Treat for shock by having the victim lie down, elevating the legs and maintaining normal body temperature.

Additional Care

- Keep an unresponsive victim in the recovery position and monitor breathing until help arrives. Be ready to give CPR if needed.

ALERT
Electrical Shock

- Do not touch a victim you think is receiving an electrical shock! First make sure the power is turned off or the person is well away from the power source. Turn off the circuit breaker and call 9-1-1.

- Note that electrical burns can cause massive internal injuries even when the external burn may look minor.

Concluding Thoughts

First aid for burns may seem complex because of the variations in care depending on the type of burn, its size and location on the body, and its depth. Most important, remember the general first aid principles for all burns:

- Act fast to stop the burning.
- Cool the area.
- Seek help.
- Protect the victim.

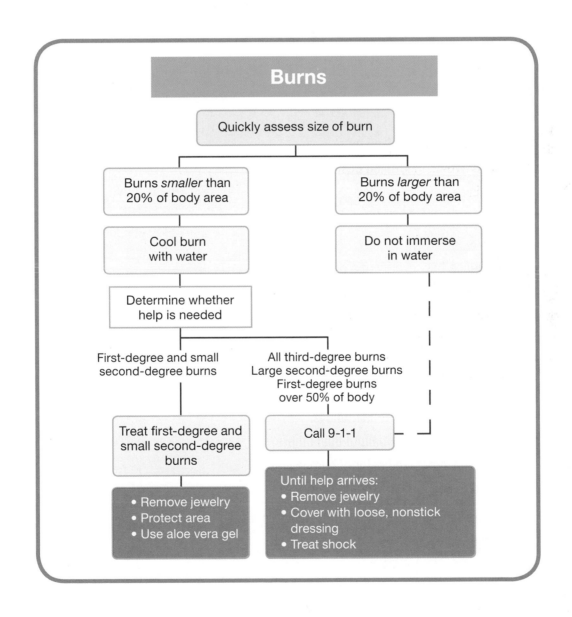

Learning Outcomes

You should now be able to do the following:

1. Explain common causes of fires and burns and how to prevent them.

2. Describe what happens to the body when it receives a burn.

3. List the differences between first-, second- and third-degree burns.

4. Describe first aid for first-, second- and third-degree heat burns.

5. Describe first aid for smoke inhalation.

6. Describe first aid for chemical burns.

7. Describe first aid for electrical burns and shocks.

Review Questions

1. Most fires occur –
   a. in the home.
   b. in the workplace.
   c. in schools.
   d. in public gathering places.

2. A first-degree burn is characterized by –
   a. the presence of white, fluid-filled blisters.
   b. pink or red skin.
   c. white, leathery areas of skin.
   d. bleeding.

3. Factors that influence the severity of a burn include –
   a. the depth of the burn.
   b. the percentage of body area burned.
   c. the location of the burn.
   d. All of the above

4. Which of the following is true about burns?
   a. The deeper the burn, the more painful it is.
   b. Third-degree burns are more painful than others.
   c. The level of pain is not an indicator of burn severity.
   d. Blisters are more painful than charred or red skin.

5. Which of the following is the best substance to put on a burn immediately after it has occurred?
   a. Antibiotic ointment
   b. Aloe vera
   c. Butter
   d. Cold running water

6. The purpose of putting a dressing over a second- or third-degree burn is to –

  a. protect the area.

  b. absorb the fluid from blisters.

  c. keep the area moist for 24 hours.

  d. prevent swelling.

7. Using icy water to cool a burn that covers 25% of the body may result in –

  a. hypothermia and shock.

  b. shock and cardiac arrest.

  c. hypothermia and severe bleeding.

  d. electrolyte imbalances and infection.

8. A ring should be removed from a burned finger because –

  a. gold and silver are toxic metals on exposed skin.

  b. swelling may cut off circulation.

  c. the ring is a likely source of infection.

  d. the ring makes it difficult to cool the burn.

9. First aid for a dry chemical burn includes –

  a. neutralizing an acid with an alkaline substance.

  b. neutralizing an alkaline burn with an acidic substance.

  c. brushing off the chemical and then flushing the skin with water.

  d. tightly taping a dressing over the burn.

10. Call 9-1-1 for –

  a. a second-degree burn larger than 10% of body surface area in an adult victim.

  b. a second-degree burn larger than 5% of body surface area in an elderly victim.

  c. a third-degree burn.

  d. All of the above

11 • Burns

Chapter 12 • Head and Spinal Injuries

Chapter Preview

- Prevention of Head and Spinal Injuries
- Assessing Head and Spinal Injuries
- Skull Fractures
- Brain Injuries
- Spinal Injuries

You have stopped by a neighborhood school on your way home to see a friend who helps coach the girls' gymnastic team. While talking in a corner of the gym, you are horrified to see a young girl on the uneven bars attempt a release move and miss the bar. You run to her and find that she is unresponsive. What should you do?

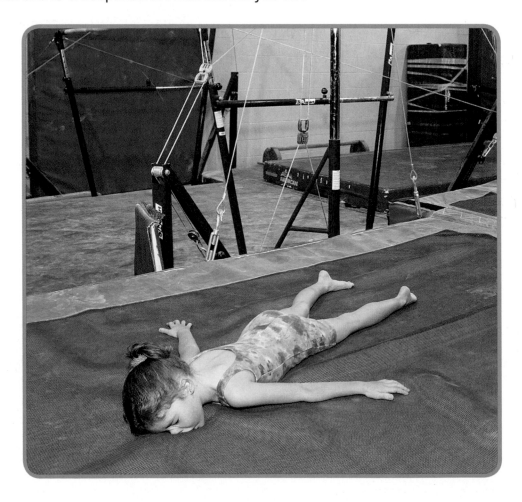

Head and spinal injuries may be life-threatening or may cause permanent damage to the brain or spinal cord, producing nervous system deficits such as paralysis. Any trauma to the head, neck or back may result in a serious injury. Injuries that cause unresponsiveness or loss of sensation in a body part are especially likely to be serious, but even injuries without immediate, obvious signs and symptoms may create a potentially life-threatening problem.

Because of the forces involved, any injury to the head may also injure the spine. Whenever you find a serious head injury, suspect a neck or back injury.

This chapter considers head and spinal injuries that involve deeper injuries to the skull or spine, including bone and nerves. **Chapter 10** describes the first aid for more superficial wounds to the head and face.

Prevention of Head and Spinal Injuries

Motor vehicle crashes are the leading cause of head and spinal injuries in people younger than 65, with about 200,000 people dying each year from brain injuries and another 500,000 hospitalized for treatment.[1] Falls are the leading cause of these injuries in people older than 65. Violence and sports and recreation activities are additional leading causes of spinal cord injuries. About 12,000 people in the United States suffer a spinal injury each year, and about 300,000 Americans live with a disability resulting from a spinal cord injury.[2]

Many head and spinal injuries can be prevented by following accepted guidelines for safety in vehicles, during recreation and at work.[3]

- Always wear safety belts and shoulder restraints in vehicles.

- Use approved car seats for infants and small children and make sure they are installed correctly (incorrect installation is a frequent cause of injury).

- Wear appropriate helmets, headgear or hard hats for bicycling, skating, skateboarding, other sports and work activities.

- At work, follow appropriate OSHA guidelines for equipment and safety practices.

- Avoid risky activities, including driving, when you are under the influence of drugs, alcohol or medications that produce drowsiness.

- Ensure that children's playground surfaces are made of a shock-absorbing material.

- Store firearms in a locked cabinet with ammunition in a separate secure location.

- Do not dive into murky or shallow water (less than 9 feet deep).

- To prevent falls, keep yourself and your house safe for children and older adults:

  - To reach high shelves, use a step stool with a grab bar.

  - Make sure all stairways have handrails.

  - Use safety gates at the top and bottom of stairs when young children are present.

  - Remove tripping hazards such as small area rugs and loose electrical cords.

  - Use nonslip mats in the tub and shower.

  - Install grab bars by the toilet and in the tub or shower.

  - Exercise regularly to improve strength, balance and coordination.

  - See an eye doctor regularly for vision checks.

  - Because falls often result from dizziness caused by medications, have your health care provider review your medications.

[1]*Physicians Desk Reference, http://www.pdrhealth.com/ disease/disease-mono.aspx?contentFileName=BHG01 NE01.xml&contentName=Brain+and+Spinal+Cord+Injury& contentId=16&TypeId=1 Accessed March 1, 2011.*

[2]*BrainandSpinalCord.org, http://www.brainandspinalcord. org/spinal-cord-injury/statistics.htm Accessed March 1, 2011.*

[3]*The Centers for Disease Control and Prevention. http:// www.cdc.gov/ncipc/pub-res/tbi_toolkit/patients/ preventing.htm Accessed March 4, 2011.*

Assessing Head and Spinal Injuries

Assessing a victim with a potential head and spinal injury begins with considering the cause of the injury and the forces involved. An understanding of the general signs and symptoms of head and spinal injuries helps you to focus the physical examination.

It is essential to recognize the possibility of a head or spinal injury immediately because the possibility of a spinal injury determines how and when a victim is positioned and moved.

Causes of Head and Spinal Injuries

Any trauma to the head may cause a head or spinal injury. In addition, spinal injuries may be caused by forces to the back, chest or even the pelvis or legs by indirect force. Common causes of head and spinal injuries include the following:

- Motor vehicle crashes (including whiplash injuries without direct impact to the head)
- Falls from a height of more than a few feet
- Diving emergencies involving impact to the head (even blows that do not cause bruises or wounds)
- Skiing emergencies and other sports injuries
- Any forceful blow to the head, neck or back

Suspect a spinal injury in an injured victim who has these risk factors:

- Victim is 65 or older
- Child older than 2 with trauma to head or neck
- Motor vehicle or bicycle crash involving driver, passenger or pedestrian
- Falls from more than the person's standing height
- Victim feels tingling in hands or feet, pain in back or neck, or muscle weakness or lack of feeling in torso or arms
- Victim is intoxicated or not alert
- Any painful injury, particularly to the head, neck or back

In addition, if you encounter an unresponsive victim with an unknown mechanism of injury, suspect a spinal injury when wounds or other injuries in the body suggest large forces were involved. If so, observe the victim carefully and thoroughly for the signs and symptoms of a head or spinal injury even as you are carrying out the initial assessment.

General Signs and Symptoms of Head and Spinal Injuries

Head and spinal injuries are closely related because a traumatic injury to one may injure the other as well. For example, a blow to the head that fractures the skull may also put enough force on vertebrae in the neck that a spinal injury occurs. Although a head injury may occur in a victim without a spinal injury and a spinal injury may occur in a victim without a head injury, the assessment of a victim with such injuries should look for both head and spinal injuries.

The general signs and symptoms of head and spinal injuries may overlap in victims with an injury of the head, neck or back. Suspect a head or spinal injury in a victim if any of these signs and symptoms is present:

- Lump or deformity in the head, neck or back
- Changing levels of responsiveness, drowsiness, confusion, dizziness (see AVPU scale in **Chapter 4**)
- Unequal pupils
- Headache
- Clear or bloody fluid from the nose or ears
- Stiff neck
- Inability to move any body part
- Tingling, numbness or lack of feeling in feet or hands

Noting any of these signs and symptoms in the initial assessment or physical examination of a victim should lead to a more specific assessment for a head or spinal injury. These specific injuries are described in following sections in this chapter.

Physical Examination of Head and Spinal Injuries

Chapter 4, "Assessing the Victim," describes general procedures for assessing all victims, including a physical examination of a victim not being treated for a life-threatening injury. In the initial assessment of an unresponsive victim, consider whether the victim may have a spinal injury based on the risk factors listed earlier and these factors:

- The cause of the victim's injuries (e.g., blow to the head, a fall, strong forces)

- Observations of bystanders at the scene who saw the injury occur

- Immediately apparent injuries and wounds (e.g., a serious head wound or the neck twisted at an unusual angle – but do not take the time to do a physical examination if the victim is not breathing

- Any observed sign of a head or spinal injury

During the initial assessment of the victim, you may have to position the victim to open the airway, to check breathing, to give CPR, to control bleeding or to allow blood, vomit or other fluid to drain from the mouth. If you suspect that the victim may have a spinal injury, take great care when moving or repositioning the victim, as described later in this chapter. Unless it is necessary, do not move the victim.

If the victim is unresponsive and the initial assessment does not reveal a life-threatening condition for which you must care, do not perform a physical examination but observe the victim for other injuries. If an unresponsive victim may have a spinal injury, do not move the victim unless it is necessary. Check only for serious injuries such as bleeding that must be controlled. Otherwise, maintain the victim's head position to prevent movement and wait for EMS professionals.

If the victim is responsive and you suspect the possibility of a spinal injury, carefully assess for the signs and symptoms of spinal injury during the physical examination. Ask the victim to stay in position and not move more than you ask during the examination, to prevent further damage to the spine.

Perform the physical examination as described in **Chapter 4**, paying particular attention to signs and symptoms of a head or spinal injury. Gently feel the skull for bumps or depressions. Check the ears and nose for blood or a clear fluid. Check the pupils of both eyes, which should be of equal size and should respond to light when you cover and uncover the eyes with your hand. Check the neck for deformity or swelling, bleeding or pain. When checking the torso, observe for impaired breathing and loss of bladder or bowel control (a sign of nerve damage). When assessing the extremities, check for sensation and the ability to move the hand or foot, comparing strength from one side of the body to the other.

If you suspect a head or spinal injury, call 9-1-1 and keep the victim still until EMS professionals arrive. Note that it can be very difficult for first aiders without advanced training to recognize a spinal injury with certainty. ***Do not depend on any specific assessment of a victim to decide whether or not the victim may have a spinal injury. Do not assume a victim without specific symptoms does not have a possible spinal injury***. Consider the forces involved in the injury and when in doubt, keep the victim's head immobile while waiting for help to arrive. With a responsive victim, encourage the victim not to move and with an unresponsive victim, hold the head in place to prevent movement.

In addition, the results of the examination are not always clear-cut. For example, even though the spinal cord may be intact, an injury may put pressure on the cord that results in limited sensation, pain or partial inability to move. If the victim can move a hand or foot only weakly, for example, assume a spinal injury has occurred.

Follow this assessment approach for all suspected cases of head or spinal injuries (see Skill: "Assessing Head and Spinal Injuries").

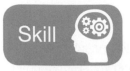

Skill — Assessing Head and Spinal Injuries

1 Check the victim's head.

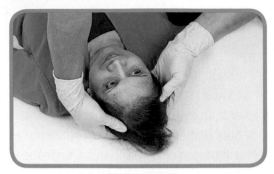

2 Check neck for deformity, swelling and pain.

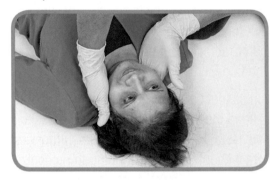

3 Touch toes of both feet and ask victim if the sensation feels normal.

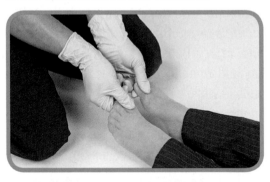

4 Ask victim to point toes.

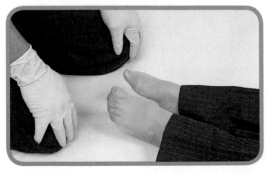

5 Ask victim to push against your hands with the feet.

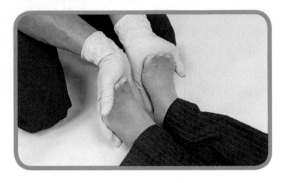

6 Touch fingers of both hands and ask victim if the sensation feels normal.

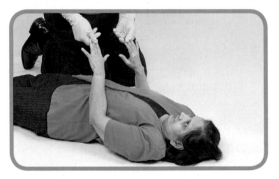

7 Ask victim to make a fist and curl (flex) it in.

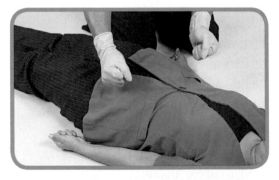

8 Ask victim to squeeze your hands.

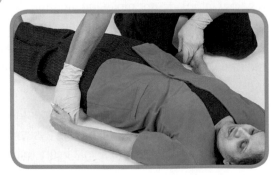

Skull Fractures

If the victim had a blow to the head, consider the possibility of a skull fracture or a brain injury. The skull is generally strong and is fractured only with severe trauma. When you find bleeding from the scalp, check carefully for a possible skull fracture before applying direct pressure to the wound. If the skull is fractured, direct pressure on the wound could push bone fragments into the brain, causing serious injury.

Feel the scalp gently for signs of a skull fracture: a depressed or spongy area or the presence of bone fragments. Blood or a clear fluid leaking from the nose or eyes may also be a sign of a skull injury. In such a case, to control bleeding, apply pressure around the wound rather than directly on it. Note that a skull fracture may occur even without an open wound.

A skull fracture is life-threatening. Call 9-1-1 immediately. Note that a skull fracture often also causes injuries to the brain (see First Aid: "Skull Fracture").

Brain Injuries

Brain injuries may occur with a blow to the head with or without an open wound. A brain injury is likely with a skull fracture. Injury results when the traumatic force is transmitted to brain tissue, causing bleeding or swelling of the brain and concussion. Brain injuries may cause a range of signs or symptoms, including headache, altered mental status, confusion or unresponsiveness; weakness, numbness, loss of sensation or **paralysis** of body areas; nausea and vomiting; seizures; and unequal pupils **(Figure 12-1)**. If breathing is impaired, the victim may need basic life support.

Call 9-1-1 for any victim with a suspected brain injury. Even if the signs and symptoms seem mild at first, swelling and/or bleeding in the brain may continue and the victim's condition may rapidly deteriorate and become life-threatening. Stay with the victim and be prepared to give basic life support if needed. With any force strong enough to injure the brain, suspect a possible spinal injury as well and support the victim's head to prevent movement while waiting for help to arrive. Because vomiting commonly occurs with brain injuries, be prepared to move the victim into the recovery position to allow fluid to drain from the mouth. Enlist the help of bystanders to keep the victim's head in line with the body whenever you move the victim (see First Aid: "Brain Injuries").

In some cases after a blow to the head the victim does not immediately have the signs and symptoms of brain injury and does not seek medical care. Signs and symptoms may appear within the next 48 hours that indicate a more serious injury. Seek medical attention immediately if any of the following late signs and symptoms occurs following a head injury:

- Nausea and vomiting
- Severe or persistent headache
- Changing levels of responsiveness
- Lack of coordination, movement problems
- Problems with vision or speech
- Seizures

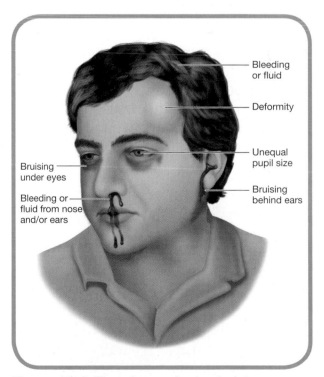

Bleeding or fluid

Deformity

Unequal pupil size

Bruising behind ears

Bruising under eyes

Bleeding or fluid from nose and/or ears

Figure 12-1 *The signs of a brain injury.*

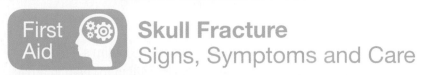

Skull Fracture
Signs, Symptoms and Care

When You See

- **A deformed area of the skull**
- **A depressed area in the bone felt during the physical examination**
- **Blood or fluid coming from the ears or nose**
- **Eyelids swollen shut or becoming discolored (bruising)**
- **Bruising behind the ears**
- **Unequal pupils**
- **Impaled object in the skull**

Do This First

1 Call 9-1-1 and stay with the victim.

2 Put a breathing unresponsive victim in the recovery position unless you suspect a spinal injury. Monitor breathing and be ready to give CPR if needed.

3 *Do not* clean the wound, press on it or remove an impaled object.

4 Cover the wound with a sterile dressing.

5 If there is significant bleeding, apply pressure only around the edges of the wound, not on the wound itself. You may use a ring dressing to apply pressure around the wound (see **Chapter 10**). Do not apply pressure if you feel bone fragments move.

6 Do not move the victim unnecessarily because there may also be a spinal injury.

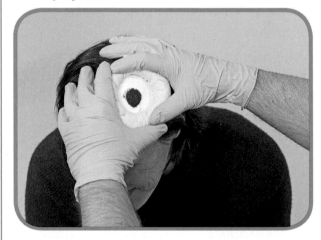

Additional Care

- Put an unresponsive victim in the recovery position (unless there may be a spinal injury).
- Do not raise the victim's legs.

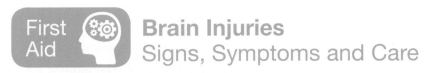

Brain Injuries
Signs, Symptoms and Care

When You See

- **A head wound suggesting a blow to the head occurred**
- **Changing levels of responsiveness, drowsiness**
- **Confusion, disorientation or memory loss about the injury**
- **Headache**
- **Dizziness**
- **Seizures**
- **Nausea or vomiting**
- **Breathing problems or irregularities**
- **Unequal pupils**

Do This First

For a responsive victim:

1 Have the victim lie down.

2 Keep the victim still and protect him or her from becoming chilled or overheated.

3 Call 9-1-1 and monitor the victim's condition until help arrives.

4 Support the head and neck, even in a responsive victim, if you suspect a spinal injury.

For an unresponsive victim:

1 Call 9-1-1.

2 Monitor the victim's breathing without moving the victim unless necessary.

3 Suspect a spinal injury and prevent movement of the head and neck.

4 Control serious bleeding and cover any wounds with a dressing.

ALERT

- Do not let the victim eat or drink anything.

Concussion

A **concussion** is a type of brain injury that involves a temporary impairment of brain function but usually not permanent damage. Usually there is no head wound and the victim may not have many of the signs and symptoms of a more serious brain injury. The victim may have been "knocked out" by a blow to the head but regained consciousness quickly. A concussion typically causes these signs and symptoms:

- Temporary confusion
- Memory loss about the traumatic event
- Brief loss of responsiveness
- Mildly or moderately altered mental status
- Unusual behavior
- Headache

Although a victim with a concussion may seem to recover quickly and to experience no signs or symptoms, it is generally difficult to determine the seriousness of the injury. More serious signs and symptoms may occur over time. Therefore, it is important to seek medical care for all suspected brain injuries. If a brain injury may be possible, call 9-1-1 and keep the victim still and give supportive care while waiting for help to arrive. In no situation should a victim with a suspected head injury, no matter how mild, continue an activity, such as a sport, in which a second injury may occur (see **Box 12-1**).

Spinal Injuries

A fracture of the neck or back is a spinal injury. These injuries are always serious because of possible damage to the **spinal cord** – the bundle of nerves that runs down from the base of the skull and through the neck to branch off to all parts of the body. As **Figure 12-2** shows, these nerves pass through openings in the **vertebrae**, the bones of the neck and back. Even a small displacement or fracture of these bones can damage the soft tissue of the spinal cord or the nerves that lead

---

BOX 12-1: SECOND IMPACT SYNDROME

The American College of Sports Medicine estimates that as many as 2 million concussions occur each year, with only 15% diagnosed.[4] Such brain injuries are more likely to occur in contact sports such as football. In the last two decades, sports physicians have become increasingly aware of the fact that a second head impact after even a mild concussion can cause severe brain swelling that may lead to death. Both high school and college football players have died of brain swelling after a second impact. In some cases the first injury was so mild that the player did not tell the coach at all before returning to play. Even mild injuries can have this cumulative fatal effect. Because an athlete with only a mild concussion may not tell anyone, statistics are lacking for how often "second impact syndrome" occurs.

The problem occurs in part because it is difficult to diagnose a concussion quickly and to know whether it is safe for the player to get back into the game. Pressure from coaches and other players to stay in the game may contribute to an athlete's not admitting to a mild injury.

There is hope, however, that the situation may improve with increased awareness of second impact syndrome among athletes, athletic trainers and coaches. In addition, a new methods have been devised for testing within minutes whether a player has a mild concussion, to prevent the athlete from returning to play and risking another injury.

[4]*Arizona Sports Concussion Center, http://www. azsportsconcussion.com/faqs.php Accessed March 4, 2011.*

Learning Checkpoint 1

1. List two or three signs of a possible skull fracture. What is one thing you should not do to stop bleeding from the head if you suspect a skull fracture?

   _____

2. True or False: You can easily distinguish a mild concussion from a serious brain injury by the signs and symptoms.

3. Check off the possible signs and symptoms of a brain injury:

   _____ Headache   _____ Fingernail beds look blue

   _____ Rapid blinking   _____ Dizziness or confusion

   _____ Memory loss   _____ Nausea and vomiting

4. The one sure way to know whether the victim has a spinal injury is –

   a. pain in the neck.

   b. headache.

   c. unresponsiveness.

   d. None of the above

5. How long after a blow to the head might signs and symptoms of a more serious injury appear?

   _____

from the cord to the body. Spinal injuries are serious because the spinal cord, unlike bones and some soft tissues, cannot grow back to heal the injury. Although medical care can improve the condition of a victim with partially damaged nerves, if the spinal cord is severed by the injury, the victim will have permanent paralysis and loss of function.

The effects of nerve damage caused by a spinal injury depend on the nature and location of the injury. In general, body functions controlled by nerves exiting the spinal cord below the level of injury may be affected. An injury to the lower spine may result in paralysis of the legs, for example, while an injury to the spinal cord at a higher level may paralyze the arms as well as the legs. If the nerves controlling the muscles involved in breathing are damaged, the victim may have a life-threatening breathing problem. Any spinal cord damage can cause permanent paralysis.

Although an injury to the spine may cause immediate nerve damage with immediate signs

and symptoms, in some cases nerve damage may not yet have occurred. For example, a fractured vertebra in the neck could put the nerves of

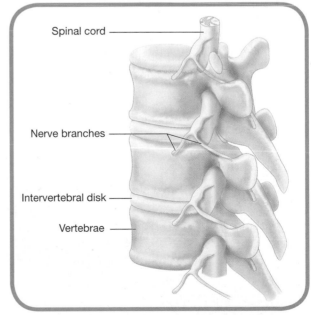

Figure 12-2 *The spinal cord passes through openings in the vertebrae. Nerve branches exit the spinal cord to reach all body areas.*

the spinal cord at risk for damage if the neck vertebrae were to move. The victim may not have signs and symptoms of a spinal injury, but if the neck were moved carelessly, fractured bone could damage nerve tissue and cause permanent paralysis or a life-threatening condition. Similarly, when signs and symptoms of spinal nerve damage are present, movement of the head or neck could make the injury worse. Therefore it is critical to prevent head and neck movement in all victims suspected of having a spinal injury.

The primary care for a suspected spinal cord injury is to prevent movement of the spine by preventing movement of the head, neck and body. Unless you must move the victim, support the victim's head in the position in which you find the victim **(Figure 12-3)**. Although it is generally better for the head to be in line with the body, *do not move the victim's head to put it in line with the body.* Damage to the spinal cord and nerves could be worsened by any unnecessary movement of the head. If the victim's head is already in line with the body when you reach the scene, support it in that position in line; this can be done with the victim lying down or sitting up. This technique is called **spinal motion restriction**, which simply means to prevent movement of the head and neck by supporting them manually in line with the body (see Skill: "Spinal Motion Restriction"). A responsive victim is likely to be in this position and you should encourage the victim not to move while you provide support. If the victim is unresponsive and must be moved in order to give CPR, keep the head in line with the body while you move the victim with assistance from others.

If a victim with a suspected spinal cord injury is wearing a helmet, the helmet should remain in place unless the victim is experiencing respiratory difficulty and the helmet prevents giving care to the victim.

While supporting the victim's head manually until help arrives, continue to maintain the victim's open airway if needed and monitor the victim's breathing (see First Aid: "Spinal Injuries").

Positioning the Victim

Generally you support the victim's head and neck in the position found. Move the victim only if absolutely necessary. If the victim is lying on his or her back and vomits, you must roll the victim onto his or her side to let the mouth drain and allow breathing. If the victim is lying on his or her side or face-down and requires CPR, you must move the victim onto his or her back.

The help of two or three others is necessary to keep the back and neck aligned during the move. The technique called a log roll is used by multiple rescuers to turn the victim while keeping the head supported in line with the body (see Skill: "Rolling

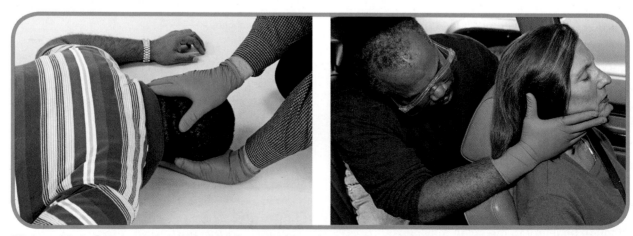

Figure 12-3 *Support the head in the position in which you find the victim.*

Skill 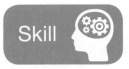 Spinal Motion Restriction

1 Ask a responsive victim what happened. If he or she has any of the risk factors, explain the need to hold the head still to prevent spinal movement and spinal cord injury. With an unresponsive victim, check for risk factors for suspected spinal injury.

2 Hold the victim's head and neck with both hands in the position found to prevent movement.

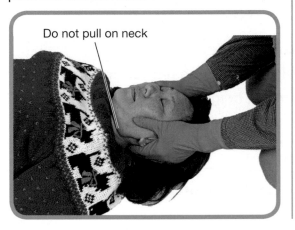

Do not pull on neck

3 Monitor the victim's breathing and be ready to provide basic life support.

4 Have someone call 9-1-1.

5 Reassure a conscious victim and tell him or her not to move.

6 Continue to stabilize the head and spine, and monitor the victim's breathing until help arrives.

a Victim with Spinal Injury [Log Roll]"). Continue to monitor the victim's breathing until help arrives.

If you are alone and the victim vomits, move him or her into the HAINES recovery position, supporting the head and neck at all times.

Injuries to Lower Back

Spinal injuries include lower back injuries that may not damage the spinal cord or be as serious as other spinal injuries. Such injuries generally occur as a result of a stressful activity rather than a traumatic injury such as a fall or blow to the head or neck. For example, the victim may have been lifting or moving a heavy object or working in an unusual position. A strained muscle or ligament may result or a disk (soft tissue between vertebrae) may be damaged. Such injuries may not be emergencies, although often they require medical attention.

Signs and symptoms of a less serious lower back injury may include sharp pain in the lower back, stiffness and reduced movement in the back and possible sharp pain in one leg. If any of the signs and symptoms of a spinal injury are present, call 9-1-1 and keep the victim from moving. Otherwise, the victim should see a health care provider.

Concluding Thoughts

Because of the risk of brain damage or paralysis, head and spinal injuries can be frightening experiences. Most important, remember that you do not have to assess the injury with certainty before acting. Any time you suspect a victim has a head or spinal injury, call 9-1-1 and keep the victim still until help arrives.

12 • Head and Spinal Injuries

First Aid
Spinal Injuries
Signs, Symptoms and Care

When You See

For a responsive victim:

- Inability to move any body part
- Tingling or a lack of sensation in hands or feet
- Deformed neck or back
- Breathing problems
- Headache

For an unresponsive victim:

- Deformed neck or back
- Signs of blow to head or back
- Nature of the emergency suggests possible spinal injury

Suspect a spinal injury in an injured victim who has these risk factors:

- 65 or older
- Child older than 2 with trauma of head or neck
- Motor vehicle or bicycle crash involving driver, passenger or pedestrian
- Fall from more than the person's standing height
- Victim feels tingling in hands or feet, pain in back or neck, or muscle weakness or lack of feeling in torso or arms
- Victim is intoxicated or not alert
- Any painful injury, particularly to the head, neck or back

Do This First

1 Ask a responsive victim what happened. If they have any of the risk factors, explain the need to hold the head still to prevent spinal movement. With an unresponsive victim, check for risk factors for suspected spinal injury.

2 Hold the victim's head and neck with both hands in the position found to prevent movement of the neck and spine.

3 Monitor the victim's breathing and be ready to give CPR if needed.

4 Have someone call 9-1-1.

Additional Care

- Reassure a responsive victim and tell him or her not to move.
- Continue to stabilize the head and spine, and monitor the victim's breathing until help arrives.

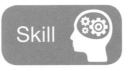
1 Hold the victim's head with hands on both sides over ears.

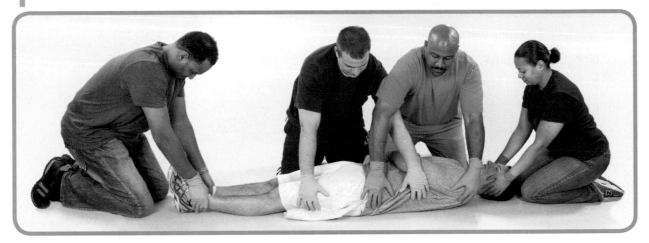

2 The first aider at the victim's head directs others to roll the body as a unit.

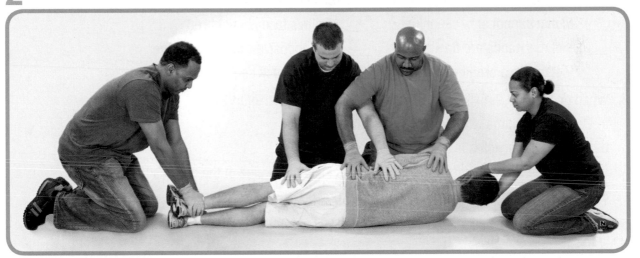

3 Continue to support head in new position on side.

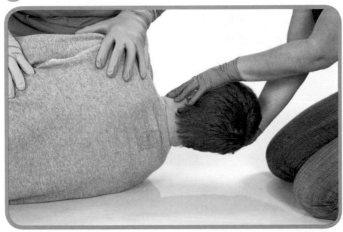

Learning **Checkpoint 2**

1. True or False: Suspect a spinal injury in any victim with a serious head injury.

2. For an unresponsive victim you suspect may have a spinal injury –
   a. immediately place the victim on his or her back in case you have to give CPR.
   b. monitor the victim's breathing in the position in which you found the victim.
   c. turn the head to one side in case the victim vomits.
   d. move all body parts to see if anything feels broken.

3. A spinal injury should be suspected in which of these situations? (Check all that apply.)
   _____ The victim fell from a roof 20 feet high.
   _____ A victim with diabetes passes out at lunch.
   _____ The victim was in a car that hit a telephone pole.
   _____ A piece of heavy equipment fell from a shelf onto the victim's head.
   _____ You find a victim slumped over in a desk chair.

4. Which of these are signs and symptoms of a spinal injury? (Check all that apply.)
   _____ Victim cannot stop coughing   _____ Victim's face is bright red
   _____ Victim's hands are tingling   _____ Unresponsive victim has a fever
   _____ Victim has a breathing problem   _____ Victim's neck seems oddly turned

5. When do you call 9-1-1 for a victim with a potential spinal injury?
   a. Call for all victims with potential spinal injury.
   b. Call only if the victim is unresponsive.
   c. Call for a responsive victim only if feeling is lost on one side of the victim's body.
   d. Call after waiting 10 minutes to see if an unresponsive victim awakes.

6. In what position do you stabilize the head of a victim with a suspected spinal injury?

   _____

7. Roll a victim with a suspected spinal injury onto his or her side only if the victim _____ .

8. In the company parking lot you see a car skid on an icy patch and smash into another car. The driver is still behind the wheel and looks dazed. Her forehead is bleeding. You ask her how she feels, and she does not answer but just stares ahead. What should you do?

   _____

   _____

Learning Outcomes

You should now be able to do the following:

1. List the signs and symptoms of head and spinal injuries.

2. Perform a physical examination of a victim with head or spinal injury.

3. Describe the first aid for a victim with a possible brain injury.

4. Explain why a victim with a possible spinal injury should not be moved unnecessarily.

5. Perform spinal motion restriction.

6. With other rescuers, perform a log roll of a victim with a spinal injury.

Review Questions

1. Assessing a victim with a potential head or spinal injury includes –

   a. considering the risk factors in an injured victim.

   b. asking the victim to turn his or her head to the side.

   c. assessing how the victim holds his or her head when sitting.

   d. comparing skin color in different parts of the body.

2. Which of the following is not a sign or symptom of a possible head or spinal injury?

   a. Unequal pupils

   b. Sudden red rash around neck

   c. Tingling in hands

   d. Headache

3. What is the best way to stop bleeding from the scalp at the site of a skull fracture?

   a. Apply direct pressure on the wound.

   b. Apply indirect pressure on the pulse point in the neck.

   c. Apply pressure only around the edges of the wound.

   d. Tightly bandage the wound but do not apply pressure at all.

4. What is the one sure way for a first aider to know whether a head injury victim has a serious brain injury?

   a. The victim feels temporarily confused.

   b. The victim is acting unusually.

   c. The victim was briefly unconscious.

   d. There is no certain way.

5. A spinal cord injury can cause –

   a. paralysis.

   b. a breathing problem.

   c. numbness in the feet.

   d. All of the above

6. You find an unresponsive victim at the base of a ladder with his head turned to one side. He is breathing normally. You should —

   a. support the head in the position found.

   b. gently move the head in line with the body.

   c. roll the victim onto his side.

   d. try to move his body in line with his head.

7. In your physical examination of a victim with a suspected spinal injury, the victim squeezes your hand only very softly with her left hand. To further assess this victim you can —

   a. squeeze her hand hard and ask what she feels.

   b. ask her to squeeze with both hands at the same time and compare them.

   c. ask her to snap her fingers with her left hand.

   d. have her clasp her hands together and pull with each, to see which arm pulls the other.

8. When might you have to move a victim with a suspected spinal injury?

   a. To position the victim for CPR

   b. To drain vomit from the victim's mouth

   c. To escape an encroaching fire

   d. All of the above

9. When should you call 9-1-1 for a suspected spinal injury?

   a. Call only if the victim is unresponsive.

   b. Call only if the victim is unresponsive or if a responsive victim is experiencing a severe headache.

   c. Call for any suspected spinal injury.

   d. Call if no one else is present to help you transport the victim to the emergency department.

Chapter 13 • Chest, Abdominal and Pelvic Injuries

Chapter Preview

- Chest Injuries
- Abdominal Injuries
- Pelvic Injuries

The car in front of you suddenly swerves to the right and runs into the back of a parked car. Fortunately, it was not moving very fast at the time. You pull over and get out to see if you can help. The driver is slumped forward against the steering wheel, apparently not wearing a safety belt and shoulder harness. As you approach, at first he seems unresponsive, but then he leans back and opens the car door. He gets out, holding his chest on one side, and staggers a few feet before you reach him. He does not seem to be bleeding but is obviously in pain. What do you do?

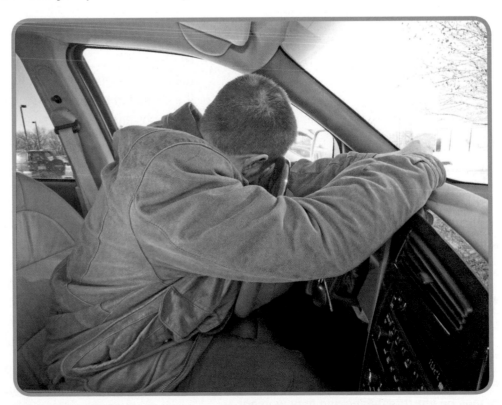

Injuries to the chest, abdomen or pelvis can result from either blunt or penetrating forces. Blunt trauma typically occurs from motor vehicle crashes, falls, industrial emergencies, fights and similar events. Open injuries can result from any object that breaks the skin, including gunshots and stab wounds. Both closed and open injuries to the chest, abdomen and pelvis can be life-threatening when bleeding is severe or internal organs are injured. Shock often occurs. Always call 9-1-1 for these injuries.

Chest Injuries

The chest contains many important structures that may be damaged from a chest injury, including the heart, lungs and large blood vessels. Trauma may injure the chest wall, including the ribs and soft tissues or structures within the chest or both. Serious chest injuries include broken ribs, objects impaled in the chest and sucking chest wounds in which air passes in and out of the chest cavity. These wounds can be life-threatening if breathing is affected. Chest injuries may result from such things as:

- Striking the steering wheel in a motor vehicle crash

- A blow to the chest

- A fall from a height

- Sports injuries

- Physical assault

- A penetrating injury or impaled object

The general signs and symptoms of a serious chest injury include:

- Breathing problems

- Severe pain

- Bruising or swelling

- Deformity of the chest

- Coughing blood

Because the condition of a victim with a chest injury may be life-threatening and may worsen over time, it is essential to continue checking the victim's breathing and provide basic life support as needed. The forces involved may also suggest the possibility of a spinal injury. In addition, specific first aid is given for the particular injury.

Closed Chest Injuries

Common chest injuries involving the lungs include pneumothorax and hemothorax, which may occur with either open or closed injuries. In a pneumothorax, air escapes from an injured lung into the thoracic cavity – the space inside the chest around the lungs – causing collapse of some or all of the lung and resulting in respiratory distress. In a hemothorax, blood from an injury accumulates in the thoracic cavity, compressing the lung and causing respiratory distress and possibly shock.

The fact that the skin is not broken in a closed chest injury does not mean that there is not serious underlying damage. Because organ damage or internal bleeding could be serious, call 9-1-1 and monitor the victim's breathing while waiting for help to arrive. In an unresponsive victim, maintain an open airway and keep checking breathing. Let a responsive victim find the position that is most comfortable and allows for easiest breathing.

Broken Ribs

Rib fractures typically result from blunt trauma to the chest. Rib fractures are more common in the lower ribs and along the side. Rib fractures usually cause severe pain, discoloration and swelling at the site of the fracture. The pain is often sharper upon breathing in and the victim may be breathing shallowly. Another sign of a rib fracture is the victim holding or supporting the area. Many rib fractures involve only the fracture, but with severe trauma there also may be injuries to the lungs or other underlying organs **(Figure 13-1)**. Because of the possibility of serious injury and the risk that the injury may become worse with movement, always call 9-1-1 for a rib fracture.

The first aid for rib fractures is primarily supportive. Let a responsive victim assume a comfortable position. The victim may sit or stand,

and often leans toward the side of the injury with an arm compressed against the rib. Use a pillow or blanket to help immobilize the area and reduce pain. Do not tightly wrap a bandage or padding around the chest, because this could restrict breathing (see First Aid: "Broken Ribs").

Flail Chest

A flail chest is the fracture of two or more ribs in two or more places **(Figure 13-2)**. Flail chest usually results from a severe blow to the chest. The injury actually separates a segment of the chest wall from the remainder of the chest.

With breathing, the flail segment moves in the opposite direction from the rest of the chest wall in what is called **paradoxical movement**. This part of the chest wall moves outward during exhalation because of the increased pressure within the chest. During inhalation the segment moves inward. The larger the flail segment, the greater the threat to the victim's respiratory function.

First aid for flail chest includes monitoring the victim's breathing and supporting the affected chest area with a bulky dressing, towel, or pillow secured with tape or bandages (see First Aid: "Flail Chest").

Impaled Object

Removing an impaled object from the chest could cause additional bleeding, injury and breathing problems. Leave the object in place and stabilize it using bulky dressings bandaged around the object, as described in **Chapter 8**. Call 9-1-1 and treat the victim for shock (see **Chapter 9**). Monitor the victim's breathing while waiting for help to arrive (see First Aid: "Impaled Object").

Sucking Chest Wound

A **sucking chest wound** is an open wound in the chest caused by a penetrating injury that lets air move in and out of the chest during breathing. When the chest expands during inhalation, the pressure inside the chest decreases and air is sucked in through the wound. When the chest contracts during exhalation, air is forced out through the wound. You may hear a gurgling or sucking sound and may see air bubbles in the blood around the wound.

A sucking chest wound can be life-threatening because breathing can be affected. First aid includes sealing the wound to help the victim

(continues on page 201)

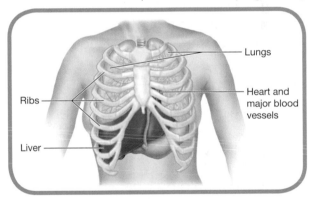

Figure 13-1 *The rib cage protects underlying organs in the chest.*

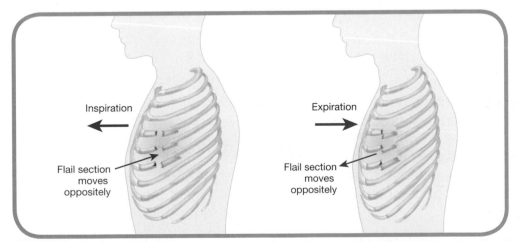

Figure 13-2 *In flail chest, a section of the chest wall moves in and out opposite to the normal motion of breathing.*

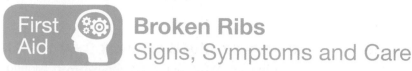

Broken Ribs
Signs, Symptoms and Care

When You See

- **Signs of pain with deep breathing or movement**
- **Victim holding ribs**
- **Shallow breathing**

Do This First

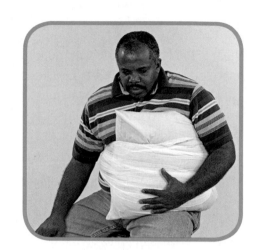

1 Help the victim to sit or stand in the position of easiest breathing.

2 Support the ribs with a pillow or soft padding loosely bandaged over the area and under the arm.

3 Call 9-1-1.

Additional Care

- Monitor the victim's breathing while waiting for help.
- If helpful, immobilize the arm with a sling and binder (see **Chapter 15**) to prevent movement and ease pain.

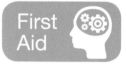

Flail Chest
Signs, Symptoms and Care

When You See

- **Victim holding ribs**
- **Shallow breathing**
- **Paradoxical movement of chest segment**
- **Severe pain**
- **Swelling or chest deformity**

Do This First

1 Help the victim sit in a comfortable position for easiest breathing.

2 Splint the flail area with a small pillow or thick padding loosely bandaged in place (but not completely around the chest).

3 Position the victim lying on the injured side to give more support to the area.

4 Call 9-1-1.

Additional Care

- If padding is not available to splint the flail area, support it with pressure from your hand.
- Monitor the victim until help arrives.

(continued from page 199)

maintain adequate respiratory function. The dressed wound should be covered with an occlusive dressing such as plastic food wrap, a plastic bag or a piece of aluminum foil. This **occlusive** dressing should be taped on three sides, with the fourth left open **(Figure 13-3)**. This prevents air from being sucked into the chest, allowing more normal breathing, while allowing allow air to escape from the wound, to prevent a buildup of pressure in the chest (see First Aid: "Sucking Chest Wound").

Abdominal Injuries

Abdominal injuries include closed and open wounds that result from a blow to the abdomen or a fall. Because large blood vessels are present within the abdomen along with many organs, injury may cause internal and/or external bleeding. The abdominal cavity is not protected from injury as the chest is by the ribs. The posterior abdomen is afforded some protection by the spine and lower part of the rib cage, but the anterior abdomen is relatively unprotected **(Figure 13-4)**. Internal organs may be damaged and organs may protrude from an open wound.

The external appearance of an injured abdomen can sometimes be deceptive, even when serious or life-threatening injuries to organs are present. Often the only indication of abdominal injury is a small bruise or wound. Because of the potential for serious injury, all abdominal wounds should be regarded as potentially life-threatening and treated accordingly.

Closed Abdominal Injury

A closed abdominal injury can threaten life because internal organs may have ruptured and there may be serious internal bleeding. Blunt abdominal trauma commonly occurs in motor vehicle crashes but may also result from sports injuries, falls, physical assault or industrial emergencies.

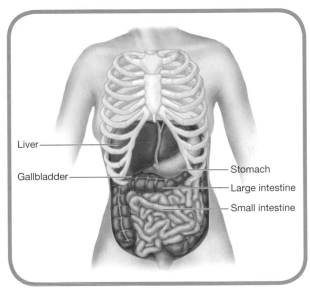

Figure 13-4 *Abdominal organs have little protection from injury.*

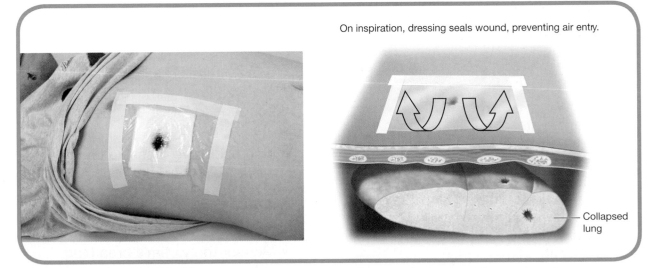

Figure 13-3 *First aid for sucking chest wound. (a) Tape only three sides to let air escape from a sucking chest wound. (b) When victim breathes in, the dressing seals the wound and prevents air entry.*

On inspiration, dressing seals wound, preventing air entry.

Collapsed lung

13 • Chest, Abdominal and Pelvic Injuries

| 201

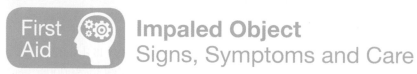

Impaled Object
Signs, Symptoms and Care

When You See

• **An object impaled in a chest wound**

Do This First

1 Keep victim still. The victim may be seated or lying down.

2 Stabilize the impaled object with bulky dressings.

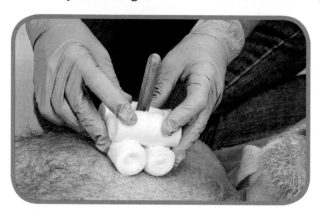

3 Bandage around the object.

4 Call 9-1-1.

Additional Care

• Reassure the victim.

• Monitor the victim's breathing until help arrives.

ALERT

• Do not give the victim anything to eat or drink.

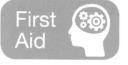

Sucking Chest Wound
Signs, Symptoms and Care

When You See

• **Air moving in or out of a penetrating chest wound**

• **Sucking sounds on inhalation**

Do This First

1 Put a thin, sterile dressing over the wound.

2 Cover the dressing with a plastic wrap or plastic bag to make an airtight seal. As the victim exhales, tape it in place on three sides, leaving one side untaped to let exhaled air escape.

3 Position victim lying down inclined toward the injured side.

4 Call 9-1-1.

Additional Care

• If the victim's breathing becomes more difficult, remove the plastic bandage to let air escape; then reapply it.

• If an occlusive dressing is not available, cover the wound with your gloved hand during inhalation to prevent air from entering the chest.

• Monitor the victim's breathing until help arrives.

• Treat the victim for shock.

Learning Checkpoint 1

1. True or False: Broken ribs are treated by taping the entire rib cage tightly.

2. Immobilize the arm of a victim with a rib fracture to –

   a. prevent movement.

   b. ease pain.

   c. help immobilize that side of the chest.

   d. All of the above

3. What should you do with a screwdriver you see embedded in the chest of an unresponsive friend after an explosion in his garage?

   _____

4. A gunshot victim has a small, bleeding hole in the right side of his chest. You open his shirt to treat the bleeding and see air bubbles forming in the hole as air escapes. How do you dress this wound?

   _____

The signs and symptoms of abdominal trauma can vary. Often, the only symptom is pain. The physical examination may reveal bruising or an obvious abdominal wound. If bleeding is severe, shock may also be present and the abdomen may appear very firm, almost rigid. Abdominal muscles may also contract to minimize movement or agitation of the affected site, a condition called guarding.

First aid for a victim with an abdominal injury includes monitoring the victim's breathing and giving supportive care as well as first aid for an open wound. Do not move the victim, who should try to avoid coughing or straining. Keep the victim warm. Do not give the victim anything to eat or drink because emergency surgery may be needed (see First Aid: "Closed Abdominal Injury").

Open Abdominal Wound

An open abdominal injury usually injures internal organs such as the intestines, liver, kidneys or stomach. A large wound in the abdominal wall may allow abdominal organs to protrude through the wound **(Figure 13-5)**; this is called evisceration. This is a serious emergency because organs can be further damaged by drying out, bleeding from associated blood vessels or infection.

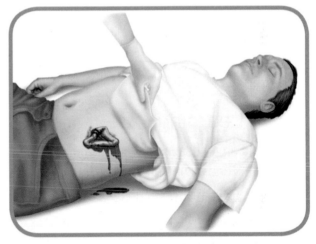

Figure 13-5 *Open abdominal wound.*

First aid includes positioning the victim as you would for a closed abdominal injury and providing wound care and treatment for shock. If abdominal organs are protruding through an open wound, do not touch them or try to push them back into the abdomen. Do not pack the wound with dressings. Instead, cover the wound with a moist, sterile dressing or a dry, nonadherent dressing and cover with an occlusive dressing or plastic wrap loosely taped in place to keep the organs from drying out (see First Aid: "Open Abdominal Wound").

First Aid

Closed Abdominal Injury
Signs, Symptoms and Care

When You See

- **Signs of severe pain, tenderness in area or victim protecting the abdomen**
- **Bruising**
- **Swollen or rigid abdomen**
- **Rapid, shallow breathing**
- **Nausea or vomiting**

Do This First

1 Carefully position the victim on his or her back and loosen any tight clothing.

2 Call 9-1-1.

3 Treat the victim for shock, monitor the victim's breathing and be ready to give CPR if needed.

Additional Care

- Continue to monitor the victim's breathing until help arrives.

ALERT

- Do not let the victim eat or drink.

Learning Checkpoint 2

1. You find an unresponsive victim who has suffered a sports injury on the ground. Which of the following are signs and symptoms he may have a closed abdominal injury? (Check all that apply.)

   _____ Bruises below the rib cage   _____ Blotchy skin around the eyes

   _____ Abrasions on the chest   _____ Swollen abdomen

   _____ Skin feels hot all over   _____ Tight skin around the neck

2. Describe the best position for a victim with either an open or closed abdominal wound.

   _____

3. True or False: To treat a victim for shock, help maintain normal body temperature.

4. If the victim has an organ protruding from an open abdominal wound, what should you do?

   a. Push the organ back into the abdomen.

   b. Spray clean water over the organ to keep it moist.

   c. Leave the wound exposed to the air.

   d. Cover the wound with a nonadherent dressing and plastic wrap.

5. In what circumstances do you call 9-1-1 for a victim with an open or closed abdominal wound?

   _____

   _____

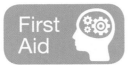

First Aid

Open Abdominal Wound
Signs, Symptoms and Care

When You See

- **Open abdominal wound**
- **Bleeding**
- **Severe pain**
- **Organs possibly protruding from wound**
- **Signs of shock**

Do This First

1 Lay the victim on his or her back and loosen any tight clothing.

2 Cover the wound with a moist, sterile dressing or a dry, nonadherent dressing.

3 Cover the dressing with a large, occlusive dressing or plastic wrap, taped loosely in place. Then cover the area with a blanket or towel to help maintain warmth.

4 Call 9-1-1.

5 Treat the victim for shock. Monitor the victim's breathing and be ready to give CPR if needed.

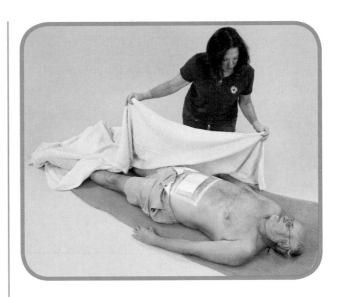

Additional Care

- Monitor the victim until help arrives.

ALERT

- Do not push protruding organs back inside the abdomen, but keep them from drying out with an occlusive dressing or plastic covering.
- Do not apply direct pressure on the wound.

13 • Chest, Abdominal and Pelvic Injuries

Pelvic Injuries

The most common pelvic injury is fracture of the pelvis. Such fractures in healthy adults are usually caused only by large forces, which are likely to cause other injuries as well. Pelvic fractures are more common in the elderly and may be caused by lesser forces, such as falls. Pelvic fractures are generally very serious. A broken pelvis may cause severe internal bleeding and organ damage. A broken pelvis can be life-threatening. With severe bleeding the victim may be in shock.

A victim with a pelvic fracture cannot move and often has severe pain. In the physical examination you may note instability in the pelvic area. The victim may be bleeding from the genitalia or rectum or leaking urine.

Because of the large forces that typically cause the injury, consider that the victim also may have a spinal injury, and support the head and neck accordingly. The care for a suspected pelvic fracture is primarily supportive. Do not move the victim or let the victim move. Take steps to minimize shock, including maintaining the victim's body temperature, but do not elevate the legs (see First Aid: "Pelvic Injuries").

Learning Checkpoint 3

1. First aid for a pelvic fracture prevents _____ of the area.

2. True or False: Internal bleeding can be severe with a broken pelvis.

3. True or False: For a victim with a broken pelvis, raise the victim's feet and legs to treat for shock.

Concluding Thoughts

Victims with serious injuries to the chest, abdomen or pelvis usually have experienced significant trauma and often there are injuries to internal organs you cannot observe. The victim may have other wounds or injuries as well, complicating the situation. Most important, ensure that 9-1-1 is called immediately to get help on the way. Then care for any life-threatening conditions first and provide specific first aid for the injuries.

Learning Outcomes

You should now be able to do the following:

1. Explain why chest injuries may be life-threatening, and list the general signs and symptoms of chest injuries.

2. Describe the specific first aid steps for broken ribs, flail chest, an impaled object in the chest and a sucking chest wound.

3. Describe the signs and symptoms of a closed abdominal injury and the first aid to give.

4. Explain how to care for an open abdominal wound.

5. Describe the signs and symptoms of a pelvic fracture and the first aid to give.

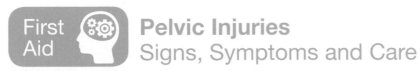
Pelvic Injuries
Signs, Symptoms and Care

When You See

- **Signs of pain and tenderness around the hips**
- **Inability to walk or stand**
- **Signs and symptoms of shock**

Do This First

1 Help the victim lie quietly on the back.

2 Call 9-1-1.

3 If help may be delayed, immobilize the victim's legs by padding between the legs and then bandaging them together, unless this causes more pain.

4 Treat the victim for shock. Monitor the victim's breathing and be ready to give CPR if needed.

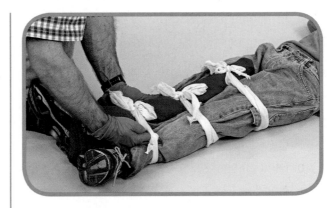

Additional Care

- Monitor the victim until help arrives.
- Care for any open wounds, such as wounds to the genitals.

Review Questions

1. Chest injuries may be life-threatening because –

   a. breathing may be affected.

   b. rib fractures usually involve nerve damage.

   c. chest abrasions can bleed heavily.

   d. All of the above

2. First aid for a rib fracture includes –

   a. tightly bandaging around the chest to prevent movement.

   b. using a pillow or blanket to help support the area.

   c. taping the arm against the side down to the waist.

   d. applying rigid splints on both sides of the thorax.

3. When should an impaled object be removed from the chest wall?

   a. Always

   b. Only when there is no heavy bleeding around it

   c. Only when air bubbles from the lungs are escaping around it

   d. Never

13 • Chest, Abdominal and Pelvic Injuries

4. The dressing and bandage over a sucking chest wound should –
   a. allow air to escape but prevent air from being sucked in.
   b. allow air to be sucked in but prevent air from escaping.
   c. allow air to flow in and out of the wound.
   d. prevent air from flowing in or out of the wound.

5. Which of the following is a sign of a closed abdominal injury with severe internal bleeding?
   a. Breathing is slow and very deep.
   b. The area of skin below the umbilicus looks red.
   c. The abdomen feels hard.
   d. The victim always has a fever.

6. The position that is usually most comfortable for a victim with an abdominal injury is –
   a. curled up on side in fetal position.
   b. lying on back.
   c. standing
   d. lying face-down.

7. Internal organs protruding from an abdominal wound should be protected by –
   a. covering them with the victim's shirt.
   b. covering them with a sterile, moist dressing.
   c. pushing them back into the body.
   d. placing the victim's hand over them.

8. What should you do if you suspect the victim has a pelvic fracture?
   a. See if the victim can stand up.
   b. Carefully roll the victim into a face-down position.
   c. Elevate the legs to prevent shock.
   d. Keep the victim still and call 9-1-1.

Chapter 14 • Bone, Joint and Muscle Injuries

Chapter Preview

- Prevention of Sports and Recreation Injuries
- Assessing Musculoskeletal Injuries
- General First Aid

- Fractures
- Joint Injuries
- Muscle Injuries

On a Saturday morning you are jogging on a trail at a local park when you see a woman jogging some distance in front of you suddenly tumble to the ground. When you reach her, she is holding her ankle, which she says really hurts. She says she came down on the side of her foot and felt her ankle twist. She thinks it is sprained, but she doesn't know what to do. How can you help?

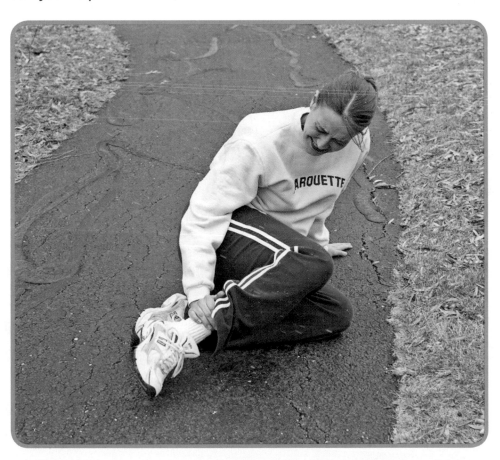

Injuries of the bones, joints and muscles are among the most common injuries in the home, at work, and during sports and recreation (Table 14-1). Injuries may result from a blow, the impact of a body part against an object or surface (as in a fall) or other forces acting on the body's bones, joints or muscles. Most sports injuries are musculoskeletal injuries. Although this chapter focuses on first aid for more serious injuries, the most common musculoskeletal injuries are less serious, such as muscle strains resulting from overexertion, and they are seldom an emergency.

This chapter covers musculoskeletal injuries to the extremities. Injuries to the skull or spine are discussed in Chapter 12, and injuries to the rib cage and pelvis are discussed in Chapter 13.

Musculoskeletal injuries are generally classified as injuries of bones (**fractures**), **joints** (dislocations and sprains) or muscles (strains, contusions, cramps). A **dislocation** is movement of a bone out of its usual position in a joint. A **sprain** is a tearing of **ligaments** in a joint. A **strain** is the tearing of a muscle or **tendon** and a **contusion** is a bruised muscle. It is not necessary to know the exact nature of the injury, however, to provide effective first aid. Remember always to first assess the victim's breathing and look for any threats to life before looking for musculoskeletal injuries.

Prevention of Sports and Recreation Injuries

Injuries from almost all sports and recreational activities are very common. Death from such injuries, although very rare, is usually caused by head injuries in victims not wearing helmets. However, emergency department visits are very common (Table 14-2). In addition to causing pain and temporary disability, sports injuries may cause long-term or even permanent disability.

Preventing sports and recreational injuries begins with the correct use of sports equipment, such as helmets and other protective gear, and following established safety guidelines for the particular sport. No sport can be made 100% safe, however,

Table 14-1: Number of occupational injuries and illnesses (in thousands) involving time away from work for selected occupations, 1995- 2001

Year End Total Cases	1995 2,040.9	1996 1,880.5	1997 1,833.4	1998 1,730.5	1999 1,702.5	2000 1,664.0	2001 1,537.6
Truck Drivers	151.3	152.8	145.5	131.8	141.1	136.1	129.1
Nursing Aides, Orderlies	100.6	93.6	91.3	84.1	75.7	74.2	71.0
Laborers, Nonconstruction	115.5	108.5	106.9	97.2	89.1	87.0	68.9
Construction Laborers	43.5	43.7	45.8	44.1	46.5	45.4	44.1
Janitors and Cleaners	52.6	46.9	45.8	44.2	43.4	40.7	38.6
Carpenters	35.0	33.5	37.1	33.0	35.0	38.3	32.7
Assemblers	55.5	44.0	44.3	43.3	40.0	38.9	31.1
Cooks	35.4	30.7	31.5	28.5	28.0	27.8	27.8
Stock Handlers and Baggers	34.7	31.9	29.2	26.3	27.3	23.8	25.7
Registered Nurses	27.8	28.9	27.3	25.0	25.7	24.5	24.7

Source: US Bureau of Labor Statistics. *http://www.bls.gov/iif/oshwc/osh/case/osnr0017.pdf. Accessed March 4, 2011.*

and specific sports have certain risks for injury – a factor that should be considered by those involved and the parents of young athletes. Sports medicine is increasingly investigating the long-term effects of some types of sports injuries, such as the potential for disabling conditions such as arthritis or pain from hairline fractures that appear years or decades after the injury.

To reduce the risk of injury, before beginning a strenuous new activity, check with a health care provider. To prevent common sprains and strains in sports and recreational activities, the following are recommended:

- Maintain a healthy, well-balanced diet to keep muscles strong.

- Maintain a healthy weight.

- Practice safety measures to help prevent falls. For example, keep stairways, walkways, yards and driveways free of clutter and salt or sand icy patches in the winter.

- Wear shoes that fit properly. Replace athletic shoes as soon as the tread wears out or the heel wears down on one side.

- Do stretching exercises daily.

- Drink enough water to stay hydrated and prevent heat exhaustion and heatstroke.

- Be in proper physical condition to play a sport.

- Warm up and stretch before participating in any sports or exercise. Use a cool-down routine afterwards.

- Schedule regular days off.

- Wear protective equipment when playing.

- Avoid exercising or playing sports when tired or in pain.

- Run on even surfaces.

Assessing Musculoskeletal Injuries

Remember to first perform the initial assessment of any victim and to care for any life-threatening conditions before performing a physical examination. Musculoskeletal injuries are usually not life-threatening, except in cases of severe bleeding, but they may nonetheless be serious and result in pain and disability.

When assessing the injury, consider the type and size of the forces involved. Ask a responsive victim what happened and what he or she felt when the injury occurred. **Figure 14-2** describes common mechanisms of injury.

If large forces were involved in the injury, consider the potential for a spinal injury and assess the victim accordingly (see **Chapter 12**). Particularly, if the victim is unresponsive, do not move him or her unnecessarily to assess a musculoskeletal injury.

Table 14-2: **Sports and Recreation Injuries Resulting in U.S. Emergency Department Visits per Year**		
Activity	**Children 5 to 14***	**All People Ages 5 to 24****
Group Sports		
Basketball	193,000	447,000
Football	186,000	271,000
Baseball/softball	116,000	245,000
Soccer	85,000	95,000
Other group sports	—	112,000
Individual Sports/Activities		
Bicycling	373,000	421,000
Ice/roller skating/boarding	99,000	150,000
Gymnastics/cheerleading	—	146,000
Playground injuries	—	137,000
Trampoline	68,000	—
Sledding/skiing/snowboarding	42,000	111,000
Water sports	—	100,000
Other individual sports/activities	—	381,000
All Sports/Recreation	—	2,616,000

Sources: *National Youth Sports Safety Foundation. Available from: http://www.nyssf.org
**National Center for Health Statistics, 2005. Available from: http://www.cdc.gov/nchs Accessed May 2006.

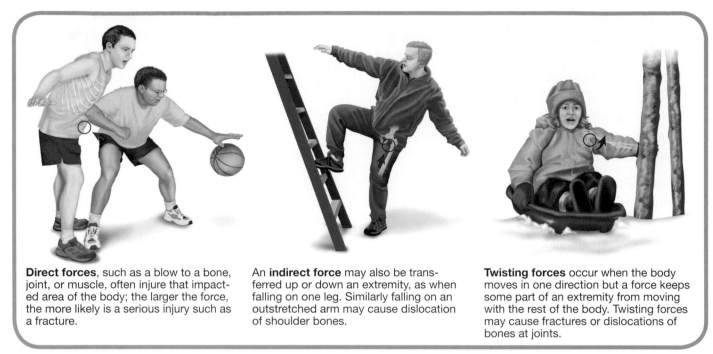

Direct forces, such as a blow to a bone, joint, or muscle, often injure that impacted area of the body; the larger the force, the more likely is a serious injury such as a fracture.

An **indirect force** may also be transferred up or down an extremity, as when falling on one leg. Similarly falling on an outstretched arm may cause dislocation of shoulder bones.

Twisting forces occur when the body moves in one direction but a force keeps some part of an extremity from moving with the rest of the body. Twisting forces may cause fractures or dislocations of bones at joints.

Figure 14-2 *Common mechanisms of injury.*

When you perform a physical examination on an injured extremity, remember to look for the following signs and symptoms **(Figure 14-3)**. Compare the injured arm or leg to the opposite one.

- Pain when an area is touched
- Bleeding or other wounds
- Swelling
- An area that is deformed
- Skin discoloration
- Abnormal sensation (numbness, tingling)
- Inability to move the area
- Difference in temperature
- Guarding: Because of pain, victim holds the area to prevent movement

In addition, with a fracture, you may hear the broken bone ends grating together, or the victim may feel them grinding together. This is called **crepitus**.

Carefully remove the victim's clothing as needed to examine an injured area and check for an open wound that may require care. Pain occurs with most musculoskeletal injuries and may be more severe with serious injuries, although less painful injuries should not be assumed to be minor. When checking for the ability to move the extremities, do not ask the victim to move an injured area that causes pain. A lack of sensation in the injured area or below it (for example, the finger or toes) may be a symptom of a serious injury involving nerve damage. Swelling occurs in most musculoskeletal injuries because of bleeding in injured tissues, but the amount of swelling is not a good indication of the severity of the injury. An obvious deformity or difference between the injured extremity and its uninjured opposite is usually a sign of a fracture or dislocation, both of which are serious injuries. Skin discoloration may include the "black and blue" color of bruising or a pale or light blue skin color (ashen in dark-skinned individuals) that, along with cool skin, may indicate a lack of blood flow below the injured area and is a sign of a serious injury.

General First Aid

Later sections in this chapter describe the specific care for fractures, dislocations, sprains, strains and other injuries. The general first aid for all

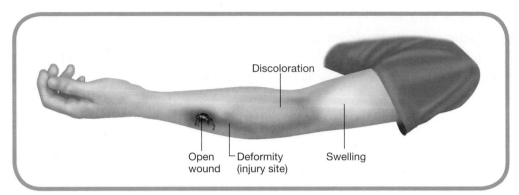

Figure 14-3 *Signs of a musculoskeletal injury.*

musculoskeletal injuries is similar, however, based on the same principles of care. You do not have to know the specific type of injury before caring for the victim. The general first aid for most bone, joint and muscle injuries involves four steps that are summarized in the acronym **RICE (Box 14-1)**:

R = Rest

I = Ice

C = Compression

E = Elevation

Rest

Any movement of a musculoskeletal injury can cause further injury, pain and swelling. With a fracture or dislocation, for example, any movement of the extremity could cause movement of the bone, further injuring soft tissues such as blood vessels and nerves around the bone. In addition, movement generally increases blood flow, which may increase internal bleeding and swelling. For serious injuries, call 9-1-1 and have the victim rest until help arrives. Usually the victim can assume whatever position is the least painful. For less serious injuries,

BOX 14-1: "RICE" AND OTHER ACRONYMS

RICE is a widely used acronym to help first aiders remember the treatment for most musculoskeletal injuries, but other acronyms also have been devised for the care of these injuries.

One that is becoming more commonly used now is PRICE, in which the P stands for "protection". This is intended to remind the first aider to protect the injured area by immobilizing it either with a splint (when appropriate) or by protecting the area from movement until the victim is seen by emergency personnel. (Some would argue that this protection is already implied by the R in RICE – resting the injured area.)

Other old standards are PIE (pressure, ice, elevation) and PIES (pressure, ice, elevation,

splinting). The P for pressure is equivalent to the C for compression – both referring to wrapping the injury. Proponents of these acronyms suggest the R in RICE for rest is not necessary because the pain and discomfort of the injury will force the victim to rest the area anyway. Still other acronyms that have been used as memory aids include ICE, ICES and PRICES. Occasionally the same acronym has been defined in different ways, such as having I stand for ice in one definition but immobilization in another and C for cold in one definition but compression in another.

What matters, of course, is remembering the first aid steps behind the acronym.

when the victim will be transported to a health care provider or home, minimize movement of the injured extremity as much as possible. For a fracture or dislocation, if medical care may be delayed or the victim must be moved, use a **splint** to immobilize the injured area, as described in **Chapter 15**.

Rest is also important for healing. The victim should follow the health care provider's advice to continue to rest the injured area after treatment.

Ice

Cold applied to a musculoskeletal injury reduces swelling, lessens pain and minimizes bruising. Broken blood vessels constrict, reducing the bleeding into tissues. Nerves are numbed by cold, thereby reducing pain. Cold also helps relieve muscle spasms.

For any musculoskeletal injury other than an open fracture, put ice or a cold pack on the injury as soon as possible. A plastic bag with an ice-water mix is preferred; a commercial cold pack or a cloth pad soaked in cold water can be used. A cold pack that undergoes a phase change (melts) is preferred to refreezable gel packs. The ice or cold pack should be wrapped in a damp cloth, or a damp cloth barrier placed between it and the skin, to prevent injury caused by cold in direct contact with the skin.

Cold works best if applied to the injury as soon as possible, preferably within 10 minutes. Apply the cold for 20 minutes (or 10 minutes if it produces discomfort), then remove it for 30 minutes. Repeat the process for 24 to 48 hours or until the victim receives medical help. For any injury for which the victim sees a health care provider, follow the provider's instructions for the use of cold (and later heat) after the injury and during the healing period **(Box 14-2)**.

Compression

Compression provides comfort and support and may prevent swelling. Compression of an injured extremity is done with an elastic roller bandage. Wrap the bandage over the injured area, starting at least 2 inches below the injury and using overlapping turns for at least 2 inches above the injury. The bandage should be firm but not so tight that it cuts off circulation. Compare the fingers or toes before the injury to those on the other extremity to ensure that circulation is not impeded by the bandage. If the fingers or toes look pale and feel cold compared with the other side or feel numb or tingling, loosen the bandage (see Skill: "Applying a Spiral Bandage," Skill: "Applying a Figure-Eight Bandage to the Wrist" and "Skill: Applying an Elastic Bandage to the Ankle").

BOX 14-2: COLD FIRST, HEAT LATER

People sometimes become confused about applying cold to an injury because they know heat is also used to treat musculoskeletal injuries. It is true that heat is beneficial for healing – just not soon after the injury.

Heat is beneficial for the healing of sprains and strains in part because it causes blood vessels to dilate or enlarge, which allows more blood to reach the injured area. This increased circulation helps speed up the body's healing processes.

But heat should not be used for about three days or until the initial swelling of the injury is diminished. Heat applied too early would have the opposite of the desired effect of cold: heat would encourage more internal bleeding because of the increased circulation, would increase swelling and would make nerve endings more sensitive to pain. Follow your health care provider's guidelines and wait at least 72 hours after the injury, or until the swelling goes down, before soaking the injured area in warm water or applying a heat pad.

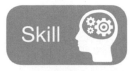
1 Anchor the starting end of the elastic roller bandage below the injured area, farther from the trunk.

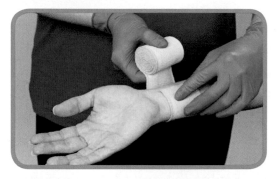

2 Wrap the bandage in spirals up the limb toward the center of the body.

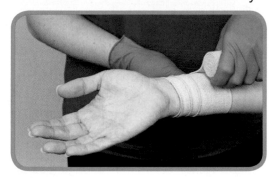

3 Fasten the end of the bandage with clips, tape or safety pins.

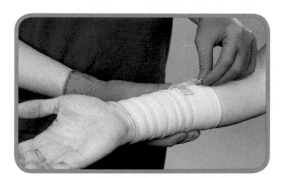

Skill 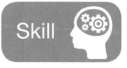 **Applying a Figure-Eight Bandage to the Wrist**

1 Anchor the starting end of the roller bandage.

2 Turn the bandage diagonally across the wrist and back around the hand.

3 Continue with overlapping figure-eight turns.

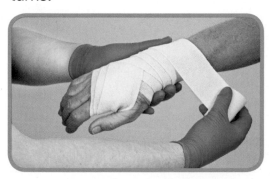

4 Fasten the end of the bandage by tying it or using clips, tape or safety pins.

14 • Bone, Joint and Muscle Injuries

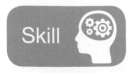

Skill   **Applying a Figure-Eight Bandage to the Ankle**

1 Anchor the starting end of the bandage.

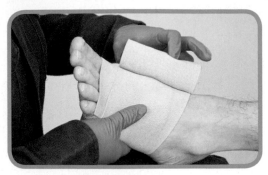

2 Turn the bandage diagonally across the top of foot and around the ankle and bring bandage the around in a figure-eight.

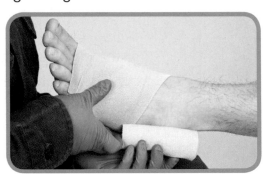

3 Continue with overlapping figure-eight turns.

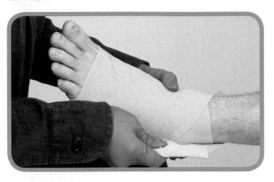

4 Fasten the end of the bandage with clips, tape or safety pins.

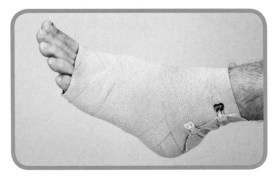

Learning Checkpoint 1

1. Use RICE for –

   a. most musculoskeletal injuries.

   b. fractures only.

   c. muscle injuries only.

   d. muscle and joint injuries only.

2. True or False: Putting a bag with an ice-water mixture or a commercial cold pack directly on the skin is the best way to relieve pain and reduce swelling.

3. What is important about how you apply a compression bandage?

   a. Using an elastic roller bandage

   b. Putting the cold pack under the bandage if needed

   c. Checking that circulation is not cut off

   d. All of the above

4. Describe the steps you would follow to use RICE for an injured ankle.

A compression bandage can also be applied around a cold pack. Remove the bandage just long enough to remove the cold pack after 20 minutes (or 10 minutes if it produces discomfort), and then rewrap it until it is time to apply cold again. Because in some cases swelling may increase after bandaging and cause the bandage to become tighter, it is necessary to continue checking the fingers or toes for circulation.

A compression bandage can be used for 24 to 48 hours as long as it is not too tight and the person can assess the injury to ensure that the bandage is not too tight.

Elevation

Elevating an injured arm or leg uses gravity to help slow the blood flow to the injury, thereby helping to minimize swelling and internal bleeding. First, apply cold and a compression bandage and then elevate the injured area above the level of the heart if possible **(Figure 14-4)**. Do not try to elevate an extremity with a suspected fracture or dislocation – or move it at all – without first splinting it as described in **Chapter 15.** In all cases, elevate the injured extremity only if moving the limb does not cause pain (see Skill: "RICE: Wrist Injury").

Fractures

A fracture is a broken bone. The bone may be completely broken with the pieces separated or still together, or it may only be cracked.

With a closed fracture the skin is not broken. Internal bleeding may occur. With an open fracture there is an open wound at the fracture site and the bone end may protrude through the wound **(Figure 14-5)**. An open fracture can be more serious because there is a greater chance of infection and more serious bleeding. **Figure 14-6** describes common types of fractures.

Although most fractures are not life-threatening, external or internal bleeding can be severe with fractures of large bones such as the femur (thigh bone). Nerves and organs nearby may also be injured. A fracture can also result in extended or

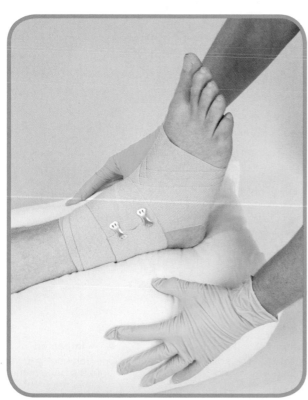

Figure 14-4 *Remember the acronym RICE for treatment of musculoskeletal injuries.*

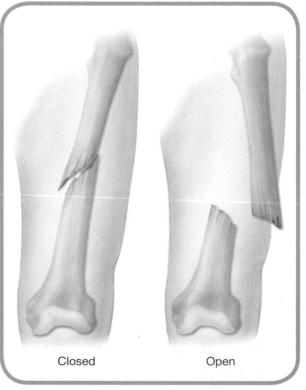

Closed   Open

Figure 14-5 *Closed and open fractures.*

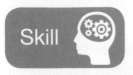

Skill — RICE: Wrist Injury

1 Rest the injured wrist.

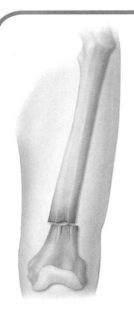

2 Put ice or a cold pack on the injured area.

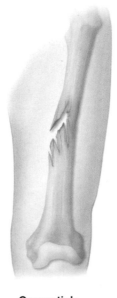

3 Compress the injured area with an elastic roller bandage.

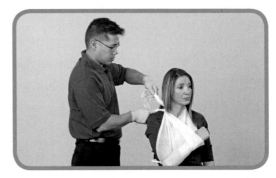

4 Elevate the injured area. Use a sling to hold the wrist in place.

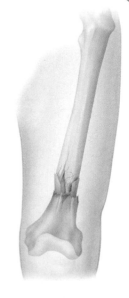

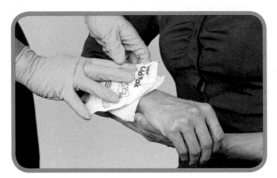
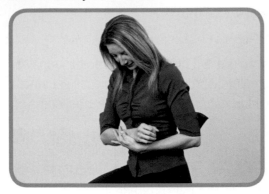
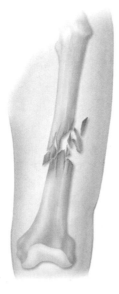
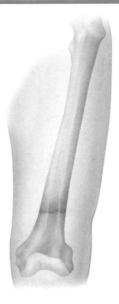
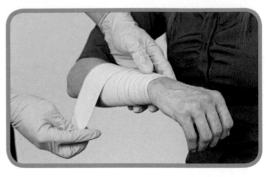

Transverse
The fracture line crosses the bone at a right angle.

Greenstick
An incomplete fracture and bending of bone that is more likely in children whose bones are soft.

Comminuted fracture
The bone is broken into more than two fragments.

Hairline fracture
The bone fragments do not separate.

Impacted
One fragment is driven into the bone of the other fragment.

Figure 14-6 *Common types of fractures.*

permanent disability. Fractures are more likely in elderly adults whose bones are often weaker due to osteoporosis, a gradual thinning of bone with aging. In more severe cases of osteoporosis, a bone may fracture with relatively little force.

A fracture causes pain, swelling, bruising, deformity and an inability to use the affected body part. You may hear or the victim may feel, the broken bone ends grating together. With severe bleeding the victim may also experience shock. With a fracture of a long bone like the femur, muscle spasms in the area may occur, possibly further damaging blood vessels or nerves. Check the victim first for any life-threatening conditions and then care for the fracture. Assess the victim's fingers or toes below the injury to determine if circulation has been disrupted; if so, call 9-1-1 immediately. Also call 9-1-1 for fractures of large bones or bones of the spine, head or trunk. The first aid for fractures includes resting and immobilizing the area, the use of ice or a cold pack, the use of a compression bandage (except for open fractures) and, when practical, elevating a splinted arm (never elevate a leg with a leg fracture). The victim needs to see a health care provider as soon as possible (see First Aid: "Fractures"). The splinting of specific injuries is described in **Chapter 15**.

Joint Injuries

In joints, bones are held in place by ligaments and other structures that allow for movement. Every joint allows a certain range of motion. Forcing a body part beyond the normal range of a joint, or in a direction in which the joint normally cannot move, causes a joint injury.

Injuries to joints include dislocations and sprains. In a dislocation, one or more bones have been moved out of their normal position in a joint; this usually involves the tearing of ligaments and other joint structures. In a sprain, the bones remain in place in the joint, but ligaments and other structures are injured. Both kinds of joint injuries often look similar to a fracture and may be just as

serious. When in doubt about the seriousness of any injury, assume the worst. Treat the injury as severe and call 9-1-1.

Dislocations

In a dislocation, one or more of the bones at the joint are displaced from their normal position when the ligaments that normally hold the bone in place are torn **(Figure 14-7)**. Dislocations typically result from strong forces and are sometimes accompanied by bone fractures or other serious injuries.

Pain, swelling and bruising usually occur. The victim is unable to use the joint because of both pain and structural damage in the joint. Because major blood vessels and nerves are located near joints in many parts of the body, a significant displacement of the bones can damage nearby nerves and cause serious bleeding. If the dislocation is severe, the joint or limb will look deformed. Dislocations can be serious because of the potential for nerve and blood vessel injury, which may be indicated by a loss of sensation or cool, pale skin in the extremity below the injury.

It is not always possible to tell a dislocation from a closed fracture, but the first aid is very similar for both. With severe bleeding, the victim may experience shock. Check the victim first for any life-threatening conditions and then care for the

(continues on page 222)

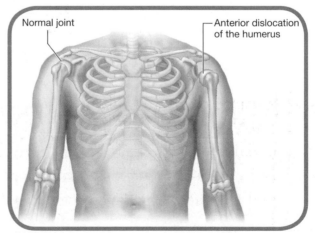

Figure 14-7 *In a dislocation, the bones at the joint are not in normal position.*

14 • Bone, Joint and Muscle Injuries

Fractures
Signs, Symptoms and Care

When You See

- **A deformed body part (compare to other side of body)**
- **Signs of pain**
- **Swelling or discoloration of skin**
- **Inability to use the body part**
- **Bone exposed in a wound**
- **Victim heard or felt a bone snap**
- **Possible signs and symptoms of shock**

Do This First

1 Immobilize the area. For an extremity, also immobilize the joints above and below the fracture.

2 Call 9-1-1 for a large bone fracture. A victim with a fracture in the hand or foot may be transported to the emergency department.

3 For an open fracture, cover the wound with a dressing and apply gentle pressure around the fracture area only if needed to control bleeding.

4 Apply RICE.

5 If help may be delayed or if the victim is to be transported, use a splint to keep the area immobilized (see **Chapter 15**). Elevate a splinted arm.

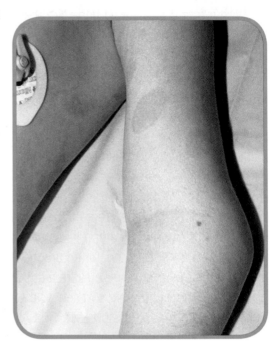

Additional Care

- Treat the victim for shock.
- Monitor the victim's breathing.
- Remove clothing and jewelry if they may cut off circulation as swelling occurs.

ALERT

- Do not try to align the ends of a broken bone.
- Do not put pressure on bone ends when controlling bleeding.
- Do not give the victim anything to eat or drink.

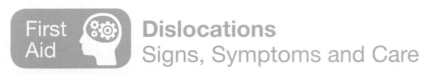
Dislocations
Signs, Symptoms and Care

When You See

- **The joint is deformed (compare to other side of body)**
- **Signs of pain**
- **Swelling**
- **Inability to use the body part**

Do This First

1 Immobilize the area in the position in which you find it.

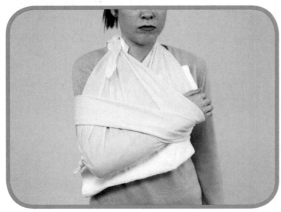

2 Call 9-1-1. A victim with a dislocated bone in the hand or foot may instead be transported to an emergency department.

3 Apply RICE, but do not use a compression bandage or elevate the injured area if moving the joint causes pain.

4 If help may be delayed or if the victim is to be transported, use a splint to keep the area immobilized in the position in which you find it (see **Chapter 15**).

Additional Care

- Treat the victim for shock if needed.
- Monitor the victim's breathing.
- Remove clothing and jewelry if they may cut off circulation as swelling occurs.

ALERT

- Do not try to put the displaced bone back in place.
- Do not let the victim eat or drink.

14 • Bone, Joint and Muscle Injuries

WHEN TO SEE A HEALTH CARE PROVIDER FOR A MUSCULOSKELETAL INJURY

Because you cannot always judge the type or severity of an injury by the signs and symptoms, you may be unsure about whether you need medical attention. You should see a health care provider if any of the following is true:

- You have the signs and symptoms of a fracture or dislocation.

- The injury causes severe pain.

- You cannot put any weight on an injured leg or walk more than a few steps without significant pain, or the leg buckles when you try to walk.

- An injured joint or the area around it is very tender to touch or feels numb.

- The injured area looks different from the same area on the other extremity (other than swelling).

- The injured joint cannot move.

- Redness or red streaks spread out from the injured area.

- An area that has been injured several times before is reinjured.

- You are unsure how serious an injury is or what treatment to give.

(continued from page 219)

dislocation. Assess the victim's fingers or toes below the injury to determine if circulation has been disrupted; if so, call 9-1-1 immediately. Except for a dislocation in the hand or foot, which can be immobilized so that the victim can be transported to a hospital, call 9-1-1 for a suspected dislocation. First aid includes resting and immobilizing the area, the use of ice or a cold pack, use of a compression bandage and, when practical, elevating a splinted hand or foot (see First Aid: "Dislocations"). The splinting of specific injuries is described in **Chapter 15**.

Sprains

A sprain is a joint injury involving the stretching or tearing of ligaments. Sprains typically occur when the joint is overextended or forced beyond the range of normal movement, as when the ankle is twisted by a sideways force on the foot. Sprains can range from mild to severe. The ankles, knees, wrists and fingers are the body parts most often sprained.

Sprains cause swelling, pain, bruising and an inability to use the joint because of the pain. The swelling may be considerable and often occurs rapidly. It can be difficult to tell a severe sprain from a fracture, but the first aid is similar for both. Check the victim first for any life-threatening conditions and then care for the sprain. Assess the victim's fingers or toes below the injury to determine if circulation has been disrupted; if so, call 9-1-1. Use RICE, immobilize the joint with a splint if the victim is to be moved and seek medical attention (see First Aid: "Sprains"). The splinting of specific sprains is described in **Chapter 15**.

REMOVING A RING

When an injury to the hand or fingers causes swelling, the victim's watch or rings can cut off circulation. Try to remove a watch and rings before swelling occurs. Removal of a ring is easier if you first soak the finger in cold water or wrap it in a cold pack, and then put oil or butter on the finger.

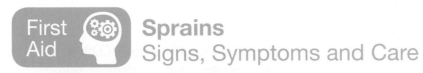

First Aid — Sprains
Signs, Symptoms and Care

When You See

- **Signs of pain**
- **Swollen joint**
- **Bruising of joint area**
- **Inability to use joint**

Do This First

1 Immobilize the area in the position in which you find it.

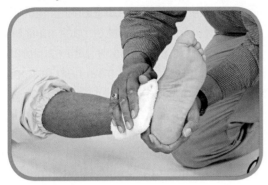

2 Apply RICE.

3 Use a soft splint (bandage, pillow or blanket) to immobilize and support the joint.

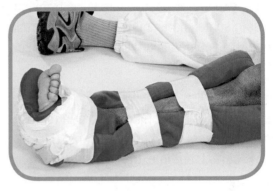

4 Seek medical attention

Additional Care

- Remove clothing or jewelry if they may cut off circulation as swelling occurs.

Learning Checkpoint 2

1. True or False: Call 9-1-1 for a fracture of a large bone such as the thigh bone.

2. When you are immobilizing a fracture injury, what body area should be immobilized?

   a. The immediate fracture area

   b. The fracture area and the joint above it

   c. The fracture area and the joints both above and below it

   d. The entire victim

3. True or False: For a fracture, you may also need to treat the victim for shock.

4. The signs and symptoms of a bone or joint injury include which of the following? (Check all that apply.)

   _____ Deformed area   _____ Pain

   _____ Small or unequal pupils   _____ Inability to use body part

   _____ Skin is hot and red   _____ Fever

   _____ Swelling   _____ Spasms and jerking of nearby muscles

5. True or False: A victim with a sprained ankle should "walk it off."

Muscle Injuries

Common muscle injuries include strains, contusions and cramps. These injuries are usually less serious than fractures and joint injuries. Muscle injuries are often easy to identify because, unlike sprains and dislocations, they do not usually involve the joint. Muscle injuries are typically caused by overexertion, careless or sudden uncoordinated movements, or poor body mechanics such as lifting a weight with back bent or twisted. Repetitive forces, as frequently occur in some sports, may also inflame or injure tendons. Repeated injury can lead to chronic problems.

Strains

A strain is a tearing of a muscle or a tendon, which connects the muscle to bone. Usually the tear is partial, but in extreme cases the muscle or tendon may tear completely. A strain occurs when the muscle is stretched too far by over-exerting the body area. The victim experiences pain, swelling and sometimes an inability to use the muscle. Back strains are common occupational injuries, and strains in extremities are common in sports. In most cases strains can be prevented by avoiding overexertion, using good body mechanics and following accepted guidelines for sports safety.

Use RICE to treat strains (see First Aid: "Strains"). Follow-up light exercise may help with healing and later muscle strengthening. With a very serious muscle or tendon tear, surgical repair may be required.

Contusions

A contusion is a bruised muscle that may result from a blow. The blow causes blood vessels within the muscle to rupture, leaking blood into the muscle tissue. This injury often occurs when the muscle is compressed between the object causing the blow and an underlying bone. Contusions cause pain, swelling and discoloration **(Figure 14-8)** and are treated with RICE (see First Aid: "Contusion"). The discoloration may persist up to a month.

Cramps

A muscle cramp is a tightening of a muscle that usually results from prolonged use but may occur with no apparent cause. Cramps are most common in the thigh and calf muscles, but they may also occur in abdominal or back muscles, in any muscle that is overused or with dehydration. These cramps are different from heat cramps, which result from fluid loss in hot environments (see **Chapter 20**). A cramp may last only a few seconds or up to 15 minutes. You may see the muscle bunching up or twitching under the skin. Cramps are treated with gentle stretching, a cold pack and massage after the cramping stops (see First Aid: "Muscle Cramp"). Cramps may be prevented with flexibility exercises and stretching before engaging in physical activity.

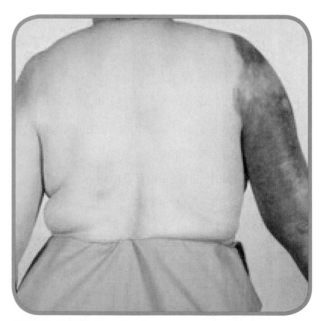

Figure 14-8 *Contusion.*

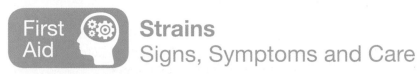

Strains
Signs, Symptoms and Care

When You See

- **Signs of dull or sharp pain when muscle is used**
- **Stiffness in the area of the injury**
- **Weakness or inability to use the muscle normally**

Do This First

1 Apply RICE.

2 Keep the cold pack on the area for 20 minutes (or 10 minutes if it produces discomfort), then remove it for at least 30 minutes.

Additional Care

- Seek medical attention if pain is severe or persistent, or if there is a significant or prolonged (3 days or more) impairment of function.

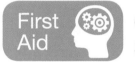

Contusion
Signs, Symptoms and Care

When You See

- **Signs of pain**
- **Swollen, tender area**
- **Skin discoloration (black and blue)**

Do This First

1 Apply RICE. Do not massage the muscle.

2 Keep the cold pack on the area for 20 minutes (or 10 minutes if it produces discomfort), then remove it for 30 minutes. Repeat the process for 24 to 48 hours as needed.

Additional Care

- Seek medical attention if pain is severe or impaired function persists.

14 • Bone, Joint and Muscle Injuries

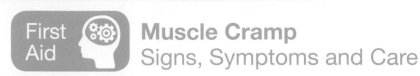

First Aid — Muscle Cramp
Signs, Symptoms and Care

When You See

- **Signs of muscle pain and tightness**

Do This First

1 Stop the activity.

2 Gently stretch out the muscle if possible.

3 Keep the cold pack on the area for 20 minutes (or 10 minutes if it produces discomfort), then remove it for 30 minutes.

4 Gently massage the muscle after active cramping stops, if this provides relief.

Additional Care

- Drink plenty of fluids such as sports drinks.

Learning Checkpoint 3

1. True or False: For a muscle strain, keep an ice pack on the injury for at least 2 hours.

2. True or False: Vigorous massage is the best treatment for a muscle contusion.

3. True or False: You can distinguish a contusion from a fracture because only a contusion causes an area of skin discoloration.

4. Name three things you can do to ease a muscle cramp.

Concluding Thoughts

Millions of people every year go to the emergency department with musculoskeletal injuries. Countless others sustain less serious injuries that do not require a health care provider's attention. Most people will experience at least one sprain or strain in their lifetime and will also care for another person with such an injury. Fortunately, most of these injuries are not life-threatening or very severe and the victim recovers well. Giving the appropriate first aid, however, is important for making a good recovery without future disability. Remember that you do not have to know the exact nature of the injury before helping: Use RICE (Rest, Ice, Compression, Elevation) for most injuries, and call 9-1-1 or seek medical attention for more serious injuries.

Learning Outcomes

You should now be able to do the following:

1. Describe ways to prevent common sports and recreational injuries.

2. Explain what to look for when assessing musculoskeletal injuries.

3. Demonstrate how to use RICE to care for a musculoskeletal injury.

4. Describe the first aid for fractures, dislocations and sprains.

5. Explain the differences among strains, contusions and cramps and describe the first aid for each.

Review Questions

1. Steps to help prevent sports and recreational injuries include –

   a. maintaining a healthy weight.

   b. wearing shoes that fit properly.

   c. wearing protective equipment.

   d. All of the above

2. What is true about swelling in most musculoskeletal injuries?

   a. Swelling occurs because of internal bleeding in tissues.

   b. Swelling occurs with all injuries except fractures.

   c. The amount of swelling indicates the seriousness of the injury.

   d. Swelling should be promoted because it aids healing.

3. Cold is best applied to a musculoskeletal injury by –

   a. an ice-water mixture.

   b. a gel pack.

   c. a bag of frozen peas.

   d. All of the above

4. Which statement is generally true of treatment for a musculoskeletal injury?

   a. Apply heat for up to 2 days, then apply cold.

   b. Apply cold for up to 2 days, then apply heat.

   c. Apply cold for the first 12 hours, then apply heat.

   d. Apply cold and heat alternating every 6 hours.

5. The purpose of using a compression bandage on a musculoskeletal injury is to –

   a. dress the injured area.

   b. cut off circulation to the area.

   c. help support injury and prevent swelling.

   d. prevent infection.

14 • Bone, Joint and Muscle Injuries

6. The most important aspect of fracture care is to –

   a. apply antibiotic ointment to an open fracture.

   b. put the bone ends together in their normal position.

   c. apply traction to prevent shortening of the limb.

   d. immobilize the area.

7. What should not be done to a dislocation?

   a. Apply ice or a cold pack on the joint.

   b. Try to move the bone ends back into their normal position in the joint.

   c. Apply a compression bandage over the joint if it is in an extremity.

   d. Prevent the victim from moving the joint.

8. To assess for circulation in the foot when the victim has an ankle injury, –

   a. check the toes for color, temperature and sensation.

   b. ask the victim to push against your hand with his or her foot.

   c. determine whether the victim can stand without feeling pain.

   d. have the victim take a few steps and report whether his or her toes tingle.

9. A strain occurs when a muscle –

   a. is bruised by a blunt blow.

   b. is separated from ligaments in a joint.

   c. is stretched too far (overexertion).

   d. becomes dehydrated.

10. First aid for a muscle cramp may include –

   a. returning to activity as soon as possible.

   b. massaging the muscle.

   c. applying a heat pad.

   d. soaking the extremity in icy water.

Chapter 15 • Extremity Injuries and Splinting

Chapter Preview

- Types of Splints
- Guidelines for Splinting
- Applying Slings
- Splinting Extremity Injuries

Your young daughter is playing with two friends on the playground while you watch from a nearby bench. While climbing up a climbing structure, she loses her grip and tumbles to the ground. Although she falls only a couple feet, she lands hard on her arm. When you reach her a few seconds later, she is crying and clutching her arm tightly. What do you do?

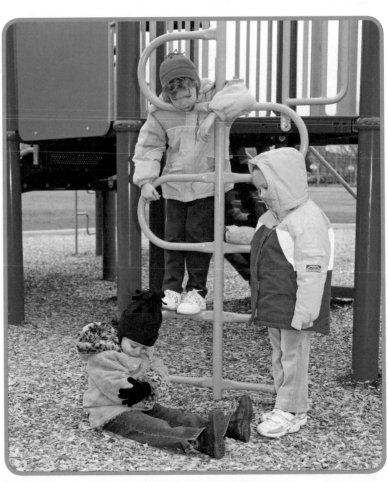

As described in **Chapter 14**, with most musculoskeletal injuries there is a risk of movement worsening the injury and causing more pain. All such injuries should be stabilized to prevent movement. When a victim has a fracture, dislocation or sprain in an arm or leg, the arm or leg may be splinted if there is a risk for moving the injured area unless help is expected within a few minutes. Always splint an extremity before transporting the victim to a health care provider or the emergency department. Splinting helps prevent further injury, reduces pain, and minimizes bleeding and swelling. Splints can be improvised when needed and tied in place with bandages, belts, neckties or strips of cloth torn from clothing.

This chapter describes splinting and other first aid for specific musculoskeletal injuries of the arms and legs. Remember always to first check the victim's breathing and provide care for life-threatening conditions. Consider the forces involved in the injury and whether a spinal injury may be present. If you suspect a spinal injury, the priority is to support the head and neck and prevent spinal movement. Because splinting a fracture may involve moving some part of the victim or may distract from care given for the spinal injury, unless multiple rescuers are present, leave an extremity injury unsplinted while waiting for help to arrive.

Types of Splints

A splint is any object you can use to help keep an injured body area from moving. Various kinds of commercial splints are available and are used by professional rescuers, but splints can also be made from many different materials at hand. There are three general types of splints **(Figure 15-1)**:

- **Rigid splints** may be made from a board, a cane or walking stick, a broom handle, a piece of plastic or metal, a rolled newspaper or magazine, or thick cardboard.

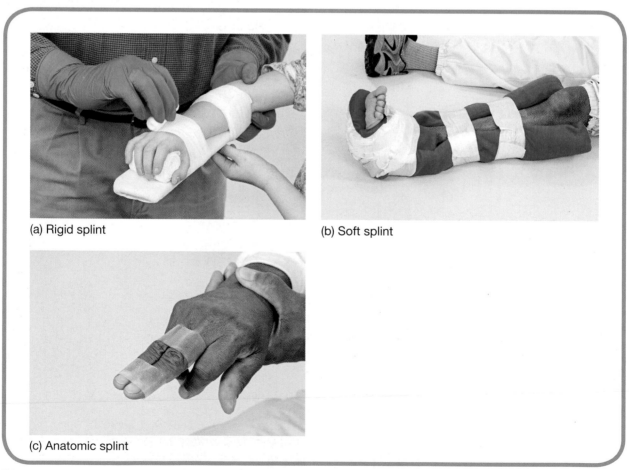

(a) Rigid splint

(b) Soft splint

(c) Anatomic splint

Figure 15-1 *Examples of general types of splints.*

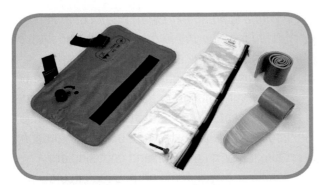

Figure 15-2 *Commercial splints.*

- **Soft splints** may be made from a pillow, a folded blanket or towel, or a triangular bandage folded into a sling.

- **Anatomic splints** involve splinting one part of the body with another part, such as an injured leg to the uninjured leg, or splinting fingers together or splinting the arm to the chest to immobilize the shoulder.

The splint is the object to which the injured extremity is secured to prevent movement. The splint is usually secured by wrapping bandages, strips of cloth (often called **cravats**), Velcro straps or other materials around the splint and extremity. Because you may have to loosen or remove a splint if it interferes with circulation to the limb, use knots that can be untied if needed. If tape is used, do not tape to the skin directly; instead, put a dressing or other material over the skin first or fold the sticky side back on itself.

In addition to common rigid and soft splints, commercial splints are available that are typically used by rescuers with more training. **Figure 15-2** shows some examples of commercial splints.

Guidelines for Splinting

Regardless of the specific type of injury and its location, always apply the following general guidelines for splinting. Later sections in this chapter show how to use these guidelines when splinting specific extremity injuries.

- *Put a dressing on any open wound before splinting the area.* This helps protect the wound, control bleeding and prevent infection.

- *Splint an injury only if it does not cause more pain for the victim.* Splinting usually involves touching and perhaps manipulating the injured area, which may cause pain and may worsen the injury. If the victim complains, stop the splinting and have the victim immobilize the area as well as possible until help arrives.

- *Splint the injury in the position in which you find it* **(Figure 15-3)**. Trying to straighten out a limb or joint will likely cause pain and could worsen the injury. Blood vessels or nerves near a fracture or dislocation, for example, could be damaged by moving the bone ends. In almost all cases the injured extremity can be splinted in the position in which you find it, as shown later in this chapter. Only if the victim is in a remote location and will not receive medical attention for a long time, or if circulation has been cut off in the extremity by the injury, should the limb be straightened (see **Chapter 23**).

- *Splint to immobilize the entire injured area.* For example, the splint should extend to the joints above and below the injured area. With a bone fracture near a joint, assume that the joint is injured, as well, and extend the splint well beyond the joint to keep it and the fracture site immobilized.

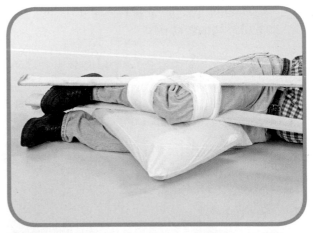

Figure 15-3 *Splint an injury in the position found, such as this knee injury. Do not try to straighten the limb to splint it.*

- *Put padding such as cloth between the splint and the victim's skin.* This is especially important with rigid splints, which otherwise may press into soft tissues and cause pain and further injury. Use whatever materials are at hand that will conform to the space between the splint and the body part. Pad body hollows and ensure that the area of the splint close to the injury is well padded.

- *Put splints on both sides of a fractured bone if possible.* If the injury makes this difficult or splinting materials are limited, splint one side.

- *Do not secure the splint on an open wound because the securing bandage or strap could cut into or irritate the wound.* Tie the bandages or other materials used to hold the splint in place on both sides of the wound.

- *Elevate the splinted extremity if possible.* Do not move the injured area to elevate it if it causes the victim pain or may worsen the injury.

- *Apply a cold pack to the injury around the splint.* Because the ice or cold pack must be removed after 20 minutes, it should not be positioned inside the splint. Placing it inside would require removal and repositioning of the splint. This may cause pain and movement in the injured area. Splint the injury first and then position the cold pack as close to the injury as possible around the splint **(Figure 15-4)**.

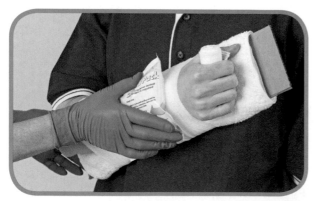

Figure 15-4 *Apply a cold pack to the injured area around the splint.*

- *With a splinted extremity, do not completely bandage over the fingers or toes, and check them frequently to make sure circulation is not cut off.* To be effective, the splint must be tied firmly enough to the extremity to prevent movement but not so tight that circulation is cut off. Swelling, pale or bluish discoloration, tingling or numbness, and cold skin are signs and symptoms of reduced circulation. If any of these occurs, the splint should be removed or the bandages holding the limb to the splint should be loosened. Periodically check for adequate circulation.

Applying Slings

A **sling** is a device used to support and immobilize the upper extremity. A sling may be used for most upper extremity injuries, including those to the shoulder, upper and lower arm, elbow, and wrist. When available, a sling is best made from a large, triangular bandage, but improvised slings can be made from many other materials, such as strips of cloth torn from clothing, neckties and so on. Cloth or soft, flexible material is generally best.

A sling is used to prevent movement of the arm and shoulder, thereby preventing a worsening of the injury, helping to limit pain, and elevating the extremity to help control bleeding and swelling. In some instances a binder is used along with the sling. A binder (or swathe) is an additional supportive bandage or cloth tied over the sling and around the chest to provide additional support (see Skill: "Applying an Arm Sling and Binder").

Follow these guidelines when using a sling:

- *Splint the injury first, when appropriate.* A fracture of the upper or lower arm or a dislocation of the elbow or wrist should be splinted to prevent movement of the area. Then a sling is applied to provide additional support and to keep the injury elevated.

- *If you splint the injury in the position found, and this position makes the use of a sling impossible or difficult, do not try to use a sling.*

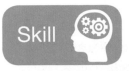

Skill   Applying an Arm Sling and Binder

1 Secure the point of the bandage at the elbow. Use a safety pin or tie the point at the elbow.

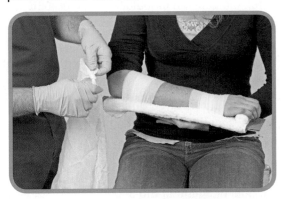

2 Position the triangular bandage.

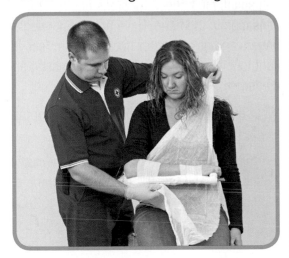

3 Bring up the lower end of the bandage to the opposite side of the neck.

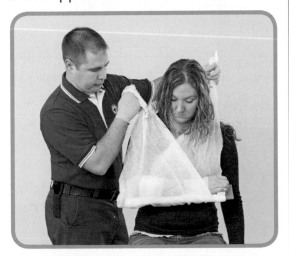

4 Tie the ends. Pad under the knot.

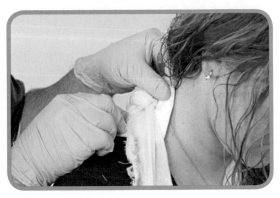

5 Tie a binder bandage over the sling and around the chest.

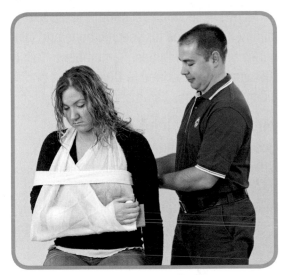

- *Do not move the arm into position for a sling if this causes the victim more pain.* If so, splint the arm in the position found, not using a sling, and have the victim immobilize it until help arrives.

- *A cold pack can be used inside the sling.* Follow the standard guidelines for applying and removing the cold pack and then reapplying it later (see **Chapter 14**).

- *Do not cover the fingers inside the sling.* Ensure circulation in the extremity periodically by checking the fingers for color, temperature and normal sensation.

Splinting Extremity Injuries

The following sections describe first aid and splinting techniques for specific bone and joint injuries of the extremities. Remember to follow the RICE acronym described in **Chapter 14** and the splinting guidelines listed earlier.

Upper Extremity Injuries

Upper extremity injuries include fractures, dislocations and sprains of the shoulder, upper arm, elbow, lower elbow, wrist and hand. Remember the general principle to splint only if help will be delayed and there is a risk of the injured area moving (or a victim with an injured hand or foot is to be transported).

Shoulder Injuries

Shoulder injuries can fracture the clavicle (collar bone), the scapula (shoulder blade) or joint structures. The clavicle is the most frequently fractured bone in the body. Victims have pain and cannot use the shoulder, which often is lower than the opposite shoulder. Swelling and tenderness are present. Fractures of the scapula are very rare. Dislocations of the shoulder are common and cause pain, deformity of the shoulder and an inability to move it.

The goal of splinting the shoulder is to stabilize the area from the trunk to the upper arm with a soft splint. First check for signs of circulation and sensation in the hand. Have the victim wiggle the fingers and ask whether he or she can feel your light touch on the palm. Then apply a sling and binder.

1. Use a soft, not rigid, splint for shoulder injuries. Do not move the extremity.

2. Check for signs of circulation and sensation in the hand and fingers. If they are absent, call 9-1-1 for immediate care.

 Learning Checkpoint 1

1. You encounter a victim with an obviously fractured forearm. What materials might you be able to find around the home that you can use to make a rigid splint?

   _____

2. When using splints, which of the following are actions you should take? (Check all that apply.)

   _____ Put a heating pad on the area.   _____ Pad the splint.

   _____ Straighten out a limb before splinting it.   _____ Put a cold pack around the splint.

   _____ Dress an open wound before splinting.   _____ Splint in the position found.

3. List signs that circulation has been cut off in an extremity below the splint:

   _____

4. Name two things you should *not* do when contemplating putting a victim's arm in a sling:

   _____

3. Pad the hollow between the body and the arm with a small pillow or towels, and apply a sling and binder to support the arm and immobilize it against the chest if this does not cause pain **(Figure 15-5)**. If moving the arm closer to the chest causes pain, use a larger pillow between the arm and the trunk.

4. Follow the general guidelines for safe splinting. Check the fingers periodically for circulation.

Upper Arm Injuries

Fractures of the **humerus**, the bone of the upper arm, cause pain, swelling and deformity of the arm. Fractures near the shoulder should be treated in a manner identical to shoulder injuries, with soft splinting.

The goal of splinting the upper arm is to stabilize the bone between the shoulder and the elbow by using a rigid splint on the outside of the arm and placing the wrist in a sling. The fracture site can then be further secured by applying a wide binder around the arm and chest. Be careful not to apply the binder directly over the fracture site.

1. Check for signs of circulation and sensation in the hand and fingers. If they are absent, call 9-1-1 for immediate care.

2. Apply a rigid splint along the outside of the upper arm, tied above and below the injury.

3. Support the wrist with a sling and then apply a wide binder to support the arm and immobilize it against the chest **(Figure 15-6)**. If it causes pain to raise the wrist for a sling, a long, rigid splint may be used that supports the arm in a straighter position.

4. Follow the general guidelines for safe splinting. Check the fingers periodically for circulation.

Elbow Injuries

The elbow can be injured by a blow or force that moves the joint beyond its normal limits. Sprains and dislocations are the most common injuries to the joint itself. Fractures of the bones above or below the elbow are also common. Nerves and arteries pass close to the bones of the elbow and may also be injured. Usually the victim is unable to move the joint and may say the joint is "locked."

The goal of splinting the elbow is to stabilize the joint from the upper arm to the forearm in the position in which you find it. If the elbow is bent, a soft splint with sling and binder may be sufficient, but a rigid splint provides greater stability. If the elbow is straight, a rigid splint should be applied.

1. Check for signs of circulation and sensation in the hand and fingers. If they are absent, call 9-1-1 for immediate care.

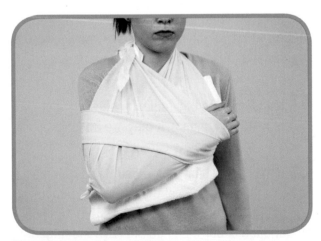

Figure 15-5 *Immobilize a shoulder injury with a sling and binder.*

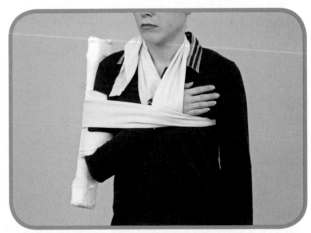

Figure 15-6 *Immobilize an upper arm injury with a splint, sling and binder.*

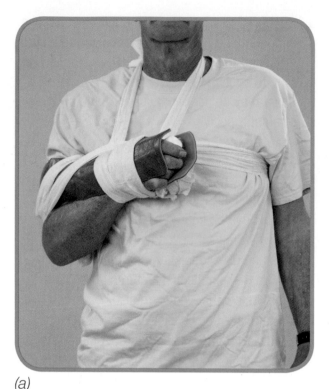
(a)

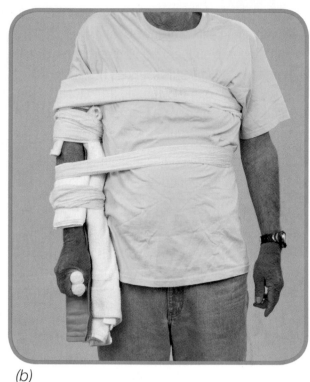
(b)

Figure 15-7 *Immobilize an elbow injury with a rigid splint in the position found. (a) Splinting a bent elbow. (b) Splinting a straight elbow.*

2. If the elbow is bent, apply a rigid splint from the upper arm to the wrist as shown in **Figure 15-7a**. If more support is needed, use a sling at the wrist and a binder around the chest at the upper arm.

3. If the elbow is straight, apply a rigid splint from the upper arm to the hand as shown in **Figure 15-7b**. If more support is needed, binders may be used around the chest and upper arm and around the lower arm and waist.

4. Follow the general guidelines for safe splinting. Check the fingers periodically for circulation.

Forearm Injuries

The forearm is frequently injured by direct blows that may fracture either or both bones. Pain, swelling and deformity typically result.

The goal of forearm splinting is to stabilize and support the area from the elbow to the hand. You may use a splint on the palm side of the forearm or on both sides. After splinting the arm, secure it with a sling and binder (see Skill: "Splinting the Forearm").

Wrist Injuries

Common wrist injuries include sprains and fractures. Movement of the wrist produces pain. Swelling, discoloration and deformity may be present.

Wrist injuries should be stabilized from the forearm to the hand. In some cases a soft splint is sufficient, with the area then elevated and supported with a sling. A rigid splint provides more support and the joint is stabilized in a manner similar to a forearm injury.

1. Check for signs of circulation and sensation in the hand and fingers. If they are absent, call 9-1-1 for immediate care.

2. Apply a rigid splint on the palm side of the arm from the forearm past the fingertips, tied above and below the wrist. If available, add a roller bandage under the fingers. Leave the fingers uncovered.

Skill 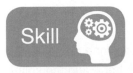 **Splinting the Forearm**

1 Support the arm above and below the injury. Check circulation.

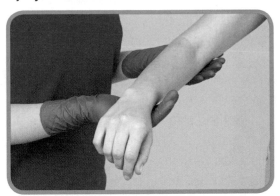

2 Position the arm on a padded rigid splint. If available, add a roller bandage under the fingers.

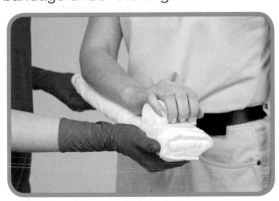

3 Secure the splint.

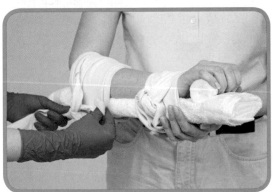

4 Check circulation.

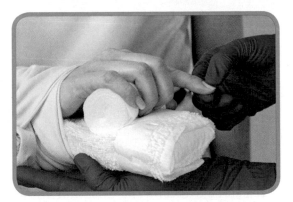

5 Put the arm in a sling and tie a binder over the sling and around the chest.

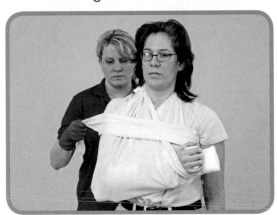

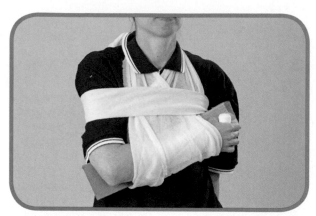

Figure 15-8 *Immobilize an injured wrist with a splint, sling and binder.*

3. Support the forearm and wrist with a sling, then apply a binder around the upper arm and chest **(Figure 15-8)**.

4. Follow the general guidelines for safe splinting. Check the fingers periodically for circulation.

Hand and Finger Injuries

The hand may be injured by a direct blow. Fractures often occur, for example, when the victim punches something with a closed fist. Pain and swelling of the hand typically result.

An injured hand may be immobilized with a soft or rigid splint. First, place a roll of gauze or similar padding in the palm, allowing the fingers to take a naturally curled position. The entire hand is then bandaged, leaving the fingers exposed if possible to check for circulation. Place a rigid splint on the palm side of the hand extending from above the wrist to the fingers, the same as for a wrist injury. Pad the area well between the hand and the splint. Then support the injury further with a sling and binder.

Finger injuries include fractures and dislocations. Both are common in both sports and industrial injuries. Often a splint is not required, but victims with a painful injury will benefit from splinting. Use a soft splint if the person cannot straighten the finger without pain. Do not try to manipulate the finger to move a bone into its normal position. Use a rigid splint such as a tongue depressor or ice cream stick secured in place with tape, or make an anatomic splint by taping the finger to an adjoining finger with gauze in between **(Figure 15-9)**.

Lower Extremity Injuries

Lower extremity injuries include fractures, dislocations and sprains of the hip, upper leg, knee, lower leg, ankle and foot. Because the bones of the thigh and lower leg are larger than those of the arm, larger forces are typically involved in these injuries. This means that there is a greater risk that a spinal injury may have occurred. Assess the victim carefully, being careful not to move the extremity. A fracture of the femur, the large bone of the thigh, can also damage the large femoral artery and cause life-threatening bleeding. Remember the general principle to splint only if help will be delayed and there is a risk of the injured area moving (or a victim with an injured foot is to be transported).

Learning Checkpoint 2

1. For an injured shoulder, use a _____ splint.

2. A splint for a fracture of the forearm should extend from the _____ to the _____.

3. Why is a binder used over a sling?

   a. To prevent movement and give additional support

   b. To pull the fractured bone ends back into position

   c. To promote good circulation

   d. All of the above

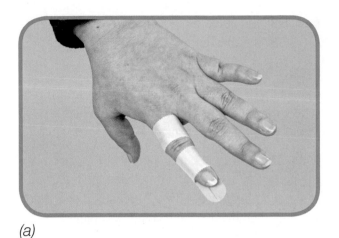

(a)

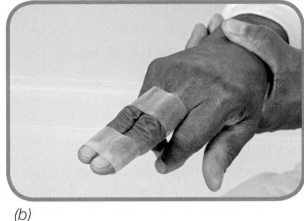

(b)

Figure 15-9 *Splint a finger injury. (a) Rigid splint. (b) Anatomic splint.*

Hip Injuries

The hip is the joint where the top of the femur meets the pelvis. Hip injuries include fractures and, less commonly, dislocations. A hip fracture is actually a fracture of the top part of the **femur**. Hip fractures are more common in the elderly, whose bones are often more brittle because **osteoporosis**, a loss of calcium from bones, is common in old age and because some older people are less stable and more likely to experience a fall. Bleeding and pain may be severe.

Hip dislocations can occur at any age. The victim feels pain and cannot move the joint. Hip dislocations result from falls, vehicular crashes and blows to the body.

First aid is similar to that for a pelvic injury, from which it is often difficult to differentiate a hip injury. Do not move the victim and immobilize the leg and hip in the position in which you find it. Call 9-1-1 immediately. Immobilize the victim's legs by padding between the legs with a soft pillow or blanket and gently bandaging them together, unless this causes more pain. Treat the victim for shock but do not elevate the legs.

Upper Leg Injuries

Fractures of the femur are serious because bleeding even with a closed injury can be profuse. The victim experiences severe pain and may be in shock. Swelling and deformity are common.

Call 9-1-1 immediately for a fracture of the femur and keep the victim from moving. If the victim is lying down with the leg supported by the ground, a rigid splint may be unnecessary. Provide additional support with folded blankets or coats to immobilize the leg in the position found. If help may be delayed, splinting can be used to stabilize the injury. To use an anatomic splint, pad between the legs, move the uninjured leg beside the injured one and carefully tie the legs together (see Skill: "Anatomic Splinting of Leg").

A rigid splint provides better support if needed:

1. Check for signs of circulation and sensation in the foot and toes.

2. If possible, put a rigid splint on each side of the leg. Pad bony areas and voids between the leg and the splints. The inside splint should extend

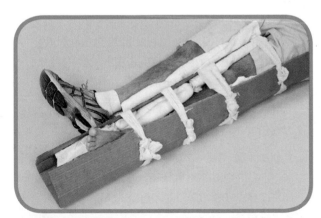

Figure 15-10 *Splinting a fractured femur.*

| 239

from the groin past the foot and the outside from the armpit past the foot.

3. Tie the splints with cravats or bandages **(Figure 15-10)**.

4. Follow the general guidelines for safe splinting. Check the toes periodically for circulation.

Knee Injuries

The most common knee injuries are sprains, but dislocations also occur. These injuries commonly result from sports injuries, motor vehicle crashes and falls. With large forces the knee can actually be dislocated, which is a serious emergency because nearby nerves and blood vessels are often injured as well. In addition, fractures of the end of the femur or the tibia or fibula (the bones of the lower leg) can be indistinguishable from other knee injuries. Dislocations of the patella (kneecap) may be mistaken for knee dislocations because they too cause the knee to appear deformed.

Knee injuries cause pain and an inability to move the knee. The knee joint may appear to be "locked." Swelling is usually present with or without bruising. With a dislocation the knee may be deformed or angulated.

Do not try to transport a victim with a knee injury; instead, call 9-1-1. With any knee injury, the knee should be splinted in the position found. A soft splint can be applied by rolling a blanket or placing a pillow around the knee. If the knee is straight, you can make an anatomical splint by tying the upper and lower leg to the unaffected leg. Rigid splints provide additional support. If the knee is straight, ideally two splints are applied along both sides of the knee. If the knee is bent, splint the joint in the position found.

1. Check for signs of circulation and sensation in the foot and toes.

2. If possible, put a rigid splint on each side of the leg in the position found. Pad bony areas and voids between the leg and the splints.

3. Tie the splints with cravats or bandages.

4. Follow the general guidelines for safe splinting. Check the toes periodically for circulation.

Lower Leg Injuries

Injuries to the lower leg commonly result from sports, motor vehicle crashes and falls. Either or both of the bones of the lower leg can be fractured.

Do not move or transport a victim with a lower leg injury. Call 9-1-1 and immobilize the leg from the knee to the ankle. Either a soft splint or a rigid splint may be used. A rigid splint is applied the same as for a knee injury; a three-sided cardboard splint can also be used **(Figure 15-11)**. Be sure not to tie the splint over the fracture site.

A leg fracture can be splinted using either a rigid splint or an anatomic splint (see Skill: "Anatomic Splinting of Leg"). A similar anatomic splint can be used for an upper leg fracture, with the bandages tied higher (including the hips).

Ankle Injuries

The most common ankle injury is a sprain, which typically occurs when the foot is forcefully twisted to one side. The victim experiences pain and swelling of the ankle. The swelling can be significant and the victim is unable to put weight on the ankle due to pain. Fracture or dislocation may also occur, often involving torn ligaments and possibly also nerve and blood vessel damage.

Usually a soft splint is best for ankle injuries, along with having the victim avoid the use of the foot and leg:

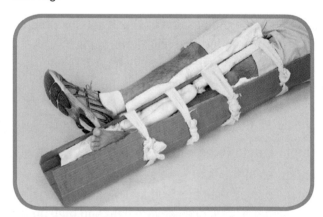

Figure 15-11 *Rigid splinting of a lower leg fracture using cardboard.*

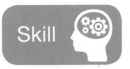 **Skill** **Anatomic Splinting of Leg**

1 Check circulation. Gently slide four or five bandages or strips of cloth under both legs. Do not put a bandage over the injury site.

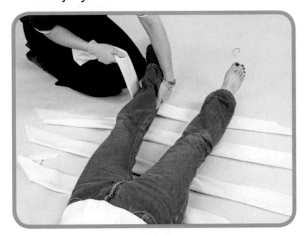

2 Put padding between the legs. Do not move the injured leg.

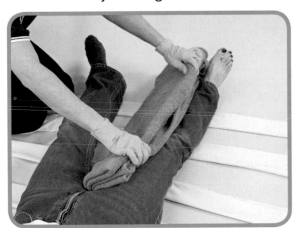

3 Gently slide the uninjured leg next to the injured leg.

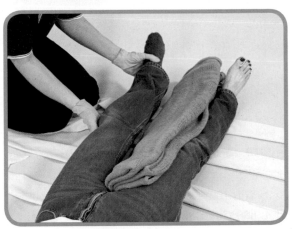

4 Tie the bandages (snug but not tight), starting in the middle, then at the lower leg and then at the top. Check circulation.

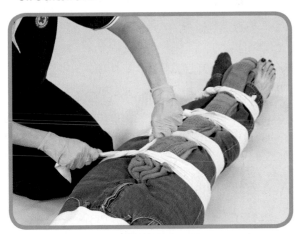

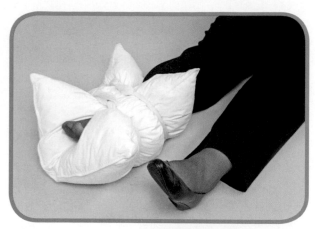

Figure 15-12 *Soft splint for an ankle injury.*

1. Gently remove the shoe to check for circulation, unless this causes significant pain.

2. Position the foot in the middle of a soft pillow and fold the pillow around the ankle.

3. Using cravats or bandages, tie the pillow around the foot and lower leg **(Figure 15-12)**.

4. Check for signs of circulation and sensation in the foot and toes. If they are absent, call 9-1-1 for immediate care.

5. Follow the general guidelines for safe splinting. Check the toes periodically for circulation.

Foot Injuries

Foot injuries most commonly result from direct blows to the foot or from falls. Foot injuries may involve almost any bone or ligament of the foot. Foot injuries should be treated identically to ankle injuries.

Fractures of the toes can be quite painful. The toe often is swollen, tender and discolored. Usually no splinting is required. If the toe is significantly bent, more than one toe is involved or the foot is very painful, a pillow splint can be used as for an ankle injury.

Learning Checkpoint 3

1. You come upon a scene where a woman on a bicycle apparently ran into a light post. She is lying on the ground and says she has severe pain in her lower leg below the knee. You cannot tell whether the bone is broken, but there is no open wound and she says she cannot move her leg. What should you do?

_____

2. A victim with a fracture of the femur may also experience what other condition?

a. Severe bleeding

b. Open or closed wound

c. Shock

d. All of the above

3. Explain when you may use two rigid splints.

_____

Concluding Thoughts

Although this chapter details how to splint all the different areas of the extremities, it is most important to remember the key principles of splinting for any body area:

- Splint only if help may be delayed (or the victim is to be transported for a hand or foot injury) and there is a risk of the area moving.

- Do not splint if it causes more pain.

- Splint an injury in the position found.

- Splint to immobilize the entire area.

- Check the circulation below the injury and splint.

- Call 9-1-1 or seek medical attention.

Learning Outcomes

You should now be able to do the following:

1. Describe the three general types of splints and how to improvise splints with common materials.

2. List the general guidelines for splinting and the use of arm slings.

3. Describe how to splint the different areas of the upper and lower extremities.

4. Demonstrate how to apply an arm sling.

5. Demonstrate how to apply a rigid splint to an injured forearm.

6. Demonstrate how to use an anatomic splint for a leg injury.

Review Questions

1. Which of the following could make an effective rigid splint?

    a. A board

    b. A rolled magazine

    c. A walking stick

    d. All of the above

2. Which statement is true about how splints should be applied?

    a. Tape the splint tightly in place.

    b. For greatest support, tie a cravat directly over the wound.

    c. Straighten the limb as much as possible before splinting.

    d. Dress an open wound before splinting the area.

3. Which is a sign of reduced circulation below an injury?

    a. Cold skin

    b. Hot skin

    c. Red skin

    d. Itching skin

4. Where is a cold pack applied to a splinted open injury?

    a. Outside the dressing but under the bandage and splint

    b. Outside the dressing and bandage but under the splint

    c. Around the splint

    d. Cold packs are not used with splints.

5. How is an injured elbow splinted when you find it in a bent position?

    a. Gently straighten the arm and use a long, rigid splint from shoulder to hand.

    b. Gently bend the elbow to 90 degrees and put it in a sling.

    c. Keep the elbow in its original bent position and use a rigid splint from the upper arm to the hand.

    d. Do not splint the arm, but bind it directly to the chest with bandages.

6. How is an injured hand positioned for splinting?

    a. Let the fingers curl naturally around a soft padding in the palm.

    b. Ask the victim to make a fist before bandaging the hand.

    c. Straighten out the fingers on the surface of a rigid splint.

    d. Keep the fingers spread wide apart with bandaging and padding between them.

7. How can you tell the difference between a hip displacement and a hip fracture?

    a. A fracture is more painful than a displacement.

    b. With a fracture, you can still move the leg, but not with a displacement.

    c. With a displacement the leg is in an unusual position, but not with a fracture.

    d. You cannot easily tell the difference between a displacement and a fracture.

8. With which of these injuries is it safe for the victim to attempt to walk?

    a. Ankle sprain

    b. Ankle displacement

    c. Ankle fracture

    d. None of the above

Chapter 16 • Sudden Illness

Chapter Preview

- General Care for Sudden Illness
- Heart Attack
- Angina
- Stroke
- Respiratory Distress

- Fainting
- Seizures
- Altered Mental Status
- Diabetic Emergencies
- Severe Abdominal Pain

Returning to your office after lunch, you find a co-worker leaning over her desk looking ill. Her breathing is labored and noisy. You ask her what is wrong and she says she doesn't know but she feels like she can't breathe. She pauses, gasping, between words. Her skin is pale. What do you do?

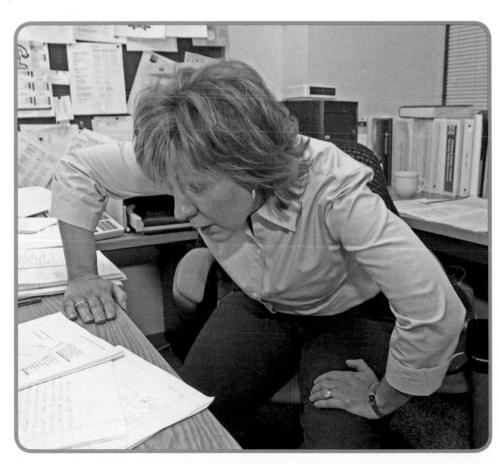

Most chapters in this text involve first aid for injuries. Illness too can cause an emergency, especially if the person becomes ill suddenly. With most illnesses, a person has time to see a health care provider long before the illness becomes an emergency, but with the specific health problems described in this chapter, the emergency may develop very quickly. Lifesaving action by first aiders and others at the scene is often needed. Because some sudden illnesses, such as a heart attack, may occur with little or no warning and can result in death within minutes if no action is taken, it is important to be aware of the common signs and symptoms and to be prepared to act any time in any place.

General Care for Sudden Illness

Many different illnesses can occur suddenly and become medical emergencies. In some cases you may know or suspect the cause of the problem, such as when a heart attack victim clutches his or her chest and complains of a crushing pressure before collapsing. In other cases neither you nor the victim may know the cause of the problem. The general first aid principles are the same for all sudden illness emergencies, however, so you do not have to know what the victim's illness is before you give first aid.

Following are common general signs and symptoms of sudden illness:

- Person feels ill, dizzy, confused or weak
- Skin color changes (flushed, pale or ashen), sweating
- Breathing changes
- Nausea or vomiting

Following are the general steps to follow for any sudden illness:

1. Call 9-1-1 for unexplained sudden illness.
2. Help the victim rest and avoid becoming chilled or overheated.
3. Reassure the victim.

4. Do not give the victim anything to eat or drink.
5. Watch for changes and be prepared to give basic life support (BLS) if needed.

In some cases of sudden illness the most difficult decision is whether to call 9-1-1. How can you tell if the illness is an emergency? Two key factors can help you decide. First, if the illness is *sudden*, it is more likely to be an emergency. Many common illnesses come on gradually. For example, with the flu a person gradually develops a headache or achy joints, fever may begin mildly and slowly rise, respiratory symptoms gradually increase, and so on. The illness seldom becomes an emergency before the person seeks health care. Problems that come on suddenly and unexpectedly often become emergencies, however, such as a sudden heart attack or asthma attack.

Second, is the illness *unexplained*? A person suddenly has an excruciating, pounding headache – but this person has never had bad headaches before and nothing special has happened today that might cause a headache. This headache is likely to be a symptom of an emergency developing. In contrast, a child who develops a "tummy ache" after gobbling down a whole carton of ice cream is unlikely to be having an emergency – unlike some victims with sudden, unexplained severe abdominal pain.

In rare instances, if you cannot decide whether someone's sudden illness might be an emergency, call 9-1-1. Tell the dispatcher exactly what you know and have observed and let the dispatcher help decide the best course of action.

In addition to these general care principles, when you can identify the specific illness, give first aid as described in the following sections.

Heart Attack

Heart attack or **acute myocardial infarction (AMI)**, involves a sudden reduced blood flow to the heart muscle. It is a medical emergency and often leads to cardiac arrest. Heart attack can

BOX 16-1: FACTS ABOUT HEART ATTACK

- More than 1,255,000 heart attacks occur a year in the United States,[1] resulting in more than 132,000 deaths.[2] Many of them could have been saved by prompt first aid and medical treatment.

- Heart attack is more likely in those with a family history of heart attack.

- One-fifth of heart attack victims do not have chest pain, but they often have other symptoms. Symptoms may be somewhat different in women and men.

- Heart attack victims typically deny that they are having a heart attack. Do not let them talk you out of getting help!

[1]*Centers for Disease Control and Prevention. http://www.cdc.gov/heartdisease/facts.htm Accessed March 29, 2011.*

[2]*Centers for Disease Control and Prevention. http://www.cdc.gov/NCHS/data/nvsr/nvsr58/nvsr58_19.pdf Accessed March 29, 2011.*

occur at any age (**Box 16-1**). Heart attack is caused by a reduced blood flow or blockage in the coronary arteries, which supply the heart muscle with blood, usually as a result of atherosclerosis (see **Chapter 5**).

Prevention of Heart Attack

Heart attack, angina and stroke are all cardiovascular diseases. **Chapter 5** describes how one can minimize the risk factors for cardiovascular disease by not smoking, eating a healthy diet low in cholesterol and salt, controlling blood pressure, maintaining a normal weight, getting exercise, and controlling stress.

First Aid for Heart Attack

The signs and symptoms of heart attack vary considerably, from vague chest discomfort (which the victim may confuse with heartburn) to crushing pain, with or without other symptoms. The victim may have no signs and symptoms at all before collapsing suddenly. Sometimes the victim has milder symptoms that come and go for two or three days before the heart attack occurs. It is important to consider the possibility of heart attack when a wide range of symptoms occurs rather than expecting only a clearly defined situation. Note that some heart attack symptoms are more common in women. Chest pain or discomfort is still the most common symptom, but women are somewhat more likely to have shortness of breath, jaw or back pain, indigestion, and nausea and vomiting.

It is important to act quickly when the victim may be having a heart attack, because deaths from heart attack usually occur within an hour or two after symptoms begin. Health care professionals can administer medications to reduce the effects of heart attack and save the victim's life – but only if EMS is involved quickly.

First aid for heart attack begins with calling 9-1-1 to get help on the way immediately. Then help the victim to rest in the most comfortable position. A sitting position is often easiest for breathing. Loosen any constricting clothing. Try to calm the victim and reassure him or her that help is on the way. Because heart attack frequently leads to cardiac arrest, be prepared to give BLS if needed (see First Aid: "Heart Attack").

In recent years the value of aspirin as a clot-preventing medication has become well known and many health care providers advise their patients who are at risk for cardiovascular disease to take one low-dose aspirin daily unless they are allergic or experience side effects such as gastrointestinal bleeding. For victims who do not need to avoid aspirin, chewing one uncoated adult aspirin or two low-dose baby aspirin is now recommended when they experience heart attack symptoms. First aiders should never on their own give aspirin or any medication to a victim, but they can encourage the victim to chew an aspirin.

Nitroglycerin is another medication of benefit for a heart attack victim who has been prescribed this drug. Nitroglycerin increases blood flow through partially restricted arteries by dilating them. Nitroglycerin is generally prescribed for angina, a condition of pain in the chest caused by narrowed coronary arteries. If the victim has nitroglycerin, you can help the person to use it. Nitroglycerin comes in small tablets that are dissolved under the tongue, tablets that dissolve in the cheek, extended-release capsules, oral sprays and extended-release patches that are applied to the chest, usually daily **(Figure 16-1)**. Follow the victim's instructions to help with the drug. The victim should be seated because dizziness or fainting may occur. Do not try to give the drug yourself if the victim is unresponsive.

Angina

Angina pectoris, usually just called angina, is chest pain caused by heart disease that usually happens after intense activity or exertion. Other factors may trigger the pain of angina, such as stress or exposure to extreme heat or cold. The pain is a sign that the heart muscle is not getting

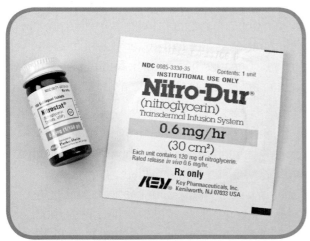

Figure 16-1 *Nitroglycerin tablets and patch.*

as much oxygen as needed, usually because of narrowed or constricted coronary arteries. The pain usually goes away after a few minutes of rest. The pain may also radiate to the jaw, neck or left arm or shoulder. People usually know when they have angina and may carry medication for it, usually nitroglycerin.

Ask if the person has been diagnosed with angina; if so, ask if the pain is like angina pain experienced in the past. If so, help the person take his or her own medication and rest. If the pain persists more than 10 minutes or stops and then returns, or if the victim has other heart attack symptoms not relieved by rest, give first aid for a heart attack.

Stroke

A **stroke**, also called a cerebrovascular accident (CVA) or a brain attack, is an interruption of blood flow to a part of the brain, which kills nerve cells and affects the victim's functioning. Stroke, like heart attack, may be caused by atherosclerosis. A blood clot may form in a brain artery or may be carried there in the blood and lodge in the artery, obstructing flow to that part of the brain. Stroke may also result when an artery in the brain ruptures or other factors impede flow. As noted in **Chapter 5**, about 795,000 people a year have a stroke, resulting in about 136,000 deaths.[3] Strokes are more common in older adults.

Because a stroke victim needs medical help immediately to decrease the chance of permanent damage, it is important to be able to identify the signs and symptoms of stroke. Stroke generally causes a sudden weakness or numbness in the face, arm or leg, especially on one side of the body; drooling; facial droop; slurred speech; and gait problems. Some stroke victims may have sudden, severe headache; vomiting; and loss of consciousness. The exact signs and symptoms vary somewhat depending on the exact site in the brain where an artery is blocked. First aiders who

[3]*American Heart Association, http://circ.ahajournals.org/cgi/ reprint/CIR.0b013e3182009701 Accessed March 29, 2011.*

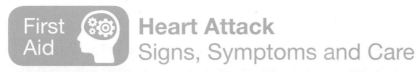

Heart Attack
Signs, Symptoms and Care

When You See

- **Complaints of persistent discomfort, pressure, tightness, ache or pain in the chest**
- **Complaints of pain spreading to neck, shoulders or arms**
- **Complaints of shortness of breath**
- **Complaints of dizziness, lightheadedness, feeling of impending doom**
- **Pale skin or sweating**
- **In women especially, symptoms include shortness of breath, indigestion, nausea or vomiting, and back or jaw pain**
- **Note that victims having a heart attack may not have all of these signs and symptoms**

Do This First

1 Call 9-1-1 immediately, even if the victim says it is not serious.

2 Help the victim to rest in a comfortable position (often sitting). Loosen any tight clothing. Keep the victim from moving.

3 Ask the victim if he or she is taking heart medication and help obtain the medication for the victim. Follow the directions on the medication.

4 Encourage the victim to chew one uncoated adult or two low-dose baby aspirin unless he or she is allergic to aspirin or cannot take aspirin for any other reason.

5 Stay with the victim and be reassuring and calming.

6 Be prepared to give CPR if the victim becomes unresponsive and normal breathing stops.

Additional Care

- Do not let the victim eat or drink anything.

are not thinking about the possibility of a stroke might attribute the victim's signs and symptoms to some other condition. Because it is so important that medical care begin as soon as possible, screening assessments have been devised to accurately identify strokes **(Box 16-2)**.

The most important thing to do for a stroke victim is to call 9-1-1 immediately to access advanced medical care. Drugs can often minimize the effects of a stroke – but only if administered very soon after the stroke. Tell the dispatcher you believe the victim has had a stroke and describe his or her signs and symptoms. Take note of the time that symptoms began, because medical treatment depends in part on how much time has passed. With the victim, be calming and reassuring, because often a stroke victim does not understand what has happened and is confused or fearful. Have the victim lie down on the back with head and shoulders slightly raised; this is often called the "stroke position." Monitor the victim and be prepared for vomiting and to give BLS if

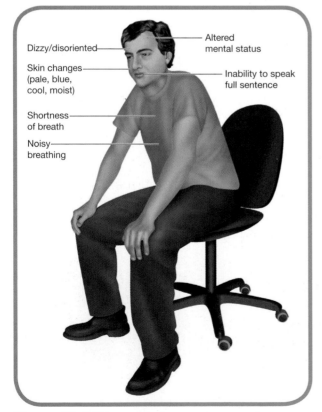

Dizzy/disoriented

Skin changes (pale, blue, cool, moist)

Shortness of breath

Noisy breathing

Altered mental status

Inability to speak full sentence

Figure 16-2 *Signs and symptoms of respiratory distress.*

needed. Move an unresponsive victim into the recovery position, with the affected side down to better maintain the airway (see First Aid: "Stroke").

Transient Ischemic Attack

A **transient ischemic attack (TIA)**, sometimes called a mini-stroke, is a temporary interruption to blood flow in an artery in the brain. A TIA produces signs and symptoms similar to those of a stroke, except they usually disappear within a few minutes. Since a person who experiences a TIA is at a high risk for a stroke, you should always call 9-1-1 for a victim who exhibits the signs and symptoms of stroke, even if they seem milder or soon disappear.

Respiratory Distress

Respiratory distress or difficulty breathing, can be caused by many different illnesses and injuries.

Prevention of Respiratory Distress

People with asthma generally have learned what factors may trigger an asthma attack so that they can try to avoid them when possible and many carry medication with them that can stop an attack when one occurs. People with other chronic respiratory problems, such as chronic obstructive pulmonary disease (COPD), should also learn to avoid situations in which respiratory difficulty may occur and should learn what actions to take if a problem does occur.

First Aid for Respiratory Distress

A victim in respiratory distress may be gasping for air, panting, breathing faster or slower than normal or making wheezing or other sounds with breathing. Typically the victim cannot speak a full sentence without pausing to breathe. The victim's skin may look pale or ashen and may be cool and moist; the lips and nail beds may be bluish. Lowered oxygen levels in the blood may make the victim feel dizzy or disoriented **(Figure 16-2)**. The victim may be sitting and leaning forward, hands on knees, in what is called the **tripod position (Figure 16-3)**.

Because respiratory distress in an infant or child may rapidly progress to respiratory arrest, it is

(continues on page 253)

BOX 16-2: THE CINCINNATI PREHOSPITAL STROKE SCALE

Among EMS professionals, the need to accurately identify a potential stroke victim is well recognized. The more quickly stroke is recognized, the more quickly the victim can be given appropriate prehospital care and rushed to a stroke center or other appropriate treatment center. Several screening processes have proved accurate in the rapid identification of stroke, and most professional rescuers now use a screening process.

A screening process can also be used effectively by lay first aiders. Emergency dispatchers who answer 9-1-1 calls in many areas are guiding callers to use such assessments. The **Cincinnati Prehospital Stroke Scale (CPSS)** is used widely and is similar to other methods. The CPSS uses three simple assessments:

1. Ask the victim to smile. In a stroke victim, often one side of the face makes a smile; the other side seems to droop.

2. Ask the victim, with eyes closed, to raise both arms out in front of the body. In a stroke victim, often one arm drifts down lower than the other in front of the body.

3. Ask the victim to repeat this sentence: "You can't teach an old dog new tricks." Often a stroke victim slurs words, uses the wrong words or cannot speak at all.

A first aider who identifies these signs of stroke in a victim and relays that information to EMS speeds the process of quickly getting the most appropriate care to the victim. The arriving EMS crew can quickly begin medical care at the scene and plan to transport the victim to the best setting for immediate care. Calling ahead helps ensure that resources are mobilized to provide advanced care on arrival.

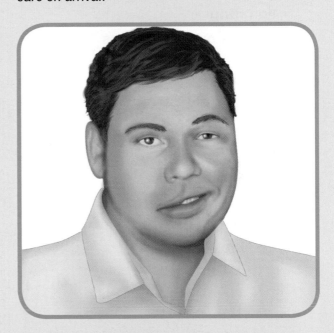

When gathering SAMPLE history information from a potential stroke victim, as explained in **Chapter 4**, try to learn the time when the signs and symptoms first occurred. Ask family members or others present at the scene as well as the victim. This information is important for the EMS treatment of the victim.

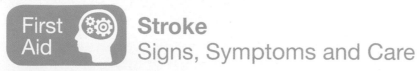

First Aid
Stroke
Signs, Symptoms and Care

When You See

Most common signs and symptoms:

- Sudden weakness or numbness of face, arm or leg, especially on one side of the body
- Drooling, facial droop or slurred speech
- Gait problems

Some stroke victims may have:

- Sudden, severe headache
- Vomiting
- Loss of consciousness

Do This First

1 Call 9-1-1.

2 Monitor the victim's breathing and be prepared to give BLS if needed.

3 Have the victim lie on his or her back with head and shoulders slightly raised.

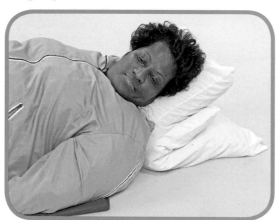

4 Loosen constrictive clothing.

3 If necessary, turn the victim's head to the side to allow drool or vomit to drain.

4 Loosen any tight clothing.

5 Be alert for the possibility of vomiting; turn the victim's head to drain the mouth.

6 Maintain the victim's normal body temperature. If necessary, maintain the victim's body heat with a blanket or coat over the victim.

Additional Care

- Keep the victim warm and quiet until help arrives.
- Put a breathing, unresponsive victim in the recovery position, with the affected side down.

ALERT

- Do not let a stroke victim eat or drink anything.

Learning **Checkpoint 1**

1. True or False: With an unknown sudden illness, do not give the victim anything to eat or drink.

2. Check off the common signs and symptoms of heart attack:

   _____ Skin red and flushed   _____ Indigestion

   _____ Tingling in fingers and toes   _____ Headache

   _____ Shortness of breath   _____ Pale skin

   _____ Chest pain or pressure   _____ Unusual cheerfulness

   _____ Sweating   _____ Dizziness

3. How do you decide if a victim's chest pain may be a heart attack or angina?

4. The immediate first action to take for a heart attack victim is _____.

5. It may be important to position a stroke victim such that –

   a. fluids drain from the mouth.

   b. the victim's head is protected from injury during convulsions.

   c. the victim can sit up even if partially paralyzed.

   d. the victim's head is lower than rest of the body.

(continued from page 250)

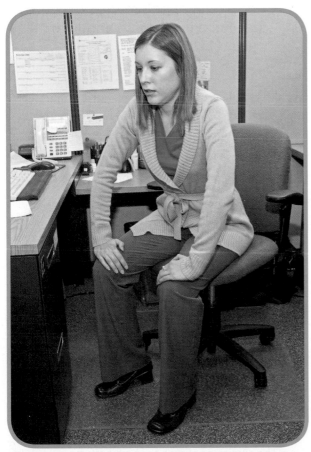

Figure 16-3 *The tripod position, commonly assumed by victims in respiratory distress.*

crucial to act quickly when an infant or child is having a problem breathing. In addition to the signs and symptoms just described, an infant or child may have obviously flaring nostrils and more obvious movements of chest muscles with the effort to breathe.

If the cause of a victim's breathing problem is not obvious, look for other signs and symptoms that may reveal the problem. Respiratory distress can be a sign of many of the injuries described in other chapters throughout this text. If you can determine the cause of a victim's breathing difficulty, give first aid for that problem. For example, a victim of a heart attack may have shortness of breath; while it is important to care for this breathing difficulty, it is most crucial to call 9-1-1 immediately for the heart attack and give the first aid described earlier.

Respiratory distress may also result from sudden illness. Asthma and chronic obstructive pulmonary disease (COPD) are two common diseases that may cause episodes of breathing difficulty. These are described in more detail in the following sections along with specific first aid steps.

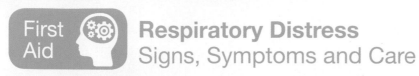

First Aid — Respiratory Distress
Signs, Symptoms and Care

When You See

- **Victim is gasping or unable to catch his or her breath.**
- **Speaking in shortened sentences**
- **Breathing is faster or slower, or deeper or shallower, than normal**
- **Breathing involves sounds such as wheezing or gurgling**
- **Victim feels dizzy or lightheaded**
- **Pale or ashen skin**

Do This First

1 Call 9-1-1 for sudden, unexplained breathing problems.

2 Help the victim to rest in the position of easiest breathing (often sitting up).

3 If the victim is hyperventilating, ask him or her to breathe slowly.

4 Ask the victim about any prescribed medicine he or she may have, and help the victim to take it if needed.

5 Stay with the victim and be prepared to give CPR if breathing stops.

Additional Care

- Calm and reassure the victim (anxiety increases breathing distress).
- Administer supplemental oxygen to the victim if available and if you are trained in its use.

In some cases you will not be able to identify the cause of a victim's respiratory distress. In this situation give the general breathing care described in First Aid: "Respiratory Distress." Call 9-1-1 for a victim of respiratory distress because this condition may progress to respiratory arrest, a life-threatening condition.

Asthma

Asthma is an increasingly common problem that will affect more than 34 million Americans in their lifetime, affecting 1 in 20 adults and 1 in 10 school-age children. Asthma attacks in the United States result in 217,000 emergency department visits a year and more than 3,300 deaths.[4] The prevalence of asthma has been increasing gradually in the United States for more than two decades. Asthma

is a chronic disease – it cannot be cured, although attacks often become less common as a child becomes older and moves through adulthood. In an asthma attack, the airway becomes narrow and the person has difficulty breathing. Many asthma victims know they have the condition and carry medication for emergency situations, typically an inhaler. They may also have learned what situations and factors can trigger an asthma attack and thus they try to avoid these **(Box 16-3)**. When left untreated, a severe asthma attack can be fatal. If a young child who is away from usual caretakers has trouble breathing, always ask if he or she has medication (see First Aid: "Asthma").

When an asthma attack occurs and the victim has an inhaler, you may assist the victim in using the inhaler under these conditions:

- The victim confirms that an asthma attack is occurring.

[4]*American Academy of Allergy, Asthma & Immunology. http://www.aaaai.org/media/statistics/asthma-statistics. asp Accessed March 1, 2011.*

BOX 16-3: ASTHMA TRIGGERS

Asthma attacks are usually triggered by some factor in the person's internal or external environment. Understanding these factors helps prevent or minimize attacks. Common triggers include:

- Respiratory infection, including the common cold (the most common cause of asthma attacks in children under age 5)
- Allergic reaction to pollen, mold, dust mites, animal fur or dander
- Exercise (especially in cold, dry air)
- Certain foods (nuts, eggs, milk)
- Emotional stress
- Medications
- Air pollution caused by such things as cigarette smoke, vehicle exhaust or fumes of cleaning products
- Temperature extremes

Knowing the specific triggers that provoke asthma can help prevent attacks. A person with asthma may have had a skin test to detect specific allergens that trigger his or her asthma. In addition to avoiding the factors just listed, follow these guidelines:

- Use a damp cloth to dust furniture and surfaces.
- Vacuum rugs frequently and when the person with asthma is not present.
- Avoid fluffy blankets and pillows that collect dust and that contain feathers.
- Enclose mattresses and pillows in plastic covers.
- Do not use air fresheners or products with strong odors.
- Use an air purifier and stay indoors when pollen counts are high.

- The victim identifies the inhaler as his or her prescribed asthma medication.
- The victim cannot self-administer the medication.

Helping a Child With an Inhaler

Parents and child care providers may need to help a small child with asthma to use an inhaler during an asthma attack. An inhaler is a device that contains and delivers the asthma medication in automatically measured doses **(Figure 16-4)**. The medication is usually a **bronchodilator**, a drug that relaxes the muscles of the airway, allowing airway passages to open wider (dilate) to make breathing easier. Always follow the health care provider's specific instructions for the inhaler. Use only the child's own prescribed inhaler. Never use an inhaler belonging to another child.

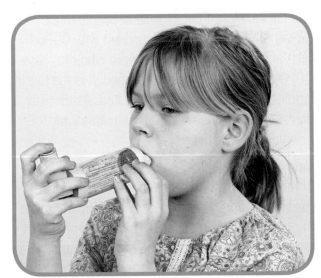

Figure 16-4 *Many people with asthma use an inhaler.*

Following are general instructions that may need modification for the specific medication device or for a particular child.

1. Remove the cap and shake the inhaler several times.

2. If a spacer is used, position it on the inhaler. (A spacer is a tube or chamber that fits between the inhaler and the child's mouth.)

3. Have the child breathe out fully through the mouth.

4. With the child's lips around the inhaler mouthpiece or the spacer, have the child inhale slowly and deeply; press the metal canister down to release one spray of medication as the child inhales. (A face mask is generally used for an infant instead of a mouthpiece.)

5. Have the child hold his or her breath for up to 10 seconds if possible and then exhale slowly. Follow the directions for the inhaler or follow the child's treatment plan to repeat doses if needed.

Chronic Obstructive Pulmonary Disease

Chronic obstructive pulmonary disease (COPD) includes emphysema, chronic bronchitis and other conditions. More than 12 million people in the United States have been diagnosed with COPD, with an estimated 12 million more who may have COPD but have not been diagnosed. It is the fourth leading cause of death in the United States.[5] These diseases may cause respiratory distress and breathing emergencies.

Emphysema is a disease that affects the alveoli of the lungs, the tiny sacs where oxygen enters the blood. The alveoli lose elasticity and decrease in number, which reduces oxygen absorption. Chronic bronchitis affects the bronchial tubes into the lungs, causing inflammation and a buildup of mucus. Both diseases are mainly caused by smoking, air pollution and other factors. Both

often become worse over time. People with these diseases often get colds and respiratory infections, and they are likely to become short of breath even with mild exertion such as walking. In advanced cases the person may need a home oxygen system.

Victims with breathing difficulty related to COPD generally have the same signs and symptoms as described earlier for respiratory distress, and the first aid care is the same. Ask the victim whether he or she has a chronic disease and give this information to the dispatcher when you call 9-1-1. If the victim has a prescribed medication to help with breathing, you may help the person to take the medication.

Hyperventilation

Hyperventilation is fast, deep breathing usually caused by anxiety or stress, although it may also be caused by some injuries or illnesses. The rapid breathing causes an imbalance in the body's levels of oxygen and carbon dioxide, which may add to the person's anxiety and cause confusion or dizziness. Numbness or tingling of the fingers, toes and lips may occur.

Hyperventilation caused by emotional stress usually does not last long or become an emergency. Help the person to calm down and relax and breathe more slowly. Do not have the person breathe into and out of a bag, which could lower the person's oxygen level too far. Breathing slowly along with the victim often helps the victim to slow his or her breathing rate.

Because rapid breathing may also be caused by injury or sudden illness, do not assume that the victim is simply hyperventilating. Look for other signs of injury or illness and ask the victim what happened to begin the problem. If there are other signs or symptoms that suggest injury or illness or if the victim's breathing does not return to normal in a few minutes, call 9-1-1 (see First Aid: "Hyperventilation").

[5]*National Heart, Lung and Blood Institute http://www.nhlbi. nih.gov/health/public/lung/copd/index.htm Accessed March 1, 2011.*

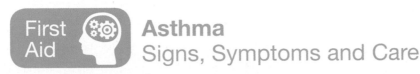

Asthma
Signs, Symptoms and Care

When You See

- **Wheezing and difficulty breathing and speaking**
- **Dry, persistent cough**
- **Fear and anxiety**
- **Gray-blue or ashen skin**
- **Changing levels of responsiveness**

Do This First

1 If the victim does not know he or she has asthma (first attack), call 9-1-1 immediately.

2 If the victim identifies the breathing difficulty as an asthma attack and has prescribed medication (usually an inhaler), help them use the medication.

- Remove the cap.
- Shake the inhaler several times.
- Connect the spacer (if needed).
- The victim places the inhaler or spacer end in mouth.
- The victim presses the metal canister down while slowly inhaling.
- Remind the victim to hold his or her breath with the medication for about 10 seconds.

3 Help the victim rest in a position for easiest breathing (usually sitting up).

Additional Care

- If needed, the victim may use the inhaler again as prescribed or directed by a medical provider.
- If the breathing difficulty persists after using the inhaler, call 9-1-1.
- If the difficulty persists, give supplemental oxygen if available and if you are trained in its use (see **Appendix A**).
- Never unnecessarily separate a child from a parent or loved one when providing care.

Fainting

Fainting is caused by a temporarily reduced blood flow to the brain. This commonly occurs in hot weather or after a prolonged period of inactivity, or from other causes such as fright, emotional shock or lack of food. A temporary drop in blood pressure caused by suddenly standing after prolonged sitting or lying down may cause dizziness or fainting, especially in the elderly. In a young, healthy, nonpregnant adult, fainting is usually not a sign of a more serious problem, unless the person faints often or does not recover quickly.

In someone who has heart disease, is pregnant or is older than 65, fainting may be a sign of a serious problem requiring immediate medical attention.

Injury may result if the fainting person falls – try to catch the person and gently lower him or her to the floor. Sometimes a person has signs or symptoms before fainting, including dizziness, sweating, nausea, blurring or dimming of vision, and generalized weakness. If fainting is anticipated, have the person sit or lie down (see First Aid: "Fainting").

First Aid

Hyperventilation
Signs, Symptoms and Care

When You See

- **Very fast breathing rate**
- **Dizziness or faintness**
- **Tingling or numbness in hands, feet and lips**
- **Muscle twitching or cramping**

Do This First

1 Make sure there is no other cause for the breathing difficulty that requires care.

2 Reassure the victim and ask him or her to try to breathe slowly.

3 Call 9-1-1 if the victim's breathing does not return to normal within a few minutes.

Additional Care

- A victim who has this problem frequently should seek medical care, because some medical conditions can cause rapid breathing.

ALERT

- Do not ask the victim to breathe into a bag or other container. A victim who repeatedly rebreathes his or her exhaled air will not be getting enough oxygen.

Learning Checkpoint 2

1. True or False: You cannot give first aid for a person with difficulty breathing unless you know the specific cause of the problem.

2. To help someone to breathe more easily, –

    a. position the victim flat on his or her back.

    b. have the victim stand, and clap him or her on the back with each breath.

    c. have the victim sit and put his or her head between the knees.

    d. let the victim find the position in which he or she can breathe most easily.

3. What is the best thing a victim with asthma can do when having an asthma attack?

   _____

4. True or False: Have a hyperventilation victim breathe into a bag to start breathing normally again.

5. When should you call 9-1-1 for a victim who seems to be hyperventilating?

   _____

Fainting
Signs, Symptoms and Care

When You See

- **Sudden, brief loss of responsiveness and collapse**
- **Pale, cool skin; sweating**

Do This First

1 Monitor the victim's breathing and be ready to give CPR if needed.

2 Lay the victim down and raise the legs 6 to 12 inches. Loosen constricting clothing.

3 Check for possible injuries caused by falling.

4 Reassure the victim as he or she recovers.

Additional Care

- Call 9-1-1 if the victim does not regain responsiveness soon or faints repeatedly. Always call 9-1-1 for all older adults, people with heart disease and pregnant women.
- Place a victim who is breathing normally but remains unresponsive in the recovery position.

ALERT

- Do not pour or splash water on the victim's face; it could be aspirated into the lungs.

Seizures

Seizures, or convulsions, result from a brain disturbance caused by many different conditions, including epilepsy, high fever in infants and young children, head injuries, low blood sugar in a person with diabetes, poisoning, and electric shock. The brain's normal electrical activity becomes out of balance, resulting in a sudden altered mental status and uncontrolled muscular contractions that cause jerking or shaking of the body. Most seizures are caused by epilepsy **(Box 16-4)**.

Prevention of Seizures

First-time seizures can seldom be prevented, but someone with a diagnosed seizure disorder usually has prescribed medication that will prevent most seizures. Sometimes specific factors may increase the risk of a seizure occurring (such as inadequate sleep or flashing lights), and the individual can learn to control these factors. Seizures caused by head injuries can be prevented by preventing injuries (see **Chapter 12**) – for example, by wearing an appropriate helmet during sports and other activities.

First Aid for Seizures

Seizures generally occur suddenly and without warning. Some victims have an unusual feeling in advance of the seizure called an aura. An aura may be a generalized sensation or a hallucinatory sensation involving any of the senses.

Seizures follow a wide variety of different patterns, depending in part on the cause. Several different patterns occur in people with epilepsy; some may have only one type of seizure, while others experience different types at different times.

BOX 16-4: FACTS ABOUT EPILEPSY

- Epilepsy and seizures affect 3 million people of all ages in the United States.

- Approximately 200,000 new cases of seizures and epilepsy occur each year.

- 10% of the U.S. population will experience a seizure in their lifetime.

- 45,000 children younger than 15 develop epilepsy each year.

- Males are slightly more likely to develop epilepsy than females.

- The incidence is greater in African-American and socially disadvantaged populations.

- In 70% of new cases, no cause is apparent.

- 50% of people with new cases of epilepsy will have seizures.

- 70% of people with epilepsy can be expected to enter remission, defined as 5 or more years seizure-free using medication.

- 75% of people who are seizure-free on medication after 2 to 5 years can be successfully withdrawn from medication.

- 10% of new patients may still have seizures despite optimal medical management.

Source: Epilepsy Foundation. http://www. epilepsyfoundation.org/about/statistics.cfm Accessed March 1, 2011.

Following are some of the more common types of seizures:

- **Complex partial seizures**. These occur in some people with epilepsy. The person is conscious but does not interact normally with others and is not in control of movements or speech. These seizures are called "partial" because only part of the brain is involved. The person seems dazed and may mumble or wander. This type of seizure is often mistaken for a behavioral problem.

- **Absence seizures**. These occur in some people with epilepsy. The person seems to stare blankly into space and does not respond to others; the seizure begins and ends abruptly, often lasting only a few seconds.

- **Generalized tonic clonic seizures**. These occur in some people with epilepsy. This type is also called convulsions or grand mal seizures. The person loses consciousness and falls; the person is at first stiff (tonic), then experiences jerking of muscles (clonic) throughout the body. Breathing may stop momentarily but restarts spontaneously.

After the seizure the person may be confused or agitated.

- **Febrile seizures**. These seizures are not related to epilepsy. Febrile seizures are caused by high fever (usually higher than 102° F) in infants or young children. The convulsions are similar to those of tonic clonic seizures and the first aid is the same, followed by measures to bring down the victim's body temperature.

The first aid for all kinds of seizures is primarily directed toward protecting the person until the seizure ends, almost always within seconds to minutes. If the person seems conscious, stay with him or her until it passes. Someone having a complex partial seizure may wander about; if the person is moving into a hazardous situation, gently guide the person away from danger. Look for a medical identification bracelet or necklace if you are unsure why the person is suddenly acting oddly. Reassure the person as the seizure ends. If the person seems agitated or angry, stay back but close enough to protect the person from danger. Never try to restrain a person who is having any kind of a seizure.

Do not put anything in the person's mouth because objects may damage teeth or other tissues during the seizure or break and obstruct the airway. Protect the head from injury with a folded jacket or soft padding. Keep track of how long the seizure lasts because 9-1-1 should be called for any seizure lasting longer than 5 minutes. There is nothing you can do to stop or shorten the seizure, but try to keep the person as comfortable as possible during the seizure. Keep bystanders away. Afterwards the person is likely to be confused or disoriented, drowsy or agitated; be reassuring and help the person to rest as needed (see First Aid: "Seizures"). Help preserve the victim's privacy and dignity. If incontinence occurs, cover the victim with a blanket or coat. Commonly the victim is unresponsive for a time after a seizure; place the victim in the recovery position and monitor breathing.

Seizures in Special Circumstances

A person who has a seizure while in the water is at risk of aspirating water into the lungs or even drowning. Because a seizure lasts only a few minutes at most, do not try to move the person from the water; instead, support him or her with the head tilted to keep water out of the mouth. After the seizure, help the person out of the water. If the person is not responsive, check for breathing and give CPR if needed.

Another special circumstance is a seizure that occurs in an airplane, motor vehicle or other confined area. If there are empty seats around the person, fold back the armrests so the person can lie on his or her side across the seats with his or her head on a cushion. If there is no room to lie down, use padding or pillows to protect the person's head from striking hard objects around the seat. Try to lean the person to one side to keep the airway open.

Altered Mental Status

Altered mental status is a phrase used to refer to a change from a person's normal responsiveness and awareness. The person may be confused, disoriented, combative, drowsy, or partially or wholly unresponsive. Altered mental status is not a condition itself but is a sign or symptom that may result from many different injuries and illnesses. Following are just a few of the many causes of altered mental status:

- Seizures
- Stroke
- Head injury
- Poisoning, drug use or overdose
- High fever
- Diabetic emergencies
- Any condition causing lowered blood oxygen levels

When you encounter someone with altered mental status, determine the nature of the problem if possible. If the victim is responsive, perform a physical examination and gather a SAMPLE history. Then give first aid for any problems found.

If the person's altered mental status is due to drug or alcohol use and the person is acting erratically or in a potentially violent manner, the situation may involve a behavioral emergency. In such cases it is important to ensure your own safety and that of other bystanders. **Chapter 21** describes how to manage behavioral emergencies. Never assume, however, that a person with altered mental status is intoxicated or is using drugs, or that someone acting strangely has a mental illness. Certain injuries and sudden illnesses such as a diabetic emergency can produce behavior that is easily mistaken for intoxication. Even if the person is intoxicated, he or she may still have an injury or illness that could become an emergency if not cared for.

Altered mental status is often a sign of deteriorating condition. If you cannot determine a cause for the person's condition or behavior or if you are unsure what to do, call 9-1-1. Describe the situation and the person's signs and symptoms to the dispatcher, who will determine the correct course of action.

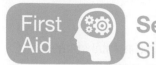

First Aid — Seizures
Signs, Symptoms and Care

When You See

- **Minor seizures: staring blankly ahead; slight twitching of lips, head, or arms and legs; other movements such as lip-smacking or chewing**
- **Major seizures: crying out and then becoming unresponsive; body becomes rigid and then shakes in convulsions; jaw may clench**
- **Fever convulsions in young children: hot, flushed skin; violent muscle twitching; arched back; clenched fists**

Do This First

1 Prevent injury during the seizure by moving dangerous objects and putting soft padding such as a jacket under the person's head. Remove eyeglasses.

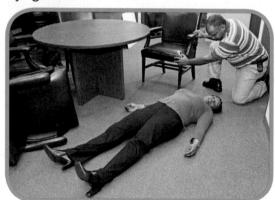

2 Loosen tight clothing around the neck to ease breathing. Check for a medical identification bracelet or necklace.

3 If vomiting occurs, gently turn the person's head to one side to help keep the airway clear.

4 After the seizure, ensure the victim's airway remains open by using the recovery position or head tilt–chin lift if needed.

5 Be reassuring as the person regains responsiveness.

Additional Care

- Check for a medical identification.
- Call 9-1-1 if the seizure lasts more than 5 minutes, if the person is not known to have epilepsy, if the person recovers very slowly or has trouble breathing or has another seizure, if the person is pregnant or is wearing a medical ID for a condition other than epilepsy, or if the person is injured.
- Place an unresponsive victim in the recovery position and monitor breathing.
- For an infant or child with fever convulsions, sponge the body with lukewarm water to help cool the victim and call 9-1-1.

ALERT

- Do not try to stop the person's movements or restrain the person.
- Do not place any objects in the person's mouth.

Diabetic Emergencies

Diabetes is actually a group of related diseases in which blood sugar (glucose) levels are not well regulated by the body. The hormone insulin, normally produced in the pancreas, is needed for body cells to be able to use glucose. When insulin levels are too low, glucose levels rise too high. The problem results if the body is not producing enough insulin or if the body does not use the insulin well – a condition called insulin resistance. Currently more than 25 million people in the United States have diabetes, about 7 million of whom have not been diagnosed.[6] The disease is chronic and incurable.

There are two primary types of diabetes. In type 1, formerly called insulin-dependent diabetes or juvenile-onset diabetes, the body does not produce enough or any insulin. The person must receive insulin by injection or a pump. In type 2 diabetes, formerly called non-insulin-dependent or adult-onset diabetes, body cells do not use insulin well. Eventually the pancreas may not produce as much insulin. Either way, blood glucose levels may be too high. More than 90% of adults who develop diabetes have type 2 diabetes, which becomes more common as one grows older or becomes more overweight. Most people with type 2 diabetes can control the problem with diet, exercise, weight control and oral medication when needed.

Blood glucose levels vary moment by moment in the body as a result of many factors including what one has eaten, when it was eaten, one's level of activity and other factors. In a person who is not diabetic, insulin maintains a dynamic balance with blood glucose to prevent levels from becoming too high or too low. People with diabetes, however, sometimes have problems maintaining this balance even with careful attention to diet, activity levels and blood glucose monitoring.

Prevention of Diabetes and Diabetic Emergencies

Diabetes is a serious and growing problem in the United States. It kills more than 70,000 people yearly, making it the sixth leading cause of death. Diabetes contributes to an additional 160,000 deaths annually from related causes.[6] In addition, diabetes causes complications throughout the body. Diabetes contributes to heart disease and stroke, is the most common cause of blindness in people 20 to 74 years old, causes severe kidney disease, and damages the nervous system. Because of resulting circulation problems, foot infections in diabetics often lead to amputation. An alarming current trend is the increasing numbers of children and adolescents who are developing type 2 diabetes related to overweight and lack of exercise.

Type 2 diabetes often can be prevented or delayed in people at a high risk for developing the problem. Diet, exercise and weight control are critical for prevention – the same lifestyle factors that can reduce one's risk for cardiovascular disease (see **Chapter 5**). For those with diabetes, careful control of their glucose levels, blood pressure and cholesterol levels along with preventive care for the eyes, kidneys and feet can help prevent complications from developing.

Diabetic emergencies can usually be prevented by careful monitoring of blood glucose levels and by controlling diet, medication use and activity levels **(Figure 16-5)**.

[6]*American Diabetes Association. http://www.diabetes.org/ diabetes-basics/diabetes-statistics Accessed March 1, 2011.*

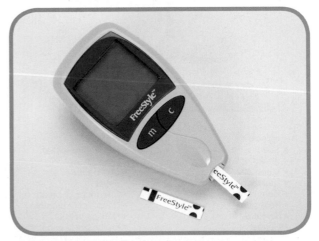

Figure 16-5 *People with diabetes often use a blood glucose monitoring system like this one to check their glucose levels using a tiny drop of blood.*

First Aid for Diabetic Emergencies

In a person with diabetes, the blood sugar level may become either too low or too high as a result of many interacting factors. Low blood sugar, called **hypoglycemia**, may result if a person takes too much insulin, does not eat enough food or the right kind of foods, or uses blood sugar too quickly through exercise or emotional stress. High blood sugar, called **hyperglycemia**, may result if a person takes too little insulin, eats too much food or the wrong kind of foods or does not use blood sugar through activity **(Figure 16-6)**. Other factors, too, can affect blood sugar levels.

Either hypoglycemia or hyperglycemia can quickly progress to a medical emergency if the person is not treated. In many cases you may know if a victim experiencing this emergency has diabetes. Both hypoglycemia and hyperglycemia cause altered mental status (drowsiness, disorientation) and a generalized feeling of sickness. When taking the SAMPLE history of any victim who suddenly feels ill, ask about diabetes or other medical conditions and look for a medical alert ID. If the victim is responsive and alert, he or she may know from experience whether the problem is hypoglycemia or hyperglycemia.

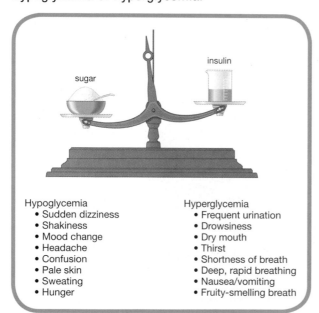

Hypoglycemia
- Sudden dizziness
- Shakiness
- Mood change
- Headache
- Confusion
- Pale skin
- Sweating
- Hunger

Hyperglycemia
- Frequent urination
- Drowsiness
- Dry mouth
- Thirst
- Shortness of breath
- Deep, rapid breathing
- Nausea/vomiting
- Fruity-smelling breath

Figure 16-6 *A diabetic emergency may result if the body's balance of insulin and blood sugar is disrupted.*

Hypoglycemia

The signs and symptoms of hypoglycemia include sudden dizziness, shakiness or mood change (even combativeness); headache, confusion and difficulty paying attention; pale or ashen skin, sweating; hunger; and clumsy, jerky movements. A seizure may occur. Although the victim may appear to be intoxicated (slurring words, staggering gait, confusion, etc.), it is important never to dismiss these symptoms without considering the possibility of a diabetic emergency.

First aid for hypoglycemia involves raising the victim's blood sugar level by giving the person food or drink that is high in glucose. Diabetics often carry glucose tablets in case of episodes of low blood sugar **(Figure 16-7)**. Glucose is quickly absorbed into the blood, quickly relieving the problem (see First Aid: "Low Blood Sugar").

Hyperglycemia

The signs and symptoms of hyperglycemia include frequent urination; drowsiness; dry mouth and thirst; shortness of breath and deep, rapid breathing; fruity-smelling breath; and nausea or vomiting. Unresponsiveness eventually occurs.

Hyperglycemia generally requires medical treatment. Hyperglycemia usually develops gradually over time, allowing the diabetic person to recognize and correct the problem. In an early stage of the problem, the victim may follow the instructions from his or her health care provider. For more significant symptoms, the victim needs medical help. The

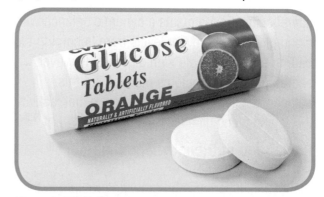

Figure 16-7 *Diabetics often carry glucose tablets in case of low blood sugar.*

Hypoglycemia (Low Blood Sugar)
Signs, Symptoms and Care

When You See

- **Sudden dizziness, shakiness or mood change (even combativeness)**
- **Headache, confusion, difficulty paying attention**
- **Pale or ashen skin, sweating**
- **Hunger**
- **Clumsy, jerky movements**
- **Possible seizure**

Do This First

1 Confirm that the victim has diabetes. Talk to the victim; look for a medical ID tag.

2 Give the victim sugar: 3 glucose tablets, ½ cup fruit juice, 1 or 2 sugar packets (but not artificial sugar or sweetener packets), or 5 to 6 pieces of hard candy. If the victim still feels ill or has signs and symptoms after 15 minutes, give more sugar.

3 Call 9-1-1 if the victim becomes unresponsive or continues to have significant signs and symptoms.

Additional Care

- If the victim becomes unresponsive or continues to have significant signs and symptoms, call 9-1-1 and monitor breathing.

ALERT

- If a diabetic victim becomes unresponsive, do not try to inject insulin or put food or fluids in the mouth.

---

victim may be taken to an emergency department, or, if he or she becomes unresponsive, call 9-1-1 (see First Aid: "High Blood Sugar").

In some situations you may know or discover the person has diabetes but not know whether the problem is high or low blood sugar. In this case, if the victim's symptoms are mild, give sugar as for low blood sugar. If it happens that the victim has high blood sugar, this additional sugar will not worsen the victim's condition, but it could solve the problem if the victim has low blood sugar. If the victim does not improve in 15 minutes, or if signs and symptoms become worse, an emergency is developing and the victim needs immediate medical attention.

Severe Abdominal Pain

Abdominal injuries were described in **Chapter 13**; always call 9-1-1 for an abdominal injury. Abdominal pain may also result from illness ranging from minor conditions to serious medical emergencies. Urgent medical care is needed for severe abdominal pain in these situations:

In adults:

- Sudden, severe, intolerable pain or pain that causes awakening from sleep
- Pain that begins in the general area of the central abdomen and later moves to the lower right

Hyperglycemia (High Blood Sugar)
Signs, Symptoms and Care

When You See

Early stage signs and symptoms:

- **Frequent urination**
- **Drowsiness**
- **Dry mouth, thirst**

Later stage signs and symptoms:

- **Shortness of breath; deep, rapid breathing**
- **Breath smells fruity**
- **Nausea or vomiting**
- **Eventual unresponsiveness**

Do This First

1 If you suspect high blood sugar, call 9-1-1 and monitor the person.

2 In the early stage, you may not be able to tell whether the victim suffers from high or low blood sugar. In this case:

- Give sugar as for hypoglycemia.
- If the victim does not improve within 15 minutes or the victim's signs and symptoms become worse, call 9-1-1.

3 In the later stage, high blood sugar is a medical emergency:

- Call 9-1-1 immediately.
- Put an unresponsive victim in the recovery position and monitor breathing.

- Pain accompanied by fever, sweating, black or bloody stool, or blood in urine
- Pain in pregnancy or accompanying abnormal vaginal bleeding
- Pain accompanied by dry mouth, dizziness on standing or decreased urination
- Pain accompanied by difficulty breathing
- Pain accompanied by vomiting blood or greenish-brown fluid

In young children:

- Pain that occurs suddenly, stops and then returns without warning
- Pain accompanied by red or purple jelly-like stool; or with blood or mucus in stool
- Pain accompanied by greenish-brown vomit
- Pain with swollen abdomen that feels hard
- Pain with a hard lump in lower abdomen or groin area

Many different factors and illnesses can result in gastrointestinal distress with or without abdominal pain. Vomiting or diarrhea may also occur from many different causes. Again, seek urgent medical care for the signs and symptoms listed here, and talk with a health care provider for other unexplained or persistent gastrointestinal distress. The following are additional key points:

- Persistent diarrhea or vomiting in an infant or small child or in an elderly or debilitated person can rapidly cause dehydration, which can become an emergency. Seek medical care immediately.
- While awaiting medical help, do not give a person with abdominal pain anything to eat or drink, as this may cause vomiting – except for clear fluids for dehydration.

Learning Checkpoint 3

1. When should you call 9-1-1 for a victim who faints?

   _____

2. True or False: When a person has fainted, lay him or her down and raise the head and shoulders 6 to 12 inches.

3. For a victim having seizures –

   a. lay the victim face down on the floor.

   b. ask others to help you hold the victim's head, arms and legs still.

   c. put something flat and soft under the victim's head.

   d. put a wooden object, such as a pencil, between the victim's teeth.

4. Name at least three situations in which you should call 9-1-1 for a seizure victim.

   _____

5. What should you do for a young child whose abdomen is swollen and feels hard?

   _____

6. Check off common signs and symptoms of a low blood sugar diabetic emergency.

   _____ Dizziness   _____ Red, blotchy skin

   _____ Hunger   _____ Sweating

   _____ Rapid deep breathing   _____ Confusion

   _____ Clumsiness   _____ Swollen legs

7. In the late afternoon you see a friend at the library who is acting oddly. She is sitting at a table staring into space, and when you ask her if she is okay, she does not seem to understand what you are saying. She looks ill, her skin is pale and she is sweating even though the room is not warm. You know this woman is diabetic and you suspect that she might have skipped lunch today. You cannot be sure whether she has low or high blood sugar. What should you do?

   _____

Concluding Thoughts

It can be a frightening experience to be with someone who is suddenly ill, especially if you do not know the cause. Remember the first steps for all first aid situations: Assess the victim and try to find out what happened. If you know the cause of the problem, give appropriate first aid; if you do not know, call 9-1-1 and give supportive care until help arrives. Reassure the victim. Help the victim to rest and to avoid getting chilled or overheated, and do not give anything to eat or drink. Stay with the person, watch for changes and be prepared to give basic life support if needed.

Learning Outcomes

You should now be able to do the following:

1. Explain why first aid is needed when someone suddenly becomes ill.

2. List the general care steps for any sudden illness.

3. Describe the signs and symptoms of, and the first aid for, each of the following sudden illnesses:

   • Heart attack

   • Angina

   • Stroke

   • Respiratory distress

   • Fainting

   • Seizures

   • Altered mental status

   • Diabetic emergencies

   • Severe abdominal pain

Review Questions

1. Common general signs and symptoms of sudden illness include –

   a. feeling ill, dizzy, confused or weak.

   b. skin color changes (flushed, pale or ashen) and sweating.

   c. breathing changes.

   d. All of the above

2. Always call 9-1-1 for a victim whose illness –

   a. occurs suddenly and without explanation.

   b. includes a fever.

   c. is chronic.

   d. involves feeling fatigued.

3. The signs and symptoms of heart attack may include –

   a. chest pain, fever and flushed skin.

   b. chest pain, headache and an inability to raise both arms.

   c. chest pain, sweating and shortness of breath.

   d. chest pain, difficulty speaking or swallowing, and vision problems.

4. The most crucial aspect of first aid for a stroke victim is –

   a. calling 9-1-1 immediately.

   b. explaining the situation to family members.

   c. elevating the victim's legs.

   d. performing a complete physical examination before calling 9-1-1.

5. Low oxygen blood levels caused by breathing difficulty may cause –

    a. heavy sweating.

    b. dizziness or disorientation.

    c. a reddish coloration of the skin.

    d. hyperactivity.

6. First aid for an asthma attack may include –

    a. calling 9-1-1 if the victim is not better in 30 minutes.

    b. asking the victim to try to breathe slowly.

    c. helping the victim to lie down with feet raised.

    d. helping the victim to use an inhaler.

7. To help a person who is hyperventilating –

    a. have the victim breathe into a paper bag.

    b. splash cold water on the victim's face.

    c. ask the victim to try to breathe slowly.

    d. ask the victim to hold his or her breath as long as possible.

8. Help to prevent injury to a person having a seizure by –

    a. putting something flat and soft under the head.

    b. putting a wooden stick between the teeth.

    c. restraining the person by holding the shoulders.

    d. having bystanders help hold the arms and legs still.

9. Altered mental status may result from –

    a. stroke.

    b. poisoning.

    c. head injury.

    d. All of the above

10. If you are unsure whether a diabetic is experiencing hypoglycemia or hyperglycemia –

    a. wait an hour to observe signs and symptoms.

    b. give sugar and monitor symptoms.

    c. call a family member of the victim to inquire.

    d. give the victim an emergency epinephrine shot in the thigh muscle.

Chapter 17 • Poisoning

Chapter Preview

- Overview of Poisoning
- Preventing Poisoning
- Swallowed Poisons
- Inhaled Poisons
- Poison Ivy, Oak and Sumac

With your young son, Danny, you are visiting a friend at her home. Danny has been playing with a toy truck on the floor, which he now pushes down the hallway into the bathroom. You start to get up to bring him back but your friend says, "That's okay, there's nothing in there he can get into." With the normal curiosity of a child, however, Danny starts looking in the bathroom drawers and soon finds a bottle of what looks to him like little candy mints. He puts a handful in his mouth – they don't taste much like mint but he chews and swallows them anyway. You see pills spilled on the floor when you walk into the bathroom. He admits he ate "some" of the pills. What do you do?

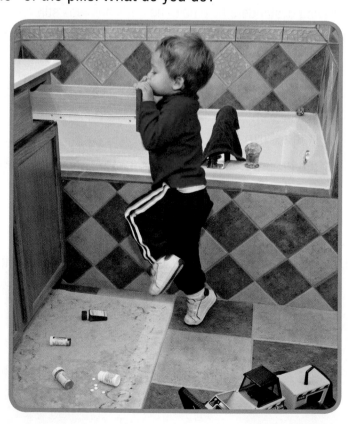

With more than 2 million poisoning incidents occurring in the United States every year, resulting in about 39,000 deaths,[1] poisoning is a huge problem in a world where so many products containing toxins are present in the home and workplace. Most poisonings are unintentional, but some victims take a poison intentionally either in a suicide attempt or to experience the effects produced by the substance. This chapter focuses primarily on unintentional poisonings. Poisoning caused by the misuse or overdose of alcohol and other drugs, including over-the-counter and prescription medications, is discussed in **Chapter 18**. Behavioral emergencies such as suicide are described in **Chapter 21**.

Virtually all poisonings can be prevented. Parents and other caretakers can protect children from poisoning by keeping them safely away from common products that are poisonous. Most adult poisonings involve the careless use or misuse of medications and cleaning products, which can be prevented by following safety guidelines.

Overview of Poisoning

A poison is any substance that enters or touches the body with effects that are injurious to health or are life-threatening. Poisons can enter the body

[1]*National Safety Council. (2011). Injury Facts®, 2011 Edition. Itasca, IL: Author.*

by being swallowed, injected (by hypodermic needle or an insect stinger), inhaled, or absorbed through the skin or mucous membranes. All too often, people think of the risk of poisoning only in terms of ingesting the substance; however, inhaling fumes from a product or spilling a chemical on unprotected skin can be just as dangerous. **Chapter 11**, (burns), describes the first aid for poisons (chemicals) that contact the skin or eyes. Injected poisons are described in **Chapters 18** (substance abuse) and **19** (insect stings). This chapter primarily discusses swallowed and inhaled poisons, along with the contact poisons of certain plants, but the prevention guidelines detailed in the next section apply to all forms of poison.

A huge percentage of poisonings occur in the home, most involving common products **(Box 17-1)**. The top 25 substances involved in poisonings are listed in **Table 17-1**. These are the most common types of products that contain poisons – a complete list of every product or substance that is poisonous would be many, many pages long. Because there are so many poisons present in so many different products, **the safest thing is to assume that *all* substances that can be swallowed, injected, breathed in or put in contact with skin are poisonous unless known to be otherwise**. Note that almost any substance

BOX 17-1: FACTS ABOUT POISONINGS

- Unintentional poisoning is second only to motor vehicle crashes as a cause of unintentional injury death.

- Among people 35 to 54 years old, unintentional poisoning causes more deaths than motor vehicle crashes.

- Unintentional poisoning causes about 708,318 emergency department visits a year.

- An estimated 71,000 children younger than 18 are seen in emergency departments each year because of medication poisonings (excluding abuse and recreational drug use). More than 80 percent of those posionings occurred because an unsupervised child found and consumed medicines.

Source: Centers for Disease Control and Prevention, Poisoning in the United States: Fact Sheet, http://www.cdc.gov/HomeandRecreationalSafety/Poisoning/poisoning-factsheet.htm Accessed March 4, 2011.

TABLE 17-1
TOP 25 SUBSTANCE CATEGORIES INVOLVED IN POISONINGS

Substance Category	All Substances	%
Analgesics	337,650	11.75
Cosmetics/Personal Care Products	222,774	7.75
Cleaning Substances (Household)	212,616	7.40
Sedative/Hypnotics/ Antipsychotics	167,916	5.84
Foreign Bodies/Toys/ Miscellaneous	125,179	4.35
Topical Preparations	116,377	4.05
Antidepressants	102,792	3.58
Cardiovascular Drugs	95,527	3.32
Antihistamines	95,304	3.32
Pesticides	92,240	3.21
Alcohol	91,973	3.20
Cold and Cough Preparations	89,722	3.12
Vitamins	73,080	2.54
Bites and Envenomations	70,857	2.46
Antimicrobials	70,592	2.46
Hormones and Hormone Antagonists	59,762	2.08
Plants	58,933	2.05
Gastrointestinal Preparations	56,635	1.97
Anticonvulsants	47,013	1.64
Stimulants and Street Drugs	46,242	1.61
Hydrocarbons	43,479	1.51
Chemicals	40,613	1.41
Arts/Crafts/Office Supplies	36,229	1.26
Electrolytes and Minerals	34,162	1.19
Fumes/Gases/Vapors	32,875	1.14

Source: American Association of Poison Control Centers http://www.aapcc.org/dnn/Portals/0/correctedannualreport. pdf Accessed March 4, 2011.

can be poisonous in doses larger than intended, including aspirin, vitamins, herbal supplements and natural remedies and prescribed or over-the-counter medication.

Poison Control Centers

A system of **Poison Control Centers (PCC)** has been developed throughout the United States to provide information and treatment advice for all types of poisonings. Presently there are 62 Poison Control Centers throughout the United States and U.S. territories. All can be reached by dialing the same telephone number: 800-222-1222, 24 hours a day. Your call will be routed to the regional PCC in your area. This telephone number should be posted by your telephone at home and in your workplace. When you are away from this number, call 9-1-1 and if necessary the dispatcher will contact the Poison Control Center. In almost all cases it is better to call the PCC in cases of poisoning than a health care provider because the PCC has the most accurate and up-to-date information. Personnel staffing each PCC have information about all known poisons and will advise you what first aid to give in each poisoning case.

The American Association of Poison Control Centers (AAPCC) provides valuable information about how to prevent poisonings as well as information about specific poisons. On request, the AAPCC will provide a list of poisonous plants in your area to help you identify threats in your yard or in places you may visit (www.aapcc.org).

Preventing Poisoning

Most poisonings occur unintentionally and can be prevented by following simple guidelines. The safety principles for preventing poisonings in children are based on keeping children away from products and substances that contain poisons and educating children on safe behaviors. Prevention principles for adults, who often use products and medications that can be poisonous, focus on safe and appropriate use, and on minimizing or eliminating the risk of unintentional exposure.

Preventing Poisoning in Children

Children younger than 6 are at the highest risk for poisoning. Children are often curious about what things taste like and will put many different substances into their mouths. Colorful product packages may attract a young child who cannot easily distinguish between food products and other products found in the home. Even if they are told to leave certain things alone, young children do not yet have the cognitive skills needed to understand why they should not eat or drink substances they find. Prevention emphasizes keeping all potentially harmful substances where children cannot get to them.

Follow these guidelines provided by the American Association of Poison Control Centers:

Household and Chemical Products

- Use safety locks on all cabinets. Store potential poisons out of reach of small children.

- Store all poisonous household and chemical products out of sight of children.

- If you are using a product and need to answer the telephone or doorbell, take the child with you. Most poisonings occur when the product is in use.

- Store all products in their original containers. *Do not* use food containers such as milk jugs or soda bottles to store household and chemical products.

- Store food and household and chemical products in separate areas. Mistaken identity could cause a serious poisoning. Many poisonous products look like and come in containers very similar to those that contain drinks or food – for example, apple juice and pine cleaner.

- Return household and chemical products to safe storage immediately after use.

- Use extra caution during mealtimes or when the family routine is disrupted. Many poisonings take place at these times.

- Pesticides can be absorbed through the skin and can be extremely toxic. Keep children away from areas that have recently been sprayed. Store pesticides in a safe place where children cannot reach them.

- Discard old or outdated household and chemical products.

- Take time to teach children about poisonous substances.

- Keep the Poison Control Center telephone number on or near your telephone.

Medicine

- Keep medicines out of sight, locked up and out of reach of children.

- Make sure all medicines are in child-resistant containers and are labeled properly. Remember that "child-resistant" does not mean childproof.

- Never leave pills on the counter or in plastic bags. Always store medicines in their original container with a child-resistant cap.

- Keep purses and diaper bags out of reach of children.

- Do not take medicines in front of children. Young children often imitate adult behaviors.

- Do not call medicine "candy". Medicines and candy look alike, and children cannot tell the difference.

- Vitamins are medicine. Vitamins with iron can be especially poisonous. Keep them locked up and out of reach of children.

- Be aware of medicines that visitors may bring into your home. Children are curious and may investigate visitors' purses and suitcases.

Plants

- Contact your local Poison Control Center for more information about toxic plants in your area. **Figure 17-1** shows three common plants that are poisonous when eaten.

- Know the names of the plants in your home and in your yard. Label all of your plants. If you are having difficulty identifying a plant, take a sample to a nursery for identification.

- Keep poisonous plants out of reach of children and pets.

- Teach your children not to eat mushrooms growing in the yard. Some of these mushrooms can be poisonous. Be aware that mushrooms are often abundant after rain.

- Teach your children not to eat leaves and berries that grow in the yard. Do not assume a plant is safe to eat if you see wild animals eating it.

- Keep children and pets away from plants that have recently been sprayed with weed killer, bug killer or fertilizer.

Preventing Poisoning in Adults

Follow these guidelines provided by the American Association of Poison Control Centers:

- Keep potential poisons in their original containers. Do not use food containers such as cups or bottles to store household and chemical products.

- Store food and household and chemical products in separate areas. Mistaken identity could cause a serious poisoning.

- Read and follow the directions and caution labels on household and chemical products before using them.

- Never mix household and chemical products together. A poisonous gas may be created when mixing chemicals.

- Turn on fans and open windows when using household and chemical products.

- When spraying household and chemical products, make sure the spray nozzle is directed away from your face and other people. Wear protective clothing –

long-sleeved shirts, long pants, socks, shoes and gloves – when spraying pesticides and other chemicals.

- Pesticides can be absorbed through the skin and can be extremely poisonous. Stay away from areas that have recently been sprayed.

- Never sniff containers to discover what is inside.

- Discard old or outdated household and chemical products.

- First aid instructions on product containers may be incorrect or outdated. Call the Poison Control Center instead for guidelines to follow if an exposure occurs.

- Keep the Poison Control Center telephone number on or near your telephone.

- Follow the prevention guidelines in **Chapter 18** to prevent unintentional poisoning by the misuse of over-the-counter and prescription medications.

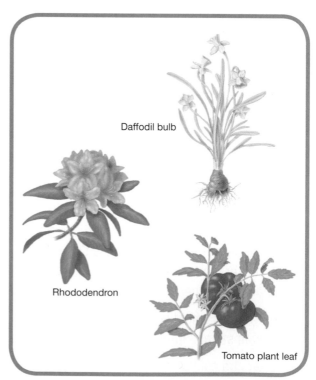

Figure 17-1 *Examples of plants that are poisonous when eaten.*

Swallowed Poisons

Most cases of poisoning involve substances that are swallowed. Depending on the poison, effects may begin almost immediately or may be delayed. First aid is most effective if given as soon as possible after the poison is swallowed, and in some cases the effects can be prevented or minimized by acting quickly. Poisoning is like sudden illness in that often there is no visible injury and you may not know immediately what happened. The victim may be unresponsive or, even if responsive, may be confused and disoriented and unable to tell you what happened. The most important aspect of first aid for a poisoning often is recognizing that a poisoning has occurred.

As you check the scene and perform your initial assessment of the victim, look around for any sign that the victim may be poisoned. Look for containers nearby or any clue that the person was using a substance or product. Ask others at the scene if anyone saw anything or knows what the person was doing when the problem occurred. If the victim is responsive and identifies a substance to which he or she was exposed, try to learn how much the person may have swallowed and how long ago.

The specific signs and symptoms of poisons depend on the substance and many other factors, although many poisons cause similar general effects:

- The victim may look and feel ill.
- The victim may have abdominal pain, feel nauseated and may vomit or have diarrhea.
- The victim may have altered mental status or become unresponsive.
- There may be burns, stains or odors around the victim's mouth.
- The pupils of the eyes may be dilated or constricted.
- The victim may be breathing abnormally.

Be aware that the condition of a poisoning victim may change rapidly.

First aid for a poisoning depends on the victim's condition. For an unresponsive victim, call 9-1-1 immediately. Check for normal breathing and provide CPR if needed. Because of the risk for vomiting, put a breathing, unresponsive victim in the recovery position and continue to monitor breathing.

If the victim is responsive, call the Poison Control Center and follow the instructions provided **(Box 17-2)**. Depending on the poison, the PCC may direct you to take any of various actions. Some poisons may be diluted by having the victim drink water or milk. For some poisons the victim may benefit from drinking a solution of activated charcoal, if available, to absorb the poison. Activated charcoal is available in a powder or liquid form without prescription and may be kept in the home medicine cabinet for use if the PCC advises it. Because none of these actions is used for all kinds of poisons, never take any of these actions unless told to do so by the Poison Control Center. The PCC will also tell you whether

BOX 17-2: CALLING THE POISON CONTROL CENTER

If possible, have the following information with you if you call a Poison Control Center for help with a suspected poisoning with any product or substance. This information will help the Center to determine the best care to provide. But do not delay a call to the PCC to look for this information if it is not readily available.

- The victim's present condition
- Name of the product and ingredients
- How much of the product was taken
- The time the poisoning happened
- Your name and phone number
- The victim's approximate age and weight

to call 9-1-1 or seek other urgent medical care for a poisoning incident (see First Aid: "Swallowed Poisons").

Note that, in the past, syrup of ipecac was used in some situations to induce vomiting in a victim of swallowed poison. Because of problems caused by this and its lack of effectiveness in most cases, PCCs no longer recommend the use of ipecac.

Food Poisoning

Food poisoning occurs after one eats food that is contaminated with microorganisms, usually bacteria or their toxins. Most cases of food poisoning are acute infections, although some bacteria make toxins that can poison a food even if the bacteria are later killed. The CDC estimates that 76 million people in the United States become sick every year from pathogens in food, and about 5,000 die.[1] Botulism is a life-threatening type of food poisoning produced by a certain bacterium present in improperly canned or preserved food.

Contamination can occur at any stage, from growing the food through processing to food preparation and delivery. Food contamination usually results from improper cooking or leaving a cooked food out for more than 2 hours at room temperature. Most bacteria grow rapidly and are undetected because they do not change the odor or taste of the food. Freezing a food will slow or stop bacteria growth but will not kill the bacteria.

Food poisoning symptoms may begin soon after eating or within a day. The most common signs and symptoms are nausea, vomiting, abdominal pain and diarrhea. Talk to your health care provider to see if treatment is needed (see First Aid: "Food Poisoning"). Seek urgent medical care if any of the following signs and symptoms occurs:

- Signs of shock: shallow breathing; cold, clammy, pale or ashen skin; shaking or chills; or chest pain

[1]*Centers for Disease Control and Prevention, http://www. cdc.gov/ncidod/eid/vol5no5/mead.htm Accessed March 11, 2011.*

- Signs of severe dehydration: dry mouth, decreased urine output, dizziness, fatigue, increased breathing rate

- Confusion or difficulty reasoning

Preventing Food Poisoning

The National Digestive Diseases Information Clearinghouse[2] recommends the following guidelines to prevent harmful bacteria from growing in food and causing food poisoning:

- Cook food long enough and at a high enough temperature to kill bacteria

- Refrigerate prepared food within 2 hours, before bacteria multiply

- Wash all raw fruits and vegetables under running water

- Never defrost food on the kitchen counter – use a refrigerator, running water or a microwave oven

- Wash your hands, utensils and surfaces with hot soapy water before and after preparing food

[2]*The National Digestive Diseases Information Clearinghouse, http://www.digestive.niddk.nih.gov/ddiseases/pubs/ bacteria_ES/index.htm#4 Accessed March 4, 2011.*

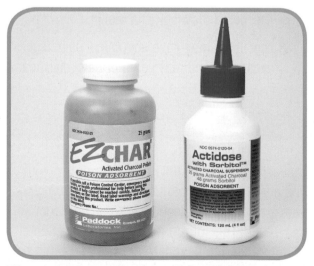

Figure 17-2 *The Poison Control Center may advise taking activated charcoal in some cases of poisoning.*

Swallowed Poisons
Signs, Symptoms and Care

When You See

- **An open container of a poisonous substance**
- **Nausea and vomiting; signs of abdominal pain or cramps**
- **Drowsiness, dizziness, disorientation or other altered mental status**
- **Changing levels of responsiveness**

Do This First

1 Determine what was swallowed, when and how much.

2 For a responsive victim, call the Poison Control Center (800-222-1222) immediately and follow the instructions given.

3 For a victim with signs of a life-threatening condition and for any unresponsive victim, call 9-1-1 and provide basic life support (BLS) as needed.

Additional Care

- Put an unresponsive victim in the recovery position and be prepared for vomiting. Monitor the victim's breathing and be ready to give CPR if needed.

- If a responsive victim's mouth or lips are burned by a corrosive chemical, rinse the mouth with cold water (do not allow the victim to swallow).

ALERT

- Do not give the victim anything to eat or drink unless instructed by the PCC or health care provider.
- Do not follow first aid instructions present on some household product labels; instead, call the PCC.

Inhaled Poisons

In both home and work settings, various gases and fumes may be present. Products such as paints, thinners and many chemicals give off fumes that can result in a poisoning if there is not enough fresh air or other protection. Some products' fumes are so toxic that a respirator must be worn when working with them, even outdoors where fresh air is plentiful. Always check product labels for health risks and safety precautions.

Inhaled poisons also include gases that may escape from pipelines or tanks being transported. Whenever you smell gas or have other evidence of a leak, stay away from the scene. Remember that not all hazardous gases or fumes can be smelled. Call 9-1-1 and let a specially trained hazardous materials team manage the situation. In such a situation do not risk your own safety in an attempt to reach a victim. **Chapter 2** describes typical hazardous scenes and the warning placards that may indicate the presence of a poisonous gas.

Smoke and fumes resulting from fires are also poisonous. Fires produce carbon monoxide and, depending on the substances being burned, may produce other highly toxic gases. **Chapter 24** describes actions to take in or near a fire.

The signs and symptoms of inhaled poisons may be similar to those of other poisons.

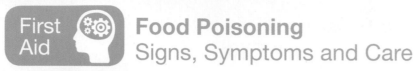

Food Poisoning
Signs, Symptoms and Care

First Aid

When You See

- **Nausea and vomiting; signs of abdominal pain or cramps**
- **Diarrhea, possibly with blood**
- **Headache or fever**

Do This First

1 Have the victim rest lying down.

2 Give the victim lots of clear liquids.

3 Seek medical attention.

Additional Care

- Check with others with whom the victim has eaten recently.

ALERT

Botulism

- Botulism is more likely to occur from the consumption of home-canned foods. If the victim experiences dizziness, muscle weakness and difficulty talking or breathing, call 9-1-1.

Breathing difficulty with or without chest pain may be present. Altered mental status may include dizziness, disorientation, headache, unresponsiveness or other symptoms.

In most cases you will not know the specific treatment for an inhaled poison. First, if it is safe for you to go to the victim, try to ensure that the victim is breathing fresh air. Move the victim outdoors or to a well-ventilated area, if possible. If the victim should not be moved because of injuries or other factors, ventilate the area. If the victim is responsive, call the PCC and follow the instructions given. If the victim is unresponsive, call 9-1-1.

The general first aid for an inhaled poison is the same as for carbon monoxide poisoning, described in the next section. Carbon monoxide is the most common gas involved in poisonings.

Carbon Monoxide

Carbon monoxide is especially dangerous because it is invisible, odorless and tasteless—and very lethal. This gas results in more fatal unintentional poisonings in the United States than any other poison. Carbon monoxide may be present from motor vehicle or boat exhaust, a faulty furnace, a kerosene heater, industrial equipment, a poorly vented fireplace, or a wood stove or fire. Exposure to large amounts causes an immediate poisoning reaction; a small leak may cause gradual poisoning with less dramatic symptoms. To prevent poisoning, carbon monoxide detectors should be installed along with smoke detectors in appropriate locations. If your carbon monoxide detector goes off, do not investigate the problem yourself; instead, leave the premises and call your furnace company or appropriate other professional.

Preventing Carbon Monoxide Poisoning

More than 15,000 cases of carbon monoxide poisoning and about 500 deaths occur each year in the United States from carbon monoxide poisoning unrelated to fires.[3] The CDC

[3]Centers for Disease Control and Prevention, http://www.cdc.gov/mmwr/preview/mmwrhtml/mm5650a1.htm Accessed March 1, 2011.

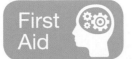
Carbon Monoxide and Inhaled Poisons
Signs, Symptoms and Care

When You See

- **Headache**
- **Dizziness, lightheadedness, confusion or weakness**
- **Nausea or vomiting**
- **Signs of chest pain**
- **Convulsions**
- **Changing levels of responsiveness**

Do This First

1 Immediately move the victim into fresh air.

2 Call 9-1-1 even if the victim starts to recover.

3 Monitor the victim's breathing and be ready to give CPR if needed.

Additional Care

- Put an unresponsive victim in the recovery position.
- Loosen tight clothing around the neck or chest.

recommends the following strategies to prevent carbon monoxide exposure in the home:

- Have your heating system, water heater, and any other gas-, oil- or coal-burning appliances serviced by a qualified technician every year.

- Install a battery-operated carbon monoxide (CO) detector in your home, and check or replace the battery when you change the time on your clocks each spring and fall.

- If your CO detector sounds, evacuate your home immediately and telephone 9-1-1.

- Seek prompt medical attention if you suspect CO poisoning and are feeling dizzy, lightheaded or nauseated.

- Do not use a generator, charcoal grill, camp stove, or other gasoline- or charcoal-burning device inside your home, basement or garage or near a window.

- Do not run a car or truck inside a garage attached to your house, even if you leave the door open.

- Do not burn anything in a stove or fireplace that is not vented.

- Do not heat your house with a gas oven.

First Aid for Carbon Monoxide Poisoning

Carbon monoxide poisoning usually causes altered mental status. Prolonged periods of exposure to CO may cause headaches, dizziness, confusion, poor judgment and sleepiness. Continued exposure brings on breathing difficulty, nausea, vomiting and heart palpitations. Exposure to high levels of CO for prolonged periods can result in seizures, unresponsiveness and death.

The most important first aid for a victim of carbon monoxide poisoning is to get the victim to fresh air, but do not risk your own health if the scene is dangerous. Call 9-1-1. If it is safe to move the victim, do so quickly. Note that even a victim who seems to recover needs medical care for the poisoning (see First Aid: "Carbon Monoxide and Inhaled Poisons").

Learning Checkpoint 1

1. Check off the common signs and symptoms of a swallowed poison.

   _____Nausea   _____Red lips

   _____Uncontrolled shaking   _____Vomiting

   _____Dizziness   _____Unresponsiveness

   _____Drowsiness   _____Hyperactivity

2. Name one action you would take for a victim of food poisoning that you would not take for a victim of swallowed poison.

   _____

3. The first thing to do for a victim of carbon monoxide poisoning is –

   a. loosen tight clothing around the neck.

   b. call 9-1-1.

   c. move the victim to fresh air.

   d. place the victim in the recovery position.

4. You are in a friend's house when you enter the kitchen and find the friend's child unresponsive on the floor. The cabinet under the sink is open and the cap is off of a bottle of a cleaning product. Describe what actions you need to take.

   _____

Poison Ivy, Oak and Sumac

Contact with poison ivy, oak and sumac causes an allergic skin reaction, called **allergic contact dermatitis**, in about half the population. A resin in the leaves of these plants causes the reaction. These plants grow in many areas of the country but can be identified by their distinctive leaves **(Figure 17-3)**. The resin can rub off on a person's clothing and shoes and then be transferred to the skin. If someone touches the leaves and gets the resin on the fingers, touching other body areas before washing may transfer the irritating resin to other skin areas, including the face and eyes and even the genitals.

If you know you have made contact with one of these plants, wash the area as soon as possible with soap and water. Also wash clothing and wipe off shoes, because the resin on these can still cause the reaction.

The rash may appear within a few hours or up to two days after exposure **(Figure 17-4)**. The skin is red and often very itchy, and young children

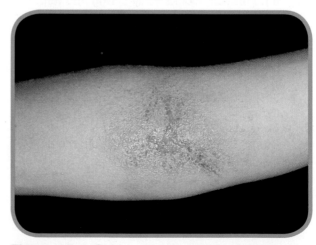

Figure 17-4 *Skin rash caused by poison ivy.*

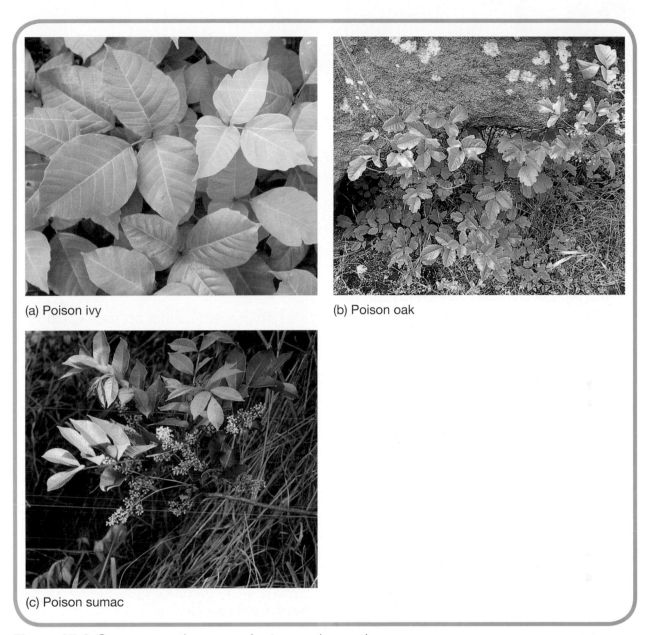

(a) Poison ivy

(b) Poison oak

(c) Poison sumac

Figure 17-3 *Common poisonous plants causing rashes.*

must be kept from scratching it because the skin easily breaks and may become infected with bacteria. Once the rash appears on the skin and has been washed, however, it cannot spread to other people. First aid is usually to control the itching, which can be intense and lasts as long as the rash persists (usually less than two weeks). Cool, wet compresses applied four times a day generally help, along with calamine lotion or a paste of baking soda and water between compresses. Make the baking soda paste just thick enough to cling to the skin without running off. Topical hydrocortisone cream or an oral antihistamine may help in more serious cases. See a health care provider if the reaction is very severe or the rash occurs around the eyes or genitals. Fever or pus oozing from the rash may indicate an infection that should also receive medical treatment (see First Aid: "Poison Ivy, Oak and Sumac").

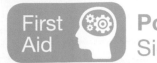

Poison Ivy, Oak and Sumac
Signs, Symptoms and Care

When You See

- **Redness and itching**
- **Rash or blisters (may weep)**
- **Possible headache and fever**

Do This First

1 Wash the area thoroughly with soap and water as soon as possible after contact.

2 For severe reactions or swelling on the face or genitals, seek medical attention.

3 Treat itching with colloid oatmeal baths; a paste made of baking soda and water; calamine lotion or topical hydrocortisone cream; and an oral antihistamine (e.g., Benadryl).

Additional Care

- To prevent further spread, wash the victim's hands, clothing and shoes (as well as pets) that came in contact with the plants.

ALERT

- Do not burn these poisonous plants to get rid of them, as smoke also spreads the poisonous resin.

Learning Checkpoint 2

1. True or False: Never put water on a site of contact with poison ivy because of the risk of spreading the rash further.

2. When should a person with a poison ivy or oak rash see a health care provider?

_____

3. Which of the following can help reduce the itching of poison ivy?

   a. Hydrocortisone cream

   b. Rubbing alcohol

   c. A paste made with dishwasher detergent

   d. All of the above

Concluding Thoughts

Remember that a poison is any substance that is injurious to health after it enters the body. In addition to those substances we all think of as obvious poisons, alcohol and drugs can be toxic when misused or abused – prescription and over-the-counter drugs as well as illicit drugs. In fact, poisonings from medications, even everyday aspirin, are more common than poisonings caused by household products. In the next chapter you will learn about the problems of substance abuse and misuse.

Learning Outcomes

You should now be able to do the following:

1. Explain different ways poisons can enter the body.

2. List things you can do in your own home to prevent the poisoning of both children and adults.

3. Describe the role of Poison Control Centers in the treatment of poisoning.

4. Describe the first aid for swallowed and inhaled poisons.

5. List actions to take when exposed to poison ivy, oak or sumac.

Review Questions

1. Where do most poisonings occur?

    a. Industrial settings

    b. Homes

    c. Farms

    d. Day care centers

2. What group experiences the largest percentage of poisonings?

    a. Children younger than 6

    b. Children 4 to 14 years old

    c. The elderly

    d. Construction workers

3. Which of the following types of products may be poisonous?

    a. Cosmetics

    b. Vitamins with iron

    c. Arts and crafts supplies

    d. All of the above

4. The common signs and symptoms of swallowed poisonings often include –

    a. dizziness and aching in the joints.

    b. unresponsiveness and high fever.

    c. nausea and altered mental status.

    d. localized redness and swelling around the joints.

5. For a responsive child who swallowed a substance that might be poisonous, it is best to call –

    a. the Poison Control Center.

    b. the child's pediatrician.

    c. the local hospital emergency department.

    d. the child's school nurse.

6. First aid for most swallowed poisons includes –

    a. giving the victim milk to drink.

    b. inducing vomiting by any means.

    c. having the victim drink as much water as possible.

    d. calling 9-1-1 or the Poison Control Center for help.

7. When should you seek medical care for a victim who feels ill a few hours after eating food that may have been contaminated?

    a. When the victim is experiencing shaking or chills

    b. When the victim feels dizzy

    c. When the victim's skin is cold and clammy

    d. All of the above

8. What should you do for a breathing, unresponsive victim suspected of having swallowed a poison?

    a. Put the victim in the shock position with the feet raised.

    b. Put the victim on his or her back with the head raised.

    c. Put the victim in the recovery position.

    d. Put the victim in the prone position with his or her head lower than the body.

9. Exposure to carbon monoxide may cause –

    a. bleeding at mucous membranes.

    b. dizziness.

    c. dark stains around the mouth.

    d. hyperexcitability.

10. To treat the itching caused by poison ivy, what can be put on the rash?

    a. An oral antihistamine tablet crushed and mixed with water

    b. A paste of baking soda and water

    c. Lemon juice mixed with powdered sugar

    d. Antibiotic cream

Chapter 18 • Substance Misuse and Abuse

Chapter Preview

- Substance Abuse
- Prevention of Substance Abuse
- Prevention of Drug Misuse and Overdose

- Intoxication
- Drug Abuse
- Medication Overdose

You are at a friend's holiday party, where some of the guests are drinking rather heavily. At the end of the evening, when most have left, you notice a young woman alone on the sofa, apparently either sleeping or passed out. She seems to be by herself and others are saying to just leave her alone and let her "sleep it off." You are wondering if you should do something – if it could be a more serious problem – but what can you do?

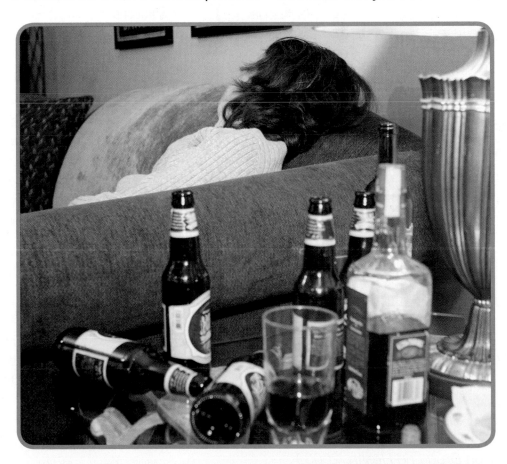

The misuse and abuse of alcohol, illicit drugs and medication is a huge problem in our society. The effects of alcohol and other drugs may cause a medical or behavioral emergency or may complicate a sudden illness or injury. In either case, first aiders need to understand the effects of alcohol and other drugs and special considerations when giving first aid to victims under the influence.

Substance Abuse

Substance abuse is a problem that occurs virtually everywhere in our society. Consider these U.S. statistics:[1]

- More than half of people 12 or older, or about 130 million, regularly consume alcohol.

- Nearly one-fourth of those, or about 59 million people, participate in binge drinking at least once a month.

- Almost 7%, or about 17 million people, routinely drink heavily.

- Over 8.7%, or 21.8 million people, use illicit drugs.

Both heavy drinking and binge drinking are most common in the late teen and early adult years and gradually taper off with age, although they remain a common behavior **(Figure 18-1)**. Although some variations in drinking habits are correlated with ethnic group, socioeconomic status and education levels, studies show alcohol use is a problem at all ages and in all groups. One common problem behavior, driving under the influence of alcohol, is practiced by about one-fourth of young adults and by high percentages of other age groups.

The popularity of alcohol may be due in part to several common myths that suggest it creates fewer risks than other drugs. Here are some facts about consumption:

- Someone drinking beer is just as likely to become impaired as someone drinking hard liquor. The amount of alcohol in a 12-ounce beer is the same as in a 5-ounce glass of wine or 1.5 ounces of 80-proof spirits.

- Heavier people are no less likely to become impaired by consuming alcohol than lighter people. Many complex factors influence a person's reaction to alcohol and these cannot easily be predicted. It is therefore unsafe to drink and drive at any time.

- From the first drink, alcohol impairs motor skills, judgment, reaction time and other abilities needed for safe driving.

The toll of alcohol abuse in society includes automobile death rates, other injuries, and huge medical costs spent on alcohol-related health problems such as liver disease and cardiovascular conditions. Millions of victims of alcohol-related

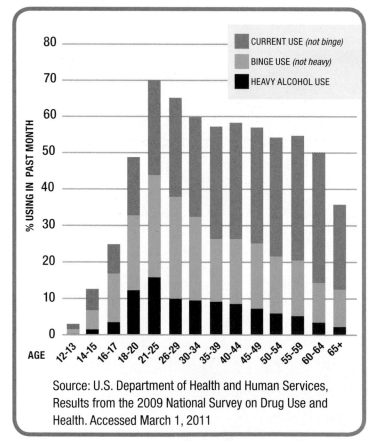

Source: U.S. Department of Health and Human Services, Results from the 2009 National Survey on Drug Use and Health. Accessed March 1, 2011

Figure 18-1 *Alcohol Use and Abuse in Different Age Groups (From the National Survey on Drug and Health, 2003.)*

[1]*U.S. Department of Health and Human Services, Results from the 2009 National Survey on Drug Use and Health. http://oas.samhsa.gov/NSDUH/2k9NSDUH/2k9ResultsP. pdf Accessed March 1, 2011.*

injuries and illnesses are brought to hospital emergency departments every year. Almost 12,000 people die each year in the United States as the result of alcohol-related motor vehicle crashes. This represents nearly one-third of all traffic deaths.[2]

Illicit drugs include marijuana, cocaine, heroin, hallucinogens, inhalants and the nonmedical use of prescription pain relievers, tranquilizers, stimulants and sedatives. Like alcohol abuse, illicit drug abuse typically begins in the preteen years, peaks in the late teen and early adult years, and gradually becomes less common thereafter. Marijuana is the most commonly used illicit drug **(Table 18-1)**.

Prevention of Substance Abuse

Because alcohol and other drug abuse typically begin at young ages, most prevention efforts focus on children and adolescents. For adults who have begun abusing alcohol and other drugs, many treatment centers and organizations have programs available. The 2009 National Survey on Drug Use and Health has identified key risk factors for developing an abuse problem, and a wide range of prevention measures have been developed to address these:

- **Substance abuse is more likely in people who perceive less risk in using the substance**. Education programs in elementary and middle schools teach students the risks of alcohol and drugs, and many public information campaigns strive to make the risks known.

- **Substance abuse is more prevalent among people with easier access to drugs and alcohol**. Law enforcement and other programs strive to reduce the availability of drugs and alcohol to young people, although most youths still report that it is easy to obtain alcohol, marijuana and other drugs.

- **Substance abuse is about five times as prevalent among youths who perceive**

that their parents would not strongly disapprove of their substance use as it is among those who feel their parents would strongly disapprove. Public education campaigns increasingly focus on the role of parents' attitudes and the need for communication with their children.

- **Substance abuse is more prevalent among people whose peers do not express disapproval about substance abuse**.

- **Substance abuse is about twice as prevalent among youths who dislike school**. Many schools have adopted programs aimed at increasing student satisfaction levels and building the self-esteem of students related to their schooling.

- **Substance abuse is more prevalent among youths who engage in delinquent behaviors such as fighting, stealing or carrying weapons**.

- **Substance abuse is about twice as prevalent among youths who do not attend religious services or youth activities such as sports, band and other after-school activities**. Recognizing this, many schools and communities have increased the availability of programs for youth.

Table 18-1: Illicit Drug Use in the United States

Drug	Number of Users (in past month)
Marijuana	16.7 million
Cocaine	1.6 million
Hallucinogens	1.3 million
Methamphetamine	502,000
Prescription drugs used illicitly	7.0 million

Source: U.S. Department of Health and Human Services, Results from the 2009 National Survey on Drug Use and Health. http://oas.samhsa.gov/NSDUH/2k9NSDUH/2k9ResultsP.pdf Accessed March 1, 2011.

[2]*National Highway Traffic Safety Administration http://www-nrd.nhtsa.dot.gov/Pubs/811155.pdf Accessed March 1, 2011.*

- **Substance abuse is less prevalent among youths who have participated in drug, tobacco or alcohol prevention programs outside of school.**

- **Substance abuse is less prevalent among youths who report that their parents always or sometimes monitored their behaviors, such as studying and doing household chores, than among youths whose parents "seldom" or "never" engaged in such behaviors.**

The 2009 National Survey on Drug Use and Health showed that prevention programs are having a positive effect. Youths exposed to substance abuse prevention messages in or outside of school, who have talked with their parents about the dangers of drug and alcohol use, and who have participated in various special programs are all less likely to use or abuse alcohol and other drugs. But as the earlier statistics show, abuse remains a huge problem and clearly more efforts are needed both to understand the many complex factors involved in substance abuse behavior and to develop prevention strategies to successfully counter those factors.

Prevention of Drug Misuse and Overdose

Substance abuse is the intentional and often frequent nonmedical use of a substance for its effects, typically without regard for potential negative health effects. **Substance misuse**, in contrast, may involve using a drug for an unintended purpose or using it in larger amounts than prescribed, including unintentional misuse. Misuse may occur, for example, if a person takes more of a medication than prescribed either by mistake or from a false belief that more of the medication is better. Because misuse, like abuse, can lead to a drug **overdose**, it is important to take steps to prevent it:

- Use medications only as prescribed, and read product information.

- Keep all medications in their original, clearly labeled containers. Check the label before taking the medication. (Never take a medication in the dark.) Help the elderly organize their medications to prevent accidental overdose.

- If a person's judgment may be diminished by a medical or other condition, make sure that the person cannot unintentionally use too much of any prescribed or over-the-counter medication.

- Read and follow the directions and warnings on the label before taking any medicine.

- If you have any questions about the intended use of your medicine, contact your doctor.

- Some medicines are dangerous when mixed with alcohol. Consult your doctor or pharmacist.

- Be aware of potential drug interactions. Some medicines interact dangerously with food or other medicines. Your doctor should be made aware of all medicines, prescription or over-the-counter, you are currently taking. Talk to your doctor before taking any natural or herbal supplements.

- Dispose of old and outdated medicines. Some medications can become dangerous or ineffective over time.

- Never share prescription medicines. Medicines should be taken by the person to whom they are prescribed and for the reason prescribed.

- Remember that any over-the-counter drug, including herbal supplements, vitamins and natural remedies, can be toxic in doses larger than recommended in the product information.

Intoxication

Excessive alcohol consumption causes problems that may lead to a medical emergency. In addition to the problems caused by intoxication, the person may have an injury or sudden illness requiring care. Remember to not assume that a victim is experiencing signs and symptoms only as a result of intoxication. In some cases, someone who

Learning Checkpoint 1

1. The most commonly abused drugs in the United States are –

    a. alcohol and marijuana.

    b. marijuana and cocaine.

    c. cocaine and pain relievers.

    d. heroin and hallucinogens.

2. Substance abuse efforts should focus on people in what age group(s)?

    _____

3. Put a check mark next to all actions that are appropriate for helping to prevent the misuse of prescribed drugs.

    _____ Take medications only when you feel the symptoms for which the medication is prescribed.

    _____ Read product information that comes with prescription medications.

    _____ Keep medications in their original labeled containers.

    _____ Use medications prescribed for someone else only when you are certain you have the same condition as the person with the medication.

    _____ Ensure that a person with diminished judgment cannot unintentionally take too much medication.

behaves as if intoxicated may not have consumed alcohol at all but may be experiencing a problem such as a diabetic emergency that causes altered mental status.

Drinking a large amount of alcohol in a short period of time can lead to alcohol poisoning, which may result in unresponsiveness, seizures or death. Alcohol has depressant effects on the respiratory system and can cause an overdose similar to that of depressant drugs. First aid focuses on ensuring that the person receives medical care if needed and protecting the person from injury due to the intoxication (see First Aid: "Intoxication").

Alcohol Withdrawal

Someone who drinks heavily for a long time may develop a physical **dependence** on alcohol. **Withdrawal** from alcohol dependence may then cause delirium tremens (sometimes called "the DTs"), an altered mental status characterized by confusion, disorientation, agitation and altered perception such as hallucinations or illusions (see First Aid: "Alcohol Withdrawal").

Drug Abuse

Illicit drugs and prescription drugs used for non-medical purposes cause a wide variety of effects, depending on the type of drug and the amount used **(Figure 18-2)**. The primary effects of drugs commonly abused are described in **Table 18-2**. You do not need to know the type of drug taken in order to care for the victim. Consider the possibility of drug abuse or overdose whenever a victim's behavior or signs and symptoms cannot otherwise be explained. Observe the scene for drug **paraphernalia**, such as

(continues on page 291)

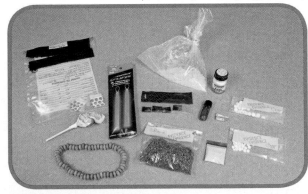

Figure 18-2 *Illicit drugs.*

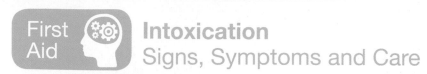

First Aid

Intoxication
Signs, Symptoms and Care

When You See

- **Smell of alcohol about the person**
- **Flushed, moist face**
- **Vomiting**
- **Slurred speech or staggering**
- **Rapid heart rate**
- **Impaired judgment and motor skills**
- **Agitated or combative behavior**
- **Changing levels of responsiveness, coma**

Do This First

1 Check for injuries or illness. Do not assume alcohol is the factor, or the only factor, involved.

2 For a responsive intoxicated person:

a. Stay with the person and protect him or her from injury (take away car keys).

b. Do not let the person lie down on his or her back.

c. Care for any injuries.

d. Calm and reassure the person.

e. If you have any doubt about whether the person may be injured or ill, may have consumed a dangerous amount of alcohol, or may injure themself or others, call 9-1-1 and let the dispatcher decide what help is needed.

3 For an unresponsive intoxicated person:

a. Position the victim in the recovery position (preferably on the left side to reduce the risk of vomiting); be prepared for vomiting.

b. Monitor the victim's breathing and be prepared to provide BLS if necessary.

c. Call 9-1-1 if the victim's breathing is irregular, if seizures occur or if the victim cannot be roused (coma).

4 For an injured intoxicated person:

a. Because alcohol may keep the person from feeling pain, do not rely on the victim's perception of an injury to guide your care.

b. Give first aid as you would if the victim were unresponsive, based on your assessment of the signs of injury or illness rather than reported symptoms.

c. If the mechanism of injury suggests the victim could have a spinal injury, do not move the victim; instead, keep the head aligned with the body.

Additional Care

- In a cold environment an intoxicated person is likely to experience hypothermia because dilated peripheral blood vessels allow the body's heat to escape more easily. Take steps to keep the victim warm (see **Chapter 20**).

ALERT

- Intoxication makes some people hostile and violent. Stay a distance away and call law enforcement if the person threatens violence.

(continued from page 289)

needles and syringes; eyedroppers; burnt spoons; straws or rolled-up dollar bills used for snorting; pipes; glass bulbs; razor blades; paper or plastic bags reeking of inhalants; or bottles of pills; powder or liquid (**Figure 18-3**).

First Aid for Drug Abuse or Overdose

The signs and symptoms of drug abuse and overdose vary widely, depending on the type and amount of the substance taken, but first aid should always follow the same general principles (see **Table 18-2**). Remember that a drug overdose is a type of poisoning. If you know the drug or other substance taken, call the Poison Control Center (PCC) and follow the instructions given (see **Chapter 17**). Otherwise, call 9-1-1 and provide supportive care and give first aid for any injuries until help arrives (see First Aid: "Drug Abuse or Overdose").

In some cases the victim may become violent or suicidal or may act bizarrely under the influence of the drug. Remember the general rule to never enter

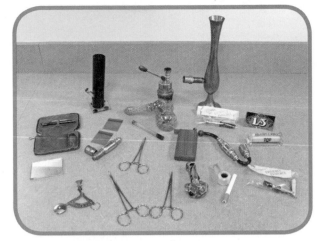

Figure 18-3 *Drug paraphernalia.*

a scene that is dangerous; withdraw from the scene if a victim's behavior becomes threatening. Note that when illegal drugs are involved, this is also a crime scene: be very careful to avoid potential dangers. **Chapter 21**, "Behavioral Emergencies," provides more information about dealing with victims who act in unusual or unpredictable ways.

METHAMPHETAMINE USE

The last two decades saw a huge increase in the abuse of methamphetamine. According to the 2004 National Survey on Drug Use and Health, 1.4 million people in the United States used methamphetamine at least once in the previous year. In 2009 this number dropped slightly to 1.2 million, but this is still a huge problem.

Methamphetamine is also known as meth, speed, crank, crystal and other street names. Methamphetamine is a powerful central nervous system stimulant with no medical uses. The many long-term health effects of methamphetamine include cancer, brain damage, heart problems, birth defects and miscarriage. The drug can also cause aggression and violence.

Methamphetamine is easily produced in illegal labs that have become increasingly common throughout the United States and now number in the thousands. Methamphetamine can be made

from common household and over-the-counter drugs such as decongestants. In addition to the dangers of the drug, the labs themselves raise many public health concerns because of the toxic wastes and poisonous fumes they produce. Fires and explosions are common. Meth labs may be set up in rental units, motel rooms, abandoned buildings, and even campgrounds and rest areas. Warning signs may include blacked-out windows, a strong odor of solvents, unusual nighttime activity, and excessive or unusual trash. Lab supplies often include pill bottles, jars, plastic tubing, metal cylinders and camp stoves. Meth labs are frequently abandoned, leaving behind potentially explosive and toxic chemicals. Never approach a suspected meth lab site, but report your suspicions to local law enforcement. Because of the chemicals involved, a hazmat team response is required.

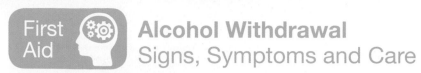

First Aid

Alcohol Withdrawal
Signs, Symptoms and Care

When You See

- **Hand trembling, head shaking**
- **Nausea or vomiting**
- **Seizures**
- **Hallucination, irrational fears or extreme confusion**
- **Unusual behavior**

Do This First

1 Call 9-1-1.

2 Give first aid as for an intoxicated victim, including the use of the recovery position for an unresponsive victim and monitoring breathing.

Additional Care

- Stay with the victim and protect him or her from injury until help arrives.

Table 18-2: Effects of Commonly Abused Drugs

Drug Class or Type	Septic Drugs	Examples of Street Names	Common Effects
Marijuana	Marijuana, hashish	Grass, pot, dope, weed, bamba, ganja, joint	Elation, relaxation, dizziness, distorted perceptions, hunger, fast pulse
Narcotics	Heroin, morphine, codeine, oxycodone (OxyContin, Percocet, Percodan)	H, horse, junk, stuff, smack, scag, poppy, ox, OCs, perc	Euphoria or stupor, depressant effects, dizziness, pain relief, muscle relaxation, impaired judgment, slowed respiration, coughing and sniffing, contracted pupils, slurred speech
Hallucinogens	LSD, PCP, mescaline, psilocybin	Acid, purple hearts, angel dust, peyote mushrooms	Stimulant effects, hallucinations, disorientation, anxiety, paranoia, trance-like state, euphoria, dilated pupils, fast pulse
Inhalants	Amyl nitrite, butyl nitrite, nitrous oxide, many solvents and common household products	Sniffing, huffing, snorting, bagging	Mood alterations, depressant or stimulant effects, nausea, excitability, slurred speech, impaired coordination
Stimulants	Amphetamine, methamphetamine, dextroamphetamine, cocaine and crack cocaine, designer drugs such as "ecstasy"	Speed, bennies, uppers, pep pills, white crosses, dex, ice, crank, rock, coke, snow, flake	Increased mental alertness, physical energy, talkativeness, restlessness, irritability or aggressive behavior, dilated pupils, increased respiration and blood pressure
Sedatives, depressants, tranquilizers	Barbiturates, benzodiazepines, muscle relaxants	Downers, goofballs, reds, ludes	Decreased mental alertness, relaxation, dizziness, slurred speech, dilated pupils, nausea and vomiting, delusions, slowed respiration and pulse

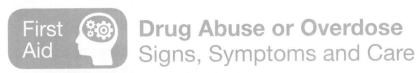

Drug Abuse or Overdose
Signs, Symptoms and Care

When You See

- **Unusual or erratic behavior**
- **The signs and symptoms of drug abuse**
- **Drug paraphernalia**

Do This First

1 Call 9-1-1 for serious signs and symptoms or call the Poison Control Center for instructions if you know the substance taken.

2 Some drugs cause violent behavior. If the victim demonstrates a potential for violent behavior, withdraw and wait for help to arrive.

3 Put an unresponsive victim in the recovery position (preferably on the left side to reduce the risk of vomiting), monitor breathing and give BLS as needed.

4 Check the victim for any injuries requiring care and provide care for any condition that occurs (seizures, shock, cardiac arrest, etc.).

5 Try to keep the victim awake and talking.

6 Keep the victim from harming himself or herself or others.

7 Question the victim and others present at the scene about the drug or substance used, the amount used, and when it was used. Give this information to arriving EMS personnel.

Additional Care

- Try to keep the victim calm.

ALERT

- Do not try to induce vomiting, which may cause further harm and is unlikely to help the victim.
- Some drugs make people hostile and violent. Stay a safe distance away and call law enforcement if you feel threatened.

18 • Substance Misuse and Abuse

Medication Overdose

Although many drug overdoses occur in people intentionally abusing drugs, overdose may also result from drug misuse, including unintentional drug poisoning caused by taking too much of a prescription or over-the-counter medication. A person having an overdose of a prescription medication may experience a wide range of behaviors and symptoms, depending on the drug.

Drug withdrawal can also be an emergency. In some cases it is impossible to know whether behaviors or symptoms are caused by drugs or by an injury or sudden illness. While caring for the victim, try to determine what drug the person may have taken: ask family members or others present at the scene, and look for pill bottles or other evidence of medications taken (see First Aid: "Medication Overdose").

Learning Checkpoint 2

1. Describe what to do for an intoxicated person who "passes out."

   _____

2. How is alcohol similar to narcotic drugs in high doses?

   a. Both stimulate the user to increased mental alertness.

   b. Both are depressants and can lead to impaired respiration or coma.

   c. Both can cause dangerously high blood pressure and internal bleeding.

   d. All of the above

3. Check off appropriate actions to take for a person with a drug or medication overdose.

   _____ Position an unresponsive victim on the back with legs raised (shock position).

   _____ Call 9-1-1 or the Poison Control Center.

   _____ Restrain a potentially violent person to prevent self-injury.

   _____ Check for injuries that may require first aid.

   _____ Induce vomiting if the person is responsive.

   _____ Try to keep the person awake and talking.

   _____ Try to find out what the person took.

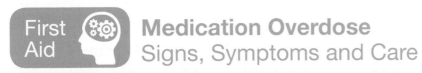

First Aid

Medication Overdose
Signs, Symptoms and Care

When You See

- **Very small or large pupils of the eye**
- **Stumbling, clumsiness, drowsiness or incoherent speech**
- **Difficulty breathing (very slow or fast)**
- **Irrational or violent behavior**
- **Changing levels of responsiveness**

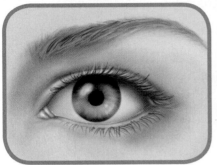

Normal

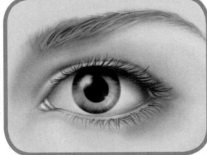

Dilated

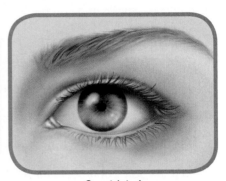

Constricted

Do This First

1 Put an unresponsive victim in the recovery position, monitor breathing and be prepared to give BLS as needed. Call 9-1-1.

2 For a responsive victim, first be sure that it is safe to approach the person. If the victim's behavior is erratic or violent, call 9-1-1 and stay a safe distance away.

3 Try to find out what drug the victim took. If there is evidence of an overdose, call 9-1-1.

4 If symptoms are minor and you know the substance taken, call the Poison Control Center and follow the instructions given.

5 If the victim vomits, save a sample for arriving medical personnel.

Additional Care

- Monitor the victim's condition while waiting for help.
- Provide care for any condition that occurs (seizures, shock, cardiac arrest, etc.).

18 • Substance Misuse and Abuse

Concluding Thoughts

Although substance abuse is a huge problem in our society, do not jump to the conclusion that someone who is behaving oddly must be on drugs. Remember that many illnesses and injuries also cause altered mental status that may lead to unusual behaviors. Take the time to assess the victim and situation and to call for help and give first aid when needed. Whenever giving first aid it is important not to be judgmental – a state of mind that could lead to not providing the best care for a person in need.

Learning Outcomes

You should now be able to do the following:

1. Explain actions that can be taken to help prevent youth from abusing drugs and other substances.

2. Describe specific steps for preventing someone from unintentionally misusing or overdosing on a medication.

3. List the steps of first aid for alcohol intoxication and alcohol withdrawal.

4. Describe the effects of commonly abused drugs.

5. List the steps of first aid for drug abuse or overdose.

6. List the steps of first aid for medication overdose.

Review Questions

1. To help prevent drug misuse or overdose in an elderly person who is taking prescription medications, –

    a. consult with a health care provider or pharmacist before allowing the person to drink alcohol while using the drug.

    b. always have the person take all medications at the same time.

    c. have the person drink lots of water while taking the medications.

    d. monitor the person continually for 2 hours after each dose.

2. Substance abuse prevention programs involve –

    a. youths at risk.

    b. parents and families.

    c. schools and communities.

    d. All of the above

3. Alcohol poisoning may cause –

    a. diabetes.

    b. seizures.

    c. heart attack.

    d. anaphylaxis.

4. Assessment of an intoxicated victim's injuries depends mostly on –

    a. the visible signs of injury.

    b. the victim's mental status when first encountered.

    c. the victim's reported symptoms.

    d. how much alcohol the victim drank.

5. Alcohol withdrawal in a dependent person may cause –

    a. anaphylaxis.

    b. permanent psychosis.

    c. hallucinations.

    d. circulation problems.

6. You are giving first aid to a man who seems mildly "high." He tells you he took two "percs." To determine how best to treat him, whom should you call for more information?

    a. Law enforcement personnel

    b. A family member

    c. The Poison Control Center

    d. The federal drug information website

7. First aid for a drug overdose is generally the same as first aid for –

    a. poisoning.

    b. stroke.

    c. diabetic coma.

    d. hypothermia.

8. A drug overdose may occur with –

    a. illicit drugs.

    b. nonprescription medication.

    c. small amounts of some substances.

    d. All of the above

Chapter 19 • Bites and Stings

Chapter Preview

- Animal Bites
- Human Bites
- Snake Bites
- Spider Bites
- Tick Bites
- Mosquito Bites
- Bee and Wasp Stings
- Scorpion Stings
- Marine Bites and Stings

You are at the beach boardwalk with your family on a bright summer day. The girls are thirsty, so Mom opens a carton of juice and pours it into cups, trying to ignore a wasp that has appeared and is buzzing around the juice. As the toddler takes her first sip, she slaps at the wasp, which stings her lip. Her juice spills everywhere, she is screaming with pain and the wasp now is nowhere to be seen. What, if anything, should you do?

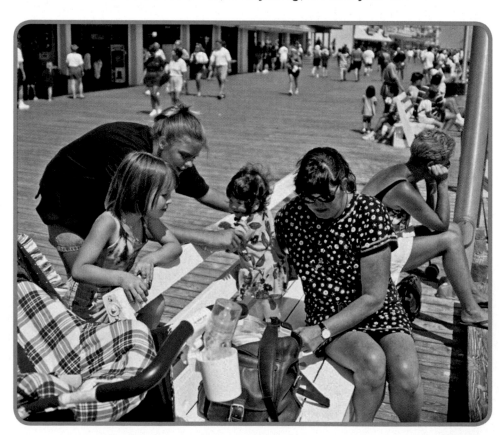

Millions of people every year are bitten or stung by animals, snakes, spiders, insects and marine life, making this a significant first aid issue. Fortunately, the majority of cases are not medical emergencies, but often medical treatment is needed for bleeding, wound care, or to treat infection or a reaction to an injected poison. In some cases, particularly when the victim is allergic, a medical emergency does occur, and appropriate, timely first aid is needed.

Animal Bites

Millions of people are bitten by dogs in the United States every year, followed by a large number of cat bites and a much lower number of bites from other domestic or wild animals. More than 32,000 dog bites are serious enough to require emergency department treatment and, on average, about 30 people a year die from dog bites.[1] Most victims are young children who often have not learned how to act around dogs and other animals. With an estimated 68 million pet dogs in the United States, it is crucial that children as well as adults learn how to safely interact with dogs as well as other animals kept as pets **(Box 19-1)**. In general, most bites occur to the arm or hand, followed by the leg or foot, but in children younger than 4, many sustain injury to the head or neck – an often dangerous injury.

Animal bites can be serious for three reasons. Depending on the location and depth of the bite injury, bleeding can be serious. Control bleeding from an animal bite as you would bleeding caused by other injuries (see **Chapter 8**). Second, because bacteria are present in animals' mouths, there is a risk that the wound will become infected. Even a small wound from a dog bite can become infected; the bites of cats have an even higher risk. Give wound care to prevent infection (see **Chapter 10**) and consult with your health care provider to see if additional measures may

[1]*National Safety Council. Injury Facts®, 2011 Edition. Itasca, IL: Author.*

be needed. Finally, the bite of any animal, even a house pet, carries the risk of **rabies**. This risk is much higher with wild animals, as most pets are vaccinated against rabies, but the risk is present with all animals.

In many other countries, dog bites are the most common source of rabies and any dog bite should immediately be examined by a health care provider. Caused by a virus that can be transmitted by saliva into the blood of a bite victim, rabies remains a major threat in all areas of the United States even though vaccinations and other precautions, have made it very rare in humans. Because rabies is fatal unless vaccination injections are given early, every bite from a mammal, domestic or wild, must be considered serious. Unless the bite occurs from your own pet and you are certain the animal's rabies vaccination is current, all dog and other animal bites should be reported to your local public health department or animal control office. Because the threat of rabies is so serious, many states have laws that require quarantining or observing any biting animal – even one with a current vaccination – to ensure that there is no risk for the bite victim. In most locations, any wild animal that bites a person is assumed to have rabies, unless the animal can be caught or killed and its brain examined for the virus.

First aid for the bite of any animal focuses on controlling bleeding and on wound care to prevent infection. Flush the wound well and apply a sterile dressing (see **Chapter 10**). Seek medical attention immediately for a puncture wound, a wound to the head or neck, and any bite wound from an animal that is not your own pet. Even with a superficial wound caused by the bite of your own pet, it is a good idea to contact your health care provider to see whether medical treatment may be needed. In all cases observe the wound carefully over the next few days for any signs of infection (see First Aid: "Animal Bites").

BOX 19-1: PREVENTING DOG BITES

The CDC recommends the following to prevent dog bites and rabies:[2]

Before you bring a dog into your household:

- Consult with a professional (e.g., veterinarian, animal behaviorist or responsible breeder) to learn what breeds of dogs are the best fit for your household.

- Dogs with histories of aggression are not suitable for households with children.

- Be sensitive to cues that a child is fearful or apprehensive about a dog. If a child seems frightened by dogs, wait before bringing a dog into your household.

- Spend time with a dog before buying or adopting it. Use caution when bringing a dog into a household with an infant or toddler.

If you decide to bring a dog into your home:

- Spay/neuter your dog (this often reduces aggressive tendencies).

- Never leave infants or young children alone with a dog.

- Don't play aggressive games with your dog (e.g., wrestling).

- Properly socialize and train any dog entering your household. Teach the dog submissive behaviors (e.g., rolling over to expose the abdomen and giving up food without growling).

- Immediately seek professional advice (e.g., from veterinarians, animal behaviorists or responsible breeders) if the dog develops aggressive or undesirable behaviors.

To help prevent children from being bitten by dogs, teach the following basic safety tips and review them regularly:

- Do not approach an unfamiliar dog.

- Do not run from a dog or scream.

- Remain motionless (e.g., "be still like a tree") when approached by an unfamiliar dog.

- If knocked over by a dog, roll into a ball and lie still (e.g., "be still like a log").

- Do not play with a dog unless supervised by an adult.

- Immediately report stray dogs or dogs displaying unusual behavior to an adult.

- Avoid direct eye contact with a dog.

- Do not disturb a dog that is sleeping, eating or caring for puppies.

- Do not pet a dog without allowing it to see and sniff you first.

- If bitten, immediately report the bite to an adult.

[2]*Centers for Disease Control and Prevention, http://www.cdc.gov/HomeandRecreationalSafety/Dog-Bites/biteprevention.html Accessed March 29, 2011.*

Human Bites

Small children often bite others when angry or acting out. Human bites are rarer among adults, but the same result may occur in a fight if someone's knuckles strike another person's teeth and break the skin. Because our mouths harbor many bacteria, a bite from a human can cause an infection the same as an animal bite. Because many of the pathogens that are harmless in the mouth can cause serious infection if they enter the blood, all human bites should be seen by a health care provider (see First Aid: "Human Bites").

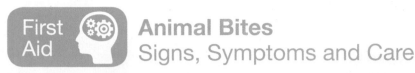

Animal Bites
Signs, Symptoms and Care

When You See

- **Any animal bite**

Do This First

1 Clean the wound with large amounts of warm or room-temperature water with or without soap (except when bleeding is severe).

2 Control bleeding.

3 Cover the wound with a sterile dressing and bandage (see **Chapter 10**).

4 The victim should see a health care provider or go to the emergency department right away.

Additional Care

- Report all animal bites to local animal control officers or police. The law requires certain procedures to be followed when rabies is a risk.

- An antibiotic ointment may be applied to a shallow wound (but not a puncture) before dressing it, if the victim is not allergic to the antibiotic.

ALERT

- Do not try to catch any animal that may have rabies, but note its appearance and describe it to the health care provider.

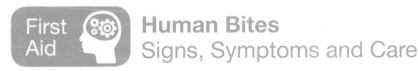

Human Bites
Signs, Symptoms and Care

When You See

- **A human bite**
- **Open puncture wound**
- **Bleeding**

Do This First

1 Clean the wound with large amounts of warm or room-temperature water with or without soap (except when bleeding is severe).

2 Control bleeding.

3 Cover the wound with a sterile dressing and bandage (see **Chapter 10**).

4 The victim should see a health care provider or go to the emergency department right away.

Additional Care

- If any tissue has been bitten off, bring it with the victim to the emergency department.

Learning Checkpoint 1

1. To minimize the risk of rabies from an animal bite, you should take which action?

   a. See a health care provider immediately.

   b. See a health care provider if you experience heavy salivation 5 to 7 days after the bite.

   c. Capture the animal and take it to a veterinarian for examination.

   d. Soak the wound area with rubbing alcohol.

2. Why can a human bite lead to a serious medical condition?

Snake Bites

Poisonous snakes in North America include rattlesnakes, copperheads, water moccasins (cottonmouths), coral snakes and exotic species kept in captivity **(Figure 19-1)**. An estimated 7,000 to 8,000 bites from venomous snakes occur every year in the United States,[3] causing an average of 7 or 8 deaths annually.[4] World travelers should be aware, however, that snake bites in many other countries are more common and more lethal, causing about 30,000 deaths annually worldwide.

Snake bite statistics in the United States reveal an interesting pattern. Most venomous snake bites occur in adolescent and young adult males and most of these occur on the hands and arms. Alcohol is often involved, and many of these victims were trying to handle the snake to impress their friends by handling or molesting the snake. Clearly the first step in preventing snake bite is to avoid a snake when one is seen **(Box 19-2)**.

Even with venomous snakes, in about half of bite cases the snake does not inject venom. In all, the risk of a lethal snake bite is very low. Nonetheless, people who live or work in areas where venomous snakes are common should take preventive steps and know what first aid to give in case a bite occurs. Venomous snakes are most common in the Southeast and the Southwest United States. Rattlesnake bites cause most snake bite deaths.

Unless you are absolutely certain that a victim's snake bite was from a nonpoisonous snake, treat all snake bites as potentially dangerous. First, calm the victim and have the victim remain still. Anything that increases the heart rate, including strong emotions and physical movement, will speed the spread of the venom. Try to identify the snake species or be able to describe it to responding EMS personnel, because **antivenin** (antidote to the poison) is available in many areas where snake bites are common. Call 9-1-1. Wash the bite area and remove any constrictive jewelry or clothing from the limb, which will likely swell (see First Aid: "Snake Bites").

Many of the traditional myths and techniques for managing snake bites do not, in fact, improve the victim's condition or minimize the risk. Do not try to suck out the venom, do not cut across the fang holes in an attempt to remove the venom and do not put a tourniquet on the limb. In addition, do not put ice on the bite because of the potential for injuring tissues further with the cold.

For venomous snake bites, it is now recommended that a bitten extremity be wrapped snugly but not tightly with an elastic bandage; you should be able to insert one finger under the bandage. Wrap the entire length of the extremity, wrapping away from the body toward the end of the limb, to reduce the spread of the venom by slowing lymph flow.

[3]*Centers for Disease Control and Prevention, http://www. cdc.gov/niosh/topics/snakes/ Accessed March 5, 2011.*

[4]*National Safety Council. Injury Facts®, 2011 Edition. Itasca, IL: Author.*

(continues on page 304)

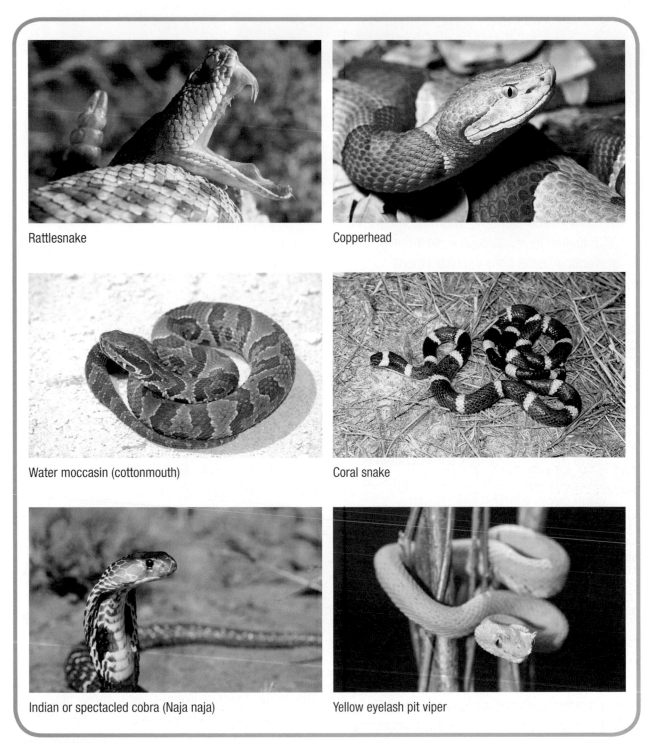

Rattlesnake

Copperhead

Water moccasin (cottonmouth)

Coral snake

Indian or spectacled cobra (Naja naja)

Yellow eyelash pit viper

Figure 19-1 *Examples of poisonous snakes.*

BOX 19-2: PREVENTING SNAKE BITES

- Stay away from areas known to have snakes.

- If you see a snake, reverse your direction and retrace your steps, watching for other snakes.

- Stay away from underbrush areas, fallen trees and other areas where snakes may live.

The Arizona Poison and Drug Information Center (APDIC)[5] makes these additional recommendations for preventing snake bites in areas where venomous snakes are common:

- Leave wild animals alone. 50% to 70% of reptile bites managed by the APDIC were provoked by the person who was bitten — that is, someone was trying to kill, capture or harass the animal.

- Be aware of peak movement times. During the hottest months, snakes will be most active at night. They may be encountered during the day in spring and fall or during a warm day in winter.

- Watch where you put your hands and feet. Try to keep your hands and feet out of crevices in rocks, wood piles and deep grass. Always carry a flashlight and wear shoes or boots when walking after dark.

- Dead snakes can bite. Never handle a venomous reptile, even after it is dead. Reflex strikes with injected venom can occur for several hours after death.

- Install outdoor lighting for yards, porches and sidewalks. If you see a venomous reptile in your yard, it is probably just "passing through." However, if you are concerned about a dangerous animal in your yard, seek professional assistance in removing it.

[5]*Arizona Poison and Drug Information Center, http://www.pharmacy.arizona.edu/centers/arizona-poison-drug-information-center/venomouscreatures/rattlesnake Accessed March 5, 2011.*

(continued from page 302)

The extremity should also be immobilized and the victim should receive medical attention as soon as possible.

Spider Bites

Many types of spiders bite, but in the United States only the venom of the black widow and brown recluse spiders is serious and sometimes fatal. The black widow often has a red hourglass-shaped marking on the underside of the abdomen. The brown recluse has a violin-shaped marking on its back **(Figure 19-2)**. Reliable statistics are not available for how many spider bites occur every year, but in recent years only 4 to 10 deaths have resulted from venomous bites, mostly from black widow spiders.[6] The venom of the brown recluse

[6]*National Safety Council. Injury Facts®, 2011 Edition. Itasca, IL: Author.*

spider can cause severe tissue damage but rarely causes death.

Both species are more common in warm climates and generally live in areas that are dry and undisturbed. Outside the home, they are often found in woodpiles, sheds or debris. Inside the home they may live in closets, rarely used cabinets, attics, crawl spaces and similar areas. Because these spiders are small and usually not seen before the bite occurs, preventive steps are important in areas where these spiders are known to live **(Box 19-3)**.

Although the signs and symptoms of the bites of these two spiders vary, the first aid is the same. A black widow bite causes immediate pain, swelling and redness at the site, followed later by sweating,

(continues on page 306)

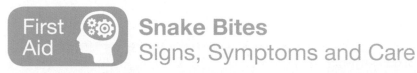

First Aid

Snake Bites
Signs, Symptoms and Care

When You See

- **Puncture marks on skin**
- **Complaint of pain or burning at bite site**
- **Redness and swelling**
- **Depending on species: difficulty breathing, numbness or muscle paralysis, nausea and vomiting, blurred vision, drowsiness or confusion, weakness**

Do This First

1 Have the victim lie down and stay calm. (Do not move the victim unless absolutely necessary.) Keep the bitten area immobile and below the level of the heart.

2 Call 9-1-1.

3 Wash the bite wound with large amounts of warm or room temperature water with or without soap.

4 Wrap the extremity with a snug but not tight elastic bandage. Wrap away from the body toward the end of the limb. The pressure is sufficient if the bandage is snug but a finger can be slipped under it.

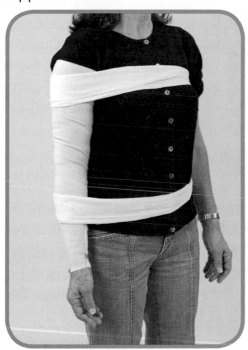

5 Remove jewelry or tight clothing before swelling begins.

Additional Care

- Do not try to catch the snake, but note its appearance and describe it to the health care provider.
- Monitor the victim's breathing and be ready to give CPR if needed.

ALERT

- Do not put a tourniquet on the victim.
- Do not cut open the wound to try to drain out the venom or try to suck out the venom.
- Do not put ice on the bite.

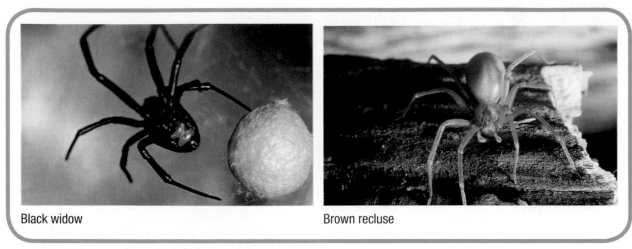

Black widow   Brown recluse

Figure 19-2 *Poisonous spiders.*

BOX 19-3: PREVENTING SPIDER BITES

Neither black widow nor brown recluse spiders attack humans: they bite defensively when someone comes too close. Preventing these and other spider bites involves two types of actions: avoiding bites in places where spiders are likely and controlling spider populations.

Avoiding Spider Bites

- Wear gloves and a long-sleeved shirt when cleaning basement or attic areas, seldom used closets, sheds or garages, and similar areas where spiders may live. Wear gloves when gathering wood from a woodpile.

- Before putting on long clothing or shoes that have been unused for a time, shake them out. Consider storing clothing and shoes in sealed plastic bags or boxes.

- Check inside tents, sleeping bags and other seldom-used equipment before using.

- Before sleeping in a bed that has not been used in a while, carefully check between the covers.

Controlling Spider Populations

- Use appropriate pesticides or spider traps (glue traps) in areas where spiders or their nests have been identified.

- Thorough, routine housecleaning helps control spider populations. Vacuum up webs and egg sacs when they are seen and dispose of the vacuum bag.

- Reduce clutter in storage areas.

- Repair or seal off openings in screens, windows, chimneys and other openings through which spiders may enter the home.

- Clean up any debris around the home where spiders may breed.

(continued from page 304)

nausea, stomach and muscle cramps, headache, dizziness or weakness, and possible difficulty breathing. A brown recluse bite causes more slowly developing pain or stinging at the site, followed later by blistering at the site, fever, chills, nausea or vomiting and joint pain; an open sore at the site will continue to grow without medical treatment.

With either bite, the victim needs emergency medical care. An antivenin is available for black widow spider bites. Wash the wound with soap and water to help prevent infection and apply ice or a cold pack. Keep the bite area below the level of the heart (see First Aid: "Spider Bites").

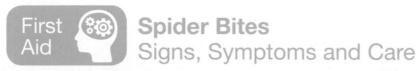

Spider Bites
Signs, Symptoms and Care

When You See

For black widow bite:

- **Complaint of pain or burning at bite site**
- **Red skin at site**
- **After 15 minutes and up to several hours: sweating, nausea, stomach and muscle cramps, increased pain at site, dizziness or weakness, and difficulty breathing**

For brown recluse bite:

- **Stinging sensation at site**
- **Over 8 to 48 hours: increasing pain, blistering at site, fever, chills, nausea or vomiting, joint pain, open sore at site**

Do This First

1 If the victim has difficulty breathing, call 9-1-1 and be prepared to give CPR if needed. Call 9-1-1 immediately for a brown recluse spider bite.

2 Keep the bite area below the level of the heart.

3 Wash the area with soap and water.

4 Put ice or a cold pack on the bite area (with a damp cloth or paper towel between the cold pack and the skin).

Additional Care

- Try to safely identify the spider for the health care provider.
- If 9-1-1 was not called, the victim should go to the emergency department.

Tick Bites

Tick bites are not poisonous but can transmit serious diseases such as Rocky Mountain spotted fever or **Lyme disease (Figure 19-3).** Ticks cannot fly but will crawl up clothing or body areas that touch the ground, or will fall off vegetation that one brushes against. Ticks may also be brought into the home in the fur of a dog or other pet that has picked up a tick outside. For guidelines to prevent tick bites see **Box 19-4**.

The tick usually crawls to an unexposed part of the body and bites into the skin, embedding its mouthparts in the skin to avoid being brushed off **(Figure 19-4)**. Because ticks are very small

and often seek unexposed areas to bite, such as the scalp, an embedded tick may not be found unless you search diligently. If not detected and removed, the tick may remain in the skin for days. A careless attempt to remove a tick may result in breaking off its body and leaving the head or mouthparts embedded in the skin, which could lead to infection. Remove a tick correctly by pulling gently but steadily with fine-tipped tweezers until the tick lets go. Then wash the area well and apply an antibiotic cream.

Medical treatment is not usually needed for tick bites. In areas where Lyme disease occurs frequently, talk with your health care provider

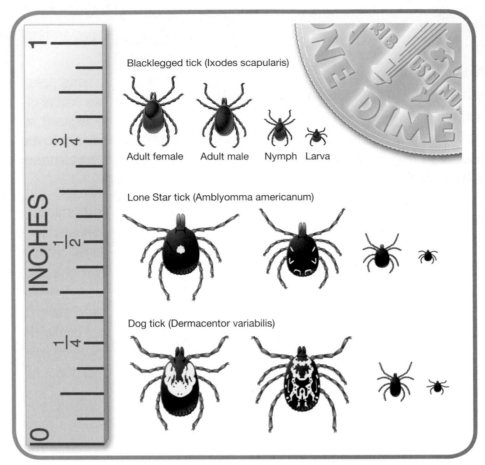

Figure 19-3 *Common types of ticks found in the United States. Only the blacklegged tick carries Lyme disease in the United States.*

about whether treatment may be beneficial. Most important, following a tick bite you should watch for the development of the signs and symptoms of Lyme disease. Lyme disease often produces a characteristic "bull's eye" rash **(Figure 19-5)** typically 7 to 14 days after the bite, but sometimes as soon as 3 days or as long as 30 days later. Other nonspecific symptoms include fever, headache, fatigue, muscle and joint pain, or other flulike symptoms (see First Aid: "Tick Bites").

Mosquito Bites

With the spread of **West Nile virus (WNV)** throughout the United States, mosquitoes are now a greater public health issue. WNV is a bloodborne disease that is a seasonal epidemic in many parts of North America **(Figure 19-6)**. According to the Centers for Disease Control (CDC), 981 human

cases were reported nationwide in 2010, causing 45 deaths.[7] A low percentage of people infected with WNV develop severe illness, however, and more than half have no signs and symptoms at all. WNV is spread mostly by the bite of infected mosquitoes, which often transmit the virus from infected birds.

In the eastern United States, eastern equine encephalitis (EEE) is another serious mosquito-borne infection that is fatal in 33% of those infected. Fortunately, there are only an average of 6 human cases of EEE annually in the U.S.[8] EEE transmission is prevented the same as WNV – by preventing mosquito bites.

[7]*Centers for Disease Control and Prevention, http://www.cdc.gov/ncidod/dvbid/westnile/surv&controlCaseCount 10_detailed.htm Accessed March 2, 2011.*

[8]*Centers for Disease Control and Prevention, http://www.cdc.gov/easternequineencephalitis/tech/epi.html#map Accessed March 5, 2011.*

Tick Bites
Signs, Symptoms and Care

When You See

- **Tick embedded in skin**

Do This First

1 Remove the tick by grasping it close to the skin with tweezers and pulling very gently to "tent" the skin until the tick lets go. Avoid pulling hard or jerking, which may leave part of the tick embedded in the skin. Keep the tick for later identification.

2 Wash the area with soap and water.

3 Put an antiseptic such as rubbing alcohol on the site. Apply an antibiotic cream if the victim is not allergic to the antibiotic.

Additional Care

- Seek medical attention if a rash appears around the site or the victim later experiences fever, headache, chills, muscle and joint pain, or other flulike symptoms.

ALERT

- Do not try to remove an embedded tick by covering it with petroleum jelly, soaking it with bleach, burning it away with a hot pin or other object, or similar methods. These methods may result in part of the tick remaining embedded in the skin.

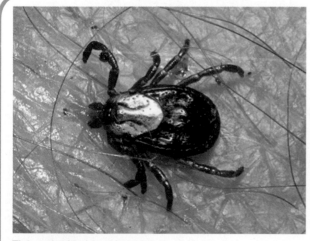 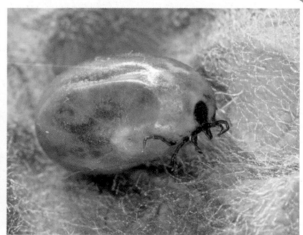

Tick embedded in skin   Tick engorged

Figure 19-4 *Tick bite.*

BOX 19-4: LYME DISEASE

Lyme disease, spread by ticks, is a potentially serious bacterial infection that has become a serious problem in many parts of the United States. Of the 23,305 reported cases in 2005[9], most were in the Northeast or Upper Midwest, although as the figure shows, people living in many other areas are at some risk. Lyme disease is a bacterial infectious disease that first causes fever, chills and other flulike symptoms and often much later causes heart and neurological problems. The longer the tick remains on the body, the greater the chance of transmitting the disease. Look for a "bull's-eye" rash that appears around the bite site 3 to 30 days later. Get medical attention if you have this rash or flulike symptoms or joint pain after a tick bite.

- Keep lawns mowed, brush cleaned up and woodpiles stacked off the ground.
- Wear socks with shoes or boots. Tuck long pants into socks.
- Wear light-colored clothing, which makes it easier to see ticks before they reach your skin. Tuck your shirt into your pants.
- Do not lay clothing or towels on the ground.
- Walk in the middle of paths, away from tall grass and underbrush.
- Comb or brush your hair after being in an infested area.
- Check your body everywhere when bathing or showering, including your neck and scalp.

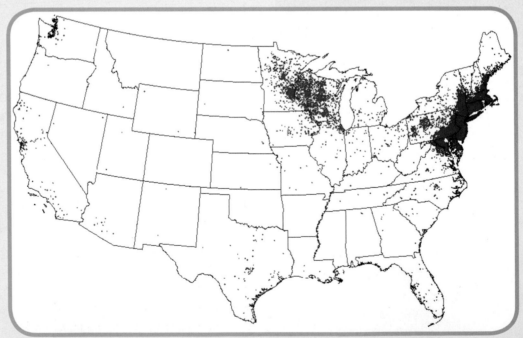

1 dot placed randomly within county of residence for each reported case.

[9]*Centers for Disease Control and Prevention, http://www.cdc.gov/nczved/divisions/dvbid/resources/lyme_brochure.pdf Accessed March 29. 2011.*

Learning Checkpoint 2

1. List three key actions to take for a victim of a snake bite.

   _____

2. Check off situations in which you should call 9-1-1 for a spider bite.

   _____ All spider bites   _____ If there is any pain at the bite site

   _____ Any spider bite in a diabetic victim _____ If the victim has trouble breathing

   _____ Any brown recluse spider bite   _____ If you have no ice to put on the bite

3. A tick is best removed from the skin using _____.

4. A prominent initial sign of Lyme disease following a tick bite is –

   a. pain and burning at the site.

   b. a bull's-eye rash.

   c. high fever within 24 hours.

   d. All of the above

Many affected states and communities have expanded mosquito control programs, but in many areas people still need to take precautions to prevent mosquito bites. The best way to avoid WNV is to prevent mosquito bites in these ways:

- Wear long-sleeved shirts and pants.

- Use an insect repellent when outside in areas where mosquitoes are common **(Box 19-5)**.

- Be aware of peak mosquito hours (from dusk to dawn).

- Mosquito-proof your home by draining standing water around your home and installing or repairing screens.

- Report dead birds to local authorities.

- Support local mosquito control programs.

Bee and Wasp Stings

Bee, wasp and other insect stings are not poisonous but can cause life-threatening allergic reactions, called anaphylaxis, in victims who have severe allergies to them. Venomous insects include honeybees, bumblebees, hornets, wasps, yellow jackets and fire ants. There are no reliable statistics about how many stings occur every year, but 3% of

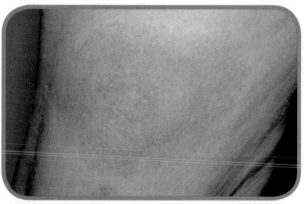

Figure 19-5 *"Bull's-eye" rash characteristic of Lyme disease.*

adults and 0.4% to 0.8% of children are allergic to stinging insects to the extent that a life-threatening reaction could occur.[10] In recent years, 52 to 82 deaths have occurred as a result of these stings.[11] Many people have very serious or life-threatening reactions and about 50 people die every year from allergic reactions to insect stings.

Chapter 9 discusses anaphylactic shock and the first aid to give. Often, someone who knows he

[10]*American Academy of Allergy, Asthma & Immunology. http://www.aaaai.org/media/statistics/allergy-statistics. asp Accessed March 5, 2011.*

[11]*National Safety Council. (2011). Injury Facts®, 2011 Edition. Itasca, IL: Author.*

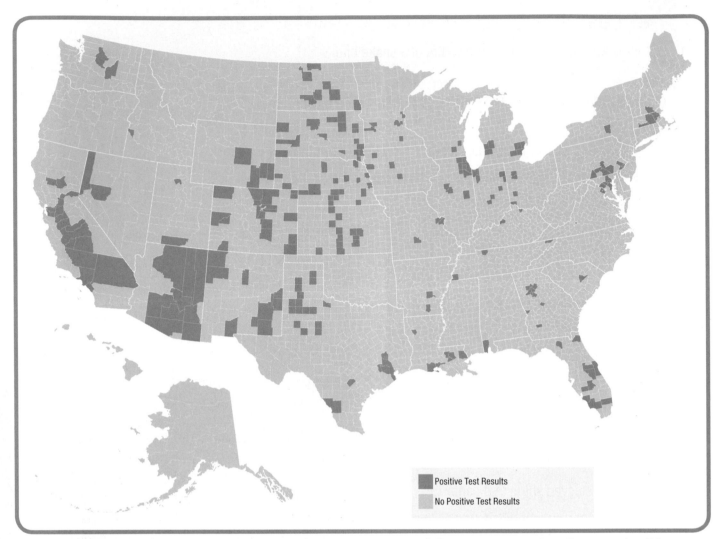

Positive Test Results

No Positive Test Results

Figure 19-6 *2004 West Nile virus activity in the United States reported to Centers for Disease Control (CDC).*

or she is allergic to bee or wasp stings carries an emergency epinephrine auto-injector to use if stung. **Chapter 9** also describes steps you can take to prevent insect stings.

In most cases, a bee or wasp sting causes pain but is not an emergency or serious problem. If present in the skin after the sting, the stinger can be scraped away with a rigid piece of plastic such as a credit card. The area is washed to prevent infection and a cold pack is applied to reduce the pain and swelling. Always observe for the signs of an allergic reaction and if they appear call 9-1-1 immediately and prepare to treat anaphylactic shock. Some sting victims who do not have allergic reactions may

have other delayed symptoms that include fever, rash, joint pain and swollen glands (see First Aid: "Bee and Wasp Stings").

Scorpion Stings

In Southwestern and Southern states, thousands of scorpion stings occur every year, but few become emergencies **(Figure 19-7)**. The great majority of scorpion species are not venomous. Even the sting of the poisonous bark scorpion, found in the Southwest, is seldom fatal. In one report, only 4 deaths resulted from scorpion stings in an 11-year period in the United States. In other countries stings are more common; in Mexico, for example, as many as 1,000 people are believed to

BOX 19-5: CDC RECOMMENDS MOSQUITO REPELLENTS

CDC recommends using products that have been shown to work in scientific trials and that contain active ingredients that have been registered with the US Environmental Protection Agency (EPA) for use as insect repellents on skin or clothing. When EPA registers a repellent, it evaluates the product for efficacy and potential effects on human beings and the environment. EPA registration means that EPA does not expect a product, when used according to the instructions on the label, to cause unreasonable adverse effects to human health or the environment.

Of the active ingredients registered with EPA, CDC believes that two have demonstrated a higher degree of efficacy in the peer-reviewed, scientific literature. Products containing these active ingredients typically provide longer-lasting protection than others:

- DEET (N,N-diethyl-m-toluamide)
- Picaridin (KBR 3023)

Oil of lemon eucalyptus, a plant-based repellent, is also registered with EPA. In two recent scientific publications, when oil of lemon eucalyptus was tested against mosquitoes found in the United States, it provided protection similar to repellents with low concentrations of DEET.

Source: http://www.cdc.gov/ncidod/dvbid/westnile/qa/ insect_repellent.htm Accessed March 1, 2011.

die every year from scorpion stings.[12] Scorpions are more active at night, and most stings occur during the warm summer months. People can avoid scorpions in areas where they are common by not walking barefoot or in sandals, and by shaking out clothing and shoes before putting them on.

Scorpion stings are most dangerous for infants, young children and the elderly. When death does occur, it is usually the result of anaphylactic shock caused by the victim's reaction to the venom. The victim of a sting should always be observed for this potential reaction. The more usual symptoms, however, consist of pain at the site along with numbness and tingling. More serious symptoms include nausea and vomiting, breathing difficulty, fever, convulsions, and in children, hyperactivity.

The first aid for a scorpion sting is similar to the first aid for a wasp or bee sting. The Arizona Poison and Drug Information Center, which manages thousands of stings a year, says most stings in healthy adults can be managed safely at home. Wash the area and apply a cold pack. Monitor the victim's symptoms and seek medical attention for signs and symptoms beyond those at the sting site. Seek urgent medical attention for a sting in a child or elderly person. Antivenin for scorpion stings may be available in some areas (see First Aid: "Scorpion Stings").

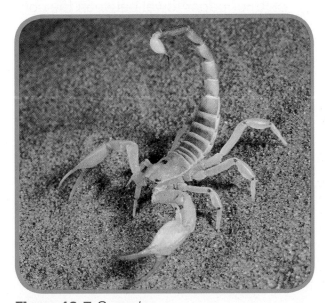

Figure 19-7 *Scorpion.*

[12]WebMD. http://emedicine.medscape.com/ article/168230-overview Accessed March 2, 2011.

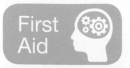

Bee and Wasp Stings
Signs, Symptoms and Care

When You See

- **Complaints of pain, burning or itching at sting site**
- **Redness or swelling**
- **Stinger possibly still in skin**

Do This First

1 Remove stinger from skin by scraping it away gently with a piece of plastic such as a credit card (not a knife blade). Call 9-1-1 if victim has known allergy to stings.

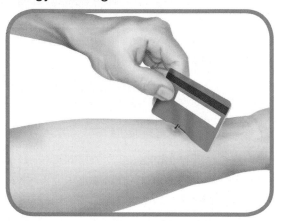

2 Wash the area with soap and water.

3 Put ice or a cold pack on the sting site for up to 20 minutes (with a damp cloth or paper towel between the cold pack and the skin).

4 Watch the victim for 30 minutes for any signs or symptoms of allergic reaction (difficulty breathing, swelling in other areas, anxiety, nausea or vomiting); if any of these occur, call 9-1-1 and treat for anaphylactic shock.

Additional Care

- An over-the-counter oral antihistamine may help reduce discomfort.
- For an insect sting in the mouth, have the victim suck on ice to reduce swelling. Call 9-1-1 if breathing becomes difficult.
- Do not let the victim scratch the sting; this increases swelling and itching and the risk of infection.

Marine Bites and Stings

Biting marine animals include sharks, barracudas and eels, although such bites are generally rare. The first aid for marine bites is essentially the same as for bleeding and wound care. For a bite that causes severe bleeding:

1. Stop the bleeding.
2. Treat for shock.
3. Summon help from lifeguards.
4. Call 9-1-1.

Stings from marine life are much more common than bites. Stinging marine life include jellyfish, Portuguese man-of-war, corals, spiny sea urchins, anemones and stingrays. Most stings are like bee or wasp stings: painful but not dangerous, except in the very rare few people who may experience an allergic reaction or severe toxic reaction. Even the venomous sting of the Portuguese man-of-war, although it can be very painful and can cause other symptoms, is rarely an emergency or life-threatening.

Scorpion Stings
Signs, Symptoms and Care

When You See

- **The scorpion sting with its tail**
- **Complaints of severe burning pain at sting site; later, numbness, tingling**
- **Possible nausea, vomiting**
- **Hyperactivity in a child**
- **Possible signs of shock, breathing difficulties**

Do This First

1 Call 9-1-1 if the victim has a problem breathing or severe symptoms.

2 Monitor the victim's breathing and be prepared to give CPR if needed.

3 Carefully wash the sting area.

4 Put ice or a cold pack on the area for up to 20 minutes (with a damp cloth or paper towel between the cold pack and the skin).

5 Seek urgent medical attention unless the symptoms are very mild.

Additional Care

- Keep the victim still.

Most marine stings can be prevented by paying attention to your environment. Warnings are generally posted on public beaches when Portuguese man-of-wars are present in the water or you may see their blue floats washed up on the beach or floating in the water **(Figure 19-8)**. Long tentacles streaming from the floating body are the source of stings; these tentacles can break off and continue to cause stings in the water or on the beach. Do not touch a jellyfish or Portuguese man-of-war on the beach. In more isolated areas, check the water around you frequently, and if there are known risks, wear a wetsuit for skin protection. Do not swim or snorkel in shallow water where you may bump into coral, urchins or anemones. Watch the area in front of you when walking in shallow water where stingrays may be present, and shuffle your feet to scare them away. Do not let small children play in such areas. If you have ever had an allergic reaction to any marine sting, talk with your health care provider about an allergy kit.

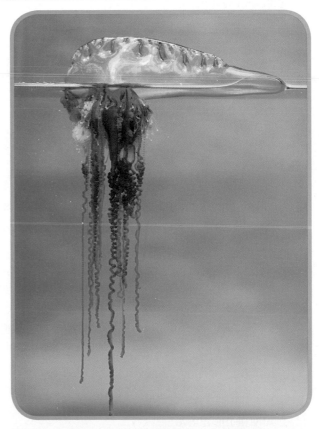

Figure 19-8 *Portuguese man-of-war.*

Jellyfish or Portuguese man-of-war stings cause an immediate intense pain and burning that may last for hours. The stinging may continue after the initial contact; the application of vinegar has been shown to inactivate the venom. Red welts usually appear on the skin, often in a row caused by a tentacle. In most cases these are the only symptoms. If a severe toxic or allergic reaction occurs after any marine sting, however, the victim may experience difficulty breathing, swelling of the throat, signs of shock, muscle paralysis, seizures or unresponsiveness. If any of these signs and symptoms occurs, or if the victim is a young child or is stung on the face or eyes, call 9-1-1.

Give this first aid for jellyfish and Portuguese man-of-war stings:

1. Wash the sting area with vinegar (4% to 6% acetic acid) as soon as possible, for at least 30 seconds or longer, to inactivate the venom. Remove any remaining tentacles.

2. If vinegar is unavailable, use a mix of baking soda and water.

3. To reduce pain, immerse the area in water as hot as can be tolerated (113° F or 45° C) for at least 20 minutes or as long as pain is felt. If pain returns on removal from the hot water, immerse the area again.

4. If hot water is unavailable, use a dry hot pack (preferable) or a dry cold pack to reduce pain.

5. Do not use meat tenderizer, a fresh water wash, commercial aerosol products or a pressure bandage.

6. Call 9-1-1 if –

   • The victim is very young or very old.

   • A sting near the mouth is causing swelling.

   • The sting involves a large area of the body, the face or genitals.

   • The victim experiences serious signs and symptoms such as difficulty breathing or swallowing or chest pain.

   • The sting is from a box jellyfish (rare in United States).

To care for urchin or stingray puncture wounds:

1. Relieve the pain by immersing the injured part in hot water for 30 minutes. Make sure the water is not so hot that it causes a burn.

2. Wash the wound with soap and water, and apply a dressing.

3. Seek medical attention.

 Learning Checkpoint 3

1. A bee's stinger can be removed from the skin using: _____.

2. A co-worker was stung by a honeybee near the flower garden by the office building's entrance. As she tells you about this, you see that her face is turning red, the skin around her eyes and mouth looks puffy, and she seems short of breath. What are the most important actions to take first? Why?

   _____

3. What substance should be put on a jellyfish sting?

   a. Boiling water

   b. Ketchup or mayonnaise

   c. Vinegar or baking soda

   d. Any of the above

Concluding Thoughts

Bites and stings are common occurrences, but fortunately they seldom become emergencies. First aid in most cases is as simple as pain relief and wound care, along with observing for more serious signs and symptoms and then seeking medical care. For those who are often outdoors where most bites and stings occur, prevention is important. Most important, people who are known to be allergic to bee stings or other stings or bites should carry an emergency epinephrine kit and follow precautions when in areas where stings or bites are likely.

Learning Outcomes

You should now be able to do the following:

1. List guidelines for preventing common bites and stings.

2. Explain the risk of infection from common types of bites and stings.

3. Describe the first aid care to give in cases of bites and stings that do not involve severe symptoms or an allergic reaction.

4. List signs and symptoms for which you should call 9-1-1 after a bite or sting.

5. Describe how to remove an embedded tick and the stinger from a bee or wasp.

Review Questions

1. Possible rabies infection should be a consideration with –

    a. only wild animal bites.

    b. only dog bites if you do not know the owner.

    c. snake bites.

    d. all animal bites from mammals.

2. Seek immediate medical attention for –

    a. a puncture wound from an animal bite.

    b. a bite to the head or neck.

    c. a bite wound from an animal that is not your own pet.

    d. All of the above

3. Why should all bites from a human be seen by a health care provider?

    a. Many pathogens in the mouth can cause serious infection.

    b. Later bleeding is likely even if it is controlled at first.

    c. Many humans are carriers of the rabies virus.

    d. Saliva is acidic and may cause tissue damage.

4. First aid for snake bite includes –

    a. sucking the venom from the bite holes.

    b. applying a tourniquet.

    c. washing the wound with soap and water.

    d. applying a hot compress on the area.

5. When should you seek urgent medical care for a brown recluse spider bite?

    a. Only if the victim is known to be allergic

    b. With all victims bitten

    c. Only if the victim develops a breathing problem

    d. Only if the victim develops fever and chills

6. The best way to remove a tick embedded in the skin is to –

    a. pull it out with tweezers.

    b. burn it with a needle sterilized in a flame.

    c. cover it with petroleum jelly.

    d. cover it with an alcohol-saturated dressing.

7. Which of the following is the most important reason to prevent mosquito bites?

    a. Mosquito bites always cause infections when scratched.

    b. Many people have allergic reactions to mosquito bites.

    c. Mosquito bites can cause infection with West Nile virus.

    d. Multiple mosquito bites can add up to cause toxic effects.

8. When should 9-1-1 be called for a bee sting?

    a. Always

    b. When a child younger than 8 is stung

    c. When the victim has a known allergy

    d. When the bee was particularly aggressive before the sting

9. Which statement is true about scorpion stings?

    a. Almost all scorpion species are venomous.

    b. Scorpion stings are very rarely fatal.

    c. Scorpion stings are likely to cause anaphylaxis.

    d. The venom from a scorpion sting is easily washed out of the bite.

10. When can the tentacles of a Portuguese man-of-war sting?

    a. When the Portuguese man-of-war is floating in the water

    b. When the Portuguese man-of-war is washed up on the sand

    c. When the tentacles are detached from the body

    d. All of the above

Chapter 20 • Cold and Heat Emergencies

Chapter Preview

- Body Temperature
- Cold Emergencies
- Heat Emergencies

After several days of bitterly cold weather, you wonder how your elderly neighbor is coping with the cold, so you stop by his house. You have to ring the door several times before he answers, and when you step inside, it feels very cold inside his house. You ask why it is so cold, and he mumbles that with rising fuel prices, he can't afford to turn the thermostat any higher. You follow him into the living room, where he stumbles before sitting on the sofa. You notice that he is shivering. You ask if you can get him a blanket and he is slow to respond and his words are slurred. Is he experiencing a problem? What should you do?

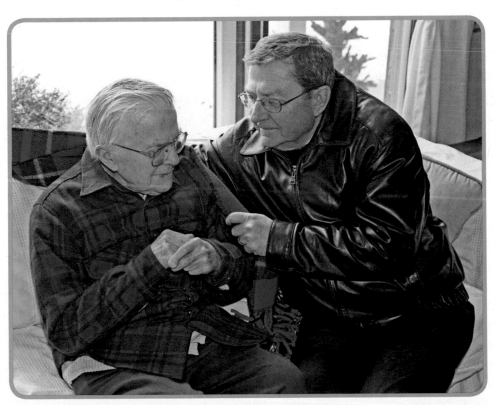

In temperature extremes or as a result of injury or illness, the body may not be able to successfully maintain its normal temperature, which can lead to medical problems. Often cold- and heat-related injuries begin gradually, but if a person remains exposed to an extreme temperature or engaged in strenuous activity, an emergency can develop. Untreated, either a cold or a heat emergency can lead to serious injury or death.

Body Temperature

A fairly constant internal body temperature is necessary for body systems to function. The body has several mechanisms to create heat or to lose heat when necessary. In most environments these mechanisms, along with protective clothing and shelter from temperature extremes, work well and body temperature is not a health issue. When exposed to environmental temperature extremes for an extended time, however, these mechanisms cannot maintain a constant internal temperature indefinitely, particularly if the victim is injured or in poor health. Infants and the elderly also are more susceptible to temperature extremes.

Mechanisms for Staying Warm

Most of the body's heat is produced by metabolic processes that break down nutrients to release energy for use by the body. About 60% of the energy in the food we eat is released as heat within the body and this heat energy in most environments is sufficient to keep the body at the optimal temperature, averaging 98.6° F. The contraction of muscle tissue also produces heat. Shivering is an involuntary movement of muscles to produce additional heat when the body needs it.

The body also has mechanisms to conserve heat when needed. Much of the body's heat is lost to a cooler environment through the process of radiation – heat radiates out from the skin in the same way that you can feel heat radiating from a hot surface. Skin temperature is normally much cooler than the body's internal temperature. If the body is losing too much heat by radiation, blood vessels in the skin contract (**vasoconstriction**)

so that less internal heat is brought by the blood to the skin to radiate away. Minimizing heat loss helps the body to conserve its heat when necessary. We also have learned behaviors to minimize heat loss, such as putting on more clothing or moving to a warmer environment.

Mechanisms for Staying Cool

Cold is the absence of heat, not a positive quality in itself – the body cannot make cold to cool the body when a very hot environment or prolonged exertion threatens to raise body temperature. Nor can the body shut down its own heat-producing processes, as cells continue to need energy to survive and function. Therefore, the body must lose internal heat when necessary to prevent overheating. A primary heat loss mechanism is dilation of blood vessels (**vasodilatation**) to bring more blood to the skin. The skin becomes warmer as the blood carries heat out from the body's core, and more heat is then radiated from the body. Sweating is a second mechanism. Sweat evaporates from the skin's surface, cooling the skin and helping to dissipate the heat brought to the surface by the blood. We also have learned behaviors to promote heat loss when needed, such as removing clothing to allow more heat to radiate away, getting out of the sun to avoid absorbing more radiated heat, spraying or wiping the body with water to help cool the skin by evaporation, or moving inside to a cooler environment where we can radiate heat more effectively.

The Body in Temperature Extremes

The body's normal heat production, heat conservation and heat loss mechanisms, regulated by the nervous system, usually cope well with changes in environmental temperatures to maintain a constant internal temperature. With extended exposure to temperature extremes, however, these mechanisms are not enough to maintain a normal body temperature.

With prolonged exposure to cold, especially when wet (because water conducts heat away from the body much faster than does air), not enough heat can be conserved in the body and shivering cannot produce enough extra heat to keep the body warm. The person develops hypothermia, a potentially life-threatening condition. Because some cellular processes cannot occur at too low a temperature, organ systems gradually begin to fail, leading eventually to death.

With prolonged exposure to heat, the body eventually cannot lose enough heat to maintain a normal temperature. Profuse sweating in an attempt to cool the body frequently leads to dehydration, which reduces blood volume and blood pressure. Even when the environment is not very hot, a long period of physical exertion, such as that which accompanies endurance sports, can lead to dehydration caused by prolonged sweating. Without sufficient fluid, the body cannot cool itself adequately. Heatstroke occurs when the body temperature rises; sweating stops as the body tries to conserve its remaining fluid. Without treatment, organ damage eventually occurs, followed by death.

Hypothermia and heatstroke are the most dangerous temperature injuries. Because both develop gradually and worsen with continued exposure, the signs and symptoms of a developing problem must be recognized early and the condition corrected before it becomes life-threatening. The first aid for these and other cold and heat emergencies is described in this chapter.

Hypothermia and heatstroke can happen to anyone in certain conditions. Generally a healthy adult is most at risk after prolonged exposure to significant temperature extremes, such as being immersed in cold water or engaging in strenuous activities in the heat without drinking enough fluid. A number of factors, however, increase the risk for cold and heat injuries **(Box 20-1)**.

BOX 20-1: RISK FACTORS FOR COLD AND HEAT INJURIES

- **Age:** Young children and the elderly are at greatest risk. Young children are at risk because their shivering produces less heat due to smaller muscle mass. They also have less body fat than others, making them more likely to lose heat. Older people are at a greater risk because their lower metabolic rate can result in a failure to maintain a normal body temperature, even indoors, when the air temperature falls under 64° F. It is also believed that older people may not perceive cold as well as younger people do and they may be slower to act to compensate for the cold. Older adults are also more likely to have a chronic illness such as diabetes that increases the risk for hypothermia.

- **Illness or injury:** Many injuries and chronic health problems, particularly those affecting circulation or the heart, increase one's susceptibility to heat and cold injuries. For example, a victim in shock often produces insufficient body heat; for this reason shock treatment usually includes keeping the victim warm. The body responds less well to heat and cold with diabetes, infection, burns, head injuries and other conditions.

- **Mental impairment:** People with cognitive disabilities are less likely to take action to prevent hypothermia when they are exposed to cold.

- **Dehydration:** Not drinking enough fluid makes one more susceptible to both heat and cold emergencies.

- **Body type:** People with little body fat have a greater risk of hypothermia, as body fat has an insulating effect to slow environmental cooling. People with a large arount of body fat have a greater risk of experiencing a heat emergency.

(continues)

BOX 20-1: RISK FACTORS FOR COLD AND HEAT INJURIES (continued)

- **Activity:** People who work outdoors in hot environments, such as construction workers or athletes in training, are more likely to experience a heat emergency if they do not take precautions such as resting and drinking fluids. People who work or participate in outdoor recreation in extreme cold are at greater risk for hypothermia, especially if they are not dressed properly or are in situations where they may not be able to reach shelter.

- **Drugs and medications:** Many medications and drugs increase the risk for heat and cold injuries. Alcohol dilates blood vessels, making hypothermia more likely because heat is lost more quickly; alcohol is also a diuretic (increases urination), so the person becomes dehydrated more quickly and is more susceptible to heatstroke. Caffeine is also a diuretic. Alcohol and some other abused drugs can suppress shivering, thereby reducing heat production, and can prevent surface blood vessels from constricting, thereby allowing more heat loss than normal. Many prescription medications also can increase a person's susceptibility to either heat or cold emergencies. Commonly used psychiatric medications,

for example, predispose people to heat and cold emergencies because of the drug's physiological mechanisms. Finally, alcohol and drugs that affect the user's judgment and reasoning often lead to the person taking risks or entering situations where a heat or cold emergency is more likely, such as falling into cold water or going into a freezing environment without adequate protection.

- **Environmental variables:** The risk of hypothermia is increased by becoming wet from rain or immersion in water. Water conducts heat away from the body much more quickly than heat can be radiated into the air. Wind also increases heat loss through the "wind chill" effect. The wind chill chart in **Figure 20-1** shows how the effects of cold increase with wind; for example, a temperature of 0° F with a wind of 20 mph has a wind chill effect of − 22° F. High humidity increases the risk of heat emergencies because sweat evaporates more slowly and provides less cooling effect, as shown in the heat index chart **(Figure 20-2)**. For example, an air temperature of 90° F with a humidity of 90% has the same effect on the body as an air temperature of 122° F.

Cold Emergencies

Exposure to cold temperatures can cause either **frostbite**, which is localized freezing of skin and other tissues or **hypothermia**, which is lowering of the whole body's temperature.

Frostbite

Frostbite is the freezing of skin or deeper tissues. Frostbite occurs when the temperature is 32° F or colder. It usually happens to exposed skin areas on the head or face, hands or feet. Wind chill increases the risk of frostbite. Severe frostbite kills

tissue and can result in gangrene and having to amputate the body part.

The first aid for frostbite involves removing the affected area from the cold as soon as possible and protecting the area until the victim receives medical treatment. In special circumstances the body part may be rewarmed — but only under certain conditions. If the frostbitten area is at any risk of being refrozen, it should not be rewarmed, because warming followed by freezing increases the tissue damage. If the extrication, rescue or transport of

(continues on page 324)

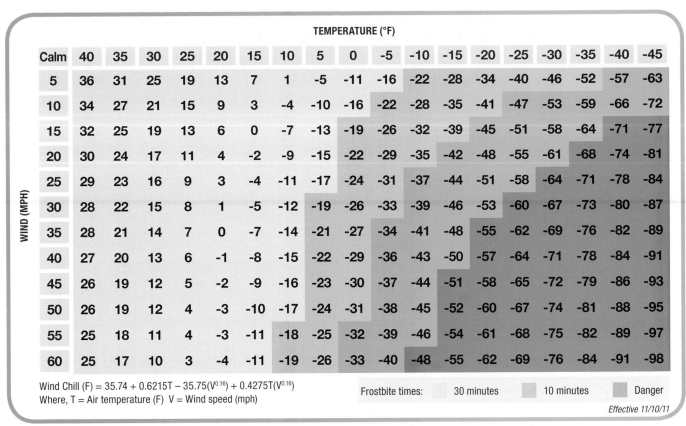

Figure 20-1 *Wind chill. (National Oceanic and Atmospheric Administration)*

Source: National Weather Service, http://www.nws.noaa.gov/om/windchill/ Accessed March 5, 2011.

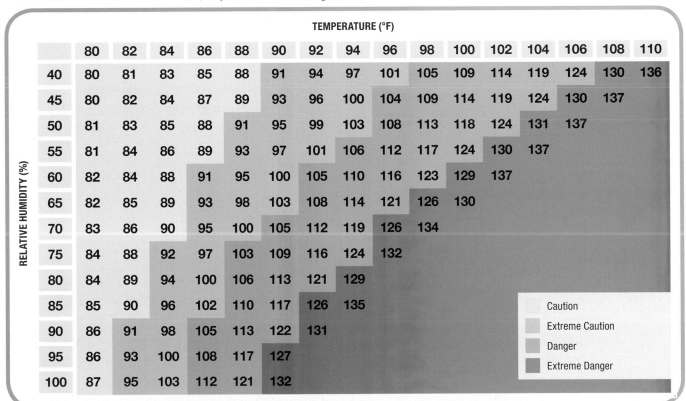

Figure 20-2 *Heat index. (National Weather Service)*

Source: National Weather Service, http://www.weather.gov/om/heat/index.shtml Accessed March 5, 2011.

20 • Cold and Heat Emergencies

(continued from page 322)

a frostbite victim may subject the area to cold again, do not warm it but let health care or EMS professionals treat the frostbite. In a situation where help will be delayed, and only if refreezing can be prevented, then severe frostbite can be rewarmed by immersing the area in lukewarm – not hot – water for 20 to 30 minutes. Never apply a direct heat source to frostbitten skin, such as heat lamp, hot water bottle or heating pad, because of the risk of additional tissue damage (see First Aid: "Frostbite").

Hypothermia

When the body cannot make heat as fast as it loses it in a cold environment, hypothermia develops. In hypothermia, body temperature drops below 95° F. It does not have to be freezing cold for hypothermia to occur. Hypothermia can occur at almost any cool temperature if the body is unprotected, especially if the victim is wet, exposed a long time or unable to restore body heat because of a medical condition. An average of about 600 individuals die each year in the United States of hypothermia, about half of them older than 65.[1] Because hypothermia alters a person's mental status, an affected victim may not take corrective actions to avoid continued exposure to cold **(Box 20-2)**.

Hypothermia is a progressive problem, as the victim transitions from simply feeling cold

[1]*Centers for Disease Control and Prevention, http://www. cdc.gov/mmwr/preview/mmwrhtml/mm5308a2.htm Accessed March 3, 2011.*

to mild hypothermia and, without the condition being relieved, to more serious symptoms and possibly to death. This progression may occur gradually, over hours or even days or very quickly, especially with a wind chill or if the victim is wet.

Preventing Hypothermia

When planning to be outdoors for a long time, be prepared for a cold emergency:

- Check the weather forecast before going outdoors for an extended period.

(continues on page 326)

BOX 20-2: FACTS ABOUT HYPOTHERMIA

- Hypothermia occurs more easily in elderly or ill people.

- People under the influence of alcohol or drugs are at greater risk for hypothermia.

- A person immersed in cold water cools 30 times faster than in cool air.

- Victims in cold water are more likely to die from hypothermia than to drown.

- Victims in cardiac arrest after immersion in cold water have been resuscitated after a long time underwater – don't give up!

Learning Checkpoint 1

1. True or False: Rubbing frostbitten fingers is the best way to warm them.

2. Frostbitten skin usually has what color(s)?

_____

3. A friend stops by your house after being outside for some time, complaining of being very cold. He has lost his hat, and his ears are white and hard and he says he has no feeling in them. Describe three actions to take for this man's frostbite.

_____

_____

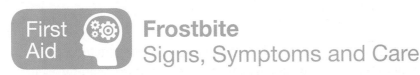

Frostbite
Signs, Symptoms and Care

When You See

- **Skin looks waxy and white, gray, yellow or bluish.**
- **The area is numb or feels tingly or aching.**
- **Severe frostbite:**
  - **The area feels hard**
  - **May become painless**
  - **After warming, the area becomes swollen and may blister**

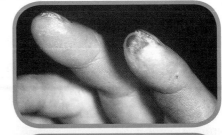

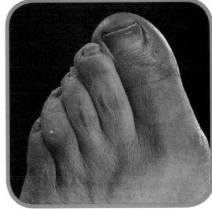

Do This First

1 Move the victim to a warm environment. Do not let the victim walk on frostbitten feet. Check the victim also for hypothermia.

2 Remove wet clothing and constricting items such as jewelry.

3 Protect between fingers and toes with dry gauze. Protect the area from being touched or rubbed by clothing or objects.

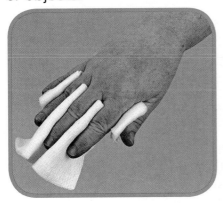

4 Seek medical attention as soon as possible.

5 Warm the frostbitten area in luke warm water (99° F to 104° F or 37° C to 40° C) for 20-30 minutes <u>only</u> if medical care will be delayed and if there is no danger of the skin refreezing.

6 Protect and elevate the frostbitten area.

Additional Care

- The victim may choose to take aspirin (adults only), acetaminophen or ibuprofen for pain.
- Drink warm liquids but not alcohol.
- Prevent the area from refreezing.

ALERT

- Do not rub frostbitten skin because this can damage the skin.
- Do not rewarm frostbitten skin if it may freeze again, which could worsen the injury.
- Do not use a fire, heat lamp, hot water bottle or heating pad to warm the area.
- After rewarming, be careful not to break blisters.

20 • Cold and Heat Emergencies

(continued from page 324)

- Take along extra clothing, socks, a sleeping bag or survival bag (see hypothermia blanket in **Chapter 23**).

- Have high-energy food bars and warm drinks.

- Do not use tobacco or consume alcohol or caffeine, which increase heat loss.

In addition, dress for the cold:

- Wear layers of clothing that do not retain moisture (wool or polypropylene).

- Choose a coat with a windproof and waterproof outer layer.

- Wear a hat (up to 50% of body heat is lost from the head).

- Use rain gear to avoid becoming wet.

During cold periods, check on people who are at risk for hypothermia:

- Check on older family members, friends and neighbors to ensure that the home is kept warm.

- Be familiar with the signs and symptoms of early hypothermia so you can recognize the problem and seek treatment.

- Employees of public health facilities, detoxification centers, shelters for the homeless and similar facilities should be educated to recognize hypothermia so victims receive appropriate treatment early.

First Aid for Hypothermia

Because hypothermia may begin gradually, it is crucial to recognize the first signs and symptoms in order to take early action. Shivering, numbness, lethargy, poor coordination and slurred speech are early manifestations. Victims of early or mild hypothermia often experience the "umbles": mumbles, fumbles and stumbles. Infants may have bright red skin and little energy. As body temperature drops, hypothermia progresses and becomes more serious. Shivering typically stops and the victim may not even feel cold. Check the victim's skin temperature under clothing at the abdomen; cool skin here often indicates hypothermia.

Breathing becomes shallow and mental status continues to deteriorate. In severe cases, the victim becomes unresponsive and may stop breathing.

First aid for hypothermia begins with removing the victim from the cold. Remove wet clothing and cover the victim with blankets or warm clothing. Call 9-1-1, and in severe cases be prepared to give basic life support. Do not try to actively warm the victim with a heat source except when far from medical care, because a heart rhythm disturbance may result.

A hypothermia victim who is not breathing may still be resuscitated. Handle the victim gently, but provide CPR or other care as needed while waiting for help to arrive (see First Aid: "Hypothermia").

Heat Emergencies

Heat illnesses can result when people become overheated in a hot environment. Generally there are three types of heat illnesses:

- **Heat cramps** are the least serious and usually first to occur.

- **Heat exhaustion** develops when the body becomes dehydrated in a hot environment.

- **Heatstroke**, with a seriously high body temperature, may develop from heat exhaustion. It is a medical emergency and, if untreated, usually causes death.

Most heatstroke deaths occur from exposure to a high temperature for a sustained period. Most heat-related deaths occur during hot weather, but heatstroke also affects people in settings where heat is generated, such as furnace rooms, factories or vehicles. Over the last two decades an average of 400 heat-related deaths a year have occurred in the United States, about half of these related to hot weather.[2] In one heat wave alone, in Chicago in 1995, 465 people died of heat emergencies.[3] Extreme heat is defined as

[2]*Centers for Disease Control and Prevention, http://www.cdc.gov/mmwr/preview/mmwrhtml/mm5126a2.htm Accessed March 3, 2011.*

[3]*Centers for Disease Control and Prevention, http://www.cdc.gov/mmwr/preview/mmwrhtml/00038443.htm Accessed March 3, 2011.*

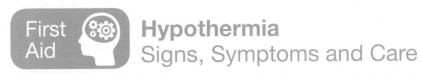

Hypothermia
Signs, Symptoms and Care

When You See

- **Shivering; may be uncontrollable (but stops in severe hypothermia)**
- **Victim seems apathetic, confused or irrational; may be belligerent**
- **Lethargy, clumsy movements, drowsiness**
- **Pale, cool skin – even under clothing (check abdomen)**
- **Slow breathing**
- **Changing levels of responsiveness**

Do This First

1 Check for responsiveness and normal breathing, and call 9-1-1. Except in mild cases, the victim needs immediate medical care.

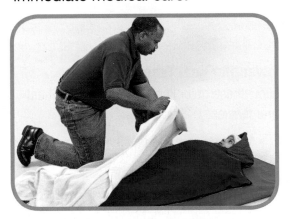

2 Provide CPR if the victim is unresponsive and not breathing normally.

3 Quickly move the victim out of the cold. Remove any wet clothing.

4 Warm the victim with blankets or warm clothing.

5 <u>Only</u> if the victim is far from medical care, use active rewarming by putting the victim near a heat source and putting warm water in containers against the skin.

6 Monitor breathing and be ready to give CPR if needed.

Additional Care

- Give warm (not hot) drinks to an alert victim who can easily swallow, but do not give alcohol or caffeine.
- Stay with the victim until he or she reaches a health care provider or help arrives.

ALERT

- Do not immerse a victim of hypothermia in hot water because warming them too rapidly can cause heart problems.
- Do not rub or massage the victim's skin. Be very gentle when handling the victim.

20 • Cold and Heat Emergencies

Learning Checkpoint 2

1. True or False: Hypothermia occurs only when the air temperature is below freezing.

2. True or False: A hypothermia victim who is generating heat by shivering still needs first aid and warming.

3. A hypothermic victim is brought into a ski lodge to be warmed. It will help to –

   a. give him a warm rum drink.

   b. have him take off his outer clothes and sit close to the fire.

   c. send him to a hot shower.

   d. remove his damp clothing and warm him with a blanket.

4. You are on a backpacking camping trip in the mountains and are caught in an unexpected snowstorm. On the way back down the mountain, about 4 miles from your car, you encounter a teenager sitting in the snow. His clothes are snowy and damp. He is lethargic and seems very confused. You call for help on your cell phone, but it will be at least 2 hours before the rescue team arrives. Using typical camping gear, what first aid can you give this victim?

---

temperatures that rise 10 degrees or more above the normal high temperature for the region and last several days to several weeks. As noted earlier in this chapter, many factors can increase the risk for developing a heat illness, including old age or infancy/youth, obesity, certain medical conditions such as heart disease, the use of certain medications, drinking alcohol, not drinking enough fluid and strenuous activity in a hot environment.

Like hypothermia, heatstroke is a progressive disease. In the mild stage (heat exhaustion), the victim is becoming dehydrated and the body is unable to cool itself. If the condition is not corrected, with continuing exposure to heat the victim's body temperature begins to rise and more serious symptoms occur, potentially leading to death. Prevention of life-threatening heatstroke depends on recognizing the early signs and symptoms and providing care before the condition becomes more serious.

Preventing Heat Emergencies

Follow these guidelines to help prevent heat emergencies:

- In hot environments, wear loose, lightweight clothing.

- Rest frequently in shady or cool areas.

- Drink adequate fluids before, during and after activity, but avoid alcohol and caffeine. Prehydrating is especially important before an endurance sport activity.

- For sports and endurance activities that may last longer than short periods of time, sports drinks that replace depleted electrolytes are generally better than water, but in most other situations adequate water consumption will prevent heat exhaustion.

- Avoid exertion if you are overweight or elderly.

- When new to a hot area, take several days (up to a week to 10 days) to gradually acclimate to heat and humidity before engaging in strenuous activity.

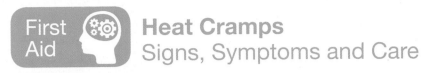

First Aid — Heat Cramps
Signs, Symptoms and Care

When You See

- **Signs of muscle pain, cramping or spasms**
- **Heavy sweating**

Do This First

1 Have the person stop the activity and sit quietly in a cool place.

2 Give a sports drink or water.

3 Have the person avoid strenuous activity for a few hours to prevent progression to heat exhaustion or heatstroke.

Additional Care

- For abdominal cramps, continue resting in a comfortable position.
- For leg cramps, stretch the muscle by extending the leg and flexing the ankle. Massage and ice the muscle.
- Seek medical attention for a victim who has heart problems or is on a low-sodium diet, or if the cramps do not subside within an hour.

- During heat waves, check on elderly friends, family and neighbors, particularly those who live alone or have a mental impairment, and if necessary move them to an air-conditioned area.

- Do not leave children alone in a vehicle. Make sure they cannot lock themselves into an enclosed space.

- Use sunscreen because sunburn causes a loss of body fluid as well as skin damage.

Heat Cramps

Activity in a hot environment may cause painful cramps in muscles, called **heat cramps**, often in the lower legs or abdominal muscles. The muscle cramps result when sweating lowers the body's sodium levels. Heat cramps may occur along with heat exhaustion and heatstroke (see First Aid: "Heat Cramps").

Heat Exhaustion

Activity in a hot environment usually causes heavy sweating, which may lead to dehydration and depletion of salt and electrolytes in the body if the person does not get enough fluids. This dehydration can lead to **heat exhaustion**.

A victim of heat exhaustion is usually sweating and the skin is pale or ashen, moist and often cool. Other signs and symptoms include thirst, fatigue and muscle cramps. Late signs and symptoms include headache or dizziness; fainting; nausea or vomiting; and fast, shallow breathing.

First, move the victim from the heat to rest in a cool place. Loosen or remove unnecessary clothing and help cool the victim's body with wet cloths, sponging the skin with cool water or spraying the skin with water and fanning the area. Give the victim a sports drink or water to drink. The victim's condition should improve within 30 minutes. If it does not, or if the victim has a heart condition or high blood pressure, seek medical attention immediately. Remember that if unrelieved, heat exhaustion may develop into heatstroke, a life-threatening emergency (see First Aid: "Heat Exhaustion").

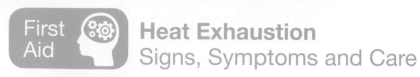

First Aid
Heat Exhaustion
Signs, Symptoms and Care

When You See

- **Sweating, pale or ashen, moist skin (often cool)**
- **Thirst**
- **Fatigue**
- **Muscle cramps**

Later signs and symptoms:

- **Headache, dizziness or fainting**
- **Nausea or vomiting**
- **Fast, shallow breathing**

Do This First

1 Move the victim from the heat to rest in a cool place. Loosen or remove outer clothing.

2 Cool the victim with one of these methods:

- Put wet cloths on the forehead and body.
- Sponge the skin with cool water.
- Spray the skin with water from a spray bottle and then fan the area.

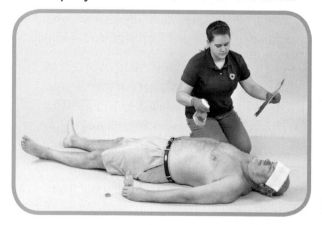

3 Give a sports drink or water to drink.

Additional Care

- Seek medical care if the victim's condition worsens or does not improve within 30 minutes.
- Seek urgent medical attention if the victim has a heart condition or high blood pressure.

ALERT

- Do not give salt tablets to a heat exhaustion or heatstroke victim. Use a sports drink instead (if the victim is awake and alert).
- Do not give liquids containing caffeine or alcohol.
- If the victim is lethargic, nauseous or vomiting, do not give any liquids.

Learning **Checkpoint 3**

1. True or False: For abdominal heat cramps, the best care is vigorous massage and stomach kneading.

2. To treat heat cramps:

   a. Immerse the victim in a bathtub of cold water.

   b. Give a sports drink or water to drink.

   c. Keep the victim very active until the cramp works itself out.

   d. Do not let the victim eat or drink anything.

3. True or False: Give salt tablets to victims who have both heat cramps and heat exhaustion.

4. Heat exhaustion begins when a person in a hot environment is not getting enough

   _____ .

5. List three possible ways to cool a victim who has heat exhaustion.

   _____

   _____

6. On a hot day you join a friend on the athletic field who has been working out for a couple of hours. He is sitting on the grass in the sun. He is sweating heavily and says he has a headache and feels nauseous. Someone has already given him a sports drink. What should you do now? List in correct order the first four actions you would take.

   _____

   _____

Heatstroke

Heatstroke is a life-threatening emergency that is more common during hot summer periods. It may develop slowly over several days or more rapidly when engaged in strenuous activity in the heat. The victim may be dehydrated and not sweating when heatstroke gradually develops or he or she may be sweating heavily from exertion. Heatstroke causes a body temperature of 104° F or higher and is different from heat exhaustion, although it may develop from untreated heat exhaustion (see First Aid: "Heatstroke"):

- In heatstroke the victim's skin is flushed and feels very hot to the touch; in heat exhaustion the skin may be pale or ashen and clammy.

- In heatstroke the victim becomes very confused and irrational and may become unresponsive or have convulsions; in heat exhaustion the victim is dizzy or tired or may be irritable or have a headache.

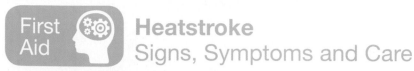

First Aid

Heatstroke
Signs, Symptoms and Care

When You See

- **Skin is flushed, dry and hot to the touch; sweating usually has stopped**
- **Fast breathing**
- **Headache, dizziness, confusion**
- **Irrational behavior**
- **Possible convulsions or unresponsiveness**

Do This First

1 Call 9-1-1.

2 Move the victim to a cool place.

3 Remove outer clothing.

4 Immediately cool the victim with any means at hand, preferably by immersing the victim up to the neck in cold water (with the help of a second rescuer). Other methods include wrapping the victim in a wet sheet kept wet; sponging the victim with cold water; spraying the skin with water and fanning the area; or applying ice bags or cold packs beside the neck, armpits and groin).

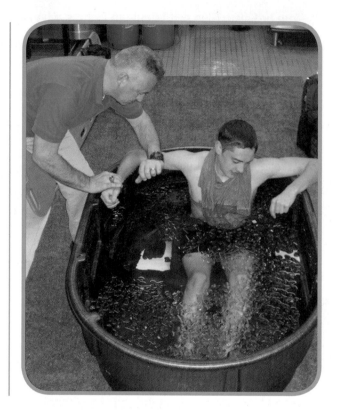

Additional Care

- Monitor the victim's breathing and be ready to give CPR if needed.
- Put an unresponsive victim in the recovery position and monitor breathing.
- Protect a victim having convulsions from injury (see **Chapter 16**).

ALERT

- Do not apply rubbing alcohol to the victim's skin.
- The victim should not take pain relievers or salt tablets.
- Do not give any beverage containing caffeine or alcohol.
- Do not let the victim use tobacco.
- If the victim is nauseated or vomiting or experiencing diminished mental status, do not give liquids.

Learning **Checkpoint 4**

1. True or False: It is safe to drive a heatstroke victim home after you have given first aid and cooled his or her body down to 100° F, as long as the victim is feeling better.

2. In what situation should you call 9-1-1 for a heatstroke victim?

   _____

3. Describe how a heatstroke victim's behavior may be different from the way in which that person usually behaves.

   _____

4. Your softball game happens to fall on the hottest day of the year. Your coach knows you have first aid training and asks you to help out to make sure none of the students has problems with heat exhaustion or heatstroke.

   a. To be prepared for these possibilities, what things should you make sure are present at the ball field?

   _____

   b. You decide to give a safety talk to your team before the game begins. What would you tell them about how to prevent heat emergencies? What signs and symptoms of a potential problem should players watch out for in others on their team?

   _____

   c. Despite these precautions, by the seventh inning the center fielder seems to be showing signs and symptoms of heatstroke. What is the first step you should take?

   _____

Concluding Thoughts

Heat and cold emergencies can be prevented by following commonsense guidelines and taking steps in extreme temperatures to maintain normal body temperature. Recognizing the early signs and symptoms of both heat and cold emergencies is important to keep these conditions from worsening. When heat or cold illness does occur, act quickly to get medical attention before the emergency becomes life-threatening. Be sure to take special precautions when engaged in activities in rural or wilderness areas where a victim cannot be easily or quickly reached by EMS professionals. **Chapter 23** describes these extra preparations to prevent these emergencies from occurring in such situations.

Learning Outcomes

You should now be able to do the following:

1. Describe the different types of cold and heat emergencies and what you can do to prevent them.

2. Explain factors that may make a person more susceptible to a cold or heat emergency.

3. List the signs and symptoms and first aid for:

   - Frostbite
   - Heat exhaustion
   - Hypothermia
   - Heatstroke
   - Heat cramps

Review Questions

1. Muscle contraction produces –

    a. heat.

    b. heat loss.

    c. vasoconstriction.

    d. vasodilation.

2. Heat and cold emergencies are more likely to occur in –

    a. the elderly.

    b. people with certain chronic diseases.

    c. infants.

    d. All of the above

3. First aid for frostbite includes –

    a. rapid rewarming using a heat lamp or heating pad.

    b. protecting the area from rubbing or constricting jewelry.

    c. vigorously rubbing the area.

    d. running very hot water over the affected area for 10 minutes.

4. To help prevent hypothermia when outdoors in frigid temperatures –

    a. drink lots of coffee or hot tea.

    b. wear thick boots because most heat loss is through the feet.

    c. try to stay dry.

    d. drink alcohol to stay warm.

5. The signs and symptoms of hypothermia include –

    a. apathy or confusion.

    b. red, blotchy skin.

    c. talkativeness.

    d. perceptions of being overly warm.

6. First aid for severe hypothermia includes –

    a. putting the victim in a hot shower.

    b. massaging the victim all over.

    c. calling 9-1-1.

    d. giving CPR regardless of whether the victim is breathing.

7. In what order do heat illnesses typically progress with continued activity in a hot environment?

    a. Heat cramps -> heatstroke -> heat exhaustion

    b. Heat cramps -> heat exhaustion -> heatstroke

    c. Heat exhaustion -> heat cramps -> heatstroke

    d. Can occur in any order

8. First aid for heat cramps includes –

  a. vigorously exercising the muscle.

  b. drinking a sports drink or water.

  c. applying a compression bandage.

  d. splinting the extremity until the cramps pass.

9. The late signs and symptoms of heat exhaustion include –

  a. headache, dizziness, fainting.

  b. constipation or diarrhea.

  c. extreme excitability.

  d. cold, tingling fingers or toes.

10. How can you cool down someone who is experiencing heatstroke?

  a. Immerse the victim up to the neck in cold water.

  b. Spray the victim with cold water.

  c. Put ice bags or cool packs beside the neck, armpits and groin area.

  d. Any of the above

Chapter 21 • Behavioral Emergencies

Chapter Preview

- Emotional and Behavioral Responses to Injury and Illness
- Victims with Emotional Problems
- Behavioral Emergencies

- Abuse
- Sexual Assault and Rape

Your boss has asked to meet with you and another employee, Meg, the woman in charge of order fulfillment. There have been several problems with important orders lately, and as the meeting explores ways to prevent future problems, Meg becomes increasingly emotional and defensive. You know she has been under a lot of stress lately, and you've overheard gossip that she has some personal problems, but that doesn't seem to account for how worked up she is becoming in this meeting. Finally, when the boss asks if she will be able to solve the order problems, Meg seems to explode, rising from her chair with her hands in fists. You are alarmed and wonder what you can do before the situation is completely out of control or even becomes violent.

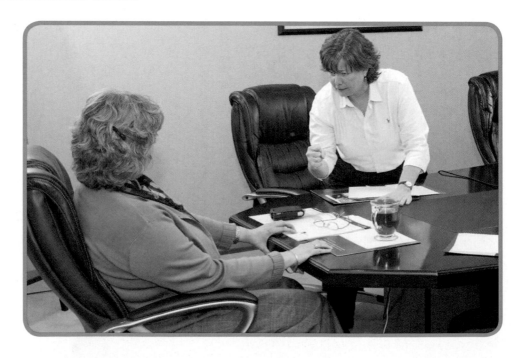

The process of giving first aid is sometimes complicated by the victim's behavior. Many injuries and medical emergencies may cause altered mental status, which can lead to a victim acting in unusual or unpredictable ways. Injury and illness also typically cause emotional responses that may affect how first aid must be given. Other victims may have emotional problems such as panic reactions or depression that also must be addressed when giving first aid. **Behavioral emergencies** involve situations in which the victim's behavior, whether caused by the injury or illness or by personality or mental health factors, results in or complicates an emergency situation. Abuse and rape are additional behavioral situations.

Emotional and Behavioral Responses to Injury and Illness

Injury, sudden illness and other emergencies typically lead to strong emotional reactions in those involved. Normal reactions include fear, anxiety and apprehensiveness. In addition to the physical effects of the injury or illness itself, which may include altered mental status, normal emotional reactions may cause other stress-related physical signs and symptoms such as trembling or shakiness, feelings of nausea, a fast heartbeat and breathing, and perspiration.

Victims with pre-existing emotional problems or mental illness are more likely to have more severe reactions. They may overreact, panic and act wildly, speak incoherently, become argumentative or withdrawn, or become violent.

There is no clear-cut line between "normal" and "abnormal" responses to injury and sudden illness. Think of these responses as a continuum from normal to abnormal, with a wide range of behaviors in the middle. It is important not to judge a victim's behavior too quickly but rather to assess the situation. For example, a person who is usually calm and rational may become seemingly irrational and act inappropriately when in great pain. In such a case accept the victim's

emotional state and address his or her concerns while providing first aid. At the other extreme, a person who is usually quick to anger and aggressive may respond to the stress of an injury with violent behavior. In this case it may become more important to protect yourself and others at the scene.

Your decision on how to approach a victim in a potential behavioral emergency depends on understanding normal versus abnormal reactions and an assessment of the victim's emotional and mental condition. Always remember your own safety – Do not approach a victim who may become violent. Call 9-1-1 and stay at a safe distance until help arrives.

Altered Mental Status

As noted in previous chapters, altered mental status, or altered responsiveness, may result from many different injuries and illnesses. The brain requires a steady level of oxygen for normal functioning, and any injury or illness that affects oxygenation may affect the victim's mental status – and therefore his or her behavior. Lowered levels of responsiveness may result from significantly reduced oxygen levels. Mental status may suddenly or gradually diminish. The victim may first feel dizzy, drowsy, disoriented or confused. The victim may suddenly or eventually become completely unresponsive. Often in such cases, the appropriate first aid is to care for the underlying cause of the altered mental status **(Box 21-1)**.

Even small oxygen reductions can cause other reactions. A victim may respond to reduced brain oxygen with extreme anxiety and panic, even potential violence. In such cases, in addition to providing first aid, you also need to calm the victim and possibly prevent further injury caused by the victim's behavior. You may need to protect yourself as well. For example, near-drowning victims who are panicking as they desperately fight for air often behave irrationally and may grab onto a rescuer so forcefully that both lives are threatened.

Typical Emotional Reactions

As noted earlier, typical reactions to injury, sudden illness and other emergencies include fear, anxiety and apprehensiveness. The sight of their own blood makes many people panic. It is difficult to think clearly when in great pain. A victim with a serious injury may overreact and be fearful of dying. A victim may be unable to act, seemingly frozen by emotional shock, or may be acting irrationally and out of control. Any of these reactions can complicate the process of giving first aid for the victim's injury or illness.

Because emotional stress can have negative physical effects on the body, it may be just as important to address the victim's emotional reaction as it is to care for the physical injury or illness. The victim needs to be calmed and reassured.

Reassuring and Calming Victims

How you act in the face of the victim's emergency can dramatically affect how the victim responds. If you react negatively, your words, gestures or facial expressions may increase the victim's stressful response rather than diminish it. You may show your own concern or fear about the emergency. You may act impatiently if the victim is not immediately cooperative. If you show a lack of self-confidence in your ability to manage the emergency and provide first aid, the victim's level of stress may increase. Any of these reactions will only increase the problem.

Instead, take steps to calm and reassure the victim, following these guidelines **(Figure 21-1)**:

1. Tell the victim who you are and say you are there to help. Avoid seeming judgmental.

2. Do not assume the victim is intoxicated, using drugs or otherwise impaired, as the victim's behavior may result from a medical condition. Even if you smell alcohol on the victim's breath, do not assume a problem is due only to intoxication – you could overlook a serious injury.

3. Reassure the victim that help is on the way (after 9-1-1 has been called).

4. Ask the victim for his or her name and use it when speaking to him or her.

5. If possible, try to involve any of the victim's friends or family members present at the scene.

6. Let the victim tell you what he or she thinks is wrong.

7. Let the victim know you understand his or her concerns.

8. Make eye contact with the victim and stay at the victim's eye level.

9. Speak in a caring, reassuring voice, but do not give false assurances or lie about the victim's condition.

10. Do not argue with the victim. Show that you understand the victim's concerns by repeating or rephrasing what the victim tells you.

11. If the victim seems irrational or delusional, do not make statements to support their false beliefs, but do not challenge them, either.

BOX 21-1: CAUSES OF ALTERED MENTAL STATUS

- Respiratory emergencies
- Cardiac emergencies
- Poisoning
- Head injuries
- Seizures
- Diabetic emergencies
- Stroke
- High fever
- Substance abuse
- Drug overdose
- Heat or cold emergencies

12. Stay a safe distance away from the victim until your help is accepted. If the victim does not accept your help, do not try to restrain or force care on him or her. Withdraw if the scene seems unsafe or if the victim may become violent.

13. Tell the victim what you plan to do before doing it.

14. Move calmly and slowly, touching the victim only as necessary.

Victims With Emotional Problems

Some victims have pre-existing emotional problems that may present greater challenges than the emotions normally provoked by emergencies. Two common problems are anxiety/panic and depression.

Anxiety and Panic

Although it is normal to feel fear and apprehension when injured or suddenly ill, some people are prone to extreme **anxiety** and may have a **panic attack**. A panic attack is a sudden, overwhelming fear that is excessive for the situation. Signs and symptoms of extreme anxiety include:

- Agitation, inability to hold still, rapid movements, pacing
- Speaking very fast or not making sense
- Inability to judge the situation accurately
- Rapid emotional changes, crying, hysteria, anger
- A desire to leave the scene or not wait for medical help
- Fast heartbeat and breathing
- Difficulty breathing, dizziness, trembling

With a victim exhibiting signs and symptoms of extreme anxiety or panic, it is important to remain calm and patient at all times. Any attempt you make to restrain the person or to shock the person out of this behavior will likely worsen the situation. Often the panic will begin to ease in a few minutes because the physiological response of the body is self-limiting.

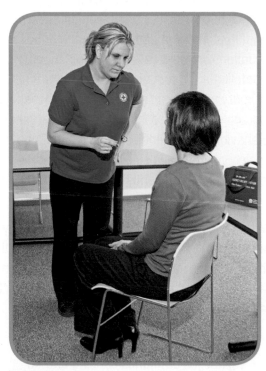
(a)

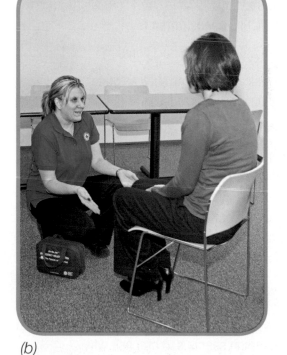
(b)

Figure 21-1 (a) When trying to calm an emotional victim, be careful not to assume a position that may seem threatening. (b) Stay a comfortable distance away and use accepting, nonthreatening body language.

Follow the guidelines given earlier for calming and reassuring victims. Recognize that an individual prone to extreme anxiety or panic may need more time to calm down and may suddenly experience renewed anxiety. Continue to use the calming techniques while providing first aid. Be empathetic and gentle, and always explain what you are doing. Avoid touching the victim without first explaining what you are about to do and why. Allow victims to keep talking about what they are feeling and to express their concerns.

Depression

Victims who experience depression also require special attention. Major **depression** is a common psychological illness, affecting an estimated 10% of Americans chronically. It occurs in people of all ages, is most prevalent in relatively young people and is about three times as common in women as in men.[1] Common signs and symptoms of depression include:

- Frequent feelings of sadness
- Loss of energy
- Feelings of hopelessness or worthlessness
- Difficulty concentrating
- Difficulty making decisions
- Physical symptoms such as abdominal pain, insomnia, appetite loss or recurrent headaches
- Thoughts of death or suicide

Someone experiencing depression often acts withdrawn, apathetic and subdued. Although the person may not resist your first aid care, he or she may not cooperate and may not offer information that would help you assess the situation. Therefore, it is important to make an effort to communicate with a victim who seems depressed. Follow these guidelines:

1. Encourage the victim to talk. Acknowledge that the person seems sad and ask why.

[1] *American Public Health Association, http://www.ncbi. nlm.nih.gov/pmc/articles/PMC1349333 Accessed March 5, 2011.*

2. Be reassuring and sympathetic.

3. Show the victim that you care about him or her as a person. Helping to make the person comfortable, offering a drink of water or a blanket and providing other comforts can encourage the victim to open up and talk about the problem.

4. If the victim is crying, do not try to make him or her stop. Allow the person to work through the emotion.

5. If the victim complains about something in his or her life, listen sympathetically but do not offer false reassurances such as saying, "Everything will be just fine" or "I'm sure that problem won't last long." Instead, talk about resources you are aware of to help people with problems such as the victim's.

6. Be alert to the possibility of suicide (see later section on "Suicidal Feelings").

Behavioral Emergencies

The previous sections have focused on interacting with victims of injury or sudden illness who are experiencing normal or abnormal emotional reactions. In most cases those reactions complicate the first aid problem but are not the primary problem. In some cases, however, the person's behavior constitutes the emergency. Behavioral emergencies include situations in which victims have suicidal feelings or the potential to act violently in a way that may harm themselves or others.

When a victim's behavior becomes obviously abnormal, remember not to assume simply that the person is intoxicated or under the influence of a drug. Many different factors can radically change a person's behavior, including:

- The stress of the situation
- Illnesses or injuries causing altered mental status
- Mental illnesses

BOX 21-2: SUICIDE RISK FACTORS AND WARNING SIGNS

Risk Factors

- Mental disorders, including depression
- History of substance abuse
- Feelings of hopelessness
- Recent emotional crisis or painful illness
- Impulsive or aggressive tendencies
- Past attempts at suicide

Warning Signs

- Talking about suicide (It is a myth that people who talk about it rarely act upon the threat)
- Comments about feeling hopeless or worthless
- Taking risks that could cause death, such as driving too fast
- Loss of interest in one's past activities
- Suddenly and unexpectedly seeming calm or happy after being sad

Suicidal Feelings

More than 33,000 individuals committed suicide in the United States in a recent year. Suicide is the third leading cause of death among people 15 to 24 years old. Men are about five times more likely to commit suicide than women,[2] although women report attempting suicide three times more often than men. Overall, suicide is the 11th leading cause of death for among people 10 and older.[3] Drug overdose (see **Chapter 18**) is the most common method used by females, and firearms are the method used most by men.[4]

The risk factors and signs of potential suicides are listed in **Box 21-2.** Research has shown that most people who commit suicide communicated their desire to others, although not always in an obvious way. Anyone who makes comments suggestive of suicidal feelings should be taken seriou sly.

[2]National Safety Council [NSC]. (2011). Injury Facts®, 2011 Edition. Itasca, IL: Author.

[3]Centers for Disease Control and Prevention, http://www.cdc.gov/violenceprevention/suicide/statistics/leading_causes.html Accessed March 3, 2011.

[4]Centers for Disease Control and Prevention, http://www.cdc.gov/violenceprevention/suicide/statistics/mechanism01.html Accessed March 3, 2011.

Follow these guidelines if you are caring for a person who may be suicidal or whose injury may have been self-inflicted:

1. Take the person seriously and listen to what he or she is saying. Ask what the person is planning to do. Talk calmly and supportively.

2. Do not try to argue the person out of committing suicide, but let him or her know that you understand and care. Do not give false reassurances.

3. Seek help. Call 9-1-1 if appropriate and involve friends or family members if possible in any care given.

4. Do not leave the person alone unless your own safety is threatened.

5. Remove any weapons, drugs or medications that might be used in a suicide attempt. Do not let the person drive.

6. If the person has a firearm and is threatening violence, withdraw, call 9-1-1, and wait for help to arrive and handle the situation. (See following section on "Violent Behavior.")

7. Give first aid and other care as appropriate.

Violent Behavior

In any behavioral emergency, consider the potential for violence. The person may threaten violence to themself or others on the scene. Following are signs that violent behavior may occur:

- The person is holding a weapon or any object that might be used as a weapon.

- The person is in a threatening or bullying posture, has his or her hands in fists, or is pacing and waving his or her arms around **(Figure 21-2)**.

- The person is threatening, verbally abusing or yelling at you or someone else.

- The person is uncontrollably angry, kicking or throwing things.

- The person seems to be hallucinating or yelling at someone not present.

- The person is known to have committed violent acts in the past.

If you think the person may commit an act of violence, follow these guidelines:

1. Do not enter the scene if your safety is at risk. Encourage others at the scene to withdraw.

2. Call 9-1-1.

3. Do not try to restrain the person unless you have had special training and have assistance from others. Monitor the situation from a safe distance and wait for help to arrive.

4. While waiting for help, do the following if it is safe to remain with the person:

   - Talk to the person calmly and quietly and listen to what he or she has to say. Do not argue or be falsely reassuring, which the person may perceive as condescending or patronizing behavior. Try to divert the person from any violent action by keeping him or her talking.

   - Do not move about or do anything the person may perceive as threatening.

- Offer to give first aid if the person calms down, but do not try to do anything without the person's consent.

- Maintain an open exit from the room or scene; do not let a potentially violent person get between you and the door.

Abuse

Abuse is the intentional inflicting of injury or suffering on someone under the abuser's power, such as a child, spouse or elderly parent. In some cases a victim needs first aid for injuries sustained in an abuse incident. In other cases abuse may become apparent when a victim is being treated for another injury or sudden illness. In still other cases you may encounter a victim of abuse who does not have a present injury requiring first aid. In all situations, and in incidents of sexual abuse or rape, you need to be sensitive to the victim's emotional status and aware of special issues for handling the situation.

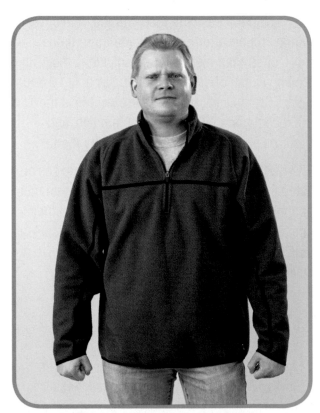

Figure 21-2 *An emotional person is potentially violent.*

Learning Checkpoint 1

1. Normal responses to many injuries and sudden illnesses include –

    a. trembling or shakiness.

    c. altered mental status.

    b. fear, anxiety.

    d. All of the above

2. Check off any of the following conditions that may cause altered mental status:

    _____Respiratory emergencies   _____Cardiac emergencies

    _____Poisoning   _____Head injuries

    _____Seizures   _____Diabetic emergencies

    _____Stroke   _____High fever

    _____Drug overdose   _____Heat or cold emergencies

3. Describe at least five things you can do to help calm an emotional victim.

    _____

4. True or False: Never acknowledge that a depressed person seems sad, but be cheerful and pretend nothing is wrong.

5. True or False: People who talk about committing suicide rarely act upon the threat.

6. You see an injured victim who is shouting and making threatening gestures and you realize he is potentially violent. Number the following actions in the order in which you should take them:

    _____ Talk to the person calmly and quietly, and try to divert the person from any violent action by keeping him or her talking.

    _____ Call 9-1-1.

    _____ Do not enter the scene if your safety is at risk. Encourage others at the scene to withdraw.

Prevention of Abuse

Many individual and cultural factors are involved in the causes of abuse. Tension, anger and frustration can grow to the point where the person in a rage commits an act of violence. In most cases this leads to a cycle of regret and promises to change, but the cycle repeats as stresses again build and lead to often increasingly violent acts.

What originally causes a person to become an abuser? Many abusers were abused themselves as children or observed abuse in their homes. Some people never develop ways to manage stress and control their feelings. Many different psychological factors are involved in why some people easily lose their temper and become violent. Unfortunately there is no simple way to predict who may become an abuser and therefore no simple way to prevent abuse from happening the first time. The cycle of repeated abuse, however, can be broken. Laws have become more protective of victims, shelters and hotlines are increasingly available for victims to break away from their abusers, and programs have been developed to help abusers learn to control impulses toward violence. Preventing abuse, therefore, begins with recognizing and acknowledging it when it occurs and understanding that resources are available for both victims and abusers. The following sections on child abuse, domestic violence, elder abuse and rape include telephone hotline numbers for finding such resources throughout the United States.

Child Abuse[5]

Child abuse and neglect are major problems in our society. Consider these statistics and facts about child abuse and neglect:

- In 2006, an estimated 905,000 children in the United States were found to be victims of child abuse and neglect.

- Children in the age group of birth to 1 year had the highest rate of victimization at 24.4 per 1,000 children of the same age group in the national population.

- Just over one-half (51.5%) of the child victims were girls and 48.2 percent were boys.

- More than 60 percent (64.1%) of victims suffered neglect. More than 15 percent (16%) of the victims suffered physical abuse.

- Less than 10 percent (8.8%) of the victims suffered sexual abuse.

- An estimated 1,530 children died from child abuse or neglect. The overall rate of child abuse fatalities was 2.04 deaths per 100,000 children.

- More than three-quarters (78.0%) of the children who died due to child abuse and neglect were younger than 4.

- Nearly 80 percent (79.4%) of perpetrators of child maltreatment were parents and another 6.7 percent were other relatives of the victim.

[5]*The information in this section on child abuse comes from The Child Welfare Information Gateway information packet "Child Abuse and Neglect." http://www. childwelfare.gov/pubs/can_info_packet.pdf Accessed March 5, 2011.*

Physical Abuse of Children

Physical abuse is physical injury (ranging from minor bruises to severe fractures or death) as a result of punching, beating, kicking, biting, shaking, throwing, stabbing, choking, hitting (with a hand, stick, strap or other object), burning or otherwise harming a child. These injuries are considered abuse regardless of whether the caretaker intended to hurt the child. "Shaken baby syndrome" is an example of usually unintended abuse: a parent or other caretaker, including baby-sitters, becomes frustrated with a crying infant and shakes the infant, potentially causing severe brain or spinal injury or death.

Following are signs of physical abuse:

The child:

- Has unexplained scalding or burns, rope burns, lacerations, bites, bruises, broken bones or black eyes.

- Has fading bruises or other marks after an absence from school or childcare.

- Seems frightened of parents and protests or cries when it is time to go home.

- Shrinks at the approach of adults.

- Reports being injured by a parent or another adult caregiver.

- Appears withdrawn or depressed and cries often – or is aggressive and disruptive.

- Seems tired often and complains of frequent nightmares.

The parent or other adult caregiver:

- Offers conflicting, unconvincing or no explanation for the child's injury.

- Describes the child with words such as "evil" or other negative terms.

- Uses harsh physical discipline with the child.

- Is known to have a history of abuse as a child.

Sexual Abuse of a Child

Sexual abuse includes any kind of sexual activity by a parent or caretaker, such as fondling a child's genitals, penetration, incest, rape, sodomy, indecent exposure or exploitation through prostitution or the production of pornographic materials.

The following are signs of sexual abuse:

The child:

- Has difficulty walking or sitting.

- Suddenly refuses to change clothing when necessary or to participate in physical activities.

- Reports nightmares or bedwetting.

- Experiences a sudden change in appetite.

- Demonstrates bizarre, sophisticated or unusual sexual knowledge or behavior.

- Becomes pregnant or contracts a venereal disease, particularly if younger than 14.

- Runs away from home.

- Reports sexual abuse by a parent or other adult caregiver.

- Seems afraid of a particular person or of being alone with that person.

The parent or other adult caregiver:

- Is unduly protective of the child or severely limits the child's contact with other children, especially those of the opposite sex.

- Is secretive and isolated.

- Is jealous or controlling with family members.

Reporting Child Abuse

Parents or other caregivers who abuse or neglect a child need help. Programs are available in most communities to provide professional help.

You should not, however, try to talk by yourself to suspected abusers in an effort to get them to seek help. Almost always the abuser will deny the problem and the situation may become worse than if you had said nothing. Instead, the single

most important thing you can do, if you suspect a child is being abused or neglected, is to report it to the proper authorities. Your report will help protect the child and get help for the family.

If you care for children as part of your job, you may be legally required to report suspected cases of child abuse or neglect. State laws vary in the specifics of who must make a report and to what agency. If this is required in your job, follow your employer's policy.

The law provides ways for private citizens to report suspected abuse or neglect, and it is important for the child's welfare that you do this even if not required to do so. Contact your local child protective services agency or police department. For more information about where and how to file a report, call the Childhelp USA® National Child Abuse Hotline (800-4-A-CHILD).

When you call to report child abuse, you will be asked for specific information, which may include:

- The child's name

- The suspected perpetrator's name (if known)

- A description of what you have seen or heard

- The names of any other people having knowledge of the abuse

- Your name and phone number

Your name will not be given to the family of the child you suspect is being abused or neglected. If you are making the report as a private citizen, you may ask to make the report anonymously, but your report may be considered more credible and can be more helpful to the child protective services agency if you give your name. Remember: Your suspicion of child abuse or neglect is enough to make a report. You do not have to provide proof. Almost every state has a law to protect people who make good-faith reports of child abuse from prosecution or liability.

Care for an Apparently Abused Child

If you suspect an injured child you are providing first aid to has been abused or neglected, do not confront the parents or ask the child direct questions about abuse. If the child needs first aid for an illness or injury, provide it as you would for any child, following standard guidelines. If you are giving first aid as part of your job, follow your employer's guidelines for documenting the care and any other actions you take. If the child tells you an injury was caused by a parent or other adult, include this information when making your report.

Spouse Abuse

Like child abuse, spouse abuse – or domestic violence – is a major problem in our society:[6]

- One in four women (25%) has experienced domestic violence in her lifetime.

- Estimates range from 960,000 incidents of violence against a current or former spouse, boyfriend or girlfriend to 3 million women who are physically abused by their husband or boyfriend per year.

- Women accounted for 85% of the victims of intimate partner violence, men for approximately 15%.

- Approximately 1 in 5 female high school students reports being physically and/or sexually abused by a dating partner.

- Women 20-24 years old are at the greatest risk of nonfatal intimate partner violence.

- Between 1993 and 2004, intimate partner violence on average made up 22% of nonfatal intimate partner victimizations against women.

- Women of all races are about equally vulnerable to violence by an intimate partner.

- Nearly 2.2 million people called a domestic violence crisis hotline in 2004 to escape crisis situations, seek advice or assist someone they thought might be victims.

[6]*Domestic Violence Resource Center, http://www.dvrc-or. org/domestic/violence/resources/C61 Accessed March 5, 2011.*

- Nearly 3 out of 4 (74%) of Americans personally know someone who is or has been a victim of domestic violence.

- On average, more than 3 women and 1 man are murdered by their intimate partners in this country every day. In 2000, 1,247 women were killed by an intimate partner.

Domestic violence and spouse abuse affect people from all races, nationalities, economic levels and religions. The three primary types of domestic violence are physical abuse, sexual abuse and rape, and verbal/emotional abuse. Physical abuse may involve hitting, slapping, punching, kicking, choking, biting and assault with objects.

Many abusive relationships continue for some time without the victim reporting the abuse to authorities. Commonly the victim stays with the abusing spouse or partner for several reasons:

- They love their partner – they only want the abuse to stop.

- They are afraid of their partner.

- They feel guilty and may blame themselves for the violence.

- They often have low self-esteem.

- They are isolated from family and friends.

- They depend emotionally and/or financially on their partner.

- They do not know their rights or that help is available.

Care for a Victim of Domestic Violence

It is seldom obvious that a victim's injuries resulted from physical abuse. Because there is often a history of abuse and physical injury, the victim may be experienced in covering up the cause of injuries. Certain signs, however, may raise a suspicion of domestic violence:

- The victim seems unusually fearful.

- The victim's account of the injury seems inconsistent or unlikely.

- The victim is uneasy in the presence of a spouse or partner.

- The victim's spouse or partner aggressively blames the woman for being injured.

If these or other signs of possible domestic violence are present, consider the possibility that the injury resulted from abuse. Follow these guidelines:

1. Provide first aid as usual for the injury. Call 9-1-1 for significant injuries and tell responding EMS personnel in private about your suspicions; they will know the correct steps to take.

2. Ensure privacy for the victim while providing care.

3. Do not directly confront the victim with your suspicions, especially if the victim's spouse or partner is present.

4. Try to involve a friend or family member of the victim in your caregiving.

5. If you are giving first aid as part of your employment responsibilities, you may be required to report suspected cases of domestic violence to authorities. Many health care workers generally are required by law to report suspected abuse. Check with your supervisor.

6. If the victim communicates information to you that suggests abuse, or if it is appropriate in your relationship with the victim to raise the issue yourself, you may choose to tell the victim that domestic violence is against the law and that help is available.

7. If you see physical abuse occurring or are certain a crime has been committed, or if the victim's partner is threatening and potentially violent, call law enforcement personnel. Withdraw from the scene to ensure your own safety. Local and state agencies are present in all 50 states to assist victims of domestic violence in many ways. Often help can be provided to the abuser so that the relationship can continue, if that is the wish of both partners. Many support groups are available to help both victims and abusers. Other assistance is available for spouses who choose to end the relationship. Victims should never feel they have no choice but to remain in an abusive relationship.

The National Domestic Violence Hotline can provide information and local contacts for those seeking help: 800-799-SAFE or www.ndvd.org.

Elder Abuse

Elder abuse is another common type of domestic violence. Typically elder abuse refers to physical, emotional or financial abuse or neglect inflicted on someone older than 60, often by someone else in the home. Over half a million elders in the United States are abused or neglected each year **(Table 21-1)**. This problem has become more common as the numbers of the elderly grow and as more elderly people live with and are often cared for by family members. In 90% of cases, the abuser is a family member, usually an adult child or spouse of the victim. Generally, the older a person is, the greater the risk of elder abuse **(Figure 21-3)**. An older adult

Table 21-1: National Estimates of the Incidence of Abuse, Neglect and Self-Neglect of People 60 Years and Older

Type of Maltreatment	Number of Victims
Abuse	402,287
Neglect	182,368
Self-neglect	138,980
Total abuse and neglect	449,924
Total abuse, neglect and self-neglect	551,011

Source: The National Elder Abuse Incidence Study. The Administration on Aging, U.S. Department of Health and Human Services. 1998. http://aoa.gov/AoARoot/AoA_Programs/Elder_Rights/Elder_Abuse/docs/ABuseReport_Full.pdf Accessed March 5, 2011. (This report remains the seminal source of data on elder abuse.)

who needs help with daily activities, who has lost bladder control or who behaves unusually because of altered mental status is more likely to be abused or neglected.

Because older adults are often frail, physical abuse is more likely to result in injury. Physical elder abuse is defined as the willful infliction of physical pain or injury, such as slapping, hitting with an object, shoving, shaking, kicking, burning, sexually molesting, force-feeding, administering of unwanted drugs or restraining the person.

The most important signs of elder maltreatment are:

- Frequent, unexplained crying
- Unexplained fear of or suspicion of particular person(s) in the home

The signs and symptoms of elder abuse are listed in **Box 21-3**.

Care for a Victim of Elder Abuse

If the signs of possible elder abuse are present, consider the possibility that the injury resulted from abuse. Follow the same general guidelines as for a victim of spouse abuse or other domestic violence. All 50 states have specific elder abuse laws. Suspected elder abuse should be reported to your state's adult protective services agency. As with reports of suspected child abuse, the information you report will be kept confidential. The state agency will investigate the case and provide services as needed for the elder and family members.

Sexual Assault and Rape

The following definitions of rape and sexual assault are from the U.S. Department of Justice's annual National Crime Victimization Survey:

Rape is forced sexual intercourse, including both psychological coercion and physical force. Forced sexual intercourse means vaginal, anal or oral penetration by the offender(s). This category includes incidents where the penetration is from a foreign object. This definition includes attempted rapes, male and female victims, and heterosexual and homosexual rape.

Sexual assault includes a wide range of victimizations, distinct from rape or attempted rape. These crimes include completed or attempted attacks generally involving unwanted

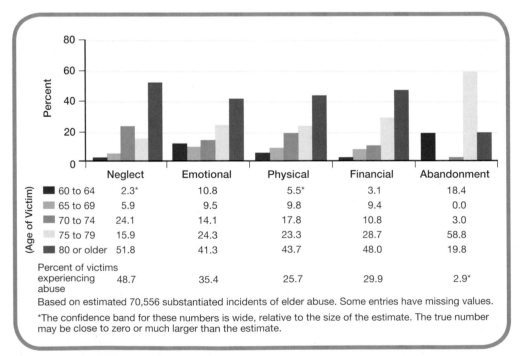

(Age of Victim)	Neglect	Emotional	Physical	Financial	Abandonment
60 to 64	2.3*	10.8	5.5*	3.1	18.4
65 to 69	5.9	9.5	9.8	9.4	0.0
70 to 74	24.1	14.1	17.8	10.8	3.0
75 to 79	15.9	24.3	23.3	28.7	58.8
80 or older	51.8	41.3	43.7	48.0	19.8
Percent of victims experiencing abuse	48.7	35.4	25.7	29.9	2.9*

Based on estimated 70,556 substantiated incidents of elder abuse. Some entries have missing values.

*The confidence band for these numbers is wide, relative to the size of the estimate. The true number may be close to zero or much larger than the estimate.

Figure 21-3 *Ages of elder abuse victims for certain types of maltreatment. (From "The National Elder Abuse Incidence Study," The Administration on Aging, U.S. Department of Health and Human Services, 1998.)*

BOX 21-3: SIGNS AND SYMPTOMS OF ELDER ABUSE AND NEGLECT

Physical Abuse

- Bruises, black eyes, welts, lacerations and rope marks

- Bone or skull fractures

- Open wounds, cuts, punctures, untreated injuries and injuries in various stages of healing

- Strains, dislocations and internal injuries/ bleeding

- Broken eyeglasses, physical signs of being subjected to punishment and signs of being restrained

- Laboratory findings of medication overdose or underutilization of prescribed drugs

- An elder's report of being hit, slapped, kicked or mistreated

- An elder's sudden change in behavior

- A caregiver's refusal to allow visitors to see an elder alone

Sexual Abuse

- Bruises around the breasts or genital area

- Unexplained venereal disease or genital infections

- Unexplained vaginal or anal bleeding

- Torn, stained or bloody underclothing

- An elder's report of being sexually assaulted or raped

Emotional/Psychological Abuse

- Emotional upset or agitation

- Extreme withdrawal, lack of communication and responsiveness

- An elder's report of being verbally or emotionally mistreated

Neglect

- Dehydration, malnutrition, untreated bed-sores and poor personal hygiene

- Unattended or untreated health problems

- Hazardous or unsafe living conditions (e.g., improper wiring, no heat or no running water)

- Unsanitary or unclean living conditions (e.g., dirt, fleas, lice on person, soiled bedding, fecal/urine smell, inadequate clothing)

- An elder's report of being neglected

Abandonment

- The desertion of an elder at a hospital, nursing facility or other similar institution

- The desertion of an elder at a shopping center or other public location

- An elder's own report of being abandoned

Self-Neglect

- Dehydration, malnutrition, untreated or improperly attended medical conditions and poor personal hygiene

- Hazardous or unsafe living conditions (e.g., improper wiring, no indoor plumbing, no heat or no running water)

- Unsanitary or unclean living quarters (e.g., animal/insect infestation, no functioning toilet, fecal/urine smell)

- Inappropriate and/or inadequate clothing, lack of necessary medical aids (e.g., eyeglasses, hearing aid, dentures)

- Grossly inadequate housing or homelessness

Source: "The National Elder Abuse Incidence Study," The Administration on Aging, U.S. Department of Health and Human Services, 1998. http://aoa.gov/AoARoot/AoA_Programs/Elder_Rights/Elder_Abuse/docs/ABuseReport_Full.pdf Accessed March 5, 2011.

21 • Behavioral Emergencies

sexual contact between the victim and offender. Sexual assaults may or may not involve force and can include such acts as grabbing or fondling. Sexual assault also includes verbal threats.

Rape and sexual assault are serious problems in our society:[7]

- 1 out of every 6 American women has been the victim of an attempted or completed rape in her lifetime (14.8% completed rape; 2.8% attempted rape).

- 17.7 million American women have been victims of attempted or completed rape.

- 2.78 million men in the U.S. have been victims of sexual assault or rape.

- 9 of every 10 rape victims were female in 2003.

- 15% of sexual assault and rape victims are younger than 12. 80% are younger than 30. 12-34 are the highest risk years.

- Victims of sexual assault are:

  - 3 times more likely to suffer from depression.

  - 6 times more likely to suffer from post-traumatic stress disorder.

  - 13 times more likely to abuse alcohol.

  - 26 times more likely to abuse drugs.

  - 4 times more likely to contemplate suicide.

Prevention of Rape and Sexual Assault

To reduce the risk of rape and sexual assault, the Rape, Abuse, & Incest National Network (RAINN) recommends these precautions:

- In a social setting, do not leave your beverage unattended or accept a drink from an open container because the drink may be drugged.

- When you go to a party, go with a group of friends. Arrive together, watch out for each other and leave together.

- Be aware of your surroundings at all times.

- Don't allow yourself to be isolated with someone you do not know or trust.

- Think about the level of intimacy you want in a relationship and clearly state your limits.

Care for a Victim of Rape or Sexual Assault

1. Be sensitive to the victim's psychological trauma. After a rape the victim may be hysterical, crying, hyperventilating or in a dazed, unresponsive state. Provide emotional support as appropriate.

2. Ensure that 9-1-1 has been called. Rape requires a coordinated response of law enforcement and EMS personnel.

3. Ensure privacy for the victim.

4. Try to involve a friend or family member of the victim in your caregiving. A first aider of the same sex may be more comforting.

5. Provide first aid as needed for any injury. Someone should stay with the victim until help arrives.

6. For legal reasons, it is important to preserve evidence of a rape. Ask the victim not to urinate, bathe or wash any area involved in the rape or assault before EMS personnel arrive. Follow-up care of rape victims usually includes a full physical examination as well as possible later testing for sexually transmitted diseases and pregnancy.

Because rape can lead to later traumatic stress and psychological problems, victims may benefit from counseling provided by rape crisis centers and support groups. To find a center in your area, call the National Sexual Assault Hotline at 800-656-HOPE or visit the RAINN website: www.rainn.org.

[7]*Rape, Abuse, & Incest National Network (RAINN) http://www.rainn.org/get-information/statistics/sexual-assault-victims Accessed March 5, 2011.*

Learning Checkpoint 2

1. If you suspect a child is being abused by a parent, the most important thing to do is –
   a. talk to the parent so he or she can get help.
   b. remove the child from the home.
   c. report the situation to authorities.
   d. talk to the spouse of the abusing parent and let him or her decide what to do.

2. Check off common characteristics of victims of domestic violence.
   _____ They love their partners.
   _____ They are not afraid of their partners.
   _____ They feel guilty and may blame themselves for the violence.
   _____ They often have low self-esteem.
   _____ They feel close to family and friends.
   _____ They depend emotionally and/or financially on their partners.

3. Elder abuse includes –
   a. sexual abuse.
   b. abandonment.
   c. neglect.
   d. All of the above

4. List six important first aid actions for a victim injured during a rape.

   _____

   _____

Concluding Thoughts

Behavioral emergencies and abuse situations are generally stressful for first aiders because of the unpredictable behavior and difficult emotions of those involved. Remember that in most cases these situations last only a few minutes before EMS professionals, or sometimes law enforcement personnel, arrive and take over. These professionals have the training to manage the situation safely and appropriately. For the few minutes you may be with a victim, be sensitive to the situation and alert for your own safety. In almost all cases you can use common sense and the general guidelines in this chapter to avoid any confrontation while providing first aid.

Learning Outcomes

You should now be able to do the following:

1. Describe common emotional and behavioral responses to injury and illness.

2. Explain how to reassure and calm an emotional victim.

3. Describe how to interact with a victim who is experiencing anxiety or depression.

4. List actions to take when dealing with a suicidal or potentially violent victim.

5. Describe appropriate care for victims of child abuse, spousal abuse, elder abuse, and sexual assault and rape.

Review Questions

1. Normal physical signs and symptoms of injury-related stress include –

   a. dry skin.

   b. nausea.

   c. slow breathing.

   d. drowsiness.

2. Altered mental status may result from any injury that causes –

   a. reduced oxygen levels.

   b. increased oxygen levels.

   c. faster heartbeat.

   d. fluid loss.

3. Why is it important to calm and reassure an emotional victim?

   a. Emotional stress has negative physical effects on the body.

   b. It is difficult to give first aid to an emotional, uncooperative victim.

   c. Calming may help prevent a victim from becoming violent.

   d. All of the above

4. True or False: Making eye contact with a victim who is irrational, delusional or potentially violent will likely upset the person and make the situation worse.

5. You should try to reassure an injured victim who is depressed by saying things such as, –

   a. "Don't worry, everything will be just fine."

   b. "Don't cry. Let's talk about more positive things in your life."

   c. "There are programs available to help you deal with problems like this."

   d. "I'm sure this problem won't last long."

6. Call 9-1-1 for –

   a. a potentially violent victim of any kind of injury.

   b. someone talking about suicide who has a bottle of pills.

   c. an injured person who is shouting at a hallucination.

   d. All of the above

7. A parent who abuses his or her child, when confronted with an accusation, is most likely to –

   a. deny the problem.

   b. admit the problem and feel relief that now he or she will get treatment.

   c. become violent and attack the accuser.

   d. blame his or her spouse for the problem.

8. Which of these statements is true?

    a. Authorities want proof of child abuse before they will take your report.

    b. A reasonable suspicion of child abuse is sufficient grounds to report to the authorities.

    c. After you report suspected child abuse, the authorities will ask you to help them "trap" the abuser to get a confession.

    d. You may be sued for making a report if your accusation turns out to be false.

9. Suspected cases of child abuse or domestic violence should be reported only by –

    a. people who have cause to suspect abuse or violence.

    b. people whose jobs require it.

    c. the victims.

    d. family members of the victims.

10. Preserving evidence of a rape includes –

    a. asking the victim not to wash until examined by a health care provider.

    b. asking the victim to avoid talking until examined by a health care provider.

    c. not allowing the victim to move at all from the position in which he or she was found.

    d. not touching the victim when giving first aid for any injuries.

Chapter 22 • Pregnancy and Childbirth

Chapter Preview

- **Prevention of Problems in Pregnancy**
- **Pregnancy and Labor**
- **First Aid in Pregnancy**
- **Childbirth**

Melanie is almost 9 months pregnant with her first baby but still a week away from her due date. You have just trimmed her hair and are blowing it dry when she suddenly gets a funny look on her face and says, "Oh, no!" Then she tells you, "My water just broke." What do you do?

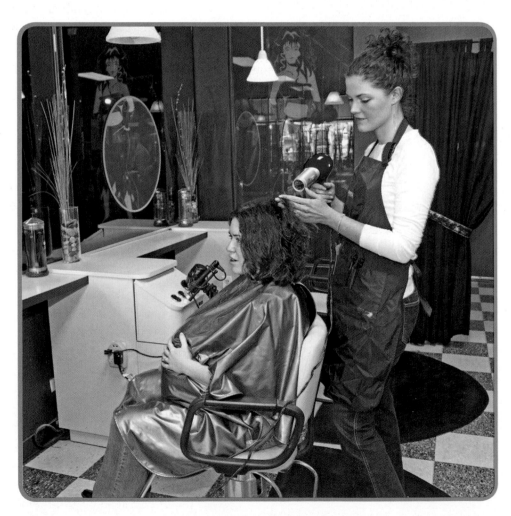

Although rare, certain health problems may occur during pregnancy that require first aid. In addition, childbirth sometimes occurs outside a planned setting. Because no one can predict in every case when labor will begin or how long it will last before the infant is delivered, a pregnant woman may find herself unable to reach the planned setting for childbirth and unattended by a doctor, midwife or other person trained in childbirth. In such a situation a first aider may be called upon to assist. This is very rarely a medical emergency because childbirth is a normal, natural process that usually takes place without problems or complications – and with only minimal assistance from others.

Prevention of Problems in Pregnancy

Preventing problems in pregnancy and maintaining good health for both the woman and the fetus begins with regular **prenatal** (before birth) care. Health care practitioners generally recommend that a woman see her health care provider as soon as she knows or suspects that she is pregnant.

The health care provider thereafter will schedule a series of regular visits to ensure the pregnancy is progressing well and to treat any complications that may arise.

Following are general guidelines many health care practitioners will recommend for pregnant women. *With any guideline, however, always follow the health care provider's specific instructions because all guidelines do not automatically apply to all pregnant women.*

- **Eat a healthy diet throughout pregnancy**. Good nutrition is important for both the woman and the developing fetus. A higher-than-usual caloric intake is usually advised, along with specific recommendations for balanced nutrition and daily supplements. Most pregnant women are advised to take folic acid (vitamin B) and iron supplements and to ensure that their diet contains sufficient calcium, protein, carbohydrates, fluids and other vitamins as well as moderate salt.

- **Accept normal weight gain**. Pregnant women should follow their health care provider's recommendations, but generally a woman of normal prepregnancy weight should gain 25 to 35 pounds gradually during pregnancy. Attempts to diet or exercise too much in an attempt to prevent weight gain are generally unhealthy for the fetus.

- **Minimize caffeine from coffee, tea and soft drinks**. Although studies do not clearly show exactly how much caffeine is safe, it has been demonstrated that high levels of caffeine are associated with higher rates of **miscarriage** and can cause other problems for the fetus.

- **Avoid alcohol entirely**. Even very small amounts of alcohol have been shown to affect fetal growth and higher levels can cause **fetal alcohol syndrome**, which causes growth deficiencies, mental retardation and other problems.

- **Stop smoking**. Cigarette smoking in pregnancy has been associated with lowered birth weight and preterm delivery.

- **Do not use illicit drugs**. Some studies suggest that marijuana use in pregnancy may have harmful effects on the fetus and drugs such as crack cocaine are known to have serious detrimental effects.

- **Get exercise**. The American College of Obstetricians and Gynecologists generally recommends 30 minutes of moderate exercise a day for most healthy pregnant women. The health care provider can recommend the most effective and safest types of exercise.

- **Get enough rest**. Sufficient sleep is important during pregnancy, as are frequent rest breaks during the day. The health care practitioner may also recommend avoidance of certain kinds of activities.

- **Prevent injury**. Avoid situations that may lead to falls, such as climbing a ladder or standing on a chair to reach a high shelf. Get help when needed, such as when getting out of a bathtub during the last weeks of pregnancy. Avoid risky sports and recreational activities.

Pregnancy and Labor

Pregnancy begins with fertilization of the woman's ovum or egg cell, by a sperm cell, in the process often called conception. Growth and development proceed in an orderly manner for about 40 weeks, when childbirth typically occurs. The pregnancy is usually considered in three stages, followed by labor and delivery.

Stages of Pregnancy

Pregnancy is often divided into three trimesters of roughly three months each. Within the first few days, the single cell that results from fertilization divides into a mass of many cells. After it implants in the uterus at five to seven days, and thereafter for the first eight weeks, the developing human is called an **embryo**; thereafter it is called a **fetus**. The embryo develops inside the **amniotic sac**, which contains **amniotic fluid** (often called "water"). The embryo is attached to the woman's **placenta**, an organ that develops in pregnancy to supply the embryo and fetus with oxygen and nutrients, via the **umbilical cord (Figure 22-1)**. By eight weeks the embryo has developed all major organ systems. Through the rest of the pregnancy it continues to grow and develop to the point where the infant can live independently outside the mother's body.

During the first trimester, although the fetus has recognizable human features and is about 2½ inches long, the pregnant woman experiences few visible changes. Her heart rate has increased by about eight beats per minute and she may experience some normal results of hormonal changes in her body, such as nausea (**morning sickness**) and breast tenderness.

During the second trimester, weeks 13 to 28, the fetus grows to a length of 12 inches. At about 18 to 20 weeks the woman may feel it moving. The woman's abdomen gradually swells, and she may experience discharge from the nipples caused by changes in the milk-producing glands.

In the third trimester (weeks 29 to 40), the fetus grows rapidly. By week 36 it is fully formed, weighs about 6½ pounds and can live outside the mother without advanced medical intervention. The head of the fetus is positioned downward in the woman's pelvis. The woman's uterus has expanded high into the abdomen and presses on the lungs, possibly causing a slight shortness of breath. The pregnant woman may also experience backache, heartburn, constipation and frequent urination.

Stages of Labor and Delivery

Labor and delivery occur in three stages, beginning with the first uterine contractions. Up to 10 days before the beginning of contractions, the mucus plug from the cervix, which had blocked the uterus from possible infection from the vagina, is released; this is sometimes called "the show" or "bloody show" but often goes unnoticed. Uterine contractions begin and eventually push the infant's head into the **cervix**, which is dilating (opening). The cervix is the lower part of the uterus opening into the vagina. Contractions gradually become stronger and more frequent. The amniotic sac ruptures either shortly before or during the first stage of labor, causing the fluid to either rush or trickle out the vaginal opening; this is often called the "water breaking." The first stage may last from a few hours to a day in a woman who has not

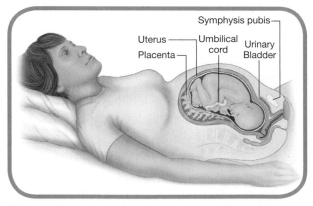

Figure 22-1 *The fetus at 8 months.*

given birth before, but sometimes occurs in only a few minutes in a woman who has given birth before. Contractions at first are usually 10 to 15 minutes apart, and shortly before childbirth they may be only 2 to 3 minutes apart.

In the second stage the infant is delivered. This stage typically lasts one to two hours but may happen more quickly in women who have given birth previously. The cervix has fully dilated and contractions are powerful and often painful. The infant's head presses on the floor of the pelvis and the woman feels a strong urge to push down. The vagina, or birth canal, stretches open as the infant's head moves out of the uterus and the top of the infant's head can now be seen; this is called **crowning (Figure 22-2)**. The vagina stretches more as the head emerges, often quickly, and the rest of the infant's body is typically pushed out very quickly **(Figure 22-3)**. The person assisting with the delivery supports the infant's head as it emerges and ensures that the umbilical cord is not wrapped around the infant's neck.

In the third stage, the placenta separates from the uterus and is delivered, usually within 30 minutes after childbirth. The uterus then contracts and seals off bleeding vessels.

First Aid in Pregnancy

Most pregnant women receive regular care and are advised by their health care providers about potential problems to watch for. Although rare, problems may occur that require emergency care and possibly first aid before the woman receives medical attention.

Vaginal Bleeding

Vaginal bleeding during pregnancy is abnormal. Bleeding may be caused by cervical growths or erosion, by a problem with the placenta or by miscarriage. In the third trimester, vaginal bleeding may be a sign of potential preterm birth. The woman should see her health care provider immediately. Call 9-1-1 for heavy bleeding. While waiting for help, calm the woman and help her into a comfortable position. Have a female assistant present if possible. Give the woman a towel or sanitary napkins to absorb the blood, but do not try to pack the vagina. Save the blood and any expelled material to give to arriving EMS personnel.

Miscarriage

Miscarriage, also called spontaneous abortion, is loss of the embryo or fetus, usually during the first 14 weeks of pregnancy. An estimated 10% to 25%

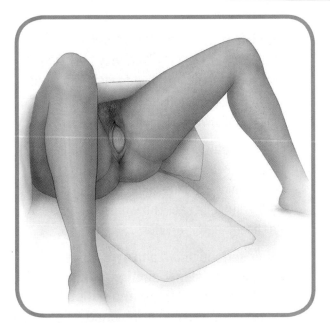

Figure 22-2 *Crowning: the infant's head begins to show.*

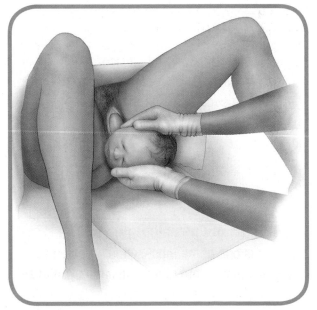

Figure 22-3 *The infant moves through the birth canal.*

Learning Checkpoint 1

1. Put a check mark before the accepted guidelines for a healthy pregnancy:

_____ Walk at least a mile a day.

_____ Minimize caffeine and alcohol consumption.

_____ Exercise to prevent weight gain.

_____ Eliminate salt from the diet.

_____ Take dietary supplements as recommended.

_____ Adopt a low-carbohydrate diet.

2. The first stage of labor begins with –

a. crowning.

b. uterine contractions.

c. cervical dilation.

d. rupture of the amniotic sac.

3. Shortly before birth occurs, contractions usually occur –

a. every 30 seconds.

b. every 2 to 3 minutes.

c. every 5 to 10 minutes.

d. between 1 to 10 minutes.

of all pregnancies end in miscarriage,[1] which is a natural way that the body manages a potential problem in the pregnancy. It may result from a genetic disorder or fetal abnormality, some factor related to the woman's health or to no known cause. Smoking and the use of alcohol or drugs are also risk factors. Most women who have a miscarriage do not have problems with later pregnancies.

The early signs of a possible miscarriage are vaginal bleeding and abdominal pain or cramping. The woman needs immediate medical attention. Give first aid for bleeding and call 9-1-1 if the bleeding is heavy. Take steps to minimize shock if bleeding is heavy (see **Chapter 9**). Because the possibility of miscarriage is usually very distressing, be calm and reassuring.

Other Signs of Possible Problems

Bleeding is one of the most serious problems during pregnancy, but other signs and symptoms may also indicate a problem. The woman should see her health care provider if she experiences any of the following:

- **Abdominal pain** which may result from miscarriage or a problem with the placenta. The woman should rest until she receives medical advice.

- **Persistent or severe headache**, especially in the last trimester, which may be a sign of a serious condition called toxemia. Toxemia may also cause unusual weight gain, blurred vision, and swollen fingers or face.

- **Sudden leaking of water from the vagina**, unless the woman is close to the time of labor, which may indicate premature rupture of the amniotic sac. The woman should see her health care provider.

- **Other serious signs and symptoms include persistent vomiting, chills and fever, convulsions, and difficulty breathing**. All should be reported immediately to a health care provider.

[1]*American Pregnancy Association, http://www. americanpregnancy.org/pregnancycomplications/ miscarriage.html Accessed March 1, 2011.*

Learning Checkpoint 2

1. Describe first aid to give a pregnant woman who has heavy vaginal bleeding.

   _____

2. The early signs of a possible miscarriage include –

   a. vaginal bleeding.

   b. high fever.

   c. altered mental status.

   d. All of the above

3. Check off the signs and symptoms that may indicate a possible problem during pregnancy:

   ____ Abdominal pain   ____ Persistent headache

   ____ Chills and fever   ____ Convulsions

   ____ Difficulty breathing   ____ Water leaking from vagina in 20th week

Choking Care for a Pregnant Woman

Do not use abdominal thrusts on a responsive pregnant woman who is choking. Instead give chest thrusts as described in **Chapter 7**.

Childbirth

In our society, childbirth has occurred predominantly in hospitals for so long that people may assume it is so difficult or dangerous that hospitals are needed. In reality, childbirth is a natural process that seldom involves complications or requires elaborate medical care. It is true that some complications are possible and that medical steps are then necessary for the health of the mother or infant. But if a woman is unable to reach medical care when contractions suggest childbirth may be imminent, this should not be a cause for panic. *The childbirth itself is not an emergency*. Nonetheless, a pregnant woman who realizes she may have her baby before reaching her planned location, and perhaps without health care providers present, is likely to be fearful and distressed. If you are helping the woman and realize that it may be you who helps deliver the infant, you are likely to experience similar emotions. Coping with these stresses may be more difficult than assisting with the childbirth itself.

Remember that once you have called 9-1-1, help is usually only minutes away. It is very unlikely that a woman close to childbirth will actually give birth before advanced care personnel arrive. Remember also that even if help is delayed or her labor advances very quickly to childbirth, in the great majority of cases there are no complications and you will be able to assist her through this process for the short time needed. It is crucial that you remain calm in order to reassure and assist the woman. Although you may be concerned about doing something wrong, try to relax and focus on the woman's need for your calm guidance to help manage her fears and the pain of labor.

Is Delivery Imminent?

Depending on how the woman's labor is progressing and the time before EMS personnel are expected to arrive, you may be assisting the woman only with labor or also with delivery. An important initial step in first aid, therefore, is assessing whether delivery may occur soon.

Remember that labor usually lasts for several hours, allowing plenty of time for the woman to be transported to the hospital or other planned childbirth location, or for other assistance to arrive. In rare cases, however, labor may proceed very quickly or transportation may be delayed. Even an expert cannot predict exactly when childbirth will occur, but the following assessments can help determine whether delivery may be imminent. If so, do not try to transport the woman; instead, prepare for childbirth.

- **Assess the contractions**. How close together are they and how long does each last? When timing contractions, time from the beginning of one contraction to the beginning of the next contraction, not the time between them. Contractions generally become stronger, last longer and come more frequently as labor progresses. If contractions are less than 5 minutes apart and each lasts 45 to 60 seconds, delivery may occur soon and you should be making preparations. When contractions are about 2 minutes apart, delivery will likely occur soon.

- **Ask the woman if she has given birth before**. First childbirths usually take longer than later ones. If she has given birth in the past, labor is likely to proceed more quickly this time. Also ask if she knows whether she may be having twins or triplets – most women have learned this during their prenatal care.

- **Check whether the amniotic sac has ruptured**. Ask the woman if her water has broken. Because this often occurs hours before delivery, however, it is not a reliable sign that childbirth is imminent.

- **Ask whether the woman feels a strong urge to push**. This may mean delivery is approaching. Similarly, a feeling that she needs to have a bowel movement may indicate the infant's head has moved to a position close to delivery.

- **If other signs are suggestive of delivery, check whether the infant's head is crowning**. If possible, ask another woman present to check this. Once the top of the head is visible through the vaginal opening during a contraction, be prepared for delivery very soon. At this point you should not be preparing the woman for transport.

Note that labor may begin potentially many weeks before the woman is due, resulting in a premature birth. Because a premature infant is more likely to need medical care after birth, it is important to recognize the first signs of labor at any point in the pregnancy and take appropriate action.

Assisting During Labor

If labor has begun but delivery is not imminent, give supportive care to the expectant mother. Follow these guidelines:

- Ensure that a plan is in place for the woman's transport to the planned childbirth location or for the arrival of the planned attendant.

- Help the woman to rest in whatever position is most comfortable for her.

- Provide any desired comfort measures, such as massaging the lower back (which may help reduce pain). Although the woman should not eat or drink, she may suck on small ice chips or have her lips moistened if her mouth is dry.

- Do not let the woman have a bath if the amniotic sac has ruptured, because of the risk of infection.

- Time the length of contractions and the interval between them and write down this information.

- Help remind the woman to control her breathing: short, quick breaths (panting) during contractions and deep, slow breaths between.

- Continue to help the woman to stay calm and provide reassurance. Anxiety and fear will only add to her pain. Regular, deep breathing in through the nose and out through the mouth may help her to relax. (Using the same technique yourself, in synch along with the woman, may help you to relax, too. If you are tense and nervous, this will make the woman more fearful.)

Assisting with Delivery

If signs are present that delivery may be imminent, prepare to assist with the delivery. Remember that childbirth is a natural process that will occur essentially by itself. Your role is simply to prepare the environment to maintain cleanliness for the mother and child, and to support both of them during and after the birth.

Preparations

Ensure that someone stays with the woman while preparations are being made. If you do not have a sterile delivery kit, you can gather household items to prepare. If possible, another woman should be present, preferably a friend or family member.

First, gather the items needed or helpful for the delivery:

- A clean blanket or coverlet

- Several pillows

- A plastic sheet (or shower curtain) or a stack of newspapers

- Clean towels and washcloths

- Sanitary napkins or pads made of clean, folded cloth

- Medical examination gloves (use clean kitchen gloves or plastic bags on your hands if gloves are unavailable)

- Plastic bags (for afterbirth and cleanup)

- Bowl of hot water (for washing)

- Empty bowl or bucket (in case of vomiting)

- Clean handkerchief (to wear as face mask)

- Eye and face protection for yourself, if available.

- Oxygen, if it is available and you have appropriate training (see **Appendix A**).

- Clean, soft towel, sheet or blanket (to wrap the newborn)

- Bulb syringe, if available (to suction infant's nose and mouth), or sterile gauze

- If help may be delayed: clean, strong string, shoelaces or cloth strips to tie the cord

- If help may be delayed: sharp scissors or knife sterilized in boiling water for 5 minutes or held over a flame for 30 seconds, to cut the cord. Prepare the birthing bed with clean sheets over a rubber or plastic sheet (or shower curtain or thicknesses of newspaper) to protect the mattress. If a bed is not present, prepare a clean place on the floor or ground, making a padded area of newspapers, clothes or blankets. Roll up your sleeves, wash your hands thoroughly for 5 minutes and put on medical examination gloves. If possible, protect your eyes, mouth and nose from likely splashes of blood and other fluids; a handkerchief can be tied over your mouth and nose.

When childbirth seems imminent, follow the steps listed in the First Aid: "Assisting with Delivery." If a telephone is available at the scene, have someone call the woman's health care provider or 9-1-1 so additional instructions can be given over the phone during or after the childbirth, if necessary.

Care of the Mother After Delivery

After the delivery, continue to support and comfort the mother. Ensure that she is warm and comfortable. She may drink water now and may find it comforting to have her face wiped with cool water. Even with a successful delivery, she and the infant should still see a health care provider because problems sometimes occur within the first 24 hours.

Care of the Newborn

Once you have determined that the newborn is breathing well, little specific care is needed. A normal newborn respiratory rate is 40 breaths per minute or more. Dry but do not try to wash the newborn, whose skin may be covered with a white, cheesy, protective coating called vernix. Ensure that the infant stays wrapped, including the head, to stay warm. Support the newborn's head if it must be moved for any reason. Continue to check the newborn's breathing.

(continues on page 364)

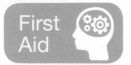

First Aid — Assisting with Delivery
Signs, Symptoms and Care

When You See

- Contractions occurring 2 to 3 minutes apart
- The woman feels a strong urge to push.
- Crowning of the infant's head

Do This First

1 Help the woman to lie on her back with knees bent and apart and feet flat on the bed. Note that she may have been trained already in other birthing positions, which are acceptable. Ensure that she is not wearing undergarments or other clothing that may get in the way. If she prefers, cover her above the knees with a blanket or sheet. Have folded towels or a blanket under her buttocks.

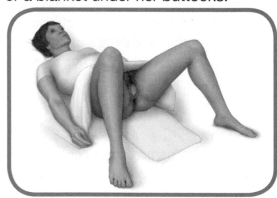

2 As the infant's head appears, have your gloved hands ready to receive and support the head, which may emerge very quickly. Check that the head is not covered by the amniotic sac; if so, pull it away as the mouth and nose emerge.

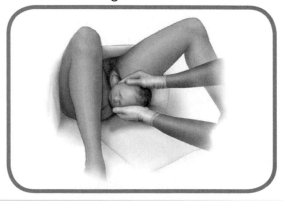

3 As the head emerges (usually face-down), support the head. Check that the umbilical cord is not wrapped around the infant's neck; if it is, see if it is loose enough to slip over the head or shoulder to prevent strangulation, but avoid putting pressure on the cord or pulling it. Use a bulb syringe to gently suck secretions from the mouth and nose, or wipe both with sterile gauze. Compress the bulb syringe before insertion.

4 After the head is out, have the woman stop pushing and breathe in a panting manner. Do not attempt to pull the infant out, but support it as its body emerges, often very quickly after the head. Usually the infant turns to the side as the shoulder emerges. Newborns are usually very slippery and should be handled carefully. Grasp the infant's feet as they emerge. If the mother is having multiple births, prepare for the delivery of the second infant. Note the time of delivery to tell medical personnel later.

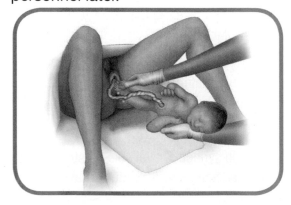

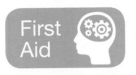
5 The newborn normally begins to cry. Hold it at the level of the woman's vagina, with head lower than the feet to allow secretions to drain from the nose and mouth. Use a bulb syringe to gently suck secretions from the mouth and then the nose, or wipe both with sterile gauze. If the infant is not crying, gently flick the bottom of its feet with a finger or gently rub its back. If he or she is still not crying, check for breathing and start CPR if needed (see **Chapter 5**).

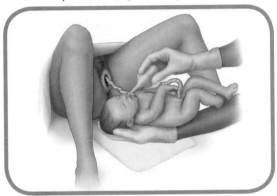

6 Gently dry and wrap the infant in a towel or blanket to prevent heat loss, keeping the cord loose. Place the infant on its side with its head low for the nose and mouth to drain. Place the infant on the mother's abdomen only after the umbilical cord has been clamped or tied.

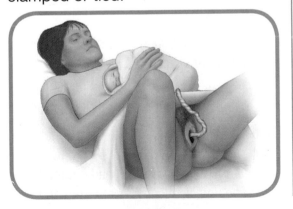

7 Stay with the mother and infant while waiting for the delivery of the afterbirth, the placenta and umbilical cord, which usually occurs with milder contractions in 10 to 30 minutes. Typically there will be a gush of blood as the placenta detaches from the uterus. Save the placenta in a plastic bag or towel because it is important for health care providers to examine it.

8 In most situations it is not necessary to tie or cut the umbilical cord, even after the placenta has been delivered, because medical help will be arriving very soon. Keep the placenta at the same level as the infant while waiting for help to arrive. If help may be delayed in a remote location, tie and cut the cord before delivery of the afterbirth. Wait until the cord stops pulsating. Then tie a tight knot around the cord about 10 inches from the infant, using string, clean shoelaces or thin strips of cloth. Tie a second knot about 7 inches from the infant, and cut the cord between the two ties with sterilized scissors or knife.

(continued)

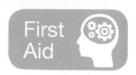

First Aid — Assisting with Delivery (continued)

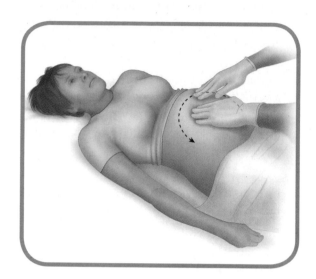

Additional Care

- The mother may continue to bleed for a time, normally up to a pint following delivery. Place sanitary napkins or folded clean cloths against the vaginal opening but do not push. Gently massage the mother's abdomen with a circular motion just below the navel to help the uterus contract to stop the bleeding.

- Ensure that the infant stays warm and continues to breathe. Skin-to-skin contact between mother and infant helps the infant to stay warm. The mother can begin nursing the infant immediately, which will help the uterus to contract and stop bleeding.

ALERT

- Do not try to delay the birth by having the woman hold her legs together or any other maneuver.
- Do not place your hands or anything else in the woman's vagina.
- Do not interfere with the childbirth or touch the infant until the head is completely out.
- Do not pull on the head or shoulders.
- Do not try to wash the infant's skin, eyes or ears.
- Do not pull on the umbilical cord in an effort to pull out the afterbirth.

(continued from page 361)

A very small or premature infant born a significant time before the mother's due date is at greater risk for complications after birth. It is crucial to keep a small newborn warm. There is also a greater likelihood that resuscitation may be needed.

Childbirth Problems

Most deliveries occur without problems or complications, but you should be prepared to manage a problem if one does occur. The most common problems involve the **presentation** of the infant (its position at emergence) or maternal bleeding after delivery.

Breech Birth

A **breech presentation** occurs when the infant's buttocks or feet appear in the birth canal rather than the head **(Figure 22-4)**. This can become an emergency because as the head enters the birth canal, the umbilical cord is squeezed and blood flow may stop. Also, if the infant's head becomes lodged in the birth canal and the infant tries to breathe, it may suffocate because the face is pressed against the vaginal wall. Medical attention may be urgently needed.

When you first see a breech presentation, move the woman to a kneeling position with her head and chest down **(Figure 22-5)**. This helps to minimize pressure on the cord and is generally the preferred childbirth position in this situation. Support the infant's body as it emerges, but do not try to pull the head out, which may cause injury and will not speed up the birth. If the head does not emerge soon after the body, you may need to open a breathing space for the infant. Carefully insert one hand alongside the infant's head, palm against the face and make a V with two fingers positioned on each side of the infant's nose. Press against the birth canal to allow air to reach the infant's nose while waiting for the head to be delivered. Check the infant immediately and be prepared to give CPR if needed.

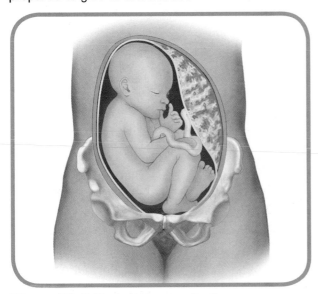

Figure 22-4 *Breech presentation.*

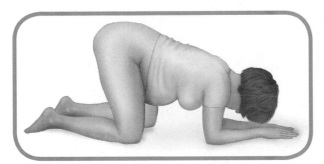

Figure 22-5 *Position for breech presentation.*

Limb Presentation

Very rarely one arm or leg may emerge first from the birth canal. This is an emergency requiring immediate medical assistance. Position the woman in the same knee-chest position as for a breech birth while waiting for help. Do not try to pull the infant out or push the arm or leg back inside the woman.

Prolapsed Cord

The umbilical cord is said to be **prolapsed** when a segment of it protrudes through the birth canal before childbirth **(Figure 22-6)**. This is an emergency because the cord will be compressed as the infant begins to move through the birth canal, cutting off blood flow. Position the woman in the knee-chest position to reduce pressure on the cord. Do not try to push the cord back inside the mother. If medical personnel have not arrived when the infant presents and begins to emerge, carefully insert your hand into the birth canal and try to separate the cord and presenting body part while allowing the birth to continue. Check the infant immediately and be prepared to give CPR if needed.

Cord Around Neck

If the umbilical cord is wrapped around the infant's neck when the head emerges, you can slip it over the head or shoulder to allow the infant to emerge

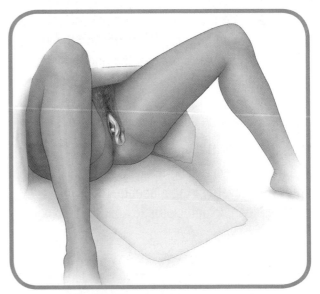

Figure 22-6 *Prolapsed cord.*

Learning Checkpoint 3

1. True or False: Childbirth is a difficult process that frequently involves complications and the need for medical treatment.

2. Put a check mark next to signs and symptoms that childbirth may occur soon:

   _____ Contractions every 10 minutes   _____ Woman feels urge to push

   _____ Amniotic sac has ruptured   _____ Infant's head is crowning

   _____ Cervix is starting to dilate   _____ Contractions are painful

3. Assisting a woman with childbirth may include –

   a. helping position the woman.

   b. supporting the infant as it emerges from the birth canal.

   c. helping secretions drain from the infant's nose and mouth.

   d. All of the above

4. List at least three things you should not do when assisting with childbirth.

   _____

5. When the umbilical cord can be seen protruding from the birth canal before childbirth occurs, what should you do?

   a. Cut the cord and wait for childbirth.

   b. Push the cord back inside the mother.

   c. Position the mother to reduce pressure on the cord.

   d. Pull on the cord to speed up the birth.

6. True or False: Some bleeding normally occurs with childbirth and delivery of the placenta.

without strangling on the cord. Rarely, it may be wrapped so tight that you cannot release the infant's head and the cord is strangling the infant and preventing emergence of the body. This is a life-threatening emergency. If medical personnel are not present, you must tie off the cord in two places and cut the cord between the two.

Bleeding After Delivery

It is normal for bleeding to occur with childbirth and with delivery of the placenta. Use sanitary pads or clean, folded cloths to absorb the blood.

Bleeding usually stops soon after the placenta is delivered. As described earlier, massage the mother's abdomen below the level of the navel, where you should feel the uterus as a mass about the size of a softball. Massage with your palms using a kneading motion. Continue massaging gently until bleeding stops.

Bleeding that persists can become an emergency. Keep the mother still and try to calm her while waiting for help to arrive. Give first aid to treat shock (see **Chapter 9**).

Concluding Thoughts

Although problems sometimes do occur during childbirth, and in such cases it is important to know what to do, remember that the overwhelming majority of births occur naturally and without problems, even when outside health care settings. Countless numbers of healthy infants have been born in taxis caught in traffic en route to hospitals and other similar places. Should you ever find yourself in such a situation, stay calm and remember the simple basics of supporting the mother and newborn through this natural process.

Learning Outcomes

You should now be able to do the following:

1. List healthy behaviors during pregnancy to prevent problems for the woman and fetus.

2. Describe the stages of pregnancy and the stages of labor and delivery.

3. Explain the first aid for vaginal bleeding during pregnancy and for possible miscarriage.

4. Describe how to assist during childbirth and care for the mother and newborn after the birth.

5. Explain actions to take in case of complications: breech presentation, prolapsed cord, the cord wrapped around the infant's head and bleeding after delivery.

Review Questions

1. During pregnancy a woman should avoid or minimize the consumption of –

    a. unsaturated fats.

    b. alcohol.

    c. artificial sweeteners.

    d. beta carotene.

2. Which sign or symptom is abnormal during pregnancy?

    a. Backache

    b. Vaginal bleeding

    c. Heartburn

    d. More frequent urination

3. When the amniotic sac ruptures after contractions begin, which of these statements is true?

    a. Childbirth may occur soon.

    b. The infant must be delivered immediately before suffocation occurs.

    c. The infant's lungs are likely to become infected if childbirth does not occur soon.

    d. The mother needs care to prevent dehydration.

4. Crowning occurs –

    a. in breech presentations.

    b. when the cord is prolapsed.

    c. when the woman pushes too hard before the delivery begins.

    d. in all normal head-first births.

5. First aid for a pregnant woman with vaginal bleeding includes –

    a. massaging the abdomen with a kneading motion.

    b. packing the vagina with a pad made from sterile dressings.

    c. absorbing the blood with a towel or sanitary napkin.

    d. controlling the bleeding with direct pressure on the abdomen.

6. A pregnant woman should see her health care provider for which of these signs and symptoms?

    a. Severe headache

    b. Difficulty breathing

    c. Abdominal pain

    d. All of the above

7. Choking care for a pregnant woman includes –

    a. abdominal thrusts.

    b. chest thrusts.

    c. back blows.

    d. abdominal thrusts and back blows.

8. During labor you can support the woman by –

    a. urging her to push with each contraction.

    b. massaging her uterus.

    c. helping her to control her breathing.

    d. holding an ice pack against her abdomen.

9. If the newborn is not crying or breathing after birth –

    a. start care for an airway obstruction.

    b. blow air into his or her mouth using the bulb syringe.

    c. flick the bottom of his or her feet with your finger.

    d. give back blows.

10. Care of the newborn includes –

    a. supporting the head when holding or moving the newborn.

    b. keeping the newborn warm.

    c. monitoring the newborn's breathing.

    d. All of the above

Chapter 23 • Remote Location First Aid

Chapter Preview

- Remote Locations
- Situations When Help May Be Delayed
- General Principles When Help Is Delayed

- Special Care for Emergencies When Help Is Delayed
- Special Wilderness Emergencies

You are on a hike with several friends and family members. About 5 miles along the trail you stop for lunch beside a river, where a friend's daughter is climbing on rocks at the water's edge. Her foot slips on a mossy patch, and she falls and strikes her head on a rock. Immediately an adult in the party helps her away from the water. Her head did not go under water, but she has a welt on her forehead and she seems groggy and mildly confused. A few minutes later she seems better, although she has a slight headache. You allow her to rest, but now you face the decision whether it is safe for her to hike back out. Unfortunately you have no means to call for help, and the terrain is too steep and rough to consider carrying her out. What should you do?

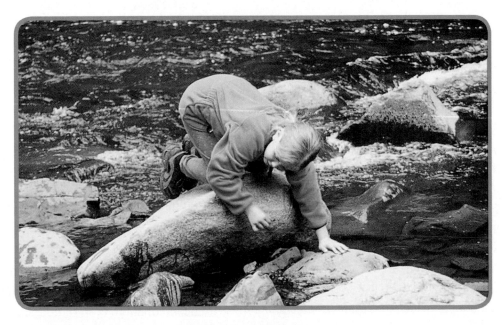

The principles of first aid described earlier in this text are based on the fact that in most locations in the United States medical help will arrive in 10 to 20 minutes, or sooner, after a call is made to 9-1-1 or the local emergency number. That means that the care first aiders give in emergencies is intended primarily to meet *short-term* goals until advanced medical personnel arrive and take over. In remote locations, however, advanced medical care may not be available for many hours or longer. In such situations you should be prepared to give additional care and, when necessary, to make decisions regarding evacuating and transporting the victim, going for help, and preparing to assist in special rescues.

Remote Locations

Being prepared for the possibility of injury or illness in a remote location is crucial. It is important to plan ahead to prevent emergencies from occurring, to be able to communicate the need for help, to have additional first aid supplies when needed, and to know how to care for a victim with common injuries and illness when more advanced medical help may be delayed. First aiders should also be prepared to manage certain types of emergencies that are more likely in remote locations, often involving extreme environmental conditions such as cold or heat or other special circumstances.

The specific issues involved in seeking medical care and caring for the victim depend on the setting where the emergency occurs, but the same general principles apply in most situations. This chapter cannot detail all procedures to follow in every possible emergency, as so many different variables are involved. For example, if a hiker in the mountains breaks his leg 20 miles from the nearest road and his only companion discovers his cell phone has no signal, the situation is different from that of an electrical power line worker who falls and breaks his leg on a rural road 40 miles from the nearest town with his partner nearby. First aiders who live, work or engage in recreational activities in remote areas should take a special remote location or wilderness first aid course and prepare for the situations in which they may find themselves.

This chapter focuses on how general principles of first aid may need to be modified when help is delayed and on other issues first aiders face in remote locations.

Situations When Help May be Delayed

Rural Areas

Rural areas include open countryside, isolated farms and ranches, and even some very small towns at a distance from medical services. The primary issue is usually only the length of time before help arrives, as roads and telephones are typically present. Any type of emergency may occur, although those working with certain types of farm equipment or in other specialized activities may face special risks. Injury prevention is especially important because an injury that may be more easily cared for in an urban area where help can be expected to arrive within minutes may become life-threatening if it takes an hour or more for help to arrive.

Hiking, Camping and Boating

Millions of people enjoy a wide range of recreational activities in natural settings far from roads, landline telephones and shelter. If an emergency occurs in such a wilderness area, you may not be able to contact EMS immediately and rescue vehicles may not be able to reach the victim. In addition to providing first aid for what may be an extended time, you may need to decide how best to shelter the victim from harsh weather and whether to send someone for help or to evacuate the victim. Again, being prepared for emergencies is crucial, but psychological and emotional issues may also become important.

Emergencies that occur when boating on remote lakes and rivers present issues similar to hiking and camping emergencies. Transportation and communication problems are likely. Boating in the ocean offshore or in remote coastal areas often

Learning Checkpoint 1

1. Name at least three different emergency situations in which rescue and medical help may be delayed.

   _____

2. Being prepared for emergencies in remote locations includes –

   a. knowing how to give first aid for an extended period.

   b. planning how to contact EMS if needed.

   c. having appropriate first aid supplies at hand.

   d. All of the above

involves different communication and rescue issues, generally involving the Coast Guard in addition to land-based EMS agencies. Like others entering remote areas, boaters need to think and plan ahead for possible emergencies and carry the appropriate first aid, communication and signaling equipment.

Natural and Other Disasters

People who live in areas that are prone to natural disasters such as hurricanes or earthquakes are generally aware of the need to be prepared. But other types of natural disasters can strike many other places, such as wildfires, floods, tornadoes and unanticipated ice storms that may close roads and cut off electricity for days. Because many natural disasters cause widespread damage and injuries, even if a hospital is not far away you may need to provide first aid in an emergency when help will be delayed. Widespread injuries may stretch emergency resources thin, increasing the time before a victim receives care. An airliner crash, industrial explosion or terrorist act may have similar effects (see **Chapter 25**).

General Principles When Help is Delayed

Preventing injury and illness when help may be delayed is especially important. This book has emphasized specific actions and guidelines for prevention and all of these apply in remote locations. People who live or work in rural areas, and those entering remote locations for recreational or other purposes, should be thinking

about safety issues at all times because of the risk that serious problems may develop if EMS cannot respond within minutes.

Regardless of the specific rural or remote location, five general principles apply whenever medical help may be delayed:

1. Be prepared for the situation. Plan for emergencies and have the right equipment and supplies.

2. Understand the psychological and emotional issues involved in a remote location emergency and be prepared to use leadership skills.

3. Know how to contact EMS or call for help by alternative means, or know how to use distress signals.

4. Know how to decide when to send someone for help versus evacuating the victim.

5. Know how to protect the victim until help arrives.

The following sections discuss these principles as they apply in different situations.

Being Prepared for the Situation

Like people who live or work in rural or remote locations, those planning a trip to remote locations should be prepared for emergencies. What will you do if someone in your group is injured and you are unable to telephone for help? Will you have the right equipment and supplies with you? Anticipating problems not only can help prevent them but also can help ensure that you are ready to act if they do occur.

Being prepared involves several guidelines that should be followed in all situations, as well as making specific preparations for the location.

1. **Do not enter remote locations alone**. All wilderness agencies and experts advise against this. Even a simple injury, such as a sprained ankle that prevents walking, can become life-threatening if you are unable to reach help. Do not assume your cell phone will bring help instantly. You may not have a signal, or rescuers may not be able to find you or reach you in time. Even a small wound can bleed severely, for example and if you are unresponsive or unable to stop the bleeding, you may go into shock rapidly and die before help arrives. Ideally, go in a group of three or more; if there are only two of you and one is injured, no one is left to help the injured person if the other has to go for help.

2. **Tell someone where you are going and when you plan to return**. If an emergency develops and you are unable to call for help, your contact person should be able to send help to you if you do not return as scheduled.

3. **Take a first aid kit equipped for possible emergencies you may face**. **Chapter 1** describes a general first aid kit. If you anticipate other types of injuries or illness because of the location you are entering, you should include additional items in your kit, including survival supplies and signaling devices.

4. **Take more food and water than you expect to need**. Any kind of emergency may delay your return, and running out of food or water would only worsen the situation. Although most people can survive a long time without food, becoming weak with hunger complicates the emergency. Anyone can rapidly become dehydrated without adequate water intake, and this can become an emergency within hours depending on the environment and the person's health status. Severe fluid loss caused by the injury, vomiting, diarrhea, excessive sweating or other conditions is a medical emergency.

5. **Expect weather emergencies**. Take extra clothing and some means to stay dry. Remember that being wet greatly increases heat loss from the body, making hypothermia a risk even at temperatures you do not consider "cold."

6. **Know where you are at all times**. Take a map along and know where you are on it. A **GPS**, a handheld location device using the satellite-based global positioning system, can show you where you are on a topographical map or water chart. If you can call for help in an emergency, you will need to be able to tell rescuers exactly where you are.

7. **Do not use alcohol or other drugs**. Alcohol and other drugs affect your physical performance and judgment, increasing the risk of injury and other emergencies.

8. **Study the location**. Be sure you are not trying to do something beyond your physical abilities. Becoming fatigued puts you at a greater risk for injury. Learn the conditions of the trail, find out whether any dangerous animals may be present and so on. Talk to local recreational groups, park rangers, the Coast Guard or other appropriate agencies.

In addition to these general principles, being prepared involves trip planning and having the right equipment and supplies, as described in the next sections.

Trip Planning

Trip planning begins with the eight general principles described in the previous section. The following are additional suggestions that depend on the specific locale.

1. Ensure that you are in good physical condition for the trip.

2. Choose the equipment you need for the setting.

3. Plan an appropriate menu with enough nutritious foods.

4. Learn the specifics of the area you plan to enter, including weather, presence of water, fire history and conditions, etc.

5. Obtain maps and guidebooks for the route you plan to take.

6. Refresh your first aid and CPR skills, if needed.

7. Plan for communications needs.

The Essential Equipment

The Wilderness Medical Society recommends a list of "10 Essentials for Outdoor Adventures." For people traveling through very isolated areas, these items should also be kept in your vehicle.

1. Map and compass

2. Flashlight or headlamp, extra batteries and bulb

3. Extra clothing including hat, gloves and rain gear

4. Sunglasses

5. Extra food and water

6. Waterproof matches in sealed container

7. Candle or fire-starter

8. Knife

9. First aid kit

10. Space blanket

Additional items that may prove useful when driving through isolated areas, especially in temperature extremes include:

- Emergency flares or bright orange "help" sign

- Sleeping bag

- Cell phone or CB radio

- Extra engine oil

- Toolkit

- Jumper cables

- Tire chains

- Shovel

- Sand (for tire traction)

- De-icer for fuel line

Remote Location First Aid Kit

If an emergency occurs in a remote location, despite the best planning and having all the appropriate equipment, the single most important item may be your first aid kit. In addition to the items listed in **Chapter 1** for a standard first aid kit, a kit carried into remote locations should have the items listed in **Box 23-1**. These should be kept also in rural location first aid kits.

Water Disinfection

Always take more water than you anticipate needing in a remote location. If you are a long distance from help or in an emergency situation where you may have to wait for some time, you may still run out of water. You should be prepared to disinfect the water found at your location. Surface water is often contaminated with bacteria, viruses or protozoa that may cause serious or life-threatening illness.

The three most common methods of disinfecting water for drinking are boiling, filtering and treating with chemicals. Boiling water effectively kills bacteria, viruses and protozoa and is often the best solution, but boiling is not always possible or practical. Many different filters are now sold in camping and specialty stores for filtering surface water. Most remove bacteria and protozoa from water but do not remove viruses. Viruses are generally rare in water that is found in wilderness areas.

Several different chemical treatments are available for disinfecting water, commonly using iodine or chlorine in tablet or liquid form. Both are generally effective for killing bacteria, viruses and some protozoa. These products must be used as directed. Before planning to use any product to obtain drinking water, it is best to learn about the characteristics of the surface water you are likely to find where you are going **(Figure 23-1)**.

In an emergency, if you have no method of disinfecting water, a difficult decision may have to be made between the risk of drinking untreated water and the risk of dehydration. Certainly it is better to be prepared and to have a disinfecting method along with other supplies and first aid items.

BOX 23-1: FIRST AID KIT FOR REMOTE LOCATIONS

- First aid guide
- Pain/anti-inflammatory medication
- Antihistamine
- Laxative
- Anti-diarrhea tablets
- Ibuprofen
- Safety pins
- Calamine lotion
- Oral decongestant
- Eye drops
- Motion sickness/anti-nausea medication
- Antifungal cream
- Antacid tablets
- Oral rehydration solution (especially for small children)

- Moleskin or Spenco 2nd Skin (for burns or open blisters)
- Oral hypothermia thermometer (to 85° F)
- Oil of cloves or other product for dental pain
- Temporary dental filling kit
- Throat lozenges
- Sunscreen and lip protection
- Sunburn lotion (aloe vera)
- Insect repellent
- SAM splint
- Sanitary napkins or tampons for bulky wound dressings
- Penlight
- Irrigation syringe
- Water purification tablets
- Sports drink containing sodium for endurance activities

Psychological Issues

Emergencies are always stressful, and in remote locations mental and emotional issues can become much more significant. The victim may not receive advanced care for many hours or days, and many decisions may be required about how best to care for the victim: whether to attempt **evacuation** or wait for help, how to provide shelter and so on. An outdoor environment often adds further stresses, such as coping with weather, temperature extremes, shortages of food or water, and other problems and uncertainties. The victim or other members of the party may not be able to cope with such stresses and may experience panic attacks, depression, denial, emotional shock or other problems that worsen the situation. In a worst-case scenario, just when cool heads and clear thinking are needed to address the emergency and first aid needs, there is a risk of the situation deteriorating because of panic, fear, confusion or indecision. Experts in wilderness survival and crisis management emphasize the importance of mental preparedness and leadership skills to be ready to act effectively in an emergency.

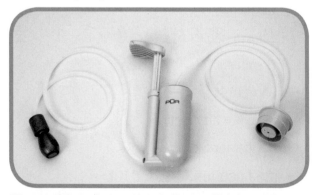

Figure 23-1 *Commercially available water purification kit and filter.*

Experts debate whether first aiders should have prescription medications for use in remote locations. One side argues that when medical help may be one or several days away, prescription medications such as a narcotic pain medication or systemic antibiotics have great value for a victim's health and well-being and may even save a life. A responsible adult can be instructed in the safe use of certain prescription medications and trusted not to misuse or abuse them. On the other side, others argue that the situations in which such medications are genuinely needed are rare and do not justify the potential for misuse or abuse.

Those planning long trips to remote locations that involve activities that put them at risk for medical emergencies are advised to talk with their health care provider about this issue. Medications that have been prescribed in such situations include cardiac emergency medications, pain medications, antibiotics, treatments for gastrointestinal infections, allergic reaction medications and others. When such prescribed medications are added to the first aid kit for remote locations, care must be taken to ensure that they are used only as directed and only in controlled circumstances.

Mental Preparedness

Being mentally prepared for an emergency in a remote location begins with first aid training and learning how best to provide care when help will be delayed. Self-confidence is important, but so is a realistic attitude about what you can and cannot do. When a life-threatening injury or illness occurs far from help, you may need to accept that you do not have the tools needed to give the victim all the help he or she needs. Yet it is equally important to not give up hope or fail to take actions that may help a victim.

Six aspects of mental preparedness are important for wilderness survival situations. They also apply in many other emergency situations.

1. Stay confident and remember your training.

2. Do not deny the seriousness of the situation, but calmly think through what you need to do.

3. Consider all your equipment and supplies as well as human resources. Be creative and improvise as necessary.

4. Stay focused on the goal and not on the hardships of the situation. Help others in the group to stay calm and act productively.

5. Remain positive but realistic.

6. Keep the faith – in yourself and in your beliefs.

Staying calm can be difficult in an emergency but is one of the most important actions one can take. If necessary, take time to control your own stress before beginning to act. Breathe deeply and slowly, and try to relax. Help others to control their fears to prevent panic, and then use your leadership skills to develop and carry out a plan.

Leadership Skills

Whenever two or more people are with a victim in an emergency, someone needs to be in charge. Often one person has more experience or training and naturally assumes leadership. In other situations, such as a group of friends going on a week-long backpacking trip, the group should discuss this before the trip begins. Who is packing the first aid kit? Who has thought about emergency communications? Advance conversations about emergency preparedness often naturally lead to consensus about who should take charge.

The most important leadership skill involves mental preparedness. Be confident and calm and help others to focus on the goal. Other leadership strategies include calmly talking through all actions with other members of the group and asking for suggestions when appropriate. Remember that you are caring not only for the victim but for other group members. Avoid rushing into decisions. The Outdoor Action Program of Princeton University describes five leadership steps when responding in an emergency:

1. Assess the situation and the victim's needs.

2. Make a plan for first aid and other needs related to rescue or obtaining medical care.

3. Delegate responsibilities to others for victim care, building shelter, handling communication or distress signals, and so on.

4. Initiate first aid care, set up camp and carry out other needed actions. Everyone in the group should participate in some useful way.

5. Continually reassess the situation and change the plan as needed. Always maintain the focus on the overall goal of getting the victim to medical care. Remember, hours or days may pass before the victim receives advanced help. During this period many decisions may be required and emotional difficulties are likely. An effective leader needs to be aware of the needs of the whole group and must work to keep up morale and prevent panic.

Calling for Help

In any emergency, one of the highest priorities is to call for help. With serious injuries or illness, medical care is needed beyond first aid. In remote locations or wilderness areas it may be more difficult to contact EMS, but with advanced planning and the appropriate equipment, help can be summoned in most situations. Communication options include cellular or satellite telephones, radios and emergency rescue beacons.

Cell Phones

Some hikers and other users of wilderness areas refuse to carry a cell phone, preferring to "get away from it all." Others take their cell phones along and assume they can simply call for help if they get lost or have any problems. Many forest rangers and park officials have received calls from hikers who were tired and lost and who expected instant help even though they had no idea where they were.

Between these two extremes, cell phones obviously have value in emergencies, although because of their limitations no one should depend entirely on a cell phone in an emergency. Cell phones are relatively fragile devices that may stop working due to temperature extremes, moisture, physical shocks or simply a dead battery. Many remote areas lack a signal. Follow these guidelines for using a cell phone in a remote area:

- Protect the phone from extreme cold, moisture and shocks.

- Pack the phone in a way that it cannot accidentally turn on and discharge the battery.

- Ensure that the battery is strong by saving the phone for emergency use.

- If you need the phone in an emergency and do not have a signal, try to get to a higher location such as a ridge top; even climbing a tree may help. Move the phone around your body, as even your own body can block a weak signal. Switch the phone from digital to analog, if you have this choice.

- Be sure you know where you are before making the call. Inexpensive handheld GPS units can provide exact longitude and latitude coordinates for rescuers.

Satellite Phones

Although still relatively expensive, satellite telephones are available for communication anywhere in the world and can be rented for special trips to very remote locations. Their use is similar to cell phones, but signal strength is not usually an issue.

Radios

Different types of radios are available for various specialized or general uses (Figure 23-2). In some areas, a handheld citizen's band (CB) radio may be able to reach authorities or other CB users, although cell phones have led to the declining use of CBs. Channel 9 is the emergency frequency for calling for help.

Family radio service (FRS) is a citizen's band frequency used by inexpensive handheld radios. Even in the best conditions, however, these radios generally transmit less than 3 miles, giving them limited use in remote locations. In areas where numbers of people are likely to be close by, however, such as ski areas, FRS radios may allow contact with others for help. They may also be useful for staying in touch when members of a group split up.

Amateur (ham) radio is another option. Portable units generally reach a significantly wider area, and more people are likely to monitor common frequencies. An FCC license is required to use ham equipment, which is also generally more expensive.

VHF radios are used on boats. Because of the lack of signal obstructions on the water, VHF (very high frequency) radios can cover up to 30 miles. Most U.S. coastal areas have coverage by Coast Guard towers. The Coast Guard monitors Channel 16 and can send a rescue ship or helicopter in an emergency. The Coast Guard recommends boaters use VHF radio rather than a cell phone to call for

help in an emergency, because their triangulation equipment can help them better determine the location of the vessel in distress and because nearby boaters also can hear the call for help and may render assistance. Although less powerful, handheld VHF radios used in smaller watercraft have enough power to summon help from the Coast Guard or other boaters in the vicinity. Larger boats often use single sideband (SSB) radio. These units use a frequency that travels greater distances beyond coastal areas.

Rescue Beacons

Emergency beacons send out a signal that is picked up by an international system of satellites. All commercial and most civil airplanes carry these beacons, known as emergency locator transmitters (ELTs), which automatically send out a signal if the aircraft crashes or has an emergency landing.

Using the same system, marine rescue beacons called **emergency position indicating radio beacons (EPIRBs)** are available for boats that leave coastal areas and cannot depend on radio transmission in an emergency. Some units are manually operated, while others automatically begin sending rescue signals upon being immersed if the boat capsizes.

In 2003 the FCC authorized the use of **personal locator beacons (PLBs)**. Hikers and other wilderness users now have the same ability to summon help from any remote location. As these units become more popular, they will become more widely available and inexpensive.

All types of rescue beacons are one-way communication devices – they function only to send an emergency signal that is received by satellites. Typically only the device's location is communicated, although one new service includes a short text message with appropriate devices. No information can be sent about the nature of the emergency, nor can the user know for certain that the signal is being received. Rescue beacons must be used only in a true emergency requiring rescue. In addition, users must register beacons, each of

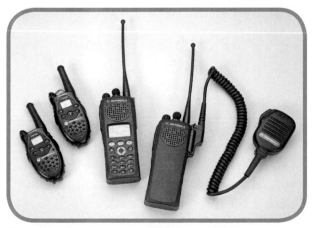

Figure 23-2 *Devices for summoning help.*

which sends out a unique signal, to help rescuers determine if an emergency has occurred when a signal is received.

Statistics are scarce for the new PLBs, but EPIRBs have led to more than 28,000 rescues worldwide, including 6,550 in the United States[1]. These included stranded hikers, shipwrecked boaters and downed pilots.

Distress Signals

If help cannot be summoned by telephone, radio or other means when rescue is required, distress signals may be used to catch the attention of passing aircraft. The following are recognized distress signals for different situations:

- At night, build three small campfires in a triangle up to 100 feet apart. Three flares can also be used or series of three flashes from a flashlight.

- In the daytime, make a large campfire and put green branches or leaves on it to create smoke. Do this in a clearing or on a hilltop.

A standard signal is to create three puffs of smoke in a row by covering and uncovering a campfire by any means available.

- Make a large X of markings in the snow or on clear ground. Green branches or bright clothing may be used. Use any material available that will contrast with the ground.

- If a passing aircraft is close enough to see you, raise both (not just one) arms above your head.

- If you have a firearm, fire three shots in a row or try three whistle blasts.

- In sunlight, use a signal mirror to flash light at a passing aircraft. The reflected beam can be aimed at the aircraft by sighting the beam past a nearby object or your own hand **(Figure 23-3)**. If you do not have a mirror, use any shiny object such as the lid from a can or a piece of glass with mud coating the back side.

[1]*NOAA Satellite and Information Service, http://www. sarsat.noaa.gov/ Accessed March 4, 2011.*

Many commercial distress signals are available, including such things as flares and aerial flare guns, strobe lights, signal flags and banners, and orange smoke signals.

Sending Someone for Help

In a situation in which an injured or ill victim cannot easily be transported to medical care and it is impossible to call for help, one or more people may need to go for help while others remain with the victim. Difficult decisions are involved, particularly in small groups with only one leader experienced in the area. Should that person be the one to go for help if he or she may get there faster or more safely, or is he or she better equipped to deal with building a camp and caring for the victim? There are no simple rules that apply in all situations, as so many different variables are involved. Most important, before decisions are made, the group should talk through the issues so that everyone understands what may be involved in both staying and going.

The person going for help must be able to communicate the group's location to rescuers. This information should be written down and carried. Unless this location is a well-known place, the person going for help must also be confident about his or her ability to lead rescuers back to the victim.

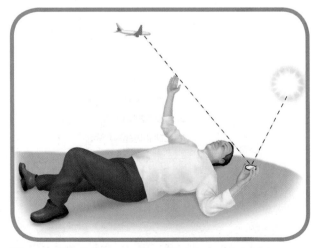

Figure 23-3 *To send a distress signal to an aircraft, aim the mirror's reflected sunlight past your fingers or a stationary object.*

Sheltering the Victim

While awaiting rescuers, a victim of injury or sudden illness needs to be protected from the environment. Unless you have camping equipment with you, you need to create an emergency shelter to keep the victim (and yourself) warm and dry. The type of shelter depends on the characteristics of the area and what materials you have with you. Look for natural shelters such as a cave or rock overhang. If you need to make a shelter, use a poncho or tarp hung over a rope or pole to make a lean-to or tent **(Figure 23-4a and b)**. If you have no waterproof material, make a lean-to from branches or poles and cover the framework with leaves, grass or other material **(Figure 23-4c)**. In swampy areas where the victim must be elevated to stay dry, cut saplings to build a "swamp bed" **(Figure 23-4d)**. A "debris hut," a tent-like structure made of branches piled over with brush, twigs and leaves, can keep you and the victim dry and warm **(Figure 23-4e)**. In a heavy snowfall, dig a pit in the snow around the base of an evergreen tree with low boughs, piling boughs against the trunk to form a snow roof as more snow falls **(Figure 23-4f)**. In a desert or on a shadeless beach, where the victim needs to be sheltered from the sun and heat, construct a shade shelter by digging a trench in cooler sand, stretching clothing or other material between mounds on each side, and anchoring the material with more sand on top at its edges **(Figure 23-4g)**.

Leaving the Victim Alone

Consider leaving a victim alone to go for help only if you are alone, you cannot communicate your need for help and it is unlikely that someone will pass your location. Because a victim's condition may deteriorate without further care, take this action only if there is no alternative. Prepare the victim as well as possible before leaving, attending to shelter and food and water needs. Leave a written note with the victim explaining when you anticipate returning with help. Carry a note on your own person also, stating the location and condition of the victim as well as your destination, in case something happens to you before you reach help.

With three or more in the group, never leave the victim alone, even when you feel sure the victim will be okay – and even if the victim agrees. Conditions may change or unanticipated things may happen.

Preparing for Rescue

Once an emergency has been communicated from the remote location to authorities such as EMS, search and rescue operations, or the Coast Guard, it is critical to remain in the same location until help arrives. You may need to help rescuers find you as they approach the area by signaling with a fire or flashlight, smoke, or a whistle. Depending on the urgency of the situation and the terrain, rescuers may arrive by vehicle, on foot or by other means.

Helicopter rescues are often used in remote areas to get a victim to advanced medical care quickly. Following are safety principles when a helicopter is arriving at your location **(Figure 23-5)**:

- A large, clear area is needed for a safe landing. Stay far back from any clearing where the helicopter is likely to land.

- The "rotor wash" (wind) from the helicopter typically exceeds 100 mph. Protect your face and the victim from injury caused by flying debris.

- Once the helicopter has landed, do not approach it until signaled to do so. The spinning tail rotor cannot be seen and you may inadvertently walk into it. Approach only in a crouch and never from an uphill side where the blade is closer to the ground.

- When making a rescue at sea or in a wilderness area where landing is impossible, the helicopter may lower a basket on a cable. Sometimes the helicopter crew lowers a two-way radio first to enable communication and give instructions for the rescue.

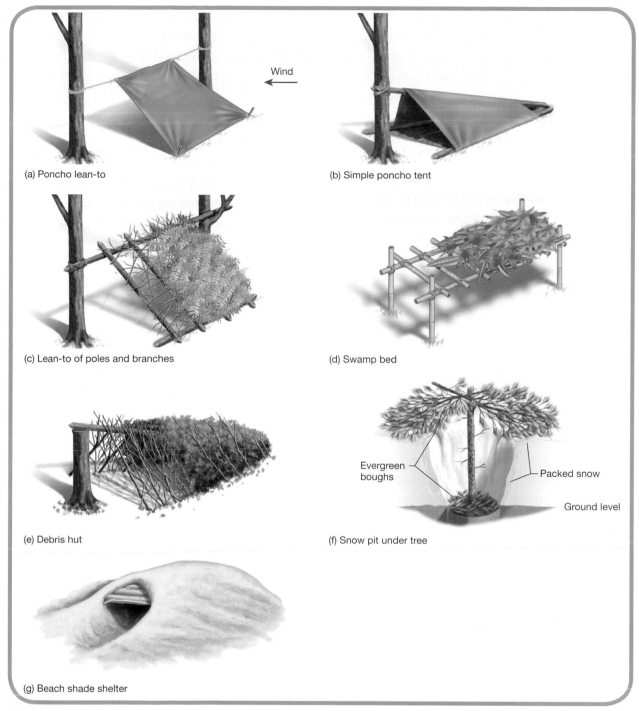

(a) Poncho lean-to

Wind

(b) Simple poncho tent

(c) Lean-to of poles and branches

(d) Swamp bed

(e) Debris hut

Evergreen boughs

Packed snow

Ground level

(f) Snow pit under tree

(g) Beach shade shelter

Figure 23-4 *Emergency shelters.*

Evacuation of Victim

Generally it is better to wait for help to come to you rather than to try to evacuate the victim yourself from a remote location. Moving the victim may worsen the victim's condition and is likely to cause additional pain. The decision to evacuate a victim depends on several key factors:

- The length of time before help can be expected to arrive
- Whether the victim's condition will be aggravated more by waiting for help than by moving the victim
- The number of people present and their ability to safely carry the victim out

- How much daylight remains and whether the weather may deteriorate

- Whether it is possible to continue giving first aid during evacuation

According to the Wilderness Medical Society, victims with the following conditions may be evacuated if help will be delayed and group members can safely carry the victim:

- A worsening condition such as a breathing problem, deteriorating mental status, shock, or recurring diarrhea or vomiting

- Severe pain

- Inability to walk

- Persistent bleeding

- Severe altitude sickness

- An infection getting worse

- Chest pain symptomatic of a cardiac condition

- Mental or behavioral disorder that threatens the safety of the victim or others

- Near drowning

- Severe burns or wounds

- Severe traumatic injury

If enough people are present, someone should be sent ahead for help, as those carrying the victim will travel more slowly.

Four or six people can carry the victim on an improvised stretcher or litter. Cut two poles from saplings and create a litter from a blanket or sleeping bag, or even two jackets or shirts as shown in **Figure 23-6**. Use other clothing to pad the litter under the victim. Use belts or rope to secure the victim in the litter and support the head and neck. During the evacuation, monitor the victim's condition and stay alert for vomiting, which can threaten the airway of a victim lying on his or her back.

Other emergency carries such as the hammock carry (see **Chapter 23**) are ineffective for the distances typically involved in remote location evacuations. In certain circumstances the two-person walking assist may be appropriate for a short distance.

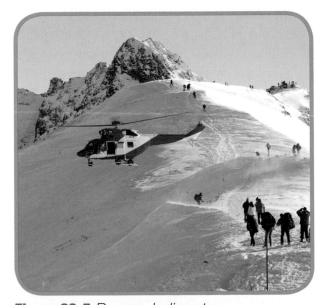

Figure 23-5 *Rescue helicopter.*

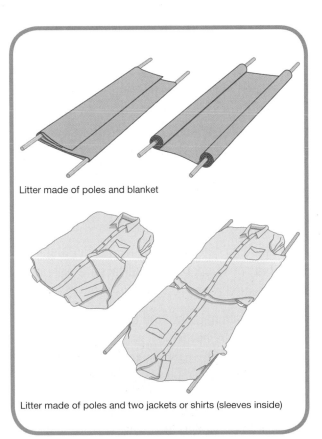

Litter made of poles and blanket

Litter made of poles and two jackets or shirts (sleeves inside)

Figure 23-6 *Emergency litters for evacuating an injured victim.*

Learning Checkpoint 2

1. Check off important principles for planning a trip into a wilderness location:

_____Do not go alone.

_____Do not go longer than three to four days.

_____Tell someone where you are going and when you will return.

_____Take more food and water than you expect to need.

_____Split up the first aid kit among three or four people in the group in case someone gets lost.

_____Do not drink more alcohol than usual.

2. True or False: When dealing with a complex emergency in a remote location, the group's leader must set the plan and resist any temptation to change it along the way.

3. Name three reasons why you should not depend on a cell phone in a wilderness location.

_____

4. Never leave a victim alone to go for help when –

   a. you cannot communicate your need for help.

   b. it is unlikely that someone will pass by your location.

   c. there are three or four people in the group.

   d. All of the above

Special Care for Emergencies When Help is Delayed

Earlier chapters describe the standard first aid for injuries and sudden illness. **This chapter describes only special considerations when help may be delayed**.

Bleeding, Wounds and Shock

Special care for bleeding may be needed in a remote location for these reasons:

- Bleeding can soon become life-threatening if it is not stopped and medical care will not be provided soon.

- A contaminated wound that a first aider may leave for medical personnel in normal situations can become seriously infected if medical care is not provided soon.

- A victim in shock caused by blood loss requires special care if medical attention is delayed, such as providing fluids if possible.

Special remote location care for bleeding, wounds and shock includes the following steps *in addition to the care described in earlier chapters*.

1. Control external bleeding as soon as possible. Maintain direct pressure as long as needed with a pressure bandage, but check for circulation below the bleeding site to avoid cutting off circulation to the limb unless absolutely necessary to control bleeding.

2. A **tourniquet** is used *only as an extreme last resort* to stop bleeding from an arm or leg to save the victim's life when medical attention will be delayed. The victim is likely to face amputation of the limb. In usual circumstances, tourniquets should be used only by rescuers trained in their use, but a wilderness setting may necessitate a decision between losing the limb or losing the person's life. To apply a tourniquet:

   - Wrap a wide belt or bandage around the limb just above the bleeding site and knot it.

- Knot a metal rod or strong stick over the first knot and twist it to tighten the constricting band until bleeding stops **(Figure 23-7)**. Note that considerable pressure may be necessary to squeeze closed the bleeding artery deep within the limb.

- Tape or fasten the rod in place to hold the pressure.

- Note the time of application to inform medical personnel.

- After 15 minutes slowly release the tourniquet pressure to see if bleeding has stopped; reapply the tourniquet if bleeding begins.

3. After stopping bleeding from a wound, you should clean the wound to prevent infection. Wash the wound with large amounts of water, if possible; then apply a sterile dressing and bandage over the wound to keep out dirt. For a deeper wound or one visibly contaminated with dirt or foreign matter, use an irrigation syringe to forcefully rinse the wound clean; if necessary, part the wound edges to allow the water to reach the bottom of the wound. Then apply a sterile dressing and bandage, applying pressure again if necessary to stop bleeding. For gaping wounds, use "butterfly" bandage strips or strips of clean tape to hold the wound closed or pack a deep wound that will not close with a dressing.

4. There is one exception to the usual care for shock caused by bleeding as described in **Chapter 9**. Normally a shock victim is not given anything to drink in the brief time before medical help arrives, but when help is delayed, the victim needs fluid. If the victim is responsive and can swallow, give water, a clear fluid or an oral rehydration solution in small amounts, frequently but only as tolerated. If the victim vomits, wait a while before giving another drink.

5. If the victim's shock resulted from dehydration, keep giving fluids slowly but steadily.

Musculoskeletal Injuries

As explained in **Chapter 15**, an injured extremity normally is splinted only if the victim is at risk for moving the injured area before help arrives. When help is delayed, especially if the victim is to be evacuated, splinting is often necessary. You may need to improvise the splint with materials at hand, such as a ski pole or a sturdy piece of wood broken from a tree branch **(Figure 23-8)**. Ideally, a first aid kit used in remote locations should include a SAM splint. When the splint will be in place for an extended time, it is essential to check circulation below the injury and to periodically loosen the splint to improve blood flow.

In very rare cases of an extremity fracture, circulation may be cut off below the injury site. If medical care is hours away and you are certain there is no circulation in the extremity below the injury, then you may try to carefully straighten the extremity to restore circulation unless this would increase bleeding. Never try to straighten a fractured limb if the victim may receive medical care within 30 minutes or if there is circulation below the injury site.

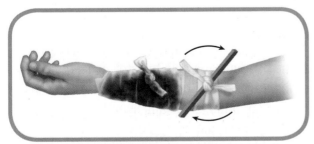

Figure 23-7 *An emergency tourniquet is used only as a last resort to stop bleeding.*

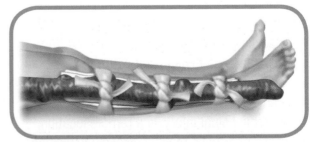

Figure 23-8 *Improvising a splint with materials at hand.*

In some cases a dislocation may impair circulation to an extremity. If you have been trained to reduce a dislocation (return bones to their normal position in the joint), and if you are sure that circulation to the extremity is cut off and the victim will not receive medical care within 30 minutes, you may then try to reduce the dislocation.

Spinal Injuries

In remote locations, three aspects of first aid in cases of suspected spinal injuries are somewhat different from the usual care described in **Chapter 12**. First, if the victim is thought to have a possible spinal injury, it may be difficult to keep the spine immobilized for an extended time. You may need to improvise with materials at hand, such as using large pieces of wood or stones padded with clothing positioned on both sides of the head to immobilize the spine of a victim who is lying down. If the victim is on the ground, you may need to put clothing or other material under the victim's body to prevent heat loss; do this by holding the head in line with the body as others roll the body to one side long enough for an insulated material to be put under the victim's body. A victim with a spinal injury should not be evacuated.

Second, although it is generally best to immobilize a victim in the position found when help will arrive soon, in remote locations it is generally better to gently place the victim in the normal position with head straight and eyes forward to prevent further injury to the spine. Do not move the victim's head, however, if it causes more pain or you feel resistance to movement.

Finally, great care is needed in assessing a possible spinal injury. When help will arrive soon, it is better to be safe than sorry, and a conservative approach is generally advised: Immobilize the victim's head and neck in line with the body, keep the victim still and wait for advanced medical personnel to determine how best to manage the possible spinal injury. In a remote location, however, other risks may be involved in waiting a long time for help, and in such cases if the

presence of a spinal injury is not obvious, the victim may be further assessed to determine whether immobilization is in fact necessary. The Wilderness Medical Associates have developed a protocol for spinal injuries in which a spine injury can be ruled out if *all* of the following criteria are met:

1. The victim is alert, sober and cooperative.

2. The victim does not feel neck or back tenderness when you press your fingers along the spine.

3. The victim does not have other injuries that mask or distract him or her from feeling the pain or tenderness of a spinal injury.

4. The victim has normal function in all four limbs:

   • The fingers of both hands can be opened and closed and the wrist moved up and down.

   • Both feet can be moved up and down and the big toe moved up and down.

   • The victim has no tingling sensation but has normal sensation in all four limbs, as determined by being able to feel a light touch and a painful pinch in all areas. One specific area may have reduced function if the cause is clearly not related to a spinal injury, such as occurs with a sprained wrist.

Head Injuries

Chapter 12 describes how when help is expected to arrive soon, it is generally best to call 9-1-1 and give supportive care while waiting for help. In a delayed help situation, especially if you cannot communicate with EMS to ask advice, you may need to make difficult decisions about whether to evacuate the victim.

A victim with a concussion caused by a blow to the head may be able to safely walk out of a remote location. The victim should be closely monitored for the signs and symptoms of a more serious brain injury, however, and should be awakened and checked every two to three hours.

A victim with a more serious head injury may have swelling or bleeding in the brain, a potentially life-threatening condition. The signs and symptoms of a brain injury are described in **Chapter 12**. A serious brain injury is unlikely to improve by itself; the victim needs immediate medical attention. If possible, call for emergency evacuation, by helicopter if available. If communication is impossible, you may face the difficult decision of whether to attempt to evacuate the victim yourself. The sooner the victim receives medical care, the better his or her chances for survival, but moving the victim over difficult terrain may worsen the condition. Either way, the victim may die. Evacuate the victim only if necessary to prevent a dangerous delay and if you can do so safely.

Abdominal Injury or Illness

A victim with an abdominal injury or severe abdominal pain needs to receive medical attention as soon as possible. As with a head injury, if communication with EMS is impossible, you must balance the risk of the victim's condition being worsened by evacuation with the risk of waiting for delayed help. A closed or open abdominal wound may progress to life-threatening shock, and abdominal pain may be a sign of appendicitis which can rapidly become an emergency.

Burns

The care for burns when help is delayed is similar to standard burn care. In addition, because a severe or large burn may cause a significant loss of body fluids, a victim who is alert should be given large amounts of water or clear fluids slowly and a little at a time to minimize shock.

Burn prevention is especially important in outdoor recreational activities such as camping. Fire is a greater risk with an outdoor campfire because of the risk of windblown sparks and the flammability of tents, sleeping bags and other camp gear. Because many of the synthetic fabrics used in such camping equipment and clothing melt when on fire, causing deeper and more serious burns when in contact with skin, water should be immediately available for dousing flames.

Sudden Illness

Special considerations may be necessary for diabetic emergencies or anaphylactic shock when help may be delayed.

A diabetic who regularly self-injects insulin or takes medication should inform others in the remote environment how to administer insulin or medication in an emergency. It is especially important that diabetics monitor their blood sugar levels and inform others of the signs and symptoms of hypoglycemia and hyperglycemia as well as what to do. Prevention is critical, but others should be prepared to take action by giving a sugar substance. If diabetic shock develops, give water and other shock care. Evacuate a victim in a diabetic crisis as quickly as possible.

Similarly, someone who has severe allergies should inform others in the group, and the first aid kit should contain emergency epinephrine such as an EpiPen if possible. Someone with severe allergies entering a wilderness location may carry up to three emergency epinephrine doses. Be sure others know where the EpiPen is kept and how to use it. A victim who develops anaphylaxis should be evacuated as quickly as possible. The protocol of the Wilderness Medical Associates calls for administering epinephrine to victims with a definite reaction marked by difficulty breathing and generalized skin redness or swelling. Although usually only one dose is needed, up to three doses may be administered if required, every five minutes if the condition is worsening or every 15 minutes if the victim's condition does not change.

Hypothermia

Hypothermia is more likely to occur during outdoor activities in cold environments, especially if one is wet or a wind is blowing. Because the body loses heat 25 to 30 times faster when immersed in cold water, hypothermia is even more likely if a victim falls into cold water.

A responsive victim of mild hypothermia, with a body temperature higher than 90° F may recover with adequate warming. Follow the standard guidelines to warm the victim. With sufficient rest and warming, in time this person may be able to walk out of the remote location.

A body temperature below 90° F indicates severe hypothermia. At this point the victim is usually no longer shivering and often has changing levels of responsiveness. This is a life-threatening emergency. It is unlikely that you will be able to fully rewarm the victim in the remote location, but make every effort to prevent further heat loss and to warm the victim as much as possible while waiting for help. Do not try to evacuate the victim by foot, as it will be difficult or impossible to keep the victim warm while being transported through a cold environment. Send someone for help immediately. Put the victim in dry clothing and inside a sleeping bag protected by shelter. The victim should be wrapped fully to prevent heat loss, including the use of a space blanket if available **(Figure 23-9)**. Avoid rough handling. Add heat with bodily contact, heating pads or hot water bottles beside the neck, armpits or groin. Whereas a hypothermia victim should not be actively rewarmed with heat sources when close to medical care, in a remote location

you may actively warm the victim with a heat source and by putting containers of warm (not hot) water against the victim's skin.

A victim in very severe hypothermia may seem to be dead. The skin is cold and blue and the victim is totally unresponsive. The internal body temperature may be lower than 85° F. Do not rush to provide CPR, however, which can lead to a life-threatening heart dysrhythmia if the victim still has a heartbeat. Assess the victim carefully. The victim may be breathing only once every 30 seconds or so. Rewarm the victim as described previously and provide CPR if the victim is not breathing.

Hypothermia caused by immersion in cold water may occur very rapidly and is often severe. These victims generally need both rewarming and CPR. Because the body's need for oxygen decreases when very cold, resuscitation may occur even after significant time in the water. Although CPR is generally not given for longer than 30 minutes in normal temperatures, victims with severe hypothermia have been given CPR for as long as three hours and recovered fully. The saying "a victim is never cold and dead, only warm and dead" reminds us to not assume a victim is dead until rewarming has occurred, because severe hypothermic victims often survive.

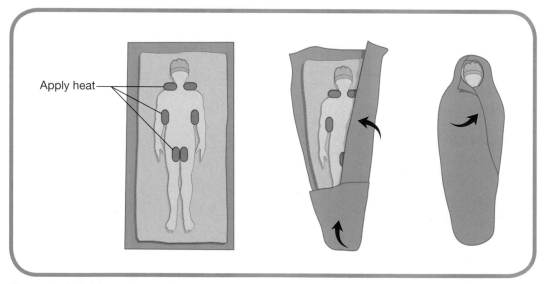

Apply heat

Figure 23-9 *Hypothermia wrap.*

Heat Emergencies

Like cold emergencies, heat emergencies such as heatstroke are more common during outdoor activities in remote locations where no relief may be possible from extreme temperatures. Prevent heat emergencies by staying out of direct sunlight, minimizing activity and staying well hydrated.

For heat exhaustion or heatstroke, cool the victim as soon as possible. If the victim is alert and not vomiting, give water or a sports drink a little at a time. A victim with heat exhaustion may be able to travel from the location after cooling and resting. The victim may remain in a weakened condition, however, and walking in continued heat may renew the problem and lead to an emergency.

Heatstroke is a life-threatening emergency. Cool the victim and evacuate if possible rather than waiting for delayed medical attention. Even if the victim seems to recover, there may be damage to internal organs.

Snake Bites

Unless you are certain the bite was from a non-poisonous snake, assume a snake bite is poisonous. Splint the limb to reduce movement and keep the area below the level of the heart.

Check the fingers or toes periodically to ensure that circulation is not impeded. Evacuate the victim as soon as possible. To be effective, antivenin must be administered within four to six hours after the bite. Other medical care may be needed.

CPR

Chapter 5 describes the standard procedures for CPR. Follow the same approach for a victim in cardiac arrest in a remote location, although in some cases the victim has smaller chances for recovery when advanced medical care cannot be given soon. CPR was developed as a short-term treatment to keep the victim alive until treated by medical professionals. Depending on the cause

 Learning Checkpoint 3

1. What is important about first aid for bleeding in a remote location?

   a. Control bleeding as quickly as possible.

   b. Use a tourniquet only as a last resort.

   c. A responsive victim in shock can drink water.

   d. All of the above

2. True or False: If you suspect a victim in a remote location may have a spinal injury, do not move him or her no matter how long you may have to wait for help.

3. True or False: In a remote location, the best thing to do for a victim believed to have a brain injury is to wait and see if the victim's condition improves.

4. On a cold day, a hiker in your group of four falls into an icy stream about a three-hour walk from the car. After being pulled out, he develops the signs and symptoms of severe hypothermia. Which is the best action to take?

   a. Immediately start hiking out – keep the person moving and he'll be okay.

   b. Send someone to get help while rest of the group works to warm the victim.

   c. Put the victim in a hypothermia wrap and carry him out.

   d. None of the above

5. Except in cases of hypothermia, drowning and lightning strike, CPR in a remote location can be stopped if the victim does not revive within _____ minutes.

of the cardiac arrest, resuscitation in a remote location may be unlikely, as when cardiac arrest is caused by a heart attack or traumatic injuries. Nonetheless, always give CPR for 30 minutes. If the victim is far from medical care and does not revive within 30 minutes *except in certain special situations*, you can stop CPR after 30 minutes.

In three types of situations victims have been successfully resuscitated after CPR was given for longer than 30 minutes: hypothermia, drowning and lightning strike. As noted earlier, victims with severe hypothermia have survived after hours of CPR. In these cases follow the standard protocol to give CPR until another trained rescuer takes over or you are too exhausted to continue.

Special Wilderness Emergencies

In addition to being prepared for an emergency in a remote location and knowing what first aid to give when help will be delayed, people entering wilderness locations where there is a risk of certain kinds of emergencies need special preparations. These special situations include:

- Ice rescue
- Snow emergencies
- Desert survival
- Lightning strikes
- Altitude sickness
- Scuba diving incidents

This text only introduces the issues involved in these situations. Special training programs are available for people planning a trip into locations where these emergencies may occur, including preparation equipment, and first aid and survival techniques.

Ice Rescue

In circumstances where EMS can be called and trained rescuers can arrive within minutes, you should never go onto ice yourself to rescue a victim. In a remote location, however, a rescuer may choose to go onto the ice as a last resort.

Lie flat with arms and legs spread to distribute your weight, and push a tree limb or other object ahead of you for the victim to grab. If at all possible, others should hold onto your legs or use clothing to fashion a rescue line if rope is not available, in case the ice breaks under you.

Snow Emergencies

Avalanches

Avalanches are a risk for backcountry trekkers and skiers. Try to avoid areas that are prone to avalanches, and talk with local officials before entering the area. Avalanche transceivers (beacons) are available that emit signals from a trapped person to transceivers carried by others in the group to help them to locate the victim. Most avalanche deaths occur by suffocation; the snow packs tightly around the victim, preventing breathing or digging out. The victim's chances of survival rapidly diminish as time passes after burial.

Call for help if someone in your group is buried by an avalanche, but time is critical and those present should begin searching for the person immediately. Start at the point where the victim was last seen and work down the slope, using a ski pole or tree branch to probe into the snow. CPR will likely be necessary.

Snow Blindness

Snow blindness is a burn on the cornea of the eyes caused by intense sunlight reflected from snow. It can be prevented by wearing dark sunglasses or goggles with UV protection. At first the eyes feel scratchy or burning sensations and become more sensitive to light. Headache may develop. Eventually the victim loses vision. First aid involves bandaging the eyes to prevent any further exposure to light. Cold compresses may ease the pain. The victim usually recovers sight in 12 to 18 hours, but if symptoms linger, medical care should be sought.

Desert Survival

Desert hiking and trekking have become more popular, exposing more people to the risks of very harsh climates. As when entering very cold climates, preparation and training are essential. Appropriate clothing is necessary for sun and heat protection, as are the right camping equipment and first aid supplies. Perhaps most important is water. Few people realize that the daily intake of water can increase to up to 3 to 5 gallons per person in extreme dry heat. Because water weighs 8 pounds per gallon, it is impractical to carry enough to sustain life for days in an emergency. Desert survival training therefore includes skills in finding and purifying water as well as techniques for building shelter, sending communications and distress signals, finding direction and traveling at night to avoid the worst heat.

Lightning Strikes

Chapter 11 lists tips to avoid being struck by lightning. About one-third of victims of lightning strike die, usually as a result of cardiac arrest. Immediate CPR is therefore critical to increase the victim's chances for survival. Remember that lightning strikes are one of the three situations (along with drowning and hypothermia) in which CPR should be continued past the 30-minute limit.

Altitude Sickness

Hikers at altitudes above 8,000 to 10,000 feet are at risk for different forms of **altitude sickness** caused by the lower concentration of oxygen. Know what symptoms to watch for and what actions to take. As many as one-fourth of people may experience altitude sickness and it is impossible to predict in advance whether one is susceptible.

Acute mountain sickness (AMS) is common and up to 75% of people will have mild symptoms after spending one or two days at above 10,000 feet. Others may experience more severe symptoms at as low as 8,000 feet. Symptoms include headache, dizziness, fatigue, shortness of breath, nausea and lack of appetite, and general malaise. Moderate AMS causes more severe headache not relieved by medication, nausea and vomiting, decreased coordination and worsening of the mild symptoms. Severe AMS causes

shortness of breath even at rest, decreasing mental status and inability to walk. Mild AMS may be overcome with acclimatization, but descent to lower altitude is the only cure for more severe symptoms. The Outdoor Action Program advises this test for a person experiencing AMS symptoms: Try to walk a straight line heel to toe (like a sobriety test). A person who has difficulty doing this should start the descent immediately before symptoms worsen.

Medication is available to treat mild to moderate symptoms in people who have experienced AMS in the past. Hikers should also maintain good hydration, as body fluid is lost more rapidly at high altitudes. New research also suggests that a high-carbohydrate diet before and during the high-altitude period may reduce the symptoms of AMS.

Two other types of altitude sickness, **high altitude pulmonary edema (HAPE)** and **high altitude cerebral edema (HACE)**, are rare but more serious. Both occur after more time at altitude and involve a fluid buildup – in the lungs in HAPE or the brain in HACE – that becomes life-threatening. A victim of HAPE experiences shortness of breath even at rest; a feeling of tightness in the chest; significant fatigue and weakness; a persistent, productive cough; and confusion or irrational behavior. A victim of HACE has significant mental signs and symptoms including headache, loss of coordination, memory loss, possible hallucinations, and psychotic confusion and coma. Any victim thought to be experiencing HAPE or HACE must be evacuated immediately down the mountain to a medical facility.

Scuba Diving

Underwater divers, as part of their scuba training and certification, learn about the risks of staying down too long or surfacing too quickly. Operators of dive boats and facilities know what signs and symptoms to look for and typically have the communications equipment and resources needed to call for professional medical help when necessary. Some divers, however, may dive on their own or accompanied by others without this training. EMS should be contacted immediately for any diver experiencing breathing difficulty, pain in joints or extremities, feelings of paralysis, tingling or numbness, significant fatigue and generalized weakness, convulsions, coma or nonresponsiveness. Decompression treatment and other specialized care may be needed.

Learning Checkpoint 4

1. In a desert or other extremely dry, hot environment, a person's daily intake of water may increase to _____ gallons.

2. Put a check mark next to the typical signs and symptoms of acute mountain sickness:

   _____ Headache   _____ Cold, dry skin

   _____ Dizziness   _____ Fatigue

   _____ Diarrhea   _____ Nausea

Concluding Thoughts

For people living or working in rural areas or visiting remote locations for any reason, the most important thing is to be aware that if an injury or sudden illness strikes, you may be on your own for a time before being rescued or reaching advanced care. This makes injury and illness prevention crucial, as is being prepared for the kinds of emergencies that are more likely to occur in the specific setting. With preparation and a healthy attitude toward minimizing the risks, you will likely be among the millions who live in remote locations or visit wilderness areas every year without incident.

Learning Outcomes

You should now be able to do the following:

1. Explain what is different about first aid principles when help may be delayed.

2. Describe common situations in which help is likely to be delayed.

3. List actions to take to be prepared for injury and illness emergencies in remote locations.

4. Describe methods by which EMS can be contacted from isolated areas.

5. Explain how to protect a victim until help arrives or how to safely transport a victim if help cannot reach the victim.

6. Describe special care for victims with common injuries and illnesses when help will be delayed.

7. Explain what to do in special wilderness emergencies such as avalanche or ice rescue, lightning strikes, altitude sickness, and scuba diving illness.

Review Questions

1. If you will be in the wilderness for several days, consider bringing along –

    a. more water than you expect to need.

    b. special medications you might need.

    c. a device for emergency communication.

    d. All of the above

2. If you need to use your cell phone to call for help while in a remote location and the signal is weak, what can you try in order to get a stronger signal?

    a. Point the antenna directly at the horizon.

    b. Move the phone around your body.

    c. Try to get near a body of water.

    d. Wrap a damp cloth around the antenna.

3. Standard distress signals involve making what number of sounds, lights or visual signals that may be heard or seen by others?

    a. 2

    b. 3

    c. 4

    d. as many as possible

4. In a remote location, leave a victim alone to go for help only if –

    a. you are alone with the victim.

    b. you cannot communicate your need for help.

    c. it is unlikely someone will pass your location soon.

    d. All of the above are true

5. Your group in a wilderness area decides to use a litter to carry an unresponsive injured victim back to safety. Which of the following is the most dangerous possibility to stay alert for as you carry the victim?

    a. Vomiting

    b. Heat exhaustion

    c. Pain caused by jiggling the litter

    d. Dehydration

6. What is different about wound care if medical attention may be delayed a day or two?

    a. Try to insert antibiotic cream into a puncture wound by any method, even cutting open the wound if necessary.

    b. Rather than covering the wound with a dressing, leave it open to "breathe" and to be able to check it frequently for signs of infection.

    c. Clean the wound after the bleeding stops, even at the risk of bleeding starting again.

    d. Use your sewing kit, if available, to stitch closed any wound.

7. A hiker in your group has experienced a blow to the head. The group cannot decide whether to send someone immediately to call for emergency evacuation or to wait and see if the victim is well enough to walk out in a few hours. Which of the following signs and symptoms may indicate a more serious brain injury requiring medical treatment as soon as possible?

    a. Unequal pupils not responding to light

    b. Headache

    c. Warm, flushed skin

    d. Bleeding of the scalp

8. Guidelines for burn prevention when camping are based in part on which of the following?

    a. Lightning strikes are very common at campsites.

    b. Tents, sleeping bags and other camping gear are often highly flammable.

    c. Campfires usually flare up several hours after going "out."

    d. Burns from boiling water are more likely when cooking over a campfire.

9. A person with diabetes who is in a group of campers in a remote location should –

    a. tell others the signs and symptoms of a diabetic emergency and what to do.

    b. bring glucose or a sugar substance to take in case of hypoglycemia.

    c. monitor his or her blood sugar levels carefully.

    d. All of the above

10. Which of these types of cardiac arrest victims have been revived when CPR lasts longer than 30 minutes?

    a. Heart attack victims

    b. Trauma victims

    c. Drowning victims

    d. Stroke victims

Chapter 24 • Rescuing and Moving Victims

Chapter Preview

- Rescuing a Victim
- Multiple Victims
- Moving Victims

You are called to the equipment room, where an employee has been found unresponsive. He is lying on the floor beneath a rack of electrical equipment that he apparently was working on. Thinking he may have been electrocuted, you first make sure the power is turned off to this equipment, and then you check him and determine he is not breathing normally. Because he is lying on his side beneath overhanging equipment, however, you cannot give him chest compressions. Given the risk of a spinal injury, you know normally that you should not move him. What should you do?

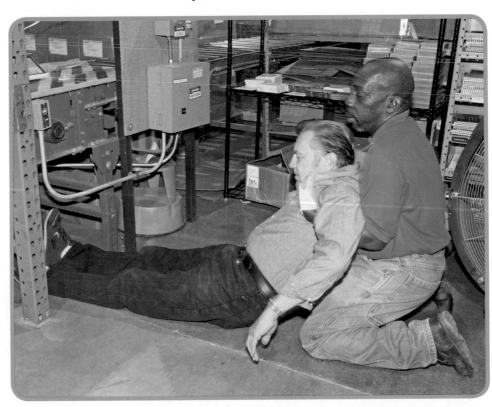

Before you can give first aid and basic life support (BLS), you have to reach the victim. If the scene is dangerous, you must stay away or take special precautions. Sometimes there is more than one victim and you have to decide whom to care for first. Sometimes the victim must be moved, if it is safe to do so, before you can give first aid. Never attempt any rescue or move a victim unless it is safe for both you and the victim.

Rescuing a Victim

Common situations involving victim rescue are fires, hazardous materials incidents, motor vehicle crashes and water rescues. Before entering any of these situations, however, be sure that it is safe to do so. If the scene is dangerous and you cannot safely approach the victim, *stay away and call for help*. The 9-1-1 dispatcher will send a crew with the appropriate training and equipment to safely reach and care for the victim. **Chapter 2** discusses scene safety in more detail. Safe rescues in most situations described in this chapter require

specialized training and gear. It is essential that you do only what you have been trained to do because otherwise you may become another victim that others will have to rescue.

Fire

If a victim needs rescue from a fire scene, do not approach unless you are certain it is safe to reach the victim. Smoke or fumes are usually present in fire situations and can easily overcome anyone entering the scene. Invisible gases resulting from fire pose a threat in both indoor and outdoor locations.

If a fire breaks out in your location, quick action is essential. Most important, evacuate others present and call 9-1-1. Do not enter an area of smoke or flames to search for victims, however, because of the high risk that you will be overcome by smoke or fumes. Do not remain in the area in an attempt to fight the fire unless the fire is very small, you have and know how to use a fire extinguisher, and you can flee safely if the fire gets out of control.

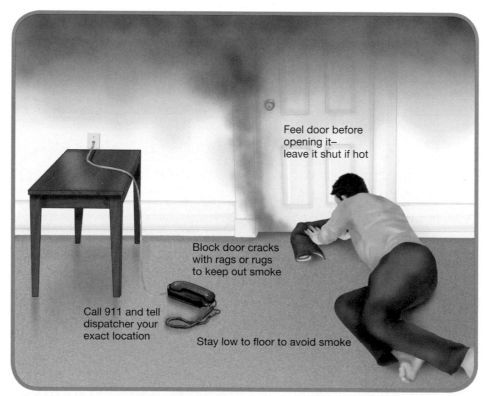

Feel door before opening it—leave it shut if hot

Block door cracks with rags or rugs to keep out smoke

Call 911 and tell dispatcher your exact location

Stay low to floor to avoid smoke

Figure 24-1 *If trapped in a building where there is a fire, take precautions to avoid smoke inhalation.*

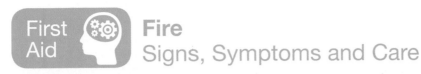

When You See

- **Flames or smoke**
- **A fire alarm sounding**

Do This First

1 Remove everyone from the area. Close doors behind you as you leave.

2 Call 9-1-1, set off alarms or follow other workplace protocols.

3 Use a fire extinguisher to combat a fire only if:
- The fire is small.
- You can easily and quickly escape the area.
- You know how to use the fire extinguisher.
- You can stay between the exit and the fire, so you can always get out safely.

4 Do not enter an area of flames and smoke in an attempt to rescue others.

5 If trapped inside:
- In a smoky room, crawl along the floor, where there is breathable air.
- Do not open a door that feels hot.
- Do not use elevators.
- If stuck inside, turn off the ventilation system, stuff towels or rags (wet if possible) into door cracks and vents, and use a phone to report your location.

ALERT

- Never put yourself at risk to rescue a victim.
- When hazards are present, leave the rescue to the professionals.
- Never try to perform any rescue technique you have not been trained to do.

If caught indoors in a smoky area, take action to avoid the smoke as much as possible by staying close to the floor (smoke rises), not opening doors, and preventing the entry of smoke through vents or door cracks (**Figure 24-1** and First Aid: "Fire"). See other guidelines in **Chapter 11**.

Hazardous Materials

Chapter 2 describes precautions to take around a spill of hazardous materials. Treat any unknown substance you see spilled as a hazard until proven otherwise. Avoid any spilled liquid or powder as well as possible fumes. Because the cleanup of hazardous materials takes special training, knowledge and equipment, leave this

to "hazmat" professionals. Do not enter a scene contaminated by hazardous materials to reach a victim. If a victim emerges from the spill area with potentially hazardous substances on clothing or skin, do not touch the victim because of the risk of contaminating yourself as well. If possible, use a water hose to wash the victim's skin and clothing before providing first aid. **Chapter 11** describes the first aid for chemicals on the skin. While waiting for help to arrive, cover a wet victim with a blanket or coats to preserve body warmth. Do not let anyone who has contacted a potentially hazardous material leave the area before EMS professionals arrive (see First Aid: "Hazardous Materials").

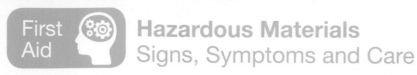

First Aid — Hazardous Materials
Signs, Symptoms and Care

When You See

- Warning signs or placards (with "flammable" or other warning terms) (see **Chapter 2**)
- Any spilled substance
- Visible vapors or fumes you can smell

Do This First

1 Stay out of the area and keep bystanders away.

2 Outside, stay upwind of the area to avoid possible fumes.

3 Call 9-1-1.

4 Approach the victim only if you are sure it is safe to do so. For a large exposure to hazardous materials, guide the victim to an emergency shower or rinse skin and clothing with a hose. Do only what you have been trained to do.

Additional Care

- If it is safe to reach the victim, move him or her away from the hazard and give first aid for a chemical burn or smoke inhalation (see **Chapter 11**).

Vehicle Crashes

Vehicle crash scenes can be extremely dangerous for rescuers because of the risks of passing traffic, fire, vehicle instability and other factors. Rescuers have been injured by unintentionally setting off an automatic airbag while trying to reach a victim. For all these reasons it is crucial to ensure that the scene is safe before approaching the vehicle and providing care for the victim.

If it is safe to reach the vehicle, do not try to remove a victim unless fire or another threat to life is likely. Call 9-1-1 as soon as you recognize a victim is present and describe the circumstances to the dispatcher so the appropriate rescue team is sent. Crash victims often have spinal or other injuries that could be made worse by moving the victim unnecessarily. Provide needed first aid through the door or window or from behind the driver's seat if the vehicle is stable and it is safe to approach (see First Aid: "Vehicle Crashes"). Because an unresponsive victim is likely to have a spinal injury, support the head and neck with your hands while waiting for help to arrive (see **Chapter 12**).

Water Rescues

Water rescues are often needed to prevent drowning. A nonswimmer may have gotten into deep water, or a swimmer may have sustained an injury or sudden illness, such as a heart attack or seizure, that prevents the person from reaching safety. Regardless of the reason, if someone in deep water cannot reach safety, immediate rescue may be required.

Preventing Drownings

As discussed in **Chapter 5**, drowning is a common cause of unintentional death in the United States, resulting in 3,700 deaths in a recent year and

(continues on page 398)

Vehicle Crashes
Signs, Symptoms and Care

When You See

- **A victim inside a motor vehicle after a crash**

Do This First

1 Stop a safe distance past the crash and turn on your vehicle's hazard lights.

2 Call 9-1-1 if you have a cell phone or ask someone else to call.

3 If available, set up warning triangles well back from the scene to warn oncoming traffic. Flares should be used only when there are no spilled chemicals and no chance of a grass fire.

4 Ensure that the scene is safe before you approach the crashed vehicle. Stay away if there are risks from passing traffic, downed electrical wires, fire or vehicle instability. Do not try to stabilize the vehicle unless you have special training.

5 If the vehicle is still running, ask the driver to turn off the ignition. If the driver is unresponsive and you can do so safely, reach in and turn off the ignition.

6 Do not try to remove a victim trapped inside a vehicle; wait for professional rescuers.

7 Assume that an unresponsive victim may have a neck injury. If the scene is safe, support the victim's head and neck with your hands.

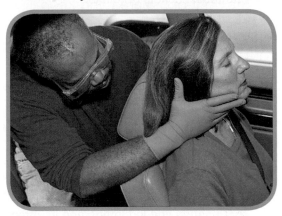

8 Do not move the victim unless there is an immediate threat of fire. If so, get several bystanders to help move the victim while you support the victim's head in line with the body the entire time.

9 Provide BLS and care for any serious injuries while waiting for help.

(continued from page 396)

about three times that many visits to emergency departments for treatment of near-drowning incidents. Near drowning can result in brain damage and other permanent disabilities. Drowning remains the second leading cause of injury-related death for children 1 to 14 years old. The CDC reports that the following are the most common risk factors for drowning:[1]

- Children younger than 1 most often drown in bathtubs, buckets or toilets.

- Among children 1 – 4 years old, most drownings occur in residential swimming pools. Most young children who drowned in pools were last seen in the home, had been out of sight less than 5 minutes and were in the care of one or both parents at the time.

- Alcohol use is involved in up to half of adolescent and adult deaths associated with water recreation. Alcohol influences balance, coordination and judgment, and its effects are heightened by sun exposure and heat.

- Boating carries risks for injury. In 2008, the U.S. Coast Guard received reports for 4,789 boating incidents; 3,331 boating participants were reported injured and 709 killed. Most boating fatalities (72%) were caused by drowning, and the remainder were due to trauma, hypothermia, carbon monoxide poisoning or other causes. Alcohol was involved in about one-fifth of reported boating fatalities. In boating deaths, 90% of victims were not wearing life jackets.

Following are guidelines to help prevent drowning by children:

- Never leave children alone near water. Do not leave small children alone in a bathtub or wading pool.

- Do not let children dive in shallow, murky or unknown water.

[1]*Centers for Disease Control and Prevention, http://www. cdc.gov/HomeandRecreationalSafety/Water-Safety/ waterinjuries-factsheet.html Accessed March 4, 2011.*

- At open waterfronts, keep children away from areas with big waves, undertows and boats.

- Both children and adults should use personal flotation devices (PFDs) on boats and around water.

- In public swimming areas, let children enter the water only where lifeguards are present.

- Make sure rescue floats and other devices are present at pools and other water areas.

- At appropriate ages children should learn from a qualified instructor to swim and to be safe in the water.

- Adult supervisors should realize that even children who can swim are not "drown-proof."

- Do not let older siblings or babysitters supervise children in the water.

- Most important, when supervising children in or near water, avoid all distractions. Do not read, eat or socialize with others. Most children drown when being "supervised" by someone who is not paying close attention.

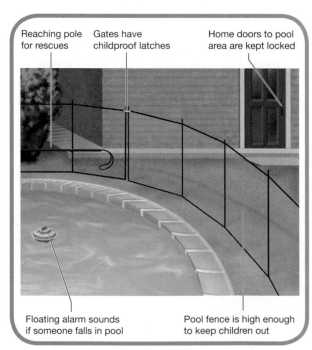

Reaching pole for rescues

Gates have childproof latches

Home doors to pool area are kept locked

Floating alarm sounds if someone falls in pool

Pool fence is high enough to keep children out

Figure 24-2 *Make a residential swimming pool safe for children with preventive devices.*

- Childproof home pools with appropriate fencing, gates, floating pool alarms and other safety devices (Figure 24-2).

Adults also should practice water safety principles to prevent drowning:

- Never drink or use other drugs when in or on the water. This includes when boating.

- Always wear a PFD when boating, even when in calm water and well away from the edge of the boat. No one ever plans to fall into the water – drowning usually occurs when the victim feels sure that a PFD is not needed.

- Dive into water only in depths of 9 feet or more when the water is clear and no obstructions are present.

- Do not swim alone.

- Consider your swimming ability before attempting a swim out to a float or boat to ensure that you are not exhausted before reaching safety. Consider waves and other conditions.

- Be aware that swimming in cold water can lead to hypothermia, which may lead to drowning.

- Be prepared for an emergency. Keep CPR skills fresh, and have a telephone handy when supervising others in the water.

Safe Techniques for Water Rescue

Rescuing someone at risk of drowning in deep water first requires recognizing that the person needs help. There are common misconceptions about how drowning victims act: you should not expect the victim to shout for help, nor is it true that "going down for the third time" is a prelude to drowning.

Recognizing a drowning situation depends on understanding three general scenarios of how people drown:

- **People who can swim**, or "dog paddle," or float well enough to keep their head above water at least for a time, may gradually or suddenly be at risk for drowning. A swimmer may become too tired to keep swimming or hypothermia may set in and weaken the victim. If the problem develops gradually, the person may be in trouble but not yet actively drowning. This type of victim may call for help in some circumstances or may be able to keep his or her head above water but unable to make progress to safety. Because it can be difficult sometimes to know whether someone in this situation needs help, it is better to offer assistance than to wait until it is obvious that the person is drowning.

- **A responsive drowning victim** cannot swim, float or tread water effectively and is at immediate risk for drowning. This victim is struggling just to keep his or her head out of the water and is in a panicked state. This victim is very unlikely to call for help. You may see the victim's face just above the surface or bobbing in and out, and his or her arms may be flailing. The victim is clearly struggling, however, rather than treading water or moving forward.

- **An unresponsive drowning victim** is no longer breathing. This victim may be a swimmer who became too exhausted to tread water or even float, a nonswimmer who can no longer keep his or her face up to breathe and has stopped struggling, or a swimmer or nonswimmer who has experienced an injury or sudden illness (such as heart attack or hypothermia) that prevented him or her from swimming or staying at the surface, resulting in submersion and respiratory arrest. Breathing stops either when water enters the lungs or when water in the larynx causes a spasm that closes the airway. When breathing stops, the victim soon becomes unresponsive. Depending on the victim's body composition and the presence or absence of air in the lungs, this victim may be floating face-down at the surface or may be underwater.

When you recognize any of these scenarios, quick action is needed to rescue the victim. Your choice of rescue technique depends on the type of situation, the equipment or objects at hand, and the circumstances. Resist the temptation to jump immediately into the water to save the victim. An actively drowning victim is in a state of panic that often leads to the victim grabbing you so forcefully and desperately that you may become a drowning victim yourself. The victim may grab your head or arms in a way that you can neither swim back to safety nor tread water to keep both of you afloat. Lifeguards receive special training in how to manage such victims: they are trained to keep a rescue tube between themselves and the victim to avoid being grabbed and also to break a victim's hold underwater should it become necessary.

Even a tired swimmer who is not yet struggling and panicking may become panicked before you reach him or her. Therefore, it is a poor choice to swim out to assist this kind of victim as well.

It may be appropriate to swim to an unresponsive victim, however, if you have no other means to get the victim quickly out of the water so that you can give CPR if needed. Similarly, a responsive small child may be rescued by an adult who is a good swimmer – although even children may cling tenaciously to one's head or arms when panicked, making a swimming rescue difficult or dangerous for the adult.

The safest and often most effective rescue technique is to reach to the victim with some object that the victim can grasp while you pull him or her to safety. The second most safe and effective technique is to throw something that floats to the victim, preferably with a rope attached for pulling the victim to safety. Third, and least safe and effective, is to go to the victim yourself. This is called the **reach-throw-go** priority, which emphasizes which techniques to try first.

"Reach" Rescue

Most public and some private pools have a rescue pole, which often has a hook at the end (called a **shepherd's crook**). This pole is usually long enough to reach a victim from the edge of the pool. Let a responsive victim hold onto it while you slowly pull the victim to the edge **(Figure 24-3)**. If the victim is unresponsive, you can hook the victim's body to pull the victim to the edge or shallow water. Unless the unresponsive victim is a small child, pulling an unresponsive victim to the edge will be faster than jumping in to tow the victim to the pool's edge.

Use anything available to reach to the victim. A residential pool may not have a reaching pole, but a broom or rake handle may work just as well. In open-water settings you may use a fishing pole, a boat's oar or even a long branch. If the victim is close enough to the pool's edge, a dock

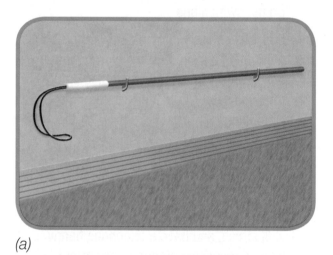

(a)

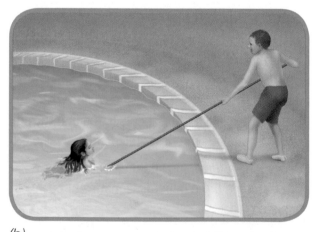

(b)

Figure 24-3 *(a) Shepherd's crook. (b) Pulling a victim to safety using a "reach" rescue.*

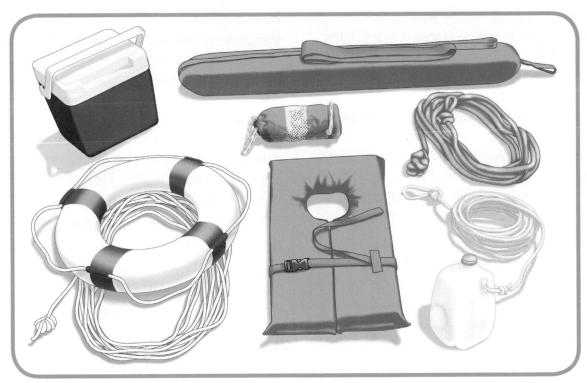

Figure 24-4 *Rescue devices and objects that can be thrown to a drowning victim.*

or the shore, you may also reach with your own body; for example, you could hold onto something secure with your arms and extend your legs on the surface to the victim.

In a natural-water setting in which the water gradually gets deeper from the shore, you may be able to reach to the victim with an object after wading a short distance into the water. If possible, stay in water shallow enough for you to stand on the bottom while reaching to the victim.

"Throw" Rescue

If you cannot reach to the victim, look for anything that floats that you can throw. Swimming pool or boating equipment may include a life ring, rescue tube, life jacket or other device **(Figure 24-4)**. Some boats carry a "throw bag", which has a coiled rope inside that uncoils when the bag is thrown to a victim while you hold the other end. If no throwable rescue device is available, look around for anything that will float – such as a buoyant seat cushion, a water jug that can be mostly emptied (keep some water inside to give it weight for throwing) or even an empty beverage cooler.

If a rope is already attached to the throwable device (or can quickly be tied on), hold it in one hand, coil the rope loosely and throw with your stronger arm. Try to throw it over the victim so that the line comes down beside the person and can be easily grasped **(Figure 24-5)**.

If you have no rope handy for the throw device, throw it to the victim anyway if it is buoyant enough to help the victim keep his or her head above water. A victim who can float by holding

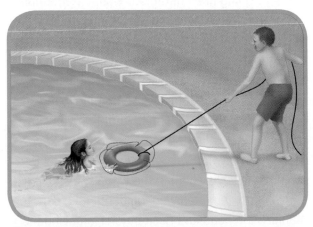

Figure 24-5 *Throw the rescue device where the victim can grab it or the rope.*

onto something can breathe more easily and may have the strength to kick to shore while holding the object. Even if the victim is too weak to do anything but just hold on, the thrown object can keep the victim safely afloat while you find a rope or something to reach with. Even if you must enter the water to go to the victim, a victim who is holding onto something that floats is much less likely to panic and grab you, and you can more easily tow the object and victim to safety.

In a natural-water setting in which the water gradually gets deeper from the shore, you may be better able to throw a rope or floating object to the victim after wading out into the water to get closer to the victim. If possible, stay in water shallow enough for you to stand on the bottom while throwing to the victim.

"Go" Rescue

As noted earlier, swimming to rescue a responsive victim is very dangerous – so much so that unless you have training, you should not attempt this except with a small child or unresponsive victim. Look for other ways to go to the victim. At a waterfront you may find a surfboard, kayak or other watercraft in which to go to the victim. Even if it is too small to support both of you, it likely has enough buoyancy to keep you both afloat until help arrives or the victim may be able to hold onto it for buoyancy while you tow him or her to shore. Wear a life jacket when entering the water or going in a boat to the victim. Remember that the victim is likely panicking, and keep the object between you and the victim so you cannot be grabbed and pulled underwater. The same is true if you decide to swim to a responsive victim: If at all possible take something with you that the victim can hold on to, and that you can release if the victim tries to grab you, and keep the object between you and the victim. Note: if an unresponsive victim in the water may have a spinal injury (e.g., a diving incident), take care to stabilize the head and neck before removing the victim from the water, if possible.

Walking Assist

Many natural bodies of water gradually get deeper away from the shore. If a responsive victim in the water is at a depth where he or she can stand or if you can assist the victim to that depth, you can help the victim to exit the water with a **walking assist (Figure 24-6)**. Put the victim's arm around your shoulder and hold it at the wrist with your hand. Put your other arm around the victim's waist and support the victim as you walk the person out of the water.

Beach Drag

An unresponsive victim who is in or can be brought to shallow water that has a gradual shoreline can be taken from the water using a **beach drag (Figure 24-7)**. Reach under the victim's shoulders and hold the victim at the armpits, resting the victim's head on your forearms (and preventing head or neck movement in case of a possible spinal injury). Then slowly back out of the water, dragging the victim out. This rescue technique is similar to the shoulder drag used to move an unresponsive victim on land from a hazardous scene, shown later in this chapter.

If Stranded in Cold Water

If you are immersed in cold water and cannot swim to safety or climb out of the water onto an overturned boat or other floating object, try to

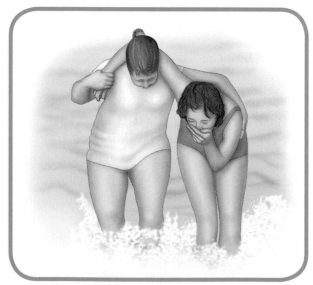

Figure 24-6 *Walking assist.*

minimize heat loss from your body while awaiting rescue. If alone, use the "heat escape lessening position" (HELP): hold your arms close to your sides, raise your knees to your chest and remain as still as possible **(Figure 24-8)**.

Two or more people together in cold water should use the "huddle position" to conserve heat: Everyone puts arms around each others' shoulders to bring the sides of their chests together (if three or more) in a tight circle **(Figure 24-9)**. Children should be sandwiched between adults.

Ice Rescue

As described in **Chapter 2**, ice rescues are very dangerous. Cold-water immersion is very serious and can quickly doom even the best swimmers. Ice rescue should be left for specially trained personnel who have the necessary safety equipment. Call 9-1-1 immediately to summon emergency personnel.

If it is safe to do so and emergency personnel will not arrive in time, you may attempt an ice rescue using the same priorities as a water rescue: reach-throw-go. Try first to reach to a victim who has broken through ice using a pole or tree limb **(Figure 24-10)**. If you cannot reach to the victim, throw a rope or any buoyant object tied

to a rope. As a last resort, throw any object that will float to help the victim stay afloat, but be aware that in icy water hypothermia sets in very quickly and the victim will not be able to hold on to an object very long. Only as an extreme last

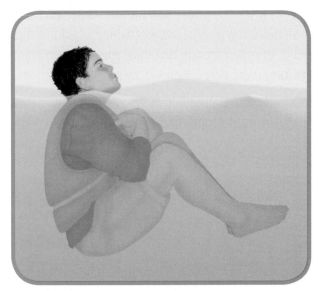

Figure 24-8 *The "HELP" position to minimize body heat loss.*

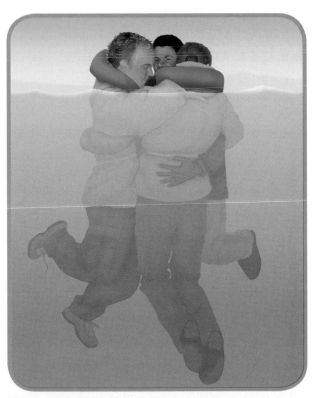

Figure 24-9 *The "huddle" position to minimize body heat loss.*

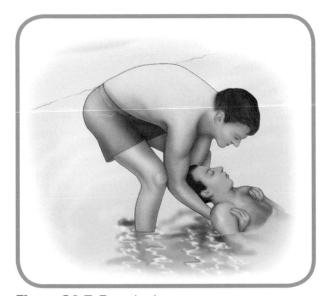

Figure 24-7 *Beach drag.*

resort should you try to go to the victim yourself. Realize that the ice may not hold your weight and that you too may become a victim. If you must go on the ice, lie down to distribute your weight over a larger surface area. Another person should hold your feet and be prepared to pull you out if the ice under you breaks. If possible, push a branch or other object ahead of you to the victim to minimize the distance you must go onto the ice.

Following ice rescue, the victim is likely to need treatment for hypothermia **(Chapter 20)**.

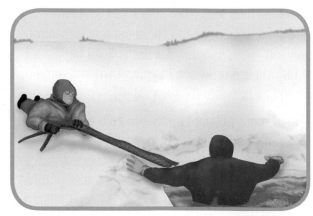

Figure 24-10 *Try to reach to a victim who has fallen through ice.*

Learning Checkpoint 1

1. During a fire, the first action to take is –
   a. get everyone out and call 9-1-1.
   b. throw water on the fire immediately.
   c. use a fire extinguisher.
   d. close all doors and windows.

2. If you are caught in a building that is on fire –
   a. stay low to the floor.
   b. feel doors before opening them.
   c. use stairs, not the elevator.
   d. All of the above

3. True or False: OSHA requires fire prevention and safety guidelines in the workplace.

4. True or False: The first action to take for a spilled dry chemical is to vacuum it up.

5. True or False: Spilled liquids may produce poisonous fumes.

6. You are the first on the scene where a car has crashed into a telephone pole. After you make sure that the scene is safe, you approach the car and find the driver alone, slumped forward against the steering wheel and unresponsive. What can you do to help?

   _____

   _____

7. The safest order in which to attempt a water rescue is –
   a. throw-reach-go.
   b. go-throw-reach.
   c. reach-throw-go.
   d. reach-go-throw.

Multiple Victims

An incident such as a car crash or a workplace explosion may involve multiple victims who need first aid. In such a case the first thing you must do, after calling 9-1-1 to get help on the way, is decide who needs your care most and who can wait until others can help. This process of setting priorities is called **triage (Figure 24-11)**.

Triage systems usually put each victim into one of four categories **(Table 24-1)**. Because the goal of triage is to determine which victim(s) require immediate care, this process should be done very quickly. As you check the scene for safety and approach, ask who can walk and have these victims move to one side – they are the third priority. Try to assess each of the remaining victims in less than a minute by checking for responsiveness, breathing and severe bleeding;

do not start to give care to any victim until you have quickly checked all victims. If a victim is very severely injured and is not breathing, and other victims require your immediate care, you should attend to others who you judge can be saved. This situation can require a difficult decision, but remember that giving BLS to an obviously dying victim may mean that someone who could have been saved may not be.

Because a victim's condition may change during the process of triage or giving care, you may have to change priorities. For example, if you are treating a second-priority victim with a fracture, another victim who at first seemed to have only minor injuries (third priority) may suddenly become unresponsive and require your immediate attention (first priority) to maintain an open airway (see First Aid: "Multiple Victims").

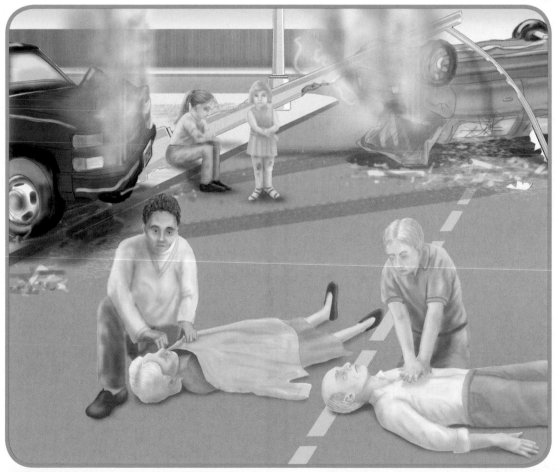

Figure 24-11 *In an emergency with multiple victims, first determine which victim is the highest priority for first aid.*

Table 24-1: Triage Priorities for Multiple Victims

Priority	Victim's Condition	Severity	Examples
First	Critical	Victims with life-threatening injuries who cannot wait for help.	Breathing problems Severe bleeding Shock Severe burn
Second	Serious	Victims with injuries that need care very soon but who may be able to wait for help.	Burns Broken bones Other injuries not severely bleeding
Third	Stable	Victims who can wait for some time.	Minor injuries Victims who can walk
Fourth	Obviously dead or dying	Victims who cannot be saved.	Not breathing with massive head or chest trauma with severe blood loss

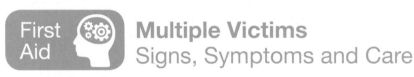

First Aid

Multiple Victims
Signs, Symptoms and Care

When You See

- **Two or more victims needing care**

Do This First

1 Call 9-1-1 immediately. Tell the dispatcher there are multiple victims.

2 Ask any victims who can walk (third priority) to move to one side. These victims do not have immediate life-threatening problems.

3 For the remaining victims, starting with unresponsive victims, quickly check for normal breathing and severe bleeding, looking for life-threatening injuries in victims who can be saved (first priority). Spend a minute or less with each victim and do not start giving care until you have checked all victims.

4 Start providing BLS to first-priority victims first. Move to second-priority victims only when the first-priority victims are stable. Ask any bystanders with first aid training to help you with other victims.

5 When help arrives, quickly tell the EMS professionals about the victims present. Offer to help them care for victims.

Learning **Checkpoint 2**

1. True or False: A victim with a broken arm is a second priority in a multiple-victim incident.

2. True or False: Victims with life-threatening injuries are first priority in a multiple-victim incident.

3. You are the lone responder at a construction site where a collapsed wall has injured four workers. Using standard triage priorities, rank these four in terms of who gets care first, second, third and fourth:

_____ a. A woman with a bruised face and abrasions on her arms, who is walking around holding her bleeding forehead

_____ b. A man on the ground with no apparent external injuries but who is unresponsive

_____ c. A man who is not breathing, whose chest has caved in under a steel beam and who is surrounded by a pool of blood

_____ d. A man sitting up and leaning against the rubble, looking very pale, who says he feels nauseous

Moving Victims

Moving an injured victim is more likely to cause further injury than not. In most cases you should wait for professionals who have training and equipment to transport the victim to advanced medical care.

In some instances, however, you must move a victim to protect him or her from a danger at the scene, such as a spreading fire, the chance of an explosion or a structure at risk of collapse **(Figure 24-12)**. *Remember: Never enter a scene*

(continues on page 410)

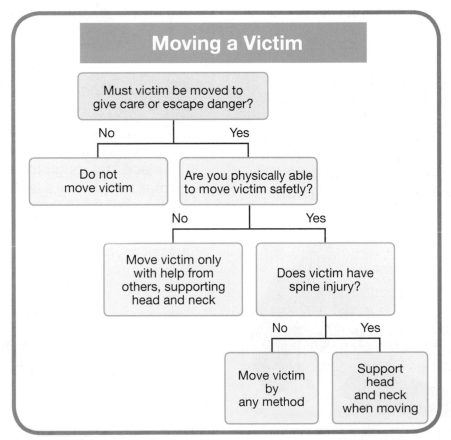

Figure 24-12 *Moving a victim.*

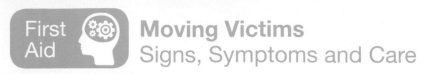

First Aid

Moving Victims
Signs, Symptoms and Care

When You See

Consider moving a victim only if:

- **Fire or explosion is likely.**
- **Poisonous fumes may be present.**
- **The structure may collapse.**
- **The victim needs to be moved into position for life-saving care such as CPR.**
- **The victim is in the way of another seriously injured victim.**

Do This First

1 Try to move the victim only if you are physically able and can do it safely.

2 Get help from others at the scene.

3 For an unresponsive victim or a victim with a spinal injury, support the head and neck in line with the body during the move.

4 Use good body mechanics.

5 If alone:

For an unresponsive victim with suspected spinal injury:

- For a short distance, use the shoulder drag (supporting the victim's head against your chest) or the clothes drag (supporting the victim's head with clothing taut between your hands).

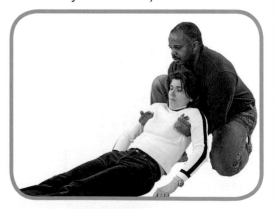

- Use the blanket drag to support the victim's head for a longer distance.

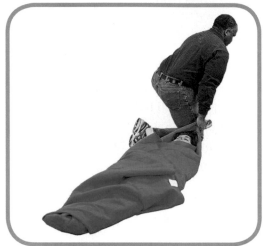

For an unresponsive victim without a spinal injury:

- The ankle drag is easier to use for short distances over a smooth surface (not rough terrain) and by a small rescuer for a large victim.

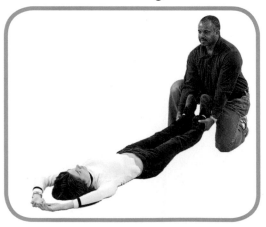

Moving Victims (continued)

For a responsive victim who can walk with help:

- Use the one- or two-person walking assist.

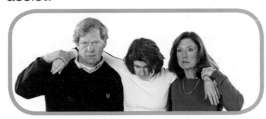

For an unresponsive victim who cannot safely be moved with a drag (if you are strong enough to lift the victim):

- Use the packstrap carry.

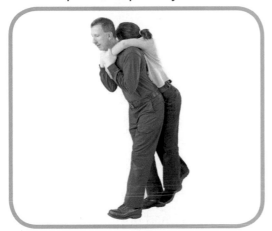

For a lighter victim or child:

- Use a cradle carry for responsive or unresponsive victims.

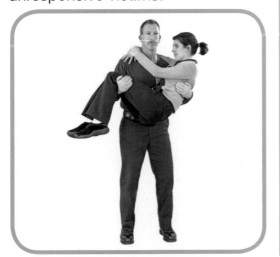

- Use a piggyback carry for responsive victims.

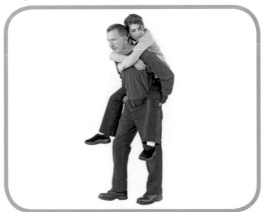

6 With the help of one or more others:

For a responsive victim:

- Use the two-person assist or two-handed seat carry.

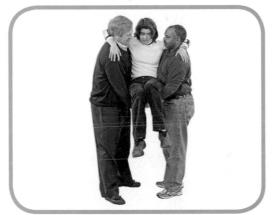

For an unresponsive victim:

- Use three to six rescuers with the hammock carry.

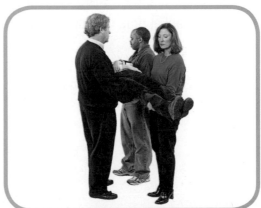

(continued from page 407)

unless you can do so safely. You may have to move one victim to reach another victim who has a life-threatening condition. You may also have to move a victim to a firm, flat surface to provide CPR. If you decide to move a victim, several factors are involved in choosing the best method (see First Aid: "Moving Victims"):

- How quickly must the victim be moved?
- Does the victim's condition affect the move (nature of injury, responsiveness, potential spinal injury, etc.)?
- Are others present who can help with the move?
- Is any equipment (e.g., stretcher) or other object (e.g., blanket) needed?
- Do you have the physical strength needed to move the victim?

Whenever you lift a victim, be sure to use good body mechanics. This means:

- Do not try to lift more weight than you can lift without straining.
- Lift with your legs instead of your back. Keep your feet shoulder-width apart with one foot in front of the other. Keep your back straight and crouch down, then lift by straightening your legs.
- Do not turn or twist your back while bearing weight.
- Bear the victim's weight as close to your trunk as possible.
- Take short steps and move forward rather than backward.

Learning Checkpoint 3

1. Check situations in which you should consider moving a victim:

_____ Fire is present   _____ Bleeding victim inside a car

_____ Cold environment   _____ Strong smell of natural gas in the room

_____ Small child with severe burns   _____ The hospital is only a short drive

_____ A victim going into shock   _____ A victim is lying on top of another

2. If you have to move an unresponsive injured victim by yourself, an effective method would be to –

  a. sling the victim over your shoulder.

  b. roll the victim over the ground like a log.

  c. grab both of the victim's wrists and pull him or her along.

  d. use a blanket drag to support the victim's head.

Concluding Thoughts

Remember that your own safety must be ensured before rescuing or moving a victim in any situation. Pause to think and plan before acting, and then move carefully to protect both yourself and the victim from further injury.

Learning Outcomes

You should now be able to do the following:

1. Describe how to rescue or care for a victim in each of the following emergencies:

   - A fire scene
   - A potential drowning situation
   - A hazardous materials incident
   - Broken ice
   - A vehicle crash

2. Describe how to prioritize care for multiple victims with different types of injuries.

3. Explain when it may be necessary to move a victim.

4. Demonstrate the following emergency moves:

   - Shoulder drag
   - Packstrap carry
   - Clothes drag
   - Cradle carry
   - Ankle drag
   - Piggyback carry
   - Blanket drag
   - Two-handed seat carry
   - Walking assist
   - Hammock carry with multiple rescuers

Review Questions

1. If the emergency scene is very dangerous, you should –

   a. run in quickly and give lifesaving care to the victim.

   b. run in quickly and pull the victim to safety.

   c. call 9-1-1 and wait for professionals with appropriate training and equipment.

   d. rescue the victim if help has not arrived 5 minutes after calling 9-1-1.

2. It is safe to enter the scene of a fire when –

   a. you can keep at least 15 feet away from flames.

   b. you can crouch below the smoke to breathe.

   c. you know a victim inside needs help.

   d. It is never safe to enter a fire scene.

3. Which of these statements is true?

   a. Poisonous fumes from a spilled substance are always visible.

   b. Poisonous fumes are not present if you see "normal" black smoke at a fire.

   c. Dangerous fumes are lighter than air and always rise to the ceiling.

   d. Invisible dangerous fumes may be present at any fire or hazardous materials spill.

4. Which action is appropriate for a victim of a vehicle crash with suspected spinal injury?

   a. Support the victim's head in place with your hands, remaining in the vehicle.

   b. Support the victim's head in place with your hands while you help the victim to exit the vehicle.

   c. Use a splint to support the victim's head while you help the victim to exit the vehicle.

   d. Use the clothes drag to support the victim's head while you pull the victim from the vehicle.

5. How can you tell if someone in the water may be drowning?

   a. The person is swimming only slowly toward a destination.

   b. The person is struggling to keep his or her mouth above the water.

   c. The person calls out for help.

   d. The person waves both arms high above his or her head.

6. Which water rescue technique should you try first?

   a. Throwing a rope to the victim

   b. Throwing the victim a ring buoy with a rope tied to it

   c. Reaching to the victim with a pole or tree branch

   d. Swimming to the victim with a flotation device

7. When you are alone and encounter a vehicle crash scene with four victims, which of these victims should you help first?

   a. The driver, who is slumped over the wheel and not breathing, his chest bloody, with a pool of blood on the seat beside him

   b. A front-seat passenger who has a cut on the forehead and a sprained wrist, who gets out of the vehicle as you approach

   c. An unresponsive rear-seat passenger with no visible injuries who is not breathing

   d. A responsive rear-seat passenger who says she thinks her leg is broken

8. How you move a victim in an emergency may depend on –

   a. whether the victim is in shock.

   b. whether others are present.

   c. whether you have medical examination gloves with you.

   d. whether the victim is wearing a medical ID.

9. Which of these emergency moves provides the best head and neck support for an unresponsive victim with a suspected spinal injury?

   a. Clothes drag

   b. Ankle drag

   c. Cradle carry

   d. Piggyback carry

10. Good body mechanics includes –

   a. lifting with your legs rather than your back.

   b. not twisting your back when carrying weight.

   c. taking short steps.

   d. All of the above

Chapter 25 • Are You Prepared?

Chapter Preview

- Before an Emergency Strikes
- After an Emergency Strikes
- Evacuation
- Natural Disasters

- Biological Threats
- Chemical Threats
- Nuclear Explosions and Radiological Contamination
- Recovering from an Emergency

It is late Saturday afternoon, and you have been so busy doing household chores that you have barely noticed the thunderstorm moving in from the west. You glance out a window and see the sky is turning black. You remember you left the car windows open and go out to raise them before the rain starts, and as you come around the corner of the house you see a funnel cloud apparently less than a mile away. What should you do?

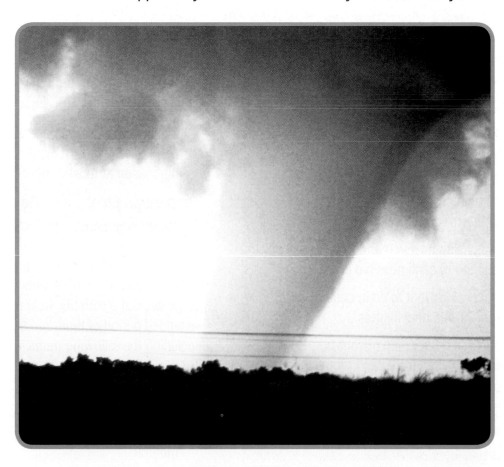

This guide[1] will help you to

- learn what to do before, during and after an emergency.

- create an emergency plan for your family.

- prepare an Emergency Go Kit.

Before an Emergency Strikes

During an emergency, you and your family may have little or no time to plan what to do next. You must learn about the things you can do to be prepared before an emergency occurs. Two actions that will help you to do this are to develop an emergency plan and to prepare an Emergency Go Kit.

Create an Emergency Plan

Part of creating your household emergency plan is to learn about the types of emergencies that may affect your community, how you will be notified of an emergency and plans that may already be in place to deal with emergencies. Determine if your community has a warning system – via television, radio or another signal – and learn what it sounds like and what to do when you hear it. Emergencies may strike when your family members are away from home, so find out about plans at your workplace, school or anywhere else you and your family spend time. Steps to take in creating a household emergency plan include:

1. Meeting with household members to discuss the dangers of possible emergency events, including fire, severe weather, hazardous spills and terrorism

2. Discussing how you and your family will respond to each possible emergency

3. Discussing what to do in case of power outages or personal injuries

4. Drawing a floor plan of your home. Mark two escape routes from each room

[1]This chapter is adapted from the "A Federal Employee's Family Preparedness Guide" prepared by the United States Office of Personnel Management, August 2005. http://www.opm.gov/emergency/pdf/NationalFamilyGuide.pdf Accessed March 1, 2011.

5. Teaching adults how to turn off the water, gas and electricity at main switches. If for any reason you turn off natural gas service to your home, call your gas utility company to restore service. *Do not attempt to restore gas service yourself*

6. Posting emergency contact numbers near all telephones and pre-programming emergency numbers into phones with autodial capabilities

7. Teaching children how and when to dial 9-1-1 to get emergency assistance

8. Teaching children how to make long-distance telephone calls and/or to use a cell phone

9. Choosing a friend or relative that all family members will call if separated (it is often easier to call out of state during an emergency than within the affected areas)

10. Instructing household members to turn on the radio for emergency information

11. Picking two meeting places:
    - A place near your home
    - A place outside your neighborhood in case you cannot return home after an emergency

12. Taking a first aid and CPR class

13. Keeping family records in a waterproof and fireproof safe. Inexpensive models can be purchased at most hardware stores.

Prepare an Emergency Go Kit

During an emergency, electricity, water, heat, air conditioning or telephone service may not work. Preparing an Emergency Go Kit ahead of time can save precious time in the event you must evacuate or go without electricity, heat or water for an extended period of time. You should consider including the following items in an Emergency Go Kit:

1. At least a three-day supply of water (one gallon per person per day). Store water in sealed, unbreakable containers. Replace every six months.

2. A three- to five-day supply of nonperishable packaged or canned food and a nonelectric can opener.

3. A change of clothing, rain gear and sturdy shoes.

4. Blankets, bedding or sleeping bags.

5. A first aid kit and prescription medications (be sure to check the expiration dates).

6. An extra pair of glasses or contact lenses and solution (be sure to check the expiration dates).

7. A list of family physicians, important medical information, and the style and serial number of medical devices such as pacemakers.

8. Special items for infants, the elderly or family members with disabilities.

9. A battery-powered radio, flashlight and plenty of extra batteries (or a hand-cranked radio and flashlight).

10. Identification, credit cards, cash and photocopies of important family documents, including home insurance information.

11. An extra set of car and house keys.

12. Tools such as screwdrivers, cutters and scissors, duct tape, waterproof matches, a fire extinguisher, flares, plastic storage containers, needle and thread, pen and paper, a compass, garbage bags and regular household bleach.

Know the Plans of Your School System

If you have a child who attends school, it is important for you to contact your school system administrators to understand fully what plans are in place to protect your child in the event of an emergency.

Be sure to keep the contact information for your child up to date. Provide your school administrators with a list of family members or caregivers whom you authorize to pick up your child or children at school.

If a dangerous substance were released in the atmosphere and posed a threat to students during the school day, it is very likely that the schools affected would shelter-in-place and protect children and staff by keeping them inside and moving them to safer areas within the school building.

Prescriptions

Store three to five days' worth of medications that are important to your health.

Include any medications that are used to stabilize a medical condition or keep a condition from worsening or resulting in hospitalization, such as medications for asthma, seizures, cardiovascular disorders, diabetes, psychiatric conditions, HIV and thyroid disorders.

Carry these with you, if possible, in a purse or briefcase in labeled containers. Rotate these medications whenever you get your prescriptions refilled. If your child takes medications, communicate with the school to discuss their emergency preparedness plans.

People with complex medication regimens should talk to their physician and pharmacist to help with emergency preparation plans. Such regimens include injectable medications, including those delivered by pumps (e.g., insulin, analgesics, chemotherapy, parenteral nutrition); medications delivered by a nebulizer (e.g., antibiotics, bronchodilators); and dialysis.

Neighbors Helping Neighbors

Working with neighbors in an emergency can save lives and property. Meet with your community members to plan how you could work together until help arrives. If you are a member of a neighborhood organization, such as a home association or crime watch group, introduce emergency preparedness as a new activity.

If You Have Pets

If you evacuate, avoid leaving family pets behind. However, keep in mind that with the exception of service animals, pets are generally not permitted in emergency shelters for health reasons.

For this reason, find out before a disaster occurs which hotels or motels (both within and outside your local area) allow pets. Determine where pet boarding facilities are located.

Create an emergency kit for your pet. This should include:

- Identification tag and rabies tags worn on a collar at all times

- Carrier or cage

- Leash

- Any medications (be sure to check expiration date)

- Newspapers and plastic bags for handling waste

- A supply of food, bottled water and food bowls

- Veterinary records (most animal boarding facilities do not allow pets without proof of vaccination)

For complete information, the American Society for the Prevention of Cruelty to Animals has an emergency preparedness guide designed specifically for pets at http://www.aspca.org/site/PageServer?pagename=emergency.

After an Emergency Strikes

Shelter-in-Place

In the event of an emergency such as the release of a hazardous material, it is not always recommended that you immediately evacuate, because leaving your house might expose you to harmful agents that have been dispersed into the air. "Sheltering-in-place," which means simply staying in your house or current location, may be the best way to avoid harm. Federal agencies have protocols in place at every agency to shelter-in-place at the workplace if circumstances warrant that action. Federal employees can ask their managers for more information about the procedures in place at their agency.

If Your Power Goes Out

1. Remain calm and assist family members or neighbors who may be vulnerable if exposed to extreme heat or cold.

2. Locate a flashlight with batteries to use until power comes back on. Do not use candles – this can cause a fire.

3. Turn off sensitive electric equipment such as computers and televisions.

4. Turn off major electric appliances that were on when the power went off. This will help prevent power surges when electricity is restored.

5. Keep your refrigerator and freezer doors closed as much as possible to keep cold in and heat out.

6. Do not use the stove to heat your home.

7. Use extreme caution when driving. If traffic signals are out, treat each signal as a stop sign – come to a complete stop at every intersection and look before you proceed.

8. Do not call 9-1-1 to ask about the power outage.

9. Listen to news radio stations for updates.

If You Need Clean Water

Flooding can cause contamination of water supplies. Contaminated water can contain micro-organisms that cause diseases such as dysentery, typhoid and hepatitis. If you think your water may be contaminated, you should purify it before using it. This includes water used for drinking, cooking, cleaning dishes or bathing. The best way to purify water is to boil it.

THINGS TO THINK ABOUT…

If any members of your household have disabilities or are elderly, find out what services may be available to aid in their care or evacuation in the event of an emergency.

Boiling

Boiling is considered the safest method of purifying water. Bring water to a boil for three to five minutes and then allow it to cool before drinking. Pouring water back and forth between two containers will improve the taste by putting oxygen back into the water.

Evacuation

If you are notified or become aware of a technological hazards emergency such as a hazardous spill/release, fire or explosion, do not panic. If you need to get out of the surrounding area or are directed to evacuate, do so immediately and:

- Take your Emergency Go Kit.
- Lock your home.
- Cover your nose and mouth with a wet cloth.
- Travel on routes specified by local authorities.
- Head upwind of the incident.

If you are sure you have time:

- Shut off water, gas and electricity before leaving.
- Post a note telling others when you left and where you are going.
- Make arrangements for your pets.

If you are instructed to stay inside and not to evacuate:

- Close and lock windows and doors.
- Seal gaps under doorways and windows with wet towels or seal with plastic and duct tape.
- Turn off ventilation systems.

Prepare Your Evacuation Routes in Advance

Many major cities have established evacuation routes that can be used to effectively move people from heavily populated areas in the event of an emergency. For instance, the city of Washington, D.C. has identified 14 major arterials that will be used for outbound traffic only. During a major event or emergency situation, radial evacuation routes featuring traffic signals will be timed. In addition, critical intersections on evacuation routes will be manned with uniformed police officers to expedite the flow of traffic and to prevent bottlenecks. Officers will be able to direct drivers to alternate routes should an emergency warrant the closing of current event/evacuation routes.

If you work or live in a heavily populated area, you should prepare in advance the best available routes for you to use in the event that you need to quickly leave the area. Contact your local police or other local emergency preparedness offices for protocols that will be in place in your area during an evacuation.

Natural Disasters

Many areas are vulnerable to a variety of types of severe weather, including thunderstorms, hurricanes, flash floods, snowstorms and tornadoes (see Appendices C, D, E and F).

It is important for you to understand the difference between a watch and a warning for severe weather. A severe storm watch means that severe weather may develop. A severe weather warning means a storm has developed and is on its way, and you should take cover immediately.

The safest place to ride out any storm is inside a secure building or well-built home. Even in a well-built apartment building, you should –

- listen to weather updates and stay informed.
- be ready to evacuate if necessary.
- keep away from windows and doors.
- have your Emergency Go Kit handy.

Tornadoes are dangerous because of their high winds and ability to lift and move heavy objects. If you receive a tornado warning, seek shelter immediately. If you are in your car:

- *Stop!* Get out and lie flat, face-down, in a low area.
- Cover your head and wait for the tornado to pass.

If you are at home:

- Go to the basement or storm shelter or rooms near the center of the house.

In a high-rise or other public building:

- Move to the interior, preferably a stairwell or hallway.

Flash flooding can be very dangerous because of strong, swift currents.

- Move immediately and quickly to higher ground. The force of six inches of swiftly moving water can knock people off their feet.

- If flood waters rise around your car, get out and move to higher ground immediately. Cars can be easily swept away in just two feet of moving water.

Biological Threats

A biological attack is the deliberate release of germs or related substances. To affect individuals adversely, these substances must usually be inhaled, be ingested or enter through cuts in the skin. Some biological agents such as smallpox can be spread from person to person, while others like anthrax do not cause contagious diseases.

Different than a conventional explosive or attack, biological attacks may not be immediately evident. Some of the normal indicators of this type of attack would be an increase in the number of illnesses reported by local health care workers or a large number of dead or sick animals throughout your area. These attacks are normally discovered by emergency response personnel in reaction to the indicators listed previously.

What Should You Do?

In the event that you witness a suspicious attack using an unknown substance, you can do a number of things to protect yourself and your family. First, leave the immediate area as quickly as possible and protect yourself by finding something to place over your nose and mouth. Any layered material such as a T-shirt, handkerchief or towel may help prevent particles of the substance from entering

your respiratory system. If you have a long-sleeved shirt or jacket, use them to cover exposed skin. They may also prevent bacteria from entering cuts you may have. If you are indoors and the suspected attack takes place outdoors, remain inside unless told otherwise by authorities. Report the attack to emergency personnel.

You can also take precautionary measures such as keeping vaccines up to date and making sure you practice good personal hygiene. A healthy body will be able to better fight any potential contamination by biological agents. In the event that anyone around you becomes ill, do not automatically assume that it is from the suspected attack, because many of the symptoms from these attacks resemble common illnesses. Seek the medical advice of your physician.

Chemical Threats

Chemical attacks differ from biological attacks in that chemical attacks use a toxic gas or liquid to contaminate people or the environment. The prevalent symptoms you would experience from a chemical attack are tightness in the chest, difficulty breathing, blurred vision, stinging of the eyes or loss of coordination. It is worth noting that the public routinely accepts the risks posed by accidental release of chemicals. The response to an emergency event involving chemicals, however, is the same regardless of whether the emergency is a result of intentional or unintentional acts.

What Should You Do?

If you witness a suspected chemical attack outdoors, move laterally or upwind from the area as quickly as possible. If you cannot leave the area, try to get inside, away from direct exposure, and follow your instructions to shelter-in-place. If you are inside and an attack occurs in your building, try to leave the area if possible. If you cannot, move to a safe location in the building and shelter-in-place.

If you experience any of the symptoms mentioned previously, try to remove any clothing you can and wash your body with water or soap and water if available. Do not scrub the area, as this may wash the chemical into the skin. Seek medical assistance as soon as possible. If you see someone experiencing the previously mentioned symptoms, keep them away from others as much as possible and try to keep them comfortable.

Although extensive decontamination requiring disrobing is a possibility, this will normally only occur if you become a casualty of the agent or are evacuated and require medical treatment in a "clean" medical facility. This procedure may be required to prevent the spread of contamination.

Nuclear Explosions and Radiological Contamination

A nuclear blast consists of tremendous thermal (heat), light and blast energy. The blast can spread radioactive waste capable of contaminating the air and surrounding landscape. While this type of attack is less likely than a biological or chemical attack, the remote possibility of its occurrence means you should be prepared.

What Should You Do?

If a nuclear explosion occurs, immediately drop and stay down until any blast wave passes over you and it is safe to get up. Debris from a nuclear explosion can cause injuries, so it is often safer to remain down until debris stops falling. Do not look at the blast. When it is safe to do so, seek shelter inside a building or basement. Because dirt or earth is one of the best forms of protection from radiation, put as much shelter between you and the potential contamination as possible. If it is safe to leave without going in the direction from which the blast came, you should decide whether to leave the area to minimize the amount of time you spend exposed to radiological contamination. You should always try to place as much shielding and distance between yourself and the contamination as possible, and to limit the amount of your exposure by leaving laterally or upwind from the area when it is safe to do so.

Dirty Bombs

Dirty bombs are regular explosives that have been combined with either radiation-causing material or chemical weapons. Although most news reports talk about radiological dirty bombs, chemical agents may be used as well. Blasts from these types of weapons normally look more like a regular explosion and the contamination spread is not often immediately noticeable. Although this type of attack normally spreads contamination over a more localized area, you should be prepared to follow many of the same procedures as listed previously.

After experiencing any of these types of attacks, tune to your local media channels for information and instructions. Emergency responders are trained and equipped to evaluate and react to threats arising from these incidents. After a nuclear blast, you may be unable to get a signal from radio or television stations for a period of time. This is expected, so be persistent.

Although radioactive, biological and chemical weapons do pose a threat, they are attacks that you and your family or fellow employees can survive if you keep a cool head and follow the instructions given by your local responders.

Recovering From an Emergency

Recovery continues even after you return home, as you and your family face the emotional and psychological effects of the event. Reactions vary from person to person, but may include:

- Restless sleep or nightmares
- Anger or desire for revenge
- Numbness or lack of emotion
- Needing to keep active, restlessness
- Needing to talk about your experiences
- Loss of appetite
- Weight loss or gain
- Headaches
- Mood swings

All of these are normal reactions to stressful events and it is important to let people react in their own way. It may be helpful to:

- Talk with your family and friends about what happened and how you feel about it and try to evaluate and plan for the chance that it could happen again.

- Volunteer at a local shelter, blood bank or food pantry to assist emergency victims.

- Consult with a counselor or faith advisor.

In particular, children may need reassurance and extra attention. It is best to encourage them to share their feelings, even if you must listen to their stories repeatedly – this is a common way for children to grasp what they have experienced. You may also want to share your feelings about the event with them.

Concluding Thoughts

Events in recent years have made everyone more aware of the possibilities of natural disasters, terrorist attacks and other emergencies involving large-scale destruction. It is important to consider the risks for disasters in your own region and to take appropriate precautions. Simple preparations can make a huge difference for your safety and well-being should such a disaster strike.

Learning Outcomes

You should now be able to do the following:

1. List general steps for what to do before, during and after an emergency.

2. Create an emergency plan for your family.

3. Prepare an Emergency Go Kit.

4. Describe specific actions to take in case of a natural disaster, chemical threat or nuclear explosion.

5. List actions to help recover from an emergency.

Resources

Department of Homeland Security: 1-800-BE-READY
FBI Joint Terrorism Task Force (24-hour line for reporting suspicious activity): (202) 278-2000
Federal Emergency Management Agency (FEMA): (202) 566-1600

Review Questions

1. Being prepared for an emergency includes knowing how to –

    a. turn off the main electricity switch in your house.

    b. inspect a backpack found in a public place for a possible bomb.

    c. defend yourself in case of personal attack.

    d. restore your natural gas service when the emergency is over.

2. Who should family members plan to call to locate each other if separated in an emergency?

    a. A nearby neighbor

    b. A local public official

    c. A distant friend or relative

    d. Federal Emergency Management Agency

3. When storing water for use after an emergency, calculate how much is needed per person per day:

    a. 1 gallon

    b. 2 gallons

    c. 3 gallons

    d. 4 gallons

4. If an emergency strikes, you should always –

    a. stay in your home except in cases of rising water or fire.

    b. drive away from your home as soon as possible following an authorized evacuation route.

    c. go to the nearest nuclear fallout shelter in your community.

    d. follow instructions from emergency officials whether and when to evacuate.

5. The safest place to be if a severe storm strikes is –

    a. inside your car in a garage.

    b. in the basement or in a room near the center of the building.

    c. near a doorway or exit for quick evacuation.

    d. in the attic or highest part of the home.

Chapter 26 • Moving Forward

Chapter Preview

- Acting with Confidence
- Key Principles of First Aid
- Prevention of Injury and Illness
- Going Forward

You are checking a co-worker's young son, who fell and hurt his arm while playing in the reception area near your office. The boy is calmer now as you check for bleeding and potential musculoskeletal injury. When you first saw the boy crying in pain, you were worried you might not know what to do or might cause him more pain when you checked his arm, but you remembered your first aid training and realized you know what to do and can act confidently.

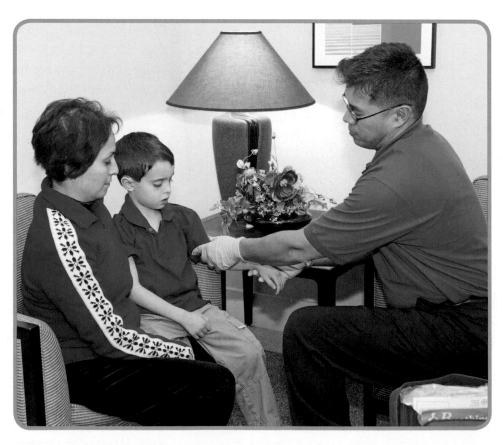

Having reached the end of this text and your first aid course, you should now feel confident that you know what to do in an emergency involving an injury or sudden illness. What is important now, as you move forward, is to remember the key principles of first aid so that you are ready to act without delay when needed.

Acting With Confidence

It is only human to be concerned that when actually confronted with an emergency, a situation that is stressful for everyone involved, you may hesitate or feel unsure exactly what to do. You may worry that you have forgotten some of the details of certain kinds of first aid. You may be fearful of or reluctant to deal with an injury involving blood or other body fluids, or with an emotional victim in pain. These are natural feelings we all share.

Nonetheless, you should feel confident in your ability to provide first aid after completing this course. Experience has shown that even first aiders with less training than you very competently provide first aid when they encounter an emergency. There are many stories in the media about lay people saving a heart attack victim, stopping life-threatening bleeding or pulling a drowning victim from the water. First aiders are often surprised how well they remember their training and are able to put their knowledge into action when suddenly called upon. Even if at some point in the future you forget some minor point, following the key principles of first aid is usually sufficient to help the victim for the few minutes before emergency medical personnel arrive.

Key Principles of First Aid

Although this text has described in some detail the first aid for all common injuries and sudden illnesses, a simple set of key principles guides one's actions in all emergencies. Remember to follow these basic principles and you will be able to render valuable aid to all victims:

- **Stay calm**. Emergencies happen without warning, giving us no time to prepare ourselves emotionally or to carefully plan out

our actions. The victim's pain and fears about what is happening, as well as the emotions of others at the scene, can cause panicky feelings that might lead to hasty or careless actions. It is very important to be calm when you respond to an emergency. Take a moment if necessary to gather your thoughts and energies. The victim and others at the scene will be reassured by your calm actions and will cope better with the situation. Remember: You have the training and know what to do until help arrives – be confident about your ability to help.

- **Call 9-1-1 for all serious emergencies and whenever in doubt**. In most areas in the United States, help is only a few minutes away once you call 9-1-1 or your local emergency number. Even if you are not near a telephone, you can shout for help and likely someone nearby will have a cell phone to call 9-1-1. Arriving EMS personnel will take over the care of the victim. If you are not sure how serious an injury or sudden illness is, call 9-1-1 anyway and tell the dispatcher the situation. Often the dispatcher can also advise you what care to give in case you are unsure what first aid is appropriate in this situation.

- **Remember your own safety**. As you take a moment to assess the situation and calm yourself before acting, remember to check the scene for any dangers before going to a help a victim. Avoid any temptation to act heroically if the scene is dangerous. Once you have called 9-1-1, personnel with special training and equipment will soon arrive who can better manage the dangers of the scene. If it is safe to give first aid, remember also to take steps to protect yourself from infectious disease.

- **Act quickly**. Although it is important to take a moment to calm yourself and plan your actions, remember that in many situations it is crucial to not delay before starting care for a life-threatening emergency. For example, a victim of cardiac arrest after a heart attack needs CPR and defibrillation immediately – every second counts once breathing and the heart stop. Call for an AED and call 9-1-1 and start CPR immediately if the victim is not breathing normally.

- **Check the victim**. Remember: First check for responsiveness, breathing and severe bleeding, and give care immediately for life-threatening problems. If there are no immediate threats, perform a physical examination and take a SAMPLE history. This information will help you to know what first aid to give and will be valuable to responding EMS professionals.

- **Do no harm**. Do only what you have learned to do. Trying some first aid technique you heard about somewhere is risky, as people often are misinformed about what first aid is safe and effective. Call 9-1-1 and give basic first aid as you have learned in this course, and nothing you do will harm the victim. Recognize your limits as a lay first aider and do not try something you have not learned to do, such as trying to rescue a victim from a hazardous situation.

- **Ask others for help**. You may be the only one at the scene of an emergency with first aid training, but bystanders are often present and will help you if asked. You may need someone to keep pressure on a wound to control bleeding, for example, while you attend to another injury. Others can call 9-1-1 or bring a first aid kit or AED. Do not hesitate to ask.

Prevention of Injury and Illness

This text has emphasized the importance of acting to prevent injury and sudden illness. Effective prevention depends on understanding that most injuries and sudden illnesses can be prevented and on adopting an attitude that motivates acting on safety principles and adopting a healthy lifestyle.

The problem in injury and illness prevention is that knowledge alone does not always translate directly into action. Everyone from school-age children to adults knows that cigarette smoking causes cancer and heart disease, yet more than one-fifth of the population still smokes. Everyone knows that safety belts and shoulder harnesses help prevent injuries in automobiles, yet every year hundreds die or are seriously injured in motor vehicle crashes because they were not properly restrained. The statistics go on and on. Taking the time to act safely and making the commitment to break unhealthy habits and adopt a healthy lifestyle requires motivation. At this point you *know* what you need to do to invest in your future health and well-being – but it is also up to you to *care* enough to make the effort.

Going Forward

As you conclude your first aid course, you probably are not thinking about future follow-up activities and refreshing your skills. It is important, however, to understand the need to stay current in your skills and knowledge, for two reasons. First, it is only human that over time we forget things and our skills become rusty. Second, new information often becomes available that changes how first aid should be given. For example, every five years an international group of emergency medical care professionals gathers to analyze the most recent research data and make recommendations for improvements in basic life support protocols. CPR techniques have changed over time and may change again in the future – and you may not learn about more effective techniques if you do not refresh your knowledge and skills.

Staying current in your knowledge and skills starts today. To help you remember what to do in different kinds of emergencies, keep this book in an appropriate place where you can consult it when needed.

You may also need additional first aid information at some future time. The Internet is an excellent source for current information, but be sure to trust only reputable websites. Much outdated or controversial information, as well as simply incorrect information, remains on private websites, but the sites for health care associations and governmental agencies generally have updated information. The agencies frequently referred to in this text, such as the Centers for Disease Control and Prevention (CDC), are excellent sources for new information.

Depending on your field of study and career plans, you may also choose to take additional advanced or specialized first aid or emergency care courses. People working in settings where they are likely to be the first trained person on the scene of an injury or sudden illness, such as law enforcement or fire personnel, health care workers and many others, may take an Emergency Medical Responder or Professional Rescuer course. The National Safety Council has more information about these and other courses (www.nsc.org).

Even if you do not move on to more advanced courses, you should still periodically renew your essential skills by taking a refresher course. Everyone needs a CPR/AED refresher course periodically. Studies have shown that lay people who do not use their CPR skills often will not be as effective when called upon to give CPR long after their training.

Concluding Thoughts

Congratulations on the completion of your first aid course! You can now be confident that at work or at play, in the privacy of your home or when interacting with others in public places, you know what to do when an emergency occurs.

Learning Outcomes

You should now be able to do the following:

1. Act with confidence if needed in an emergency.

2. List seven key principles of first aid.

3. Take steps to prevent injury and illness – both for you and for your family.

4. Describe the actions needed to stay current in your first aid knowledge and skills.

Review Questions

1. Remember that a primary goal of first aid is to –

    a. get a victim to a health care provider as quickly as possible.

    b. provide definitive medical care.

    c. provide care only for the few minutes it takes for help to arrive.

    d. administer medications as needed in an emergency.

2. When in doubt about how serious an injury or sudden illness is –

    a. always do as the victim wishes.

    b. call 9-1-1.

    c. perform an extensive physical examination.

    d. wait a few minutes to watch for changes in signs and symptoms.

3. Check the scene –

    a. as soon as you arrive at the victim's side.

    b. as you approach the victim.

    c. as soon as you have checked the victim's breathing.

    d. before you go to the victim.

4. Perform the initial assessment of a victim –

    a. for any immediate threats to life.

    b. after performing a physical examination.

    c. as you collect the SAMPLE history.

    d. by asking bystanders what happened.

5. The most important element for preventing injury and illness is –

    a. memorizing all the rules about what to do or not do.

    b. being motivated for safety and a healthy lifestyle.

    c. frequently researching the latest medical studies.

    d. taking annual courses in injury prevention.

Appendix A • Advanced Resuscitation Techniques

The skills included in this appendix are typically not taught to lay rescuers. Health care providers and rescuers at higher levels of training may be trained in some or all of these skills. As always, never attempt a skill for which you have not been appropriately trained.

This appendix discusses the following topics:

- Assessment Skills
  - Call First vs. Call Fast
  - Jaw Thrust
  - Pulse Check for Circulation
- Ventilation Skills
  - Rescue Breathing Without Chest Compressions
  - Inadequate Breathing
  - Resuscitation Masks
  - Suction Devices
  - Bag Masks
  - Supplemental Oxygen
  - Safety Around Oxygen
  - Oxygen Delivery Devices
  - Administration of Oxygen
  - Airway Adjuncts

- CPR Skills
  - Compressions for Bradycardia in Child
  - CPR
  - 2-Rescuer CPR for Adults and Children
  - 2-Rescuer CPR for Infants
- Special Resuscitation Situations
  - Trauma
  - Hypothermia
  - Near-drowning
  - Electric Shock
  - Pregnancy

Assessment Skills

Health care providers and professional rescuers with higher training follow different BLS protocols from lay first aiders and may use specialized equipment and supplies beyond basic personal protective equipment such as gloves and a resuscitation mask. Other equipment that may be of value in resuscitation situations includes suction devices, bag mask units, supplemental oxygen and airway adjuncts.

Call First vs. Call Fast

In any situation in which you recognize that a victim of injury or illness is unresponsive, if someone else is present at the scene, have that person call 9-1-1 immediately. Shout for anyone who may hear you and have them call 9-1-1 and go for an AED.

When you are alone, however, you need to decide whether to call immediately or to first begin to provide care for the victim. In **Chapter 5** you learned the general rule for lay first aiders to follow when deciding to call first or call fast (after providing 2 minutes of CPR). The guidelines are slightly different for health care providers and professional rescuers with a higher level of training. Follow these guidelines:

- Call first for a victim of any age seen to collapse suddenly. These victims are more likely to have cardiac arrest and to require defibrillation. Calling EMS immediately starts the process of getting an AED to the victim sooner.

- If the victim is found unresponsive and not breathing normally, for an adult victim you should still call first for help and an AED before providing CPR because the most likely cause is cardiac arrest. With a young child or infant victim, however, an airway obstruction is a more likely cause, so call fast after providing about 5 cycles of CPR (about 2 minutes).

- For unresponsive victims whose circumstances suggest a likely asphyxial arrest, such as a drowning victim or a victim with an airway obstruction, call fast. Give about 5 cycles of CPR (about 2 minutes) before stopping to call EMS.

Jaw Thrust

Lay rescuers are generally taught to use the head tilt–chin lift technique to open his or her airway of an unresponsive victim lying on his or her back, regardless of whether there may be a spinal injury. The jaw thrust technique, which is less likely to cause additional injury in a victim with a spinal injury, is no longer recommended to be taught to lay rescuers because it is somewhat more difficult to perform. Health care providers and professional rescuers, however, are often taught to use this technique.

With the jaw thrust, you do not tilt the head back to open the airway. Instead, only lift the jaw upward using both hands **(Figure A-1)**. If you cannot successfully open the airway with the jaw thrust, however, then switch to the head tilt–chin lift method.

Pulse Check for Circulation

Lay rescuers trained in CPR are taught to begin CPR with chest compressions immediately for an unresponsive victim who is not breathing normally. Health care and professional rescuers who are

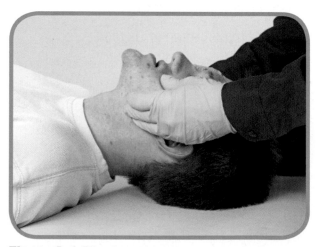

Figure A-1 *The jaw thrust.*

trained to check for a pulse should check for a pulse before beginning chest compressions – but they must do this very quickly. It is critical to use no more than 10 seconds to feel for the victim's pulse and unless a pulse is clearly found in that time, to start chest compressions immediately. If an obvious pulse is found, begin rescue breathing immediately as described in the following section.

It takes training and practice to be able to effectively and quickly locate a pulse. To check the pulse in an adult, use the **carotid pulse** in the neck. Holding the victim's forehead with one hand to keep the airway open, put the index and middle fingers of your other hand on the side of the victim's neck nearer to you. Find the Adam's apple and then slide your fingertips toward you and down the neck to the groove at the side of the neck **(Figure A-2)**. Pressing gently, feel for a pulse for at least 5 but no more than 10 seconds.

If a pulse cannot be definitely detected within 10 seconds, start CPR beginning with chest compressions.

In a child, check either the **carotid or femoral pulse**. The femoral pulse is located in the center of the groin crease **(Figure A-3)**.

To check the pulse in an infant, use the **brachial pulse** in the inside of the upper arm instead of the carotid or femoral pulse. With one hand on the infant's forehead to maintain head position for an open airway, put the fingers of your other hand about midway between the shoulder and elbow on the inside of the arm and press gently, feeling for no more than 10 seconds **(Figure A-4)**.

Lack of a definite pulse along with the absence of normal breathing signifies that the heart has stopped or is not beating effectively enough to circulate blood. If the victim lacks a pulse and is not breathing normally, start CPR beginning with chest compressions and call for an AED to be brought to the scene.

An infant or child may have a pulse under 60 beats/minute and lack adequate perfusion. This victim also needs CPR (see later section "Compressions for Bradycardia in Child").

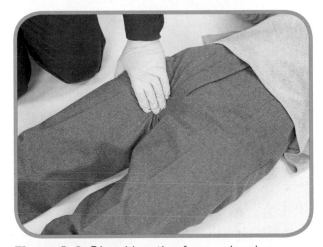

Figure A-3 *Checking the femoral pulse.*

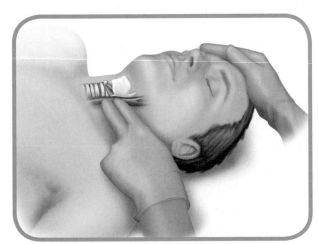

Figure A-2 *Checking the carotid pulse in an adult or child.*

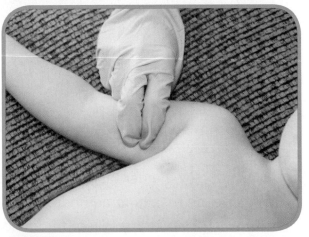

Figure A-4 *Checking the brachial pulse in an infant.*

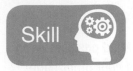

Skill Rescue Breathing

1 If the victim has a pulse but is not breathing normally, open the airway and give a breath over 1 second, watching the chest rise and letting it fall.

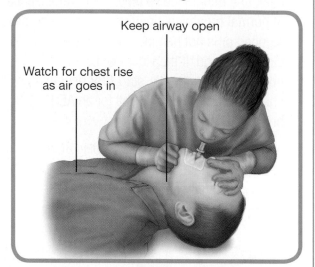

Keep airway open

Watch for chest rise as air goes in

2 If the first breath does not go in, try again to open the airway and give another rescue breath. If it still does not go in, the victim may be choking. Proceed to CPR for choking.

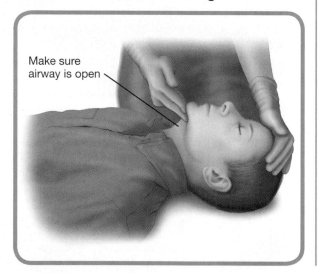

Make sure airway is open

3 If your breath goes in, continue rescue breathing. Give each breath over 1 second, at rate of 10 to 12 breaths per minute (1 breath every 5-6 seconds) for an adult; 12 to 20 breaths per minute for a child (1 breath every 3-5 seconds); or 20 breaths per minute for an infant (1 breath every 3 seconds).

4 Check the pulse about every 2 minutes (every 5 cycles of CPR). If there is no pulse, start CPR beginning with chest compressions.

ALERT

- Do not blow harder than is needed to make the chest rise.
- After each breath, remember to let the air escape and the chest fall.
- Blowing in too forcefully or for too long is ineffective and may put air in the stomach, which may cause vomiting.
- Be careful not to tilt an infant's head too far back.

Ventilation Skills

Rescue Breathing Without Chest Compressions

In some situations a victim may not be breathing adequately but may still have a heartbeat. Someone pulled from the water in a near-drowning, for example, may have stopped breathing but may still have a heartbeat. Health care providers trained in pulse checks may then find a pulse in a non-breathing victim. In this situation, chest compressions are not given while rescue breaths are provided, as described in the Skill: "Rescue Breathing."

Inadequate Breathing

In addition to giving rescue breathing to victims who are not breathing but have a pulse, health care providers and professional rescuers may use rescue breathing in cases of inadequate breathing. If an adult victim is breathing at a rate of less than 10 breaths per minute, take this as a sign of inadequate breathing – the victim is not receiving sufficient oxygen. An infant or child may have a pulse of 60 or higher per minute but may still be breathing inadequately. In a victim who is not breathing adequately, do not wait for respiratory arrest before beginning to provide rescue breaths.

Resuscitation Masks

The resuscitation mask, often called a pocket face mask or simply a face mask, seals over the victim's mouth and nose and has a port through which the rescuer blows air to give rescue breaths. A one-way valve allows the rescuer's air in through the mouthpiece, while the victim's exhaled air exits the mask through a different opening.

When using a face mask, it is essential to seal the mask well to the victim's face while maintaining an open airway. How you hold the mask depends on your position by the victim, whether the head tilt–chin lift or jaw thrust technique is used to open the airway, and whether you have one or two hands free to seal the mask. The following hand positions assume you have both hands free

Figure A-5 *(a) Face mask hand position with rescuer at victim's side. (b) Face mask hand position with rescuer at victim's head. (c) Do not tilt the head when using the jaw thrust technique for a victim with spinal injury.*

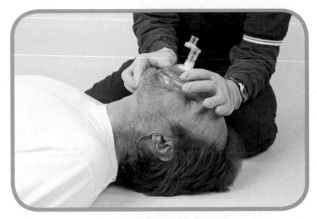

(a)

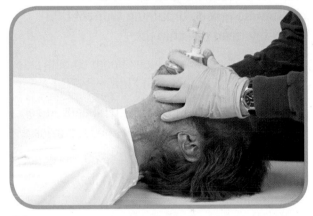

(b)

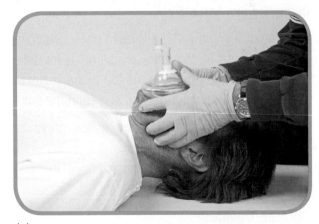

(c)

to seal the mask, whether alone at the victim's side while performing CPR or at the victim's head (alone giving only rescue breathing or with another rescuer who is providing chest compressions).

From a position at the victim's side (one rescuer giving CPR) using the head tilt–chin lift:

1. With the thumb and index finger of your hand closer to the top of the victim's head, seal the top and sides of the mask to the victim's head as shown in **Figure A-5(a)**.

2. Put the thumb of your second hand on the lower edge of the mask.

3. Put the remaining fingers of your second hand under the jaw to lift the chin.

4. Press the mask down firmly to make a seal as you perform a head tilt–chin lift to open the airway.

From a position at the top of the victim's head (two rescuers giving CPR or one rescuer performing rescue breathing without CPR) using the head tilt–chin lift:

1. Put your thumbs and index finger on both sides of the mask as shown in **Figure A-5(b)**.

2. Put the remaining finger of both hands under the angles of the victim's jaw on both sides.

3. As you tilt the head back, press the mask down firmly to make a seal as you lift the chin with your fingers.

From a position at the top of the victim's head using the jaw thrust:

1. Without tilting the victim's head back, position your thumbs on the mask the same as for the head tilt–chin lift – from the top of the victim's head, with fingers under the angles of the jaw.

2. Lift the jaw to open the airway as you press down with your thumbs to seal the mask, without tilting the head back as shown in **Figure A-5(c)**.

Suction Devices

A **suction device** is used to clear blood, vomit and other substances from a victim's airway. These devices are generally safe and easy to use. Although different types of suction devices are available, they are similar in their use. Manual devices develop suction with a hand-pumping action; other devices are powered by a battery or pressurized oxygen. Soft rubber bulb syringes are used for suctioning infants.

Suction devices for adults and children have a clear plastic tip that is inserted into the mouth or nostrils to suck out fluids and small solids. Different suction tips are available, varying from small, soft plastic tips that are more effective for fluids to larger, more rigid tips that are more effective for vomit and particulates. Some devices have a suction control port at the base of the tip that you cover with your finger to produce suction. As always, you should be familiar in advance with the specific equipment you may use in an emergency.

Suction is useful whenever a victim's airway may be obstructed – fully or in part – by body fluids, food substances or other matter. If the victim vomits when rescue breathing or CPR is underway, or if secretions or blood accumulate and impede ventilation, stop and quickly suction the mouth and/or nose and then continue resuscitation. An unresponsive breathing victim may also need suctioning to maintain an open airway. Usually you know the airway needs suctioning when you hear gurgling sounds during breathing or ventilation.

The victim's head is turned to the side to help drain vomit or fluids before suctioning. If the victim may have a spinal injury, the victim must be turned on the side with the head and body in line as a unit, with the help of other rescuers. (See Skill: "Suctioning [Adult or Child]" and Skill: "Suctioning [Infant]")

Safety precautions are necessary when suctioning. Because many suction devices generate strong suction pressures, be careful with the suction tip. Prolonged contact with mucous membranes in the mouth and nose can cause bruising, swelling and even bleeding. Never insert the suction tip farther than you can see. Prolonged suctioning can also decrease the volume of air reaching the victim's lungs. Vigorous suctioning may stimulate the victim's gag reflex, causing additional vomiting.

(continues on page 435)

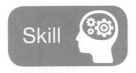
1 Confirm that the suction device is working and produces suction.

2 Turn the victim's head to one side and open the mouth (for spinal injury, support the head and turn with body as a unit).

3 Sweep out solids and larger amounts of fluid with your finger.

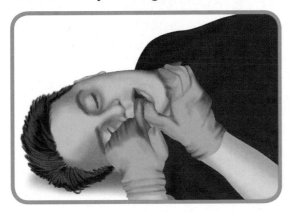

4 Determine maximum depth of insertion by measuring the catheter tip from the earlobe to the corner of the mouth.

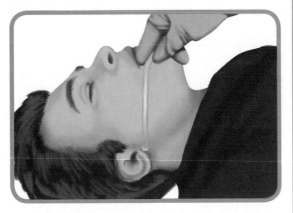

5 Turn on suction or pump the handle to create suction.

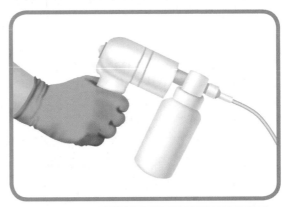

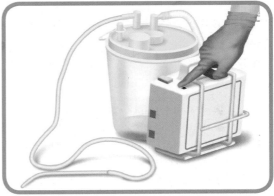

6 Insert catheter tip carefully into the mouth. Put your finger over the proximal opening to begin suctioning and move the tip about as you withdraw it.

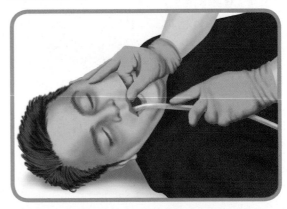

7 Reposition the victim's head with airway open, and resume rescue breathing or CPR.

A • Advanced Resuscitation Techniques

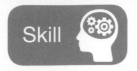

Skill — Suctioning (Infant)

1 Hold the infant in position for suctioning, with the head lower than the body and turned to one side.

2 Squeeze the suction bulb, and then gently insert the tip into the infant's mouth.

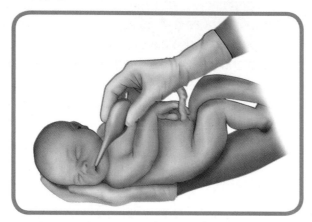

3 Gradually release the bulb to create suction as you withdraw the tip from the infant's mouth.

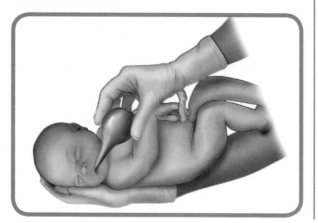

4 Move the bulb aside and squeeze it, with tip down, to empty it.

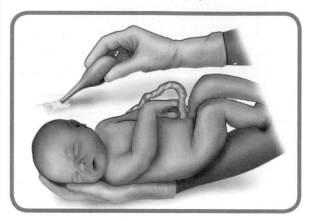

5 Repeat steps 2 through 4 until the airway seems clear, up to three times.

6 Repeat the suctioning steps for each nostril.

7 Begin or resume rescue breathing or CPR if needed.

(continued from page 432)

Be especially careful not to suction too deeply in an infant. Always suction an infant's mouth before the nostrils, because suctioning the nose may stimulate the infant to breathe in and thereby inhale fluid or secretions from the mouth.

Remember standard precautions against disease transmission through body fluids. After the emergency, dispose of any contents in the reservoir of the suction device and clean the device according to the manufacturer's recommendations.

Bag Mask

Bag mask (bag-valve-mask or BVM) units, like regular face masks, protect the first aider from disease transmission and are more effective for providing ventilations to non-breathing victims. With the BVM, the victim receives air from the atmosphere (21% oxygen) rather than air the rescuer exhales (16% oxygen). The more oxygen delivered to the lungs, the more oxygen will reach the victim's vital organs to maintain life. Several different types of BVM units are available, but each has at least three components **(Figure A-6)**:

- The self-inflating bag holds the air or oxygen that is delivered to the victim when the bag is squeezed.

- The one-way valve allows air or oxygen to flow from the bag to the victim but prevents exhaled air from returning to the bag.

- The mask is similar to a resuscitation mask and is connected to the bag and valve.

The proper size mask must be used for a proper fit. An oxygen reservoir bag may be attached to the other end of the bag when supplemental oxygen is used.

To use the BVM on a non-breathing victim, position yourself above the victim's head. Perform a head tilt and then position the mask on the victim's face. If you are alone, you need to hold the mask with one hand and squeeze the bag with the other, as shown in **Figure A-7**. To hold the mask in place with one hand, use the C-clamp technique, with thumb and index finger on the edges of the mask while the other fingers lift the jaw into the mask. If you are unable to open the airway and obtain a good seal with one hand, provide rescue breaths mouth to mask or mouth to mouth. A single rescuer skilled in its use may use a BVM when rescue breaths alone are being given.

Two-rescuer use of the BVM is recommended whenever possible because of the difficulty one person may have sealing the mask on the victim's face with one hand while squeezing the bag with the other. When a second rescuer is available to help with the BVM, one rescuer holds the mask in place using both hands as described earlier for a resuscitation mask, as shown in the Skill: "Bag Mask for Rescue Breathing (2 Rescuers)."

With the mask sealed in place, rescue breaths are delivered to the victim by squeezing the bag. Squeeze a 1-liter adult bag about ½ to ⅔ of its volume. Squeeze a 2-liter adult bag about ⅓ its

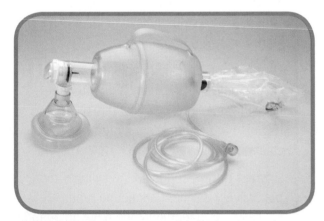

Figure A-6 *Bag mask (BVM).*

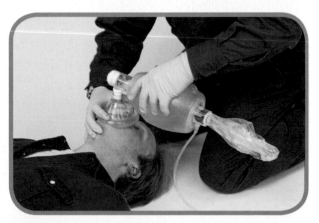

Figure A-7 *A single rescuer using a BVM for rescue breathing.*

volume. Squeeze the bag over 1 second, watching the victim's chest rise. Give a ventilation every 5 to 6 seconds in an adult (or every 3 to 5 seconds in a child or every 3 seconds in an infant), the same as with rescue breathing by mouth or resuscitation mask. If supplemental oxygen is being provided through the BVM, slightly smaller ventilations can be given.

When using a BVM, monitor the effectiveness of ventilations. Be careful to give rescue breaths at the usual rate and not to over-ventilate the victim. Watch for the rise and fall of the victim's chest and feel for resistance as you squeeze the bag. Increased resistance may mean blood or vomit is in the airway or that the airway is no longer open. A problem can also occur with sealing the mask to the victim's face, especially when a single rescuer must do this with one hand. If air is escaping around the mask, try repositioning the mask and your fingers. If you cannot obtain an adequate seal and the victim's chest does not rise with ventilations, or if there are any other problems with using the BVM, use an alternate technique, such as a resuscitation mask, instead.

If available, supplemental oxygen should be used with the BVM (see next section). An oxygen reservoir bag is attached to the valve on the bag and the oxygen tubing attached to the bag. The device is used the same way it is used to give ventilations, only now it is oxygen rather than air being delivered to the victim. The reservoir holds oxygen being delivered to the device so that the bag always fills with oxygen to be delivered in the next ventilation. When two rescuers are present, the second sets up the oxygen equipment and prepares to connect it to the BVM while the first begins providing rescue breathing with the BVM alone.

The BVM can be used for a non-breathing infant in the same manner as for an adult or child. Be sure to choose the correct size mask. Squeeze the bag only enough to make the chest rise, avoiding forceful squeezing or over-inflation that may lead to vomiting.

Supplemental Oxygen

In many emergency situations the victim will benefit from receiving **supplemental oxygen**, if available. Victims receiving basic life support are often receiving insufficient oxygen because of respiratory or cardiovascular problems. The air around us is about 21% oxygen and the air we breathe out (and into a victim's lungs during rescue breathing) is about 16% oxygen. Depending on the supplemental oxygen delivery device, the victim can receive oxygen at concentrations up to 100%.

Supplemental oxygen, when available, may be used along with other basic life support techniques, including rescue breathing and CPR. In addition, victims with serious medical conditions, including heart attack, stroke, seizures or serious injury, may benefit from supplemental oxygen (see **Chapter 16**).

The equipment involved in giving supplemental oxygen includes:

- The **oxygen source** is typically a pressurized cylinder. When full, cylinders have a pressure of 2,000 pounds per square inch (psi). They come in various sizes and are usually painted green, although some stainless steel cylinders are not.

- The **pressure regulator** reduces the pressure of oxygen leaving the tank to a safe level and has a gauge that shows the pressure remaining within the cylinder. If the gauge reads 2,000 psi, the tank is full; if it reads 1,000 psi, it is half full and so on. The pressure regulator is designed so that it works only with oxygen tanks.

- The **flowmeter**, used to adjust the rate of oxygen delivery, is usually built into the pressure regulator. The flow of oxygen reaching the victim is set by turning the calibrated flow valve.

- **Oxygen tubing** connects the cylinder to the delivery device. Connecting tubes are typically 4 to 5 feet long and have an adapter at each end.

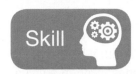
1 Rescuer 1 assembles the BVM with a mask of the correct size and puts the mask over the victim's mouth and nose.

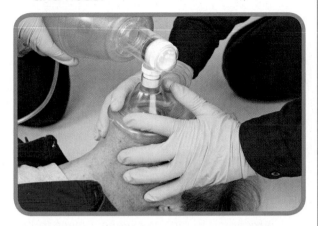

2 Rescuer 2 positions hands: thumbs and index fingers circling each side of mask, the other three fingers of each hand behind lower jawbone. Pull the jaw up into the mask instead of pushing the mask down on the jaw.

3 Rescuer 2 opens the airway and seals the mask to the victim's face.

4 Rescuer 1 squeezes the bag to provide ventilations:

  a. 1 ventilation over 1 second in adult, every 5-6 seconds.

  b. 1 ventilation over 1 second in child, every 3-5 seconds.

  c. 1 ventilation over 1 second in infant, every 3 seconds.

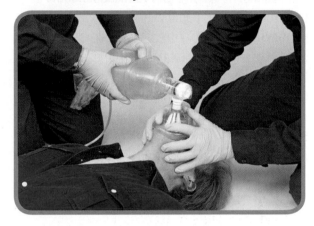

5 Recheck pulse about every 2 minutes. If no pulse, call for an AED and start CPR.

- **An oxygen delivery device**, such as a face mask or nasal cannula, provides the flowing oxygen to the victim.

Safety Around Oxygen

Although oxygen itself does not burn, it vigorously supports combustion and creates a hazardous situation if used near an ignition source. Follow these guidelines around oxygen:

- Never allow smoking or an open flame near the oxygen source.

- Never use grease, oil or adhesive tape on the cylinder, pressure regulator or delivery device, because these are combustible.

- Never expose an oxygen cylinder to a temperature above 120° F.

- Never drop a cylinder or let it fall against another object. If the valve is dislodged, the cylinder can become a dangerous projectile powered by the compressed gas.

- Never try to use a non-oxygen regulator on an oxygen cylinder.

Oxygen Delivery Devices

Many different oxygen delivery devices are available, each with certain advantages and disadvantages. The following devices are most frequently used in emergency situations:

- **Nasal cannulas**, sometimes called nasal prongs, are used on breathing victims who do not require a high concentration of oxygen. The device has two small prongs

A • Advanced Resuscitation Techniques

that fit shallowly into the nostrils. The nasal cannula is easy to use and comfortable for the victim. The oxygen concentration delivered depends on the flow rate (1 to 6 liters per minute) and the victim's breathing rate, varying from about 24% to 50% **(Figure A-8)**.

- **Resuscitation face masks** cover the mouth and nose and can be used for non-breathing victims receiving rescue breaths. Some masks have a special port for oxygen, which can be used for breathing victims who need oxygen. The mask then can be secured to the victim's head by an elastic band. A typical plastic face mask provides an oxygen concentration of 30% to 60% with a flow rate of 10 liters per minute **(Figure A-9)**.

- **Nonrebreather masks** have a mask and a reservoir bag and are used for breathing victims. The oxygen fills the reservoir, which

empties partially as the victim inhales. The victim's exhaled air escapes through a valve. With a minimum oxygen flow rate of 8 liters per minute, the oxygen concentration ranges from 80% to 95%. The flow rate is adjusted to prevent the reservoir from completely collapsing when the victim inhales. A firm mask fit is needed to prevent room air from entering the mask **(Figure A-10)**.

- **Bag masks**, as described earlier, can also deliver oxygen either through a simple connecting tube to the bag or with an oxygen reservoir. Oxygen concentrations delivered to a non-breathing victim by a BVM with a reservoir can approach 100%. A breathing victim can also use a BVM with a reservoir to receive oxygen; unless the victim is having difficulty breathing, the bag is not squeezed **(Figure A-11)**.

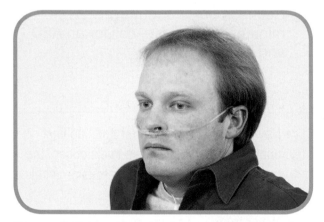

Figure A-8 *Nasal cannula.*

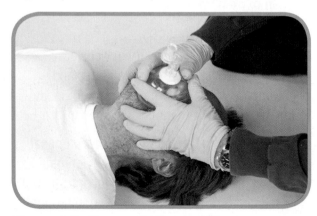

Figure A-9 *Resuscitation mask.*

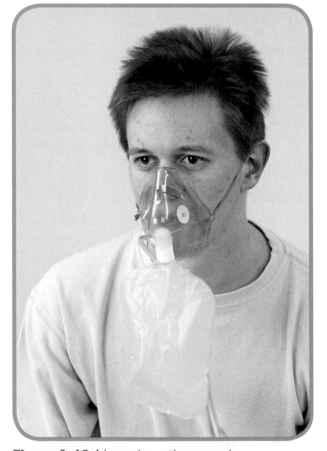

Figure A-10 *Nonrebreather mask.*

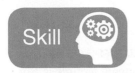
1 Check equipment: oxygen labels on the cylinder and regulator; tubing and delivery device ready.

2 Remove any protective seal, point cylinder away and open main valve for 1 second.

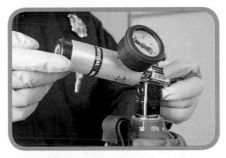

3 Remove any protective seals and attach regulator to oxygen cylinder.

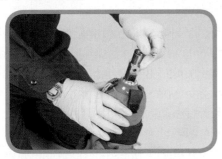

4 Open the main cylinder valve.

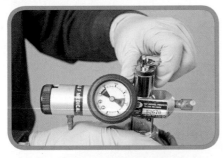

5 Check the pressure regulator gauge.

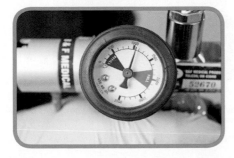

6 Attach the tubing to the flowmeter and the oxygen delivery device.

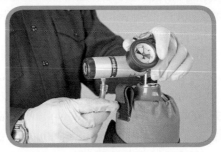

7 Set the flowmeter at the correct oxygen flow rate.
a. 1 to 6 lpm for nasal cannula
b. 10 lpm for face mask
c. 10 to 15 lpm for BVM or nonrebreather mask

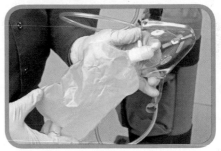

8 Confirm oxygen is flowing.

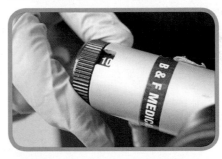

9 Position the delivery device on the victim and continue rescue breathing (or allow victim to breathe spontaneously).

10 Monitor the pressure regulator gauge and be prepared to remove the delivery device and change tanks if the pressure drops below 500 psi. Observe oxygen safety precautions.

A • Advanced Resuscitation Techniques

Administration of Oxygen

The Skill: "Oxygen Administration" describes the steps for setting up the oxygen equipment and administering oxygen to the victim. Remember to follow safety principles when working with oxygen. If you are alone with a victim, do not stop providing basic life support to set up oxygen equipment. Give rescue breathing or CPR as needed, use the AED if present and appropriate, and care for other life-threatening problems first. Wait until the victim is relatively stable and breathing independently or until another rescuer can help with the oxygen equipment. Once the victim is receiving oxygen, continue to monitor the flow of oxygen, tank pressure and flow rate, as well as the victim's condition.

Airway Adjuncts

Oral and nasal **airway adjuncts** are devices that help keep a victim's airway open during resuscitation or until the victim receives advanced medical attention. The most common cause of airway obstruction in unresponsive victims is the tongue. An airway adjunct prevents this problem and keeps the airway open more easily than head position alone while using resuscitation techniques or caring for a breathing victim. Supplemental oxygen can be given through a resuscitation mask or bag mask with an oral or nasal airway in place.

Oral Airways

Oral airways, also called **oropharyngeal airways**, are used only in unresponsive victims who do not have a gag reflex. If inserted into a responsive victim or one who still has a gag reflex, the airway adjunct can cause vomiting. The victim's airway must be opened before the airway device is inserted; the device does not open the airway itself but will help keep it open. An oral airway can be used in an unresponsive victim who is breathing or who is receiving rescue breaths.

(continues on page 443)

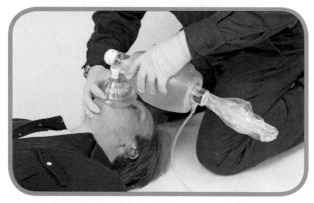

Figure A-11 *BVM with oxygen reservoir.*

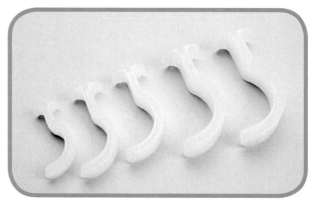

Figure A-12 *Oral airways.*

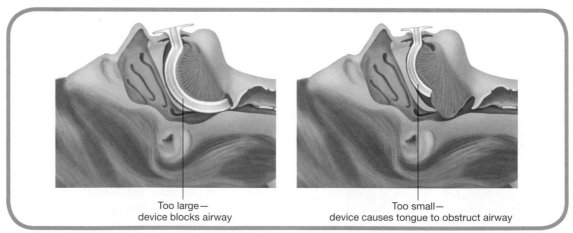

Too large—
device blocks airway

Too small—
device causes tongue to obstruct airway

Figure A-13 *An oral airway that is too large or too small will obstruct the airway.*

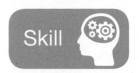

1 Choose the correct airway device size. The oral airway length should match the distance from the corner of the mouth to the tip of the earlobe on the same side of the victim's face.

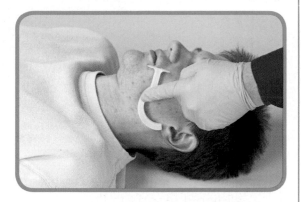

2 Open the victim's airway with head tilt–chin lift or jaw thrust and open the mouth.

3 Insert the airway device with the tip pointing toward the roof of the mouth.

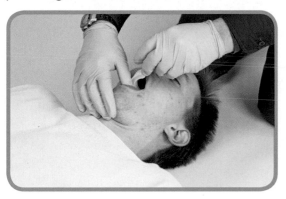

4 When tip reaches the back of the mouth and you feel resistance, rotate the airway 180 degrees.

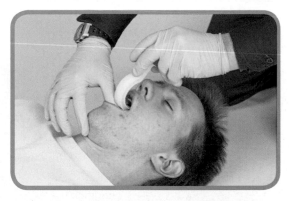

5 Continue to insert the airway device to the final position (the flange resting on the lips).

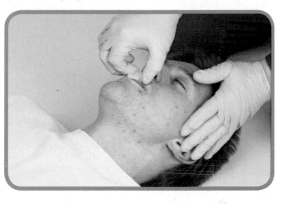

A • Advanced Resuscitation Techniques

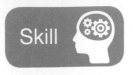

Skill Nasal Airway Insertion

1 Choose the correct nasal airway size. The nasal airway length should match the distance from the nostril to the tip of the earlobe on the same side of the victim's face.

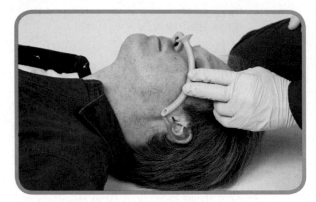

2 Coat the nasal airway with lubricant.

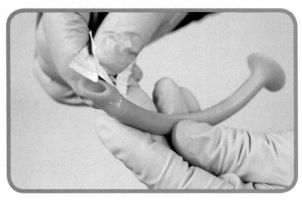

3 Insert the nasal airway in the right nostril with the bevel toward the septum.

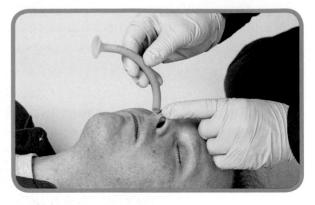

4 Insert the nasal airway straight back, sliding it along the floor of the nostril.

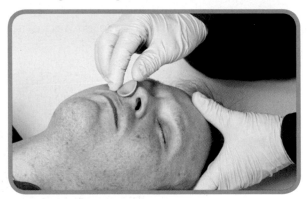

5 Insert the nasal airway until the flange rests against the nose.

(continued from page 440)

Proper placement of the oral airway is essential. An improperly placed airway device can compress the tongue into the back of the throat and further block the airway. Oral airways are curved to fit the natural contour of the mouth and are available in various sizes to ensure a proper fit **(Figure A-12)**. An airway adjunct that is too big can cause vomiting and may prevent the resuscitation mask from sealing well. An airway adjunct that is too small can slide into the back of the pharynx and obstruct the airway **(Figure A-13)**. Remember to open the victim's airway before inserting the oral airway, as described in the Skill: "Oral Airway Insertion." Periodically reassess the airway adjunct to confirm that it remains in proper position. A victim can be suctioned with an oral airway in place.

Nasal Airways

A nasal airway, like an oral airway, helps maintain an open airway **(Figure A-14)**. A nasal airway (**nasopharyngeal airway**) can be used in a victim who is responsive or who, although unresponsive, has a gag reflex. Nasal airways are also effective for unresponsive victims with mouth or jaw injuries or tightly clenched teeth that prevent the use of an oral airway. Nasal airways are less likely to cause gagging and vomiting than oral airways, but a disadvantage is that they are too narrow to suction. Insert a nasal airway as described in the Skill: "Nasal Airway Insertion," and continue to keep the victim's airway open with the head tilt–chin lift or jaw thrust. If needed, suction through a nasal airway using a small, flexible suction catheter.

CPR Skills

Compressions for Bradycardia in Child

An infant or child being given rescue breaths or oxygen may have a pulse but still have inadequate perfusion. If the pulse is under 60 beats/minute and the infant or child has signs of poor systemic perfusion (such as poor skin color), the health care provider should provide CPR with chest compressions. Do not wait for the victim to become pulseless if perfusion is poor even with ventilation (with or without supplemental oxygen).

CPR

The protocol for CPR for more highly trained health care providers differs somewhat from that for CPR by lay rescuers. Health care providers check for a pulse before beginning chest compressions.

A lone health care provider uses the same 30:2 ratio of compressions and rescue breaths for all victims. Two-rescuer CPR provided by health care providers, however, uses a 15:2 ratio for infants and children up to the onset of puberty.

Health care providers, like lay rescuers should give chest compressions at a rate of at least 100 a minute – push hard, push fast – letting the chest come all the way up between compressions. Interruptions to give rescue breaths or check the pulse should take less than 10 seconds.

Two-Rescuer CPR for Adults and Children

When two rescuers at the scene are trained in CPR, resuscitation performed by both together offers several advantages. Two-rescuer CPR –

- minimizes the time between rescue breaths and compressions, making CPR more effective.

- allows for more quickly setting up an AED **(Chapter 6)**.

- reduces rescuer fatigue.

The first rescuer begins by checking the victim for responsiveness and breathing. If the victim is not breathing normally, this rescuer checks for a pulse. Meanwhile, the second rescuer ensures that

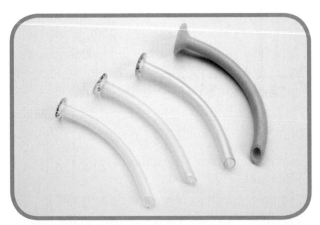

Figure A-14 *Nasal airways.*

9-1-1 has been called and an AED is on the way, then moves into position on the opposite side of the victim to give chest compressions if the victim does not have a pulse. After 30 compressions, the first rescuer gives 2 rescue breaths and CPR continues.

Two-rescuer CPR is performed in the same cycles of 30 compressions and 2 breaths for an adult (15 compressions and 2 breaths for an infant or child). One rescuer gives the chest compressions at a rate of at least 100 compressions per minute and the other rescuer gives 2 rescue breaths. The rescuer giving compressions should count aloud during the compressions and pause after the last compression to let the other rescuer give 2 breaths. See Skill: CPR for Adult or Child (2 Rescuers).

The rescuers should switch positions about every 2 minutes (about 5 cycles of 30 compressions and 2 breaths) to prevent ineffective compressions resulting from fatigue. This change should be done at the end of a full CPR cycle after breaths are given and should be accomplished in less than 5 seconds. It is recommended that positions are switched during any intervention that interrupts compressions (such as when the AED delivers a shock).

If an AED is present at the scene, the first rescuer gives both chest compressions and breaths while the second rescuer sets up the unit and attaches the pads (see **Chapter 4**). Then the rescuers resume CPR together.

Note: You may be assisting a professional with a higher level of training who places an advanced airway in the victim for ventilation. With an advanced airway in place, chest compressions are given continually at a rate of at least 100 per minute without pauses for rescue breaths. Ventilations are provided via a bag mask every 6 to 8 seconds (8 to 10 breaths per minute) while compressions are ongoing.

Transitioning from 1-Rescuer CPR to 2-Rescuer CPR

In some situations a rescuer is already giving CPR when a second rescuer arrives on the scene.

The rescuers should coordinate their actions for a smooth transition from 1-rescuer CPR to 2-rescuer CPR. The second rescuer moves into position on the other side of the victim to prepare to take over chest compressions. The first rescuer completes a series of compressions. While the first rescuer then gives 2 breaths, the second rescuer locates the correct hand position and begins compressions immediately after the second breath. For the next 2 minutes, the new rescuer gives chest compressions and the first rescuer gives the rescue breaths.

Note: If you are the first rescuer who started CPR, the arriving second rescuer may be a rescuer with a higher level of training. In such a case this rescuer assumes authority for how CPR should best be continued. If this rescuer determines your breathing or compression technique is inadequate, he or she may ask you to take on the other role – or may take over the CPR alone.

Two-Rescuer CPR for Infants

Two-rescuer CPR for an infant uses a different hand position for chest compressions from single-rescuer CPR. The rescuer giving compressions places the thumbs of both hands together in the correct position on the infant's sternum (just below the nipple line). The fingers of both hands encircle the infant's chest **(Figure A-15)**. The chest is

(continues on page 447)

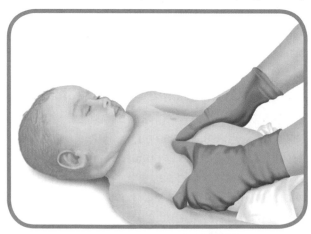

Figure A-15 *The chest-encircling hand position for infant chest compressions when two professional rescuers are giving CPR.*

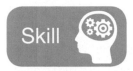

CPR for Adult or Child (2 Rescuers)

1 At the victim's head, Rescuer 1 checks for unresponsiveness and normal breathing. If the victim is not breathing, check for a pulse for no longer than 10 seconds. Rescuer 2 ensures that an AED has been summoned. At the victim's side, Rescuer 2 locates the site for chest compressions.

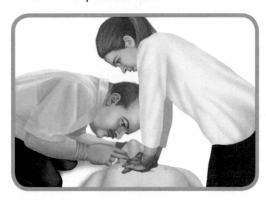

2 Rescuer 1 indicates, "No pulse." Rescuer 2 gives 30 compressions for an adult (15 for a child) at rate of at least 100 per minute, counting aloud for a fast, steady rate, then pauses.

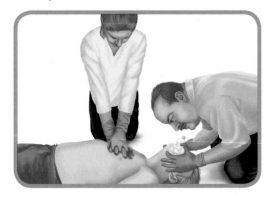

3 Rescuer 1 gives 2 breaths.

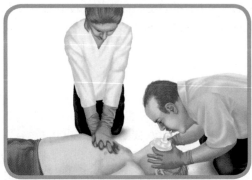

4 Rescuers continue cycles of 30 compressions for an adult (15 for a child) and 2 breaths for 2 minutes (or about 5 cycles of compressions and ventilations at a ratio of 30:2) before switching compressor and ventilator roles. The switch should be done quickly (in less than 5 seconds).

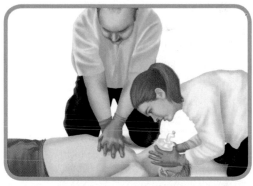

5 Rescuers continue CPR until:
- The victim is breathing normally and has a pulse
- An AED is brought to the scene and is ready to use
- Help arrives and takes over

6 a. If the victim starts breathing normally and has a pulse but is unresponsive, put the victim in the recovery position and monitor breathing and pulse.

b. For a victim who is not breathing normally and has no pulse, start the AED sequence when the AED arrives.

A • Advanced Resuscitation Techniques

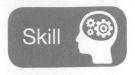

Skill — CPR for Infant (2 rescuers)

1 At the infant's head, Rescuer 1 checks for normal breathing and a pulse. At the infant's feet, Rescuer 2 positions hands in the chest-encircling position for chest compressions with both thumbs.

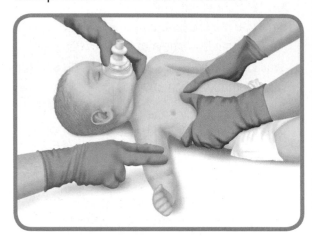

2 If pulse is absent, Rescuer 1 says, "No pulse." Rescuer 2 gives 15 chest compressions at a rate of at least 100 per minute, counting aloud for a fast, steady rate, then pauses.

3 Rescuer 1 gives 2 breaths.

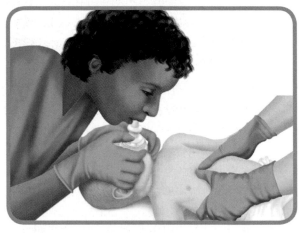

4 Rescuers continue cycles of 15 compressions and 2 breaths for about 2 minutes before switching compressor and ventilator roles. The switch should be done quickly (in less than 5 seconds). Rescuers continue CPR until:

- The infant is breathing normally and has a pulse
- More advanced help arrives and takes over

5 a. If the infant starts breathing normally but is unresponsive, hold the infant in the recovery position and monitor breathing and pulse.

b. For an infant who is not breathing normally and has no pulse, start the AED sequence when the AED arrives.

(continued from page 444)

compressed with both thumbs, as described in Skill: CPR for Infant (2 Rescuers). If you cannot encircle the infant's chest (e.g., the infant's chest is too large or the rescuer's hands are too small), use the single-rescuer method of performing compressions with 2 fingers.

Special Resuscitation Situations

In most emergencies, basic life support skills are used in the same way. A few situations, however, involve special considerations regarding the use of these skills or the approach to the victim.

Trauma

In most situations in which the victim is severely injured by blunt or penetrating trauma, problems with the airway, breathing or circulation are the result of the trauma rather than a coinciding problem. Do not assume, however, that a trauma victim has experienced *only* trauma, because another problem may have occurred first or at the same time. For example, a victim may have a heart attack and sudden cardiac arrest while on a ladder, resulting in a fall and possible fractures. A victim of drug overdose or poisoning may develop a severe breathing problem while operating machinery, causing an incident and traumatic injury. As a general rule, treat a trauma victim like any other: perform the initial assessment and give basic life support as needed.

Trauma victims generally have a "call first" rather than "call fast" status. Trauma that is severe enough to cause cardiac arrest can only be helped by invasive procedures, usually in a hospital. If the victim is to have a chance of survival, advanced care must arrive as quickly as possible so a determination can be made about the next steps. The victim needs to be transported to definitive care as quickly as possible.

Depending on the nature of the trauma, the victim may have a spinal injury as well. Any blow to the body severe enough to impact the airway, breathing or circulation is likely also to potentially injure the spine. Remember to keep the head in line with the body when positioning the victim and to use the jaw thrust technique rather than head tilt–chin lift to open the airway.

Trauma to the head or face may result in blood or other fluid blocking the airway. Check the mouth when opening the airway and if necessary wipe out any blood or vomit. With more extensive amounts of fluid, you may have to turn the victim onto one side to let it drain from the mouth. If the equipment is available and you are trained in its use, suction the victim's mouth when opening the airway.

In cases of cardiac arrest in victims with very severe trauma, local protocol may include not using the AED, as these victims seldom have a heart rhythm that can be corrected. Always follow your local protocol, and if the AED is not used, give CPR as usual while waiting for advanced help.

Hypothermia

Hypothermia is a low core body temperature as a result of exposure to a cold environment, often by immersion in cold water. Hypothermia requires special consideration when providing emergency care. Severely cold temperatures make the victim susceptible to heart rhythm problems, but a thorough assessment is important because some hypeothermia victims have been successfully resuscitated after a long period of hypothermia or immersion.

In severe hypothermia, the victim's heart may be beating very slowly or may be in arrest, and the respiratory rate may also be very slow or have stopped. For an unresponsive victim who is not breathing normally, check for a pulse no longer than 10 seconds, and if a pulse is not definitely felt, start CPR immediately. Follow local protocol for use of an AED with a hypothermia victim.

Do not delay or stop resuscitation efforts to rewarm the victim, but if possible prevent further heat loss from the victim's body. Other rescuers can remove wet clothing, for example or cover the victim with a blanket while basic life support is ongoing. Be gentle when handling or moving a hypothermic victim, because the heart is susceptible to dysrhythmias precipitated by motion or jarring.

Near-Drowning

In any situation in which a victim is in the water, ensure your own safety before attempting a rescue. It is very dangerous for an untrained rescuer to enter the water to rescue a responsive victim, who may grab the rescuer and make rescue difficult or impossible. Reach to the victim with a pole or long object, throw a rope or floating object, or go to the victim in a water-craft if possible. Beginning rescue breaths as soon as possible is a high priority for drowning victims. If you can do so, begin rescue breaths (after confirming respiratory arrest) even before removing the victim from shallow water. However, it is necessary to remove the victim from water to give CPR.

For an unresponsive victim removed from the water, consider whether the nature of the incident, such as diving in shallow or murky water or being thrown against the shore in surf conditions, suggests a possible spinal injury. If the cause of the submersion is unknown, assume the victim may have a spinal injury. Keep the head in line with the body when moving or positioning the victim and use the jaw thrust technique rather than head tilt–chin lift to open the airway.

Begin the initial assessment as usual by checking for responsiveness. Remember that this is a "call fast" rather than "call first" situation. If you are alone, give care for about 2 minutes (rescue breathing or CPR) before stopping to go for help.

Note that BLS care for a drowning victim is somewhat different from that given other victims found unresponsive. A drowning victim is more likely to have a pulse and may need only rescue breathing without chest compressions. If the victim is not breathing normally, first open the airway and give 2 rescue breaths. Then quickly check for a pulse. If the victim has a pulse but is still not breathing normally, continue with rescue breathing as described in Skill: "Rescue Breathing." If the victim does not have a pulse, then give CPR immediately, beginning with chest compressions.

Do not take any special actions to try to remove water from the victim first.

If the victim is not breathing and your rescue breaths do not make the chest rise, open the airway again and try to give 2 breaths. If your breaths still do not go in, give chest compressions for an airway obstruction.

If supplemental oxygen is available and you are trained in its use, administer oxygen to the victim. When an AED is available and ready, use it as usual. Victims have been resuscitated after being submerged in cold water for some time. If the victim may be hypothermic, follow the special considerations described earlier.

Electric Shock

Electric shock may result from a lightning strike or from contact with a source of household current or high-voltage power lines. The shock may cause the victim's breathing to stop because of paralyzed respiratory muscles and may cause cardiac arrest by disrupting the heart's electrical controls.

Remember scene safety before approaching the victim. Downed power lines, or household or industrial electrical appliances or cords may still be "live" and pose a threat to rescuers. Call 9-1-1 for downed power lines and do not try to move them yourself or to move the victim away from them. For electrical appliances, first shut the power off at the circuit breaker box or unplug the power cord if it is safe to do so.

The electric shock may cause a range of injuries in addition to effects on respiration and circulation. Especially with a high-voltage shock such as that caused by lightning, the victim may have severe burns and possible fractures due to strong muscular contractions caused by the electric shock. For a lightning strike victim, assume a possible spinal injury.

When it is safe to approach the victim, perform the initial assessment and provide care as needed. If the victim has a pulse but is not breathing, provide rescue breathing and continue to check the pulse. If the victim has no pulse, provide CPR and call for an AED. Often an electric shock causes ventricular fibrillation, in which case the AED may return the heart to a normal rhythm. If alone, first activate the emergency response system, get an AED if one is available, and then return to provide CPR.

Pregnancy

A woman in late stages of pregnancy with an airway obstruction should be given chest thrusts rather than abdominal thrusts to expel an obstructing object. A responsive victim can be given chest thrusts from behind while standing, and an unresponsive victim is given chest thrusts in the same manner as the chest compressions of CPR. Note that chest compressions should be given slightly higher on the sternum on a pregnant woman.

When a pregnant woman at a gestational age beyond 20 weeks lies on her back, the enlarged uterus may press against the inferior vena cava, the vein that returns blood to the heart from the lower half of the body. This pressure may decrease the blood flow to the heart and affect circulation to vital organs. When possible, therefore, position an injured pregnant woman lying on her left side, which reduces pressure from the uterus on the vena cava. Gently move the uterus to the left to help alleviate the pressure.

When giving CPR to a pregnant woman at a gestational age beyond 20 weeks, if possible position her for chest compressions on a firm surface that can be tilted 27 to 30 degrees such that her back is angled from the left lateral position (lying on left side).

Otherwise, perform basic life support on a pregnant woman in the same manner as for other victims, including the use of an AED in cases of cardiac arrest.

Appendix B • Performance Checklists for Skills

Participant Name _____   Date _____

Instructor Name _____

Performance Checklist: Hand Washing

Skill Step		Initial Practice		Final Performance	
		Needs Practice	Proficient	Remediate	Proficient
1	Remove any jewelry and your watch. Use a paper towel to turn on water and adjust the temperature to warm.				
2	Wet your hands to above the wrists and lather with soap. Keep your hands below your elbows throughout the hand washing process.				
3	Wash all areas of your hands and wrists. Interlace fingers to scrub between them. If your hands were exposed to infectious material, scrub beneath fingernails with a nail brush or nail stick.				
4	Rinse wrists and hands well. (Repeat soaping and washing if your hands were exposed to infectious material.)				
5	Dry hands thoroughly with paper towel and dispose of it properly. Use a new, dry paper towel to turn off the water faucet and open the door, and dispose of it properly.				
Complete Skill					

Participant Name _____   Date _____

Instructor Name _____

Performance Checklist: Putting on Gloves

	Skill Step	Initial Practice		Final Performance	
		Needs Practice	Proficient	Remediate	Proficient
1	Pull glove onto one hand.				
2	Pull glove tight.				
3	Put on other glove.				
	Complete Skill				

Participant Name _____   Date _____

Instructor Name _____

Performance Checklist: Removing Contaminated Gloves

	Skill Step	Initial Practice		Final Performance	
		Needs Practice	Proficient	Remediate	Proficient
1	With one hand, grasp your other glove at the wrist or palm and pull it away from your hand.				
2	Pull the glove the rest of the way off.				
3	Holding the removed glove balled up in the palm of your gloved hand, insert two fingers under the cuff of the remaining glove.				
4	Remove the glove by stretching it up and away from the hand and turning it inside out as you pull it off.				
5	Dispose of gloves in a biohazard container and wash your hands.				
	Complete Skill				

Performance Checklist: Initial Assessment

Skill Step	Initial Practice		Final Performance	
	Needs Practice	Proficient	Remediate	Proficient
1 Check for responsiveness and normal breathing.				
2 If the victim is unresponsive, call 9-1-1. If the victim is unresponsive and not breathing, also call for an AED and provide basic life support.				
3 If the victim is breathing, check for severe bleeding and other threats to life.				
4 Care for any life-threatening conditions before continuing to check the victim and provide other care.				
Complete Skill				

Participant Name _____   Date _____

Instructor Name _____

Performance Checklist: HAINES Recovery Position

Skill Step	Initial Practice		Final Performance	
	Needs Practice	Proficient	Remediate	Proficient
1 Extend the victim's arm that is farther from you above the victim's head.				
2 Position the victim's other arm across the chest.				
3 Bend the victim's nearer leg at the knee.				
4 Put your forearm under the victim's shoulder with your hand around the back of the neck to support the head and neck.				
5 Carefully roll the victim away from you by pushing on the victim's flexed knee and lifting with your forearm while your hand stabilizes the head and neck. The victim's head is now supported on the raised arm.				
6 While continuing to support the head and neck, position the victim's hand palm-down with fingers under the armpit of the raised arm, with forearm flat on the surface at 90 degrees to the body.				
7 Bend both legs so the victim's position is stabilized.				
8 With victim now in position, check the airway and open the mouth to allow drainage.				
Complete Skill				

Participant Name _____   Date _____

Instructor Name _____

Performance Checklist: Physical Examination

Skill Step	Initial Practice		Final Performance	
	Needs Practice	Proficient	Remediate	Proficient
If you find any problems in any body area, do not let the victim move. Wait for help.				
1 Being careful not to move the victim's head or neck, check the head.				
2 Check neck area for medical alert necklace, deformity or swelling, and pain. Do not move the neck.				
3 Check skin appearance, temperature and moisture.				
4 Check chest. Ask victim to breathe deeply.				
5 Check abdomen.				
6 Check pelvis and hips.				
7 Check upper extremities. Look for medical alert bracelet.				
8 Check lower extremities.				
Complete Skill				

Participant Name _____ Date _____

Instructor Name _____

Performance Checklist: CPR for Adults, Children and Infants (1 Rescuer)

Skill Step	Initial Practice		Final Performance	
	Needs Practice	Proficient	Remediate	Proficient
1 Determine that the victim is unresponsive, not breathing normally and is pulseless. Have someone call 9-1-1 (or call yourself if alone) and get an AED.				
2 Expose the chest. Put your hand on the lower half of the breastbone in the middle of the chest for chest compressions. For an adult, put your second hand on top of the first and interlock the fingers. For a child, use 1 or both hands. For an infant, put 2 middle fingers of 1 hand just below the nipple line.				
3 Give 30 chest compressions hard and fast at least 2 inches deep in an adult and at least ⅓ the depth of the chest in an infant (about 1½ inches) or child (about 2 inches) at a rate of at least 100 per minute. Count aloud for a steady fast rate: "One, two, three . . ." Then give 2 breaths.				
4 Open the airway and give 2 rescue breaths, each lasting 1 second, to cause a visible chest rise. (If the first breath does not go in, reposition the victim's head and try again; if the second breath does not go in, give choking care.)				
5 Continue cycles of 30 compressions and 2 breaths.				
6 Continue CPR until: • The victim wakes up • An AED is brought to the scene and is ready to use • Personnel with more training arrive and take over				
7 a. If the victim starts breathing normally but is unresponsive, put the victim in the recovery position and monitor breathing. b. If the victim is not breathing normally and has no pulse, start the AED sequence when an AED arrives.				
Complete Skill				

Participant Name _____ Date _____

Instructor Name _____

Performance Checklist: AED

	Skill Step	Initial Practice		Final Performance	
		Needs Practice	Proficient	Remediate	Proficient
1	Position the victim away from water and metal. Place the unit by the victim's shoulder and turn it on.				
2	Expose the victim's chest and quickly dry or shave the pad placement area if necessary.				
3	Apply pads to the victim's chest as shown on pads. If needed, plug the cables into the unit. *Use adult pads for a victim 8 or older. For an infant or child younger than 8, use a unit with pediatric pads if available, applied as directed by the unit. If pediatric pads are unavailable, use adult pads.*				
4	Stand clear during rhythm analysis.				
5	Follow prompts from the AED unit to do one of three things: (1) press the "shock" button, (2) stay clear while the AED automatically delivers a shock or (3) do not shock but immediately give CPR with the pads remaining in place, starting with chest compressions.				
6	Follow the AED's prompts to analyze the rhythm again after 5 cycles of CPR (about 2 minutes).				
7	Continue steps 5 and 6 until the victim wakes up or more advanced help arrives and takes over.				
8	If the victim begins breathing normally but is unresponsive, put the victim in the recovery position (with pads remaining in place) and continue to monitor breathing and pulse.				
	Complete Skill				

Participant Name _____   Date _____

Instructor Name _____

Performance Checklist: Choking Care for Responsive Adult or Child

Skill Step	Initial Practice		Final Performance	
	Needs Practice	Proficient	Remediate	Proficient
1. Stand behind an adult victim with one leg forward between the victim's legs. Keep your head slightly to one side. For a child, move down to the child's level or kneel behind the child. Reach around the abdomen.				
2. Locate the victim's navel with a finger from one hand. Make a fist with the other hand and place the thumb side of the fist against the person's abdomen just above the navel.				
3. Grasp your fist with your other hand and thrust inward and upward into the victim's abdomen with quick thrusts. Continue abdominal thrusts until the victim expels the object or becomes unresponsive.				
4. For a responsive pregnant victim or any victim you cannot get your arms around or cannot effectively give abdominal thrusts to, give chest thrusts in the middle of the breastbone from behind the victim. Avoid squeezing the ribs with your arms.				
Complete Skill				

Participant Name _____ Date _____

Instructor Name _____

Performance Checklist: Choking Care for Unresponsive Adult, Child or Infant

	Skill Step	Initial Practice		Final Performance	
		Needs Practice	Proficient	Remediate	Proficient
1	If the victim is unresponsive and not breathing normally, start CPR with 30 chest compressions at least 2 inches deep in an adult and at least ⅓ the depth of the chest in child (about 2 inches) or infant (about 1½ inches) at a rate of at least 100 per minute. Count aloud for a steady fast rate: "One, two, three, . . ."				
2	Open the airway with the head tilt–chin lift.				
3	Give 2 rescue breaths, each lasting 1 second. If the first breath does not go in and the chest does not rise, position the victim's head again to open the airway and try again.				
4	If breaths still do not go in, continue CPR with chest compressions, using a ratio of 30 compressions and 2 breaths.				
5	Look inside the mouth before giving breaths after each cycle of compressions, and remove any object you see. Then give 2 breaths.				
6	Continue CPR until: • The victim recovers and is breathing normally • Professional help arrives and takes over				
	Complete Skill				

Participant Name _____   Date _____

Instructor Name _____

Performance Checklist: Choking Care for Responsive Infant

Skill Step	Initial Practice		Final Performance	
	Needs Practice	Proficient	Remediate	Proficient
1 — Support the infant face-down by holding the head in one hand, with the torso on your forearm against your thigh. Give up to 5 back blows (slaps) between the shoulder blades with the heel of your hand.				
2 — Check for an expelled object. If not present, continue with next step.				
3 — With your other hand on the back of the infant's head, roll the infant face-up, supporting the back of the infant's head with your hand.				
4 — Give up to 5 chest thrusts with two fingers on sternum just below the nipple line, about 1 per second. Each thrust should be 1½ inches deep. Check mouth for expelled object.				
5 — Continue cycles of 5 back blows (slaps) and 5 chest thrusts and checking the mouth. If alone, call 9-1-1 after 1 minute. Continue until the object is expelled or the infant becomes unresponsive. If the infant becomes unresponsive, give CPR. Look inside the mouth before giving breaths after each cycle of compressions, and remove any object you see.				
Complete Skill				

Participant Name _____   Date _____

Instructor Name _____

Performance Checklist: Controlling Bleeding

Skill Step	Initial Practice		Final Performance	
	Needs Practice	Proficient	Remediate	Proficient
1 Put on gloves. *Improvise a barrier if no barrier is available.*				
2 Place a sterile dressing or clean cloth on the wound.				
3 Apply firm, direct pressure with your hand for about 5 minutes.				
4 Reevaluate the bleeding: If it continues, put another dressing or cloth pad on top of the first and keep applying pressure.				
5 If needed, apply a pressure bandage to keep pressure on the wound, wrapping from the end of the extremity toward the center of the body. *The pressure is sufficient if the bandage is snug but you can slip a finger under it.*				
6 If appropriate, treat the victim for shock and call 9-1-1.				
Complete Skill				

Participant Name _____   Date _____

Instructor Name _____

Performance Checklist: Applying a Pressure Bandage

	Skill Step	Initial Practice		Final Performance	
		Needs Practice	Proficient	Remediate	Proficient
1	Place a sterile dressing or clean cloth on wound. Start wrapping an elastic or self-adhering roller bandage below the wound dressing, wrapping from the end of the extremity toward the center of the body.				
2	Make several circular turns, then overlap turns by about ½ of previous turn.				
3	Work up the limb to cover the dressing completely. The pressure is sufficient if the bandage is snug but a finger can be slipped under it.				
4	Fix or tie the end of the bandage in place.				
	Complete Skill				

Participant Name _____ Date _____

Instructor Name _____

Performance Checklist: Shock Position

Skill Step	Initial Practice		Final Performance	
	Needs Practice	Proficient	Remediate	Proficient
1 — Check for responsiveness, normal breathing and severe bleeding, and care first for life-threatening injuries.				
2 — Call 9-1-1 and be ready to give basic life support if needed.				
3 — a. Position a responsive victim with trauma on his or her back using a blanket or coat as a pad. If there is no evidence of trauma, raise the legs such that the feet are 6-12 inches above the ground. b. Put a breathing, unresponsive victim (if no suspected spinal injury) in the recovery position.				
4 — Loosen any tight clothing.				
5 — Be alert for the possibility of vomiting; turn the victim's head to drain the mouth.				
6 — Maintain the victim's normal body temperature. If necessary, maintain the victim's body heat by placing a blanket or coat over the victim.				
Complete Skill				

Participant Name _____ Date _____

Instructor Name _____

Performance Checklist: Emergency Epinephrine Auto-Injector

	Skill Step	Initial Practice		Final Performance	
		Needs Practice	Proficient	Remediate	Proficient
1	Call 9-1-1.				
2	Help a responsive victim use his or her emergency epinephrine auto-injector such as an EpiPen, Ana-Kit or or TwinJect. If the victim cannot use his or her prescribed auto-injector, you may administer it yourself if permitted by state law. a. Take the auto-injector out of its case and remove the safety cap. b. To administer the medication, the victim jabs the pen tip into the outer thigh and holds it there for 10 seconds while the medication is injected. c. The medication should provide relief for 15-20 minutes.				
3	Monitor the victim's breathing and be ready to give CPR if needed.				
4	Help a responsive victim sit up in a position of easiest breathing. Put an unresponsive victim who is breathing in the recovery position.				
	Complete Skill				

Participant Name _____   Date _____

Instructor Name _____

Performance Checklist: Assessing Head and Spinal Injuries

Skill Step	Initial Practice		Final Performance	
	Needs Practice	**Proficient**	**Remediate**	**Proficient**
1 Check the victim's head.				
2 Check neck for deformity, swelling and pain.				
3 Touch toes of both feet and ask victim if the sensation feels normal.				
4 Ask victim to point toes.				
5 Ask victim to push against your hands with his or her feet.				
6 Touch fingers of both hands and ask victim if the sensation feels normal.				
7 Ask victim to make a fist and curl (flex) it in.				
8 Ask victim to squeeze your hands.				
Complete Skill				

Participant Name _____   Date _____

Instructor Name _____

Performance Checklist: Spinal Motion Restriction

Skill Step	Initial Practice		Final Performance	
	Needs Practice	Proficient	Remediate	Proficient
1 Ask a responsive victim what happened. If he or she has any of the risk factors, explain the need to hold the head still to prevent spinal movement and spinal cord injury. For an unresponsive victim, check for risk factors for suspected spinal injury.				
2 Hold the victim's head and neck with both hands in the position found to prevent movement.				
3 Monitor the victim's breathing and be ready to provide basic life support.				
4 Have someone call 9-1-1.				
5 Reassure a conscious victim and tell him or her not to move.				
6 Continue to stabilize head/spine and monitor the victim's breathing until help arrives.				
Complete Skill				

Participant Name _____   Date _____

Instructor Name _____

Performance Checklist: Rolling a Victim With Spinal Injury (Log Roll)

Skill Step	Initial Practice		Final Performance	
	Needs Practice	Proficient	Remediate	Proficient
1 Hold the victim's head with hands on both sides over ears.				
2 The first aider at the victim's head directs others to roll the body as a unit.				
3 Continue to support head in new position on side.				
Complete Skill				

Participant Name _____   Date _____

Instructor Name _____

Performance Checklist: Applying a Spiral Bandage

Skill Step	Initial Practice		Final Performance	
	Needs Practice	Proficient	Remediate	Proficient
1 Anchor the starting end of the elastic roller bandage below the injured area, farther from the trunk.				
2 Wrap the bandage in spirals up the limb toward the center of the body.				
3 Fasten the end of the bandage with clips, tape or safety pins.				
Complete Skill				

Participant Name _____   Date _____

Instructor Name _____

Performance Checklist: Applying a Figure-Eight Bandage to the Wrist

Skill Step	Initial Practice		Final Performance	
	Needs Practice	Proficient	Remediate	Proficient
1 Anchor the starting end of the roller bandage.				
2 Turn the bandage diagonally across the wrist and back around the hand.				
3 Continue with overlapping figure-eight turns.				
4 Fasten the end of the bandage by tying it or using clips, tape or safety pins.				
Complete Skill				

Participant Name _____   Date _____

Instructor Name _____

Performance Checklist: Applying a Figure-Eight Bandage to the Ankle

Skill Step	Initial Practice		Final Performance	
	Needs Practice	Proficient	Remediate	Proficient
1 Anchor the starting end of the bandage.				
2 Turn the bandage diagonally across the top of the foot and around the ankle and bring the bandage around in a figure-eight.				
3 Continue with overlapping figure-eight turns.				
4 Fasten the end of the bandage with clips, tape or safety pins.				
Complete Skill				

Participant Name _____ Date _____

Instructor Name _____

Performance Checklist: RICE: Wrist Injury

Skill Step	Initial Practice		Final Performance	
	Needs Practice	Proficient	Remediate	Proficient
1 Rest the injured wrist.				
2 Put ice or a cold pack on the injured area.				
3 Compress the injured area with an elastic roller bandage.				
4 Elevate the injured area. Use a sling to hold the wrist in place.				
Complete Skill				

Participant Name _____ Date _____

Instructor Name _____

Performance Checklist: Applying an Arm Sling and Binder

Skill Step	Initial Practice		Final Performance	
	Needs Practice	Proficient	Remediate	Proficient
1 Secure the point of the bandage at the elbow. Use a safety pin or tie the point at the elbow.				
2 Position the triangular bandage.				
3 Bring up the lower end of the bandage to the opposite side of the neck.				
4 Tie the ends. Pad under the knot.				
5 Tie a binder bandage over the sling and around the chest.				
Complete Skill				

Participant Name _____   Date _____

Instructor Name _____

Performance Checklist: Splinting the Forearm

Skill Step	Initial Practice		Final Performance	
	Needs Practice	Proficient	Remediate	Proficient
1 Support the arm above and below the injury. Check circulation.				
2 Position the arm on a padded rigid splint. If available, add a roller bandage under the fingers.				
3 Secure the splint.				
4 Check circulation.				
5 Put the arm in a sling and tie a binder over the sling and around the chest.				
Complete Skill				

Participant Name _____   Date _____

Instructor Name _____

Performance Checklist: Anatomic Splinting of Leg

Skill Step	Initial Practice		Final Performance	
	Needs Practice	Proficient	Remediate	Proficient
1 Check circulation. Gently slide four or five bandages or strips of cloth under both legs. Do not put a bandage over the injury site.				
2 Put padding between the legs. Do not move the injured leg.				
3 Gently slide the uninjured leg next to the injured leg.				
4 Tie the bandages (snug but not tight), starting in the middle, then at the lower leg and then at the top. Check circulation.				
Complete Skill				

Participant Name _____ Date _____

Instructor Name _____

Performance Checklist: Rescue Breathing

Skill Step		Initial Practice		Final Performance	
		Needs Practice	Proficient	Remediate	Proficient
1	If the victim has a pulse but is not breathing normally, open the airway and give a breath over 1 second, watching the chest rise and fall.				
2	If the first breath does not go in, try again to open the airway and give another rescue breath. If it still does not go in, the victim may be choking. Proceed to CPR for choking.				
3	If your breath goes in, continue rescue breathing. Give each breath over 1 second, at a rate of 10 to 12 breaths per minute (1 breath every 5-6 seconds) for an adult; 12 to 20 breaths per minute for a child (1 breath every 3-5 seconds); or 20 breaths per minute for an infant (1 breath every 3 seconds).				
4	Check the pulse about every 2 minutes. If victim has no pulse, start CPR beginning with chest compressions.				
Complete Skill					

Participant Name _____   Date _____

Instructor Name _____

Performance Checklist: Suctioning (Adult or Child)

Skill Step	Initial Practice		Final Performance	
	Needs Practice	Proficient	Remediate	Proficient
1 Confirm that the suction device is working and produces suction.				
2 Turn the victim's head to one side and open the mouth. For spinal injury, support the head and turn with body as one unit.				
3 Sweep out solids and larger amounts of fluid with your finger.				
4 Determine maximum depth of insertion by measuring the catheter tip from the earlobe to the corner of the mouth.				
5 Turn on suction or pump the handle to create suction.				
6 Insert catheter tip carefully into the mouth. Put your finger over the proximal opening to begin suctioning and move the tip about as you withdraw it.				
7 Reposition the victim's head with airway open and resume rescue breathing or CPR.				
Complete Skill				

Participant Name _____   Date _____

Instructor Name _____

Performance Checklist: Suctioning (Infant)

Skill Step		Initial Practice		Final Performance	
		Needs Practice	Proficient	Remediate	Proficient
1	Hold the infant in position for suctioning, with the head lower than the body and turned to one side.				
2	Squeeze the suction bulb first and then gently insert the tip into the infant's mouth.				
3	Gradually release the bulb to create suction as you withdraw the tip from the infant's mouth.				
4	Move the bulb aside and squeeze it, with tip down, to empty it.				
5	Repeat steps 2 through 4 until the airway seems clear, up to 3 times.				
6	Repeat the suctioning steps for each nostril.				
7	Begin or resume rescue breathing or CPR if needed.				
Complete Skill					

Participant Name _____   Date _____

Instructor Name _____

Performance Checklist: Bag Mask for Rescue Breathing (2 Rescuers)

	Skill Step	Initial Practice		Final Performance	
		Needs Practice	Proficient	Remediate	Proficient
1	Rescuer 1 assembles the BVM with a mask of the correct size and puts the mask over the victim's mouth and nose.				
2	Rescuer 2 positions hands: thumbs and index fingers circling each side of mask, the other three fingers of each hand behind lower jawbone. Pull the jaw up into the mask instead of pushing the mask down on the jaw.				
3	Rescuer 2 opens the airway and seals the mask to the victim's face.				
4	Rescuer 1 squeezes the bag to provide ventilations: a. 1 ventilation over 1 second in adult, every 5-6 seconds. b. 1 ventilation over 1 second in child, every 3-5 seconds. c. 1 ventilation over 1 second in infant, every 3 seconds.				
5	Recheck pulse about every 2 minutes. If no pulse, call for an AED and start CPR.				
	Complete Skill				

Participant Name _____ Date _____

Instructor Name _____

Performance Checklist: Oxygen Administration

	Skill Step	Initial Practice		Final Performance	
		Needs Practice	**Proficient**	**Remediate**	**Proficient**
1	Check equipment: oxygen labels on the cylinder and regulator; tubing and delivery device ready.				
2	Remove any protective seal, point the cylinder away and open main valve for 1 second.				
3	Remove any protective seals and attach the regulator to the oxygen cylinder.				
4	Open the main cylinder valve.				
5	Check the pressure regulator gauge.				
6	Attach the tubing to the flowmeter and the oxygen delivery device.				
7	Set the flowmeter at the correct oxygen flow rate. a. 1 to 6 lpm for nasal cannula b. 10 lpm for face mask c. 10 to 15 lpm for BVM or nonrebreather mask				
8	Confirm oxygen is flowing.				
9	Position the delivery device on the victim and continue rescue breathing (or allow victim to breathe spontaneously).				
10	Monitor the pressure regulator gauge and be prepared to remove the delivery device and change tanks if the pressure drops below 500 psi. Observe oxygen safety precautions.				
	Complete Skill				

Participant Name _____ Date _____

Instructor Name _____

Performance Checklist: Oral Airway Insertion

	Skill Step	Initial Practice		Final Performance	
		Needs Practice	Proficient	Remediate	Proficient
1	Choose the correct airway device size. (The oral airway length should match the distance from the corner of the mouth to the tip of the earlobe on the same side of the victim's face.)				
2	Open the victim's airway with head tilt–chin lift or jaw thrust, and open the mouth.				
3	Insert the airway device with the tip pointing toward the roof of the mouth.				
4	When tip reaches the back of the mouth and you feel resistance, rotate the airway 180 degrees.				
5	Continue to insert the airway device to the final position (the flange resting on the lips).				
	Complete Skill				

Participant Name _____ Date _____

Instructor Name _____

Performance Checklist: Nasal Airway Insertion

Skill Step		Initial Practice		Final Performance	
		Needs Practice	Proficient	Remediate	Proficient
1	Choose the correct nasal airway size. (The nasal airway length should match the distance from the nostril to the tip of the earlobe on the same side of the victim's face.)				
2	Coat the nasal airway with lubricant.				
3	Insert the nasal airway in the right nostril with the bevel toward the septum.				
4	Insert the nasal airway straight back, sliding it along the floor of the nostril.				
5	Insert the nasal airway until the flange rests against the nose.				
Complete Skill					

Participant Name _____ Date _____

Instructor Name _____

Performance Checklist: CPR for Adult or Child (2 Rescuers)

	Skill Step	Initial Practice		Final Performance	
		Needs Practice	Proficient	Remediate	Proficient
1	At the victim's head, Rescuer 1 checks for unresponsiveness and normal breathing. If the victim is not breathing, check for a pulse for no longer than 10 seconds. Rescuer 2 ensures that an AED has been summoned. At the victim's side, Rescuer 2 locates the site for chest compressions.				
2	Rescuer 1 indicates, "No pulse." Rescuer 2 gives 30 compressions for an adult (15 for a child) at rate of at least 100 per minute, counting aloud for a fast, steady rate, then pauses.				
3	Rescuer 1 gives 2 breaths.				
4	Rescuers continue cycles of 30 compressions in an adult (15 in a child) and 2 breaths for about 2 minutes (or after 5 cycles of compressions and ventilations at a ratio of 30:2) before switching compressor and ventilator roles. The switch should be done quickly (in less than 5 seconds).				
5	Rescuers continue CPR until: • The victim is breathing normally and has a pulse • An AED is brought to the scene and is ready to use • Help arrives and takes over				
6	a. If the victim starts breathing normally and has a pulse but is unresponsive, put the victim in the recovery position and monitor breathing and pulse. b. For a victim who is not breathing normally and has no pulse, start the AED sequence when the AED arrives.				
	Complete Skill				

Participant Name _____   Date _____

Instructor Name _____

Performance Checklist: CPR for Infant (2 rescuers)

	Skill Step	Initial Practice		Final Performance	
		Needs Practice	Proficient	Remediate	Proficient
1	At the infant's head, Rescuer 1 checks for normal breathing and a pulse. At the infant's feet, Rescuer 2 positions hands in the chest-encircling position for chest compressions with both thumbs.				
2	If pulse is absent, Rescuer 1 says, "No pulse." Rescuer 2 gives 15 chest compressions at a rate of at least 100 per minute, counting aloud for a fast, steady rate, then pauses.				
3	Rescuer 1 gives 2 breaths.				
4	Rescuers continue cycles of 15 compressions and 2 breaths for about 2 minutes before switching compressor and ventilator roles. The switch should be done quickly (in less than 5 seconds). Rescuers continue CPR until: • The infant is breathing normally and has a pulse • More advanced help arrives and takes over				
5	a. If the infant starts breathing normally but is unresponsive, hold the infant in the recovery position and monitor breathing and pulse. b. For an infant who is not breathing normally and has no pulse, start the AED sequence when the AED arrives.				
	Complete Skill				

B • Performance Checklists for Skills

Appendix C • Natural Disasters: Earthquakes

Surviving an earthquake and reducing its health impact requires preparation, planning and practice. Far in advance, you can gather emergency supplies, identify and reduce possible hazards in your home, and practice what to do during and after an earthquake. Learning what actions to take can help you and your family remain safe and healthy in the event of an earthquake.

Being Prepared

Although California has been the state most prone to serious earthquakes in recent years, many other fault zones exist in other areas of the United States. For example, geologists and seismologists have predicted a 97% chance of a major earthquake occurring in the New Madrid Seismic Zone in the central United States (including Arkansas, Missouri, Tennessee and Kentucky) between now and the year 2035. Although earthquakes with the power of the one that hit the greater Los Angeles area in January 1994 are fairly rare, less severe earthquakes can disrupt your normal living patterns and cause substantial injury.

During a major earthquake, you may hear a roaring or rumbling sound that gradually grows louder. You may feel a rolling sensation that starts out gently and, within a second or two, grows violent. Or, you may first be jarred by a violent jolt. A second or two later, you may feel shaking and find it difficult to stand up or move from one room to another.

The key to surviving an earthquake and reducing your risk of injury lies in planning, preparing and practicing what you and your family will do if it happens.

Source: Centers for Disease Control and Prevention http:// www.bt.cdc.gov/disasters Accessed March 2, 2011.

Practice Drills

By planning and practicing what to do if an earthquake strikes, you and your family can learn to react correctly and automatically when the shaking begins. During an earthquake, most deaths and injuries are caused by collapsing building materials and heavy falling objects, such as bookcases, cabinets and heating units. Learn the safe spots in each room of your home. If you have children, get the entire family to practice going to these locations. Participating in an earthquake drill will help children understand what to do in case you are not with them during an earthquake.

Make sure you and your child also understand the school's emergency procedures for disasters. This will help you coordinate where, when and how to reunite with your child after an earthquake.

During your earthquake drill:

- Get under a sturdy table or desk and hold on to it.

- If you are not near a table or desk, cover your face and head with your arms and stand or crouch in a strongly supported doorway or brace yourself in an inside corner of the house or building.

- Stay clear of windows or glass that could shatter or objects that could fall on you.

- Remember: If you are inside, stay inside. Many people are injured by falling debris at entrances of buildings.

Evacuation Plans

After an earthquake occurs, you may need to evacuate a damaged area. By planning and practicing for evacuation, you will be better prepared to respond appropriately and efficiently to signs of danger or to directions from civil authorities.

- Take a few minutes with your family to discuss a home evacuation plan. Sketch a floor plan of your home, and walk through each room and discuss evacuation details.

- Plan a second way to exit from each room or area, if possible. If you need special equipment, such as a rope ladder, mark where it is located.

- Mark where your emergency food, water, first aid kits and fire extinguishers are located.

- Mark where the utility switches or valves are located so that they can be turned off, if possible.

- Indicate the location of your family's emergency outdoor meeting place.

Establish Priorities

Take time before an earthquake strikes to write an emergency priority list, including –

- important items to be hand-carried by you.

- other items, in order of importance to you and your family.

- items to be removed by car or truck if one is available.

- things to do if time permits, such as locking doors and windows, turning off utilities, etc.

Write Down Important Information

Make a list of important information and put it in a secure location. Include on your list –

- important telephone numbers, such as police, fire, EMS and medical centers.

- the names, addresses and telephone numbers of your insurance agents, including policy types and numbers.

- the telephone numbers of the electric, gas and water companies.

- the names and telephone numbers of neighbors.

- the name and telephone number of your landlord or property manager.

- important medical information (i.e., allergies, regular medications).

- the vehicle identification number, year, model and license number of your automobile, boat, RV, etc.

- your financial institution's telephone number, and your account types and numbers.

- radio and television broadcast stations to tune to for emergency broadcast information.

Gather and Store Important Documents in a Fireproof Safe

- Birth certificates

- Ownership certificates (automobiles, boats, etc.)

- Social Security cards

- Insurance policies

- Wills

- Household inventory, including:

  - List of contents

  - Photographs of contents of every room

  - Photographs of items of high value, such as jewelry, paintings, collectors' items

Emergency Supplies

Stock up now on emergency supplies that can be used after an earthquake. These supplies should include a first aid kit; survival kits for the home, automobile and workplace; and emergency water and food. Store enough supplies to last at least three days.

First Aid Kit

Store your first aid supplies in a toolbox or fishing tackle box so they will be easy to carry and protect from water. Inspect your kit regularly and keep it freshly stocked. Note: Important medical information and most prescriptions can be stored in the refrigerator, which also provides excellent protection from fires.

Survival Kit for Your Home

Assemble a survival kit for your home with the following items:

Tools and Supplies

- Axe, shovel and broom
- Screwdriver, pliers, hammer and adjustable wrench
- Rope for towing or rescue
- Plastic sheeting and tape

Items for Safety and Comfort

- Sturdy shoes that can provide protection from broken glass, nails and other debris
- Gloves (heavy and durable for cleaning up debris)
- Candles
- Waterproof matches
- Change of clothing
- Knife
- Garden hose (for siphoning and firefighting)
- Tent
- Recreational supplies for children and adults
- Blankets or sleeping bags
- Portable radio, flashlight and extra batteries
- Essential medications and eyeglasses
- Fire extinguisher (multipurpose, dry chemical type)
- Food and water for pets
- Toilet tissue
- Cash

Survival Kit for Your Automobile

Assemble a survival kit for your automobile with the following items. Storing some of these supplies in a small bag or backpack will make

them more convenient to carry if you need to walk.

- Blankets
- Bottled water
- Change of clothes
- Coins for telephone calls
- Fire extinguisher (multipurpose, dry chemical type)
- First aid kit and manual
- Emergency signal device (light sticks, battery-type flasher, reflector, etc.)
- Flashlight with fresh batteries
- Food (nonperishable – nutrition bars, trail mix, etc.)
- Gloves
- Local map and compass
- Rope for towing, rescue, etc.
- Paper and pencils
- Premoistened towelettes
- Prescription medicines
- Battery-operated radio with fresh batteries
- Small mirror for signaling
- Toilet tissue
- Tools (pliers, adjustable wrench, screwdriver, etc.)
- Whistle for signaling
- Jumper cables
- Duct tape

Survival Kit for Your Workplace

Assemble a survival kit for the workplace with the following supplies:

- Food (nonperishable – nutrition bars, trail mix, etc.)
- Bottled water
- Jacket or sweatshirt
- Pair of sturdy shoes

- Flashlight with fresh batteries
- Battery-operated radio with fresh batteries
- Essential medications
- Blanket
- Small first aid kit
- Extra pair of eyeglasses and/or contact lens solution
- Whistle or other signaling device

Emergency Water Storage and Purification

Following are recommendations for storing and purifying water supplies:

- The minimum drinking water supply is 1 gallon per person per day. You will also need water for food preparation, bathing, brushing teeth and dishwashing. Store a three- to five-day supply of water (at least 5 gallons for each person).

- Water should be stored in sturdy plastic bottles with tight-fitting lids. Rinsed chlorine bleach bottles work well. Plastic containers for juice and milk do not work as well because they tend to crack and leak more easily.

- Stored water should be changed every 6 months.

- Avoid placing water containers in areas where toxic substances, such as gasoline and pesticides, are present. Vapors may penetrate the plastic over time.

- Do not store water containers in direct sunlight. Select a place with a fairly constant, cool temperature.

Safe Water Sources in the Home

If you do not have enough water stored, certain sources in your home may provide safe, clean water for drinking purposes.

- Water drained from the water heater faucet, if the water heater has not been damaged

- Water dipped from the tank of the toilet (not the bowl). The water in the bowl can be used for pets. Do not use water that has been chemically treated ("blue" water).

- Melted ice cubes

- Canned fruit, vegetable juice and liquids from other canned goods

- Water from the swimming pool. Use this water only after other sources of pure water are exhausted.

Unsafe Water Sources

Never use water from the following sources for drinking:

- Radiators
- Hot water boilers (home heating system)
- Water beds (fungicides added to the water or chemicals in the vinyl may make water unsafe for use)

Note: Remember that carbonated beverages do not meet drinking water requirements. Caffeinated drinks and alcohol dehydrate the body, which increases the need for drinking water.

Water for Drinking and Cooking

Safe drinking water includes bottled, boiled or treated water. Your state or local health department can make specific recommendations for boiling or treating drinking water in your area. Here are some general rules about water for drinking and cooking. Remember:

- Do not use contaminated water to wash dishes, brush your teeth, wash and prepare food, or make ice.

- If you use bottled water, make sure the seal has not been broken. Otherwise, water should be boiled or treated before use. Drink only bottled, boiled or treated water until your supply is tested and found safe.

- Boiling water kills harmful bacteria and parasites. Bringing water to a rolling boil for 1 minute will kill most organisms.

- Treat water with chlorine or iodine tablets or mix six drops (⅛ teaspoon) of unscented ordinary household chlorine bleach per gallon of water. Mix the solution thoroughly and let stand for about 30 minutes. However, this treatment will not kill parasitic organisms. Containers for water should be rinsed with a bleach solution before using and reusing. Use water storage tanks and other types of containers with caution. For example, fire truck storage tanks, as well as previously used cans or bottles, can be contaminated with microbes or chemicals.

Emergency Food

Keep foods that

- have a long storage life.

- require little or no cooking, water or refrigeration, in case utilities are disrupted.

- meet the needs of babies or other family members who are on special diets.

- meet pets' needs.

- are not very salty or spicy, as these foods increase the need for drinking water, which may be in short supply.

How to Store Emergency Food

- A disaster can easily disrupt the food supply at any time, so plan to have at least a three-day supply of food on hand.

- When storing food, it is not necessary to buy dehydrated or other types of emergency food. Canned foods and dry mixes will remain fresh for about two years.

- Certain storage conditions can enhance the shelf life of canned or dried foods. The ideal location is a cool, dry, dark place. The best temperature is 40° F to 60° F. Keep foods away from ranges or refrigerator exhausts. Heat causes many foods to spoil more quickly.

- Keep food away from petroleum products, such as gasoline, oil, paints and solvents. Some food products absorb their smell.

- Protect food from rodents and insects. Items stored in boxes or in paper cartons will keep longer if they are heavily wrapped or stored in airtight containers.

- Date all food items. Use and replace food before it loses freshness.

How to Use Emergency Food

- Use perishable food in your refrigerator or freezer before using food in your emergency supplies.

- Discard cooked, unrefrigerated foods after two hours at room temperature, regardless of appearance.

- Eat only foods that have a normal color, texture and odor.

- Discard cans that bulge at the ends or are leaking.

Preparing Food

Your ability to prepare food after an earthquake may be complicated by damage to your home and loss of electricity, gas and water. The following items will help you to prepare meals safely:

- Cooking utensils

- Knives, forks and spoons

- Paper plates, cups and towels

- A manual can and bottle opener

- Heavy-duty aluminum foil

- A gas or charcoal grill or a camp stove

- Fuel for cooking, such as charcoal. (Caution: Never burn charcoal indoors. The fumes are deadly when concentrated indoors.)

Note: Do not use your fireplace for cooking until the chimney has been inspected for cracks and damage. Sparks may escape into your attic through an undetected crack and start a fire.

Inspecting For Possible Home Hazards

An important step in earthquake preparedness is to inspect your home and its surroundings for possible hazards, and then take action to reduce those hazards. Remember: Anything can move, fall or break during an earthquake or its aftershocks.

The following is a basic checklist to help you identify and correct possible home hazards.

Rooms in the Home

Look for the following hazards in each room:

- Windows and other glass that might shatter

- Unanchored bookcases, cabinets, refrigerators, water heaters and other furniture that might topple

- Heating units, fireplaces, chimneys and stoves that could move or fall

- Areas that could be blocked by falling debris

Securing Appliances

- Secure your large appliances with flexible cable, braided wire or metal strapping.

- Install flexible gas and water connections on all gas appliances. This will significantly reduce your chances of having a major fire after an earthquake.

- Brace and support air conditioners, particularly those on rooftops.

A typical water heater weighs about 450 pounds when full. In an earthquake, the floor on which it is standing tends to move out from under the heater, often causing it to topple. The movement can also break the gas, electric and water-line connectors, posing a fire or electric shock hazard, and can shatter the glass lining within the water heater. The water tank should be well secured with bolts to wall studs.

Securing Items in the Bathroom

Replace glass bottles from your medicine cabinet and around the bathtub with plastic containers.

Hanging and Overhead Items

- Inspect and anchor overhead light fixtures, such as chandeliers.

- Move heavy mirrors and pictures hanging above beds, chairs, and other places where you sit or sleep. Otherwise, anchor these items with wire through eyescrews bolted into wall studs. Or place screws on both sides, top and bottom of the frame and screw these into the studs.

- Determine whether the full swing of your hanging lamps or plants will strike a window. If so, move them.

- Secure hanging objects by closing the opening of the hook.

- Replace heavy ceramic or glass hanging planters with lightweight plastic or wicker baskets.

Shelves, Cabinets and Furniture

- Identify top-heavy, freestanding furniture, such as bookcases and china cabinets, that could topple in an earthquake.

- Secure your furniture by using:

  - L brackets, corner brackets or aluminum molding to attach tall or top-heavy furniture to the wall

  - Eyebolts to secure items located a short distance from the wall

- Attach a wooden or metal guardrail on open shelves to keep items from sliding or falling off. Fishing line can also be used as a less-visible means of securing an item.

- Place heavy or large objects on lower shelves.

- Use Velcro-type fastenings to secure some items to their shelves.

- Secure your cabinet doors by installing sliding bolts or childproof latches.

Hazardous Materials

Identify poisons, solvents or toxic materials in breakable containers and move these containers to a safe, well-ventilated storage area. Keep them away from your water storage and out of reach of children and pets.

Inspecting And Securing Your Home's Structure

Examine the structural safety of your house. If your house is of conventional wood construction, it will probably be relatively resistant to earthquake damage, particularly if it is a single-story structure.

For information on structural safety standards and qualified contractors in your area, contact your city or county government office on community development or building code enforcement.

The following suggestions will take an investment of time and money but will add stability to your home. If you want to do the work yourself, many hardware or home-improvement stores will assist you with information and instructions.

Foundation

Check to see if your house or garage is securely fastened to the foundation. (If your house was built before 1950, it probably does not have bolts securing the wood structure to the concrete foundation.) If your house is not secured to the foundation, talk to a building contractor.

Beams, Posts, Joists and Plates

Strengthen the areas of connection between beams, posts, joists and plates using such hardware as T and L straps, mending plates, and joist hangers. Pay particular attention to exposed framing in garages, basements, porches and patio covers.

Roof and Chimney

- Check your chimney or roof for loose tiles and bricks that could fall in an earthquake. Repair loose tiles or bricks as needed.
- Protect yourself from falling chimney bricks that might penetrate the roof by reinforcing the ceiling immediately surrounding the chimney with ¾-inch plywood nailed to ceiling joists.

Learning to Shut Off Utilities

- Know where and how to shut off utilities at the main switches or valves. Check with your local utility companies for instructions.
- Teach all family members how and when to shut off utilities.

Gas

- An automatic valve (Earthquake Command System) is commercially available that will turn the gas off for you in the event of an earthquake.
- After an earthquake, do not use matches, lighters or appliances and do not operate light switches until you are sure there are no gas leaks. Sparks from electrical switches could ignite gas, causing an explosion.
- If you smell the odor of gas or if you notice a large consumption of gas being registered on the gas meter, shut off the gas immediately. First, find the main shutoff valve, located on a pipe next to the gas meter. Use an adjustable wrench to turn the valve to the Off position.

Electricity

After a major disaster, shut off the electricity. Sparks from electrical switches could pose a shock or fire hazard. Carefully turn off the electricity at the main electrical breaker in your home.

Water

Water may be turned off at either of two locations:

- At the main meter, which controls the water flow to the entire property.
- At the water main leading into the home. (Shutting off the water here retains the water supply to your water heater, which may be useful in an emergency.)

Attach a valve wrench to the water line. (This tool can be purchased at most hardware stores.) Also, label the water mains for quick identification.

During an Earthquake

Indoor Safety

There are actions you can take, even while an earthquake is happening, that will reduce your chances of being hurt. Lights may be out, and hallways, stairs and room exits may be blocked by fallen furniture, ceiling tiles and other debris. Planning for these situations will help you to take action quickly.

- If an earthquake strikes, you may be able to take cover under a heavy desk or table. It can provide you with air space if the building collapses. If you get under a table and it moves, try to move with it.

- Inner walls or door frames are the least likely structures to collapse and may also shield you from falling objects. If other cover is not available, go to an inner corner or doorway, away from windows or glass panels.

- Stay away from glass and hanging objects as well as bookcases, china cabinets or other large furniture that could fall. Watch for falling objects, such as bricks from fireplaces and chimneys, light fixtures, wall hangings, high shelves, and cabinets with doors that could swing open.

- Grab something to shield your head and face from falling debris and broken glass.

- If the lights go out, use a battery-operated flashlight. Do not use candles, matches or lighters during or after the earthquake. If there is a gas leak, an explosion could result.

- If you are in the kitchen, quickly turn off the stove and take cover at the first sign of shaking.

High-Rise Buildings

Get under a desk and stay away from windows and outside walls. Stay in the building. The electricity may go out and the sprinkler systems may come on. Do not use the elevators.

Crowded Indoor Public Places

If you are in a crowded public place, do not rush for the doorways. Others will have the same idea. Move away from display shelves containing objects that may fall. If you can, take cover and grab something to shield your head and face from falling debris and glass.

Outdoor Safety

If you are outdoors, move away from buildings and utility wires. The greatest danger from falling debris is just outside doorways and close to outer walls. Once you are in the open, stay there until the shaking stops.

Automobiles

If you are in a moving automobile, stop as quickly and safely as possible and move over to the shoulder or curb, away from utility poles, overhead wires, and under- or over-passes. Stay in the vehicle, set the parking brake and turn on the radio for emergency broadcast information. A car may jiggle violently on its springs, but it is a good place to stay until the shaking stops. If you are in a life-threatening situation, you may be able to reach someone with either a cell phone or an emergency roadside assistance phone.

When you drive on, watch for hazards created by the earthquake, such as breaks in the pavement, downed utility poles and wires, and fallen overpasses and bridges.

After an Earthquake

Aftereffects

Be prepared for additional earth movements called aftershocks. Although most of these are smaller than the main earthquake, some may be large enough to cause additional damage or bring down weakened structures.

Because other aftereffects can include fires, chemical spills, landslides, dam breaks and tidal waves, be sure to monitor your battery-operated radio or TV for additional emergency information.

Injuries

Check for injuries. Do not attempt to move injured or unconscious people unless they are in immediate danger from live electrical wires, flooding or other hazards. Internal injuries may not be evident, but they may be serious or life-threatening. If someone has stopped breathing, call for medical or first aid assistance immediately, and begin CPR if you are trained to do so. Stop a bleeding injury by applying direct pressure to the wound. If you are trapped, try to attract attention to your location.

Checking Utilities

An earthquake may break gas, electrical and water lines. If you smell gas: (1) open windows, (2) shut off the main gas valve, (3) do not turn any electrical appliances or lights on or off, (4) go outside, (5) report the leak to authorities and (6) do not reenter the building until a utility official says it is safe to do so.

- If electric wiring is shorting out, shut off the electric current at the main box.

- If water pipes are damaged, shut off the supply at the main valve.

Other Precautions

- Have chimneys inspected for cracks and damage. Do not use the fireplace if the chimney has any damage.

- Check to see if sewage lines are intact before using bathrooms or plumbing.

- Do not touch downed power lines or objects in contact with downed lines. Report electrical hazards to the authorities.

- Immediately clean up spilled medicines, drugs, flammable liquids and other potentially hazardous materials.

- Stay off all telephones except to report an emergency. Replace telephone receivers that may have been knocked off by the earthquake.

- Stay away from damaged areas. Your presence could hamper relief efforts and you could endanger yourself.

- Cooperate fully with public safety officials. Respond to requests for volunteer assistance from police, firefighters, emergency management officials and relief organizations, but do not go into damaged areas unless assistance has been requested.

Evacuating Your Home

If you must evacuate your home:

- Post a message, in a prearranged location known only to family members, indicating where you have gone.

- Confine pets to the safest location possible and make sure they have plenty of food and water. Pets will not be allowed in designated public shelters.

- Take vital documents (such as wills and insurance policies), emergency supplies and extra medications with you.

People with Special Needs

People with Disabilities

Before an earthquake:

- Write down any specific needs, limitations and capabilities that you have and any medications you take. Make a copy of the list and put it in your purse or wallet.

- Find someone (a spouse, roommate, friend, neighbor, relative or co-worker) to help you in case of an emergency. Give them the list. You may wish to provide a spare key to your home or let them know where they can find one in an emergency.

During an earthquake:

- If you are confined to a wheelchair, try to get under a doorway or into an inside corner, lock the wheels, and cover your head with your arms. Remove any items that are not securely attached to the wheelchair.

- If you are able, seek shelter under a sturdy table or desk. Stay away from outer walls, windows, fireplaces and hanging objects.

- If you are unable to move from a bed or chair, protect yourself from falling objects by covering up with blankets and pillows.

- If you are outside, go to an open area away from trees, telephone poles and buildings, and stay there.

After an earthquake:

- If you are trapped, try to attract attention to your location.

- Turn on your battery-operated TV or radio to receive emergency information and instructions.

- If you can, help others in need.

Children's Needs

Fear is a normal reaction to danger. Children may be afraid of recurrence, injury or death after an earthquake. They may fear being separated from their family or being left alone. Children may even interpret disasters as punishment for real or imagined misdeeds. Children will be less likely to experience prolonged fear or anxiety if they know what to expect before, during and after an earthquake. Talking to children openly will also help them to overcome fears.

Here are some suggestions:

- Explain that an earthquake is a natural event and not anyone's fault.

- Talk about your own experiences with natural disasters or read aloud books about earthquakes.

- Encourage your child to express feelings of fear. Listen carefully and show understanding.

- Your child may need both verbal and physical reassurance that everything will be all right. Tell your child that the situation is not permanent.

- Include your child in cleanup activities. It is comforting to the child to watch the household begin to return to normal and to have a job to do.

Note: Symptoms of anxiety may not appear for weeks or even months after an earthquake, and they can affect people of any age. If anxiety disrupts daily activities for any member of your family, seek professional assistance through a school counselor, community religious organization, your physician or a licensed mental health professional.

Appendix D • Natural Disasters: Floods

During a flood and its aftermath, there are some basic facts to remember that will help you protect your personal health and safety.

Preparing for a Flood

Here are some basic steps to take to prepare for a flood:

- Contact the local county geologist or county planning department to find out if your home is located in a flash flood-prone area or landslide-prone area.

- Learn about your community's emergency plans, warning signals, evacuation routes and locations of emergency shelters.

- Plan and practice a flood evacuation route with your family. Ask an out-of-state relative or friend to be the "family contact" in case your family is separated during a flood. Make sure everyone in your family knows the name, address and phone number of this contact person.

- Post emergency phone numbers at every phone.

- Inform local authorities about any special needs, such as elderly or bedridden people or anyone with a disability.

- Identify potential home hazards and know how to secure or protect them before the flood strikes. Be prepared to turn off electrical power when there is standing water or fallen power lines, or before your evacuation. Turn off gas and water supplies before you evacuate. Secure structurally unstable building materials.

Source: Centers for Disease Control and Prevention http://www.bt.cdc.gov/disasters Accessed March 2, 2011.

- Buy a fire extinguisher and make sure your family knows where it is and how to use it.

- Buy and install sump pumps with backup power.

- Have a licensed electrician raise electric components (switches, sockets, circuit breakers and wiring) at least 12 inches above your home's projected flood elevation.

- For drains, toilets and other sewer connections, install backflow valves or plugs to prevent floodwaters from entering.

- Anchor fuel tanks that can contaminate your basement if torn free. An unanchored tank outside can be swept downstream and damage other houses.

If you are under a flood watch or warning:

- Gather the emergency supplies you previously stocked in your home and stay tuned to local radio or television stations for updates.

- Turn off all utilities at the main power switch and close the main gas valve if evacuation appears necessary.

- Have your immunization records handy or be aware of your last tetanus shot, in case you should receive a puncture wound or a wound becomes contaminated during or after the flood.

- Fill bathtubs, sinks and plastic soda bottles with clean water. Sanitize the sinks and tubs first by using bleach. Rinse and fill with clean water.

- Bring outdoor possessions, such as lawn furniture, grills and trash cans, inside or tie them down securely.

Emergency Supplies You Will Need

You should stock your home with supplies that may be needed during the emergency period. At a minimum, these supplies should include:

- Several clean containers for water, large enough for a three- to five-day supply of water (about 5 gallons for each person)

- A three- to five-day supply of nonperishable food and a nonelectric can opener

- A first aid kit and first aid manual, prescription medicines and items for special medical needs

- A battery-powered radio, flashlights and extra batteries

- Sleeping bags or extra blankets

- Water-purifying supplies, such as chlorine or iodine tablets or unscented ordinary household chlorine bleach

- Baby food and/or prepared formula, diapers and other baby supplies

- Disposable cleaning cloths, such as baby wipes, for the whole family to use in case bathing facilities are not available

- Personal hygiene supplies such as soap, toothpaste and sanitary napkins

- An emergency kit for your car with food, flares, booster cables, maps, tools, a first aid kit, a fire extinguisher and sleeping bags

- Rubber boots, sturdy shoes and waterproof gloves

- Insect repellent containing DEET, window screens, and long-sleeved and long-legged clothing for protection from mosquitoes that may gather in pooled water remaining after the flood

Preparing to Evacuate

Expect the need to evacuate and prepare for it. When a flood watch is issued, you should:

- Fill your vehicle's gas tank and make sure the emergency kit for your car is ready.

- If no vehicle is available, make arrangements with friends or family for transportation.

- Fill your clean water containers.

- Review your emergency plans and supplies, checking to see if any items are missing.

- Tune in the radio or television for weather updates.

- Listen for disaster sirens and warning signals.

- Put livestock and family pets in a safe area. Due to food and sanitation requirements, emergency shelters cannot accept animals.

- Adjust the thermostat on refrigerators and freezers to the coolest possible temperature.

If You Are Ordered to Evacuate

You should never ignore an evacuation order. Authorities will direct you to leave if you are in a low-lying area or within the greatest potential path of the rising waters. If a flood warning is issued for your area or you are directed by authorities to evacuate the area:

- Take only essential items with you.

- If you have time, turn off the gas, electricity and water.

- Disconnect appliances to prevent electrical shock when power is restored.

- Follow the designated evacuation routes and expect heavy traffic.

- Do not attempt to drive or walk across creeks or flooded roads.

If You Are Ordered Not to Evacuate

To get through the storm in the safest possible manner:

- Monitor the radio or television for weather updates.

- Prepare to evacuate to a shelter or to a neighbor's home if your home is damaged or if you are instructed to do so by emergency personnel.

Flood Recovery

How to Avoid Illness

Always wash your hands with soap and water that has been boiled or disinfected before preparing or eating food, after toilet use, after participating in flood cleanup activities, and after handling articles contaminated with floodwater or sewage. If you receive a puncture wound or a wound contaminated with feces, soil or saliva, have a doctor or health department determine whether a tetanus booster is necessary.

How to Make Sure Your Food is Safe

Do not eat any food that may have come into contact with floodwater. For infants, use only pre-prepared canned baby formula that requires no added water, rather than powdered formulas prepared with treated water. Thawed food can usually be eaten or refrozen if it is still "refrigerator cold," or if it still contains ice crystals. To be safe, remember, "When in doubt, throw it out." Discard any refrigerated or frozen food that has been at room temperature for two hours or more as well as any food that has an unusual odor, color or texture.

How to Make Sure Your Water Is Safe

Listen for public announcements on the safety of the municipal water supply. Flooded private water wells will need to be tested and disinfected after floodwaters recede. Questions about testing should be directed to your local or state health departments.

Safe water for drinking, cooking and personal hygiene includes bottled, boiled or treated water. Your state or local health department can make specific recommendations for boiling or treating water in your area. Here are some general rules concerning water for drinking, cooking and personal hygiene: Do not use contaminated water to wash dishes, brush your teeth, wash and prepare food, wash your hands, make ice, or make baby formula. If possible, use baby formula that does not need to have water added. You can use an alcohol-based hand sanitizer to wash your hands.

- If you use bottled water, be sure it came from a safe source. If you do not know that the water came from a safe source, you should boil or treat it before you use it. Use only bottled, boiled or treated water until your supply is tested and found safe.

- Boiling water, when practical, is the preferred way to kill harmful bacteria and parasites. Bringing water to a rolling boil for 1 minute will kill most organisms.

- When boiling water is not practical, you can treat water with chlorine tablets, iodine tablets or unscented household chlorine bleach (5.25% sodium hypochlorite):

  - If you use chlorine tablets or iodine tablets, follow the directions that come with the tablets.

  - If you use household chlorine bleach, add $\frac{1}{8}$ teaspoon (about 0.75 mL) of bleach per gallon of water if the water is clear. For cloudy water, add $\frac{1}{4}$ teaspoon (about 1.50 mL) of bleach per gallon. Mix the solution thoroughly and let it stand for about 30 minutes before using it.

Note: Treating water with chlorine tablets, iodine tablets or liquid bleach will not kill parasitic organisms.

Use a bleach solution to rinse water containers before reusing them. Use water storage tanks and other types of containers with caution. For example, fire truck storage tanks and previously used cans or bottles may be contaminated with microbes or chemicals. Do not rely on untested devices for decontaminating water.

How to Handle Animals and Mosquitoes

Many wild animals have been forced from their natural habitats by flooding and many domestic animals are also without homes after the flood. Take care to avoid these animals. Do not corner an animal. If an animal must be removed, contact your local animal control authorities. If you are bitten by any animal, seek immediate medical

attention. If you are bitten by a snake, try to accurately identify the type of snake so that, if it is poisonous, the correct antivenin may be administered.

Contact local or state health and agricultural officials for state guidelines on the disposal of dead animals. Protect yourself from mosquitoes: Use screens on dwellings, wear long-sleeved and long-legged clothing, and use insect repellents that contain DEET.

How to Deal With Chemical Hazards

Be aware of potential chemical hazards you may encounter during flood recovery. Floodwaters may have buried or moved hazardous chemical containers of solvents or other industrial chemicals from their normal storage places. If any propane tanks (whether 20-pound tanks from a gas grill or household propane tanks) are discovered, do not try to move them yourself. These represent a very real danger of fire or explosion, and if any are found, police or fire departments or your state fire marshal's office should be contacted immediately. Car batteries, even those in floodwater, may still contain an electrical charge and should be removed with extreme caution by using insulated gloves. Avoid coming in contact with any acid that may have spilled from a damaged car battery.

How to Deal With Electric and Gas Utilities

Electrical power and natural gas or propane tanks should be shut off to avoid fire, electrocution or explosions until it is safe to use them. Use battery-powered flashlights and lanterns, rather than candles, gas lanterns or torches. If you smell gas or suspect a leak, turn off the main gas valve, open all windows and leave the house immediately. Notify the gas company or the police or fire department or state fire marshal's office and do not turn on the lights or do anything that could cause a spark. Avoid any downed power lines, particularly those in water. All electrical equipment and appliances must be completely dry before returning them to service. It is advisable to have a certified electrician check these items if there is any question. Also, remember not to operate any gas-powered equipment indoors.

How to Clean Up

Walls, hard-surfaced floors and many other household surfaces should be cleaned with soap and water and disinfected with a solution of 1 cup of bleach to 5 gallons of water. Wash all linens and clothing in hot water or dry clean them. For items that cannot be washed or dry cleaned, such as mattresses and upholstered furniture, air dry them in the sun and then spray them thoroughly with a disinfectant. Steam clean all carpeting. If there has been a back-flow of sewage into the house, wear rubber boots and waterproof gloves during cleanup. Remove and discard contaminated household materials that cannot be disinfected, such as wall coverings, cloth, rugs and drywall. Additional guidance is available from the Environmental Protection Agency at http://www. epa.gov/iaq/pubs/flood.html and the Federal Emergency Management Agency at http://www.fema.gov/ hazards/floods/whatshouldidoafter.shtm.

Appendix E • Natural Disasters: Hurricanes

Preparing for a Hurricane

If you are in an area that is susceptible to hurricanes, here are some basic steps to take to prepare:

- Learn about your community's emergency plans, warning signals, evacuation routes and locations of emergency shelters.

- Identify potential home hazards and know how to secure or protect them before the hurricane strikes. Be prepared to turn off electrical power when there is standing water or fallen power lines, or before your evacuation. Turn off gas and water supplies before you evacuate. Secure structurally unstable building materials.

- Buy a fire extinguisher and make sure your family knows where to find it and how to use it.

- Locate and secure your important papers, such as insurance policies, wills, licenses and stock certificates.

- Post emergency phone numbers at every phone.

- Inform local authorities about any special needs, such as elderly or bedridden people or anyone with a disability.

Emergency Supplies You Will Need

You should stock your home with supplies that may be needed during the emergency period. At a minimum, these supplies should include:

- Several clean containers for water, large enough for a three- to five-day supply of water (about 5 gallons for each person)

Source: Centers for Disease Control and Prevention (http://www.bt.cdc.gov/disasters) Accessed 2006 and March 2, 2011.

- A three- to five-day supply of nonperishable food

- A first aid kit and manual

- A battery-powered radio, flashlights and extra batteries

- Sleeping bags or extra blankets

- Water-purifying supplies, such as chlorine or iodine tablets or unscented, ordinary household chlorine bleach

- Prescription medicines and special medical needs

- Baby food and/or prepared formula, diapers and other baby supplies.

- Disposable cleaning cloths, such as baby wipes, for the whole family to use in case bathing facilities are not available

- Personal hygiene supplies such as soap, toothpaste and sanitary napkins

- An emergency kit for your car with food, flares, booster cables, maps, tools, a first aid kit, a fire extinguisher and sleeping bags

You can find more information on emergency plans and supply kits at http://www.ready.gov.

Preparing to Evacuate

Expect the need to evacuate and prepare for it. The National Weather Service will issue a hurricane watch when there is a threat to coastal areas of hurricane conditions within 24 to 36 hours.

When a hurricane watch is issued, you should:

- Fill your automobile's gas tank.

- If no vehicle is available, make arrangements with friends or family for transportation.

- Fill your clean water containers.

- Review your emergency plans and supplies, checking to see if any items are missing.

- Tune in the radio or television for weather updates.

- Listen for disaster sirens and warning signals.

- Prepare an emergency kit for your car with food, flares, booster cables, maps, tools, a first aid kit, a fire extinguisher and sleeping bags.

- Secure any items outside that may damage property in a storm, such as bicycles, grills and propane tanks.

- Cover windows and doors with plywood or boards or place large strips of masking tape or adhesive tape on the windows to reduce the risk of breakage and flying glass.

- Put livestock and family pets in a safe area. Due to food and sanitation requirements, emergency shelters cannot accept animals.

- Place vehicles under cover, if at all possible.

- Fill sinks and bathtubs with water as an extra supply for washing.

- Adjust the thermostat on refrigerators and freezers to the coolest possible temperature.

If You Are Ordered to Evacuate

Because of the destructive power of a hurricane, you should never ignore an evacuation order. Authorities will be most likely to direct you to leave if you are in a low-lying area or within the storm's greatest potential path of destruction. If a hurricane warning is issued for your area or you are directed by authorities to evacuate the area:

- Take only essential items with you.

- Leave pets indoors in a safe, covered area with ample food and water.

- If you have time, turn off the gas, electricity and water.

- Disconnect appliances to reduce the likelihood of electrical shock when power is restored.

- Make sure your automobile's emergency kit is ready.

- Follow the designated evacuation routes – others may be blocked – and expect heavy traffic.

If You Are Ordered *Not* to Evacuate

The great majority of injuries during a hurricane are cuts caused by flying glass or other debris. Other injuries include puncture wounds from debris and bone fractures.

To get through the storm in the safest possible manner:

- Monitor the radio or television for weather conditions, if possible.

- Stay indoors until the authorities declare the storm is over.

- Do not go outside, even if the weather appears to have calmed. The calm "eye" of the storm can pass quickly, leaving you outside when strong winds resume.

- Stay away from all windows and exterior doors, seeking shelter in a bathroom or basement. Bathtubs can provide some shelter if you cover yourself with plywood or other materials.

- Prepare to evacuate to a shelter or to a neighbor's home if your home is damaged or if you are instructed to do so by emergency personnel.

Hurricane Recovery

Hurricanes often cause power outages. Indoor use of portable generators, charcoal grills or camp stoves can lead to carbon monoxide poisoning. Take steps to protect your family from carbon monoxide poisoning.

How to Store Food Safely

Your refrigerator will keep foods cool for about four hours without power if it is unopened. Add a block of dry ice to your refrigerator if the electricity will be off longer than four hours.

Thawed food can usually be eaten if it is still "refrigerator cold," or refrozen if it still contains ice crystals. Discard any food that has been at temperatures greater than 40° F for two hours or more and discard any food that has an unusual odor, color or texture.

While the power is out, keep the refrigerator and freezer doors closed as much as possible to keep food cold for as long as possible.

If the power is out for longer than four hours, follow these guidelines:

- Use dry ice, if available. Twenty-five pounds of dry ice will keep a 10-cubic-foot freezer below freezing for three to four days. Use care when handling dry ice and wear dry, heavy gloves to avoid injury.

- For the freezer section: A freezer that is half full will hold food safely for up to 24 hours. A full freezer will hold food safely for 48 hours. Do not open the freezer door if you can avoid it.

- For the refrigerated section: Pack milk, other dairy products, meat, fish, eggs, gravy and spoilable leftovers into a cooler surrounded by ice. Discard this food if it is held at a temperature higher than 40° F for more than two hours.

- Use a digital quick-response thermometer to check the temperature of your food right before you cook or eat it. Throw away any food that has a temperature of higher than 40° F.

For additional information on food safety concerns following hurricanes or floods, visit the FDA website at http://www.fda.gov.

How to Make Sure Your Water Is Safe

Hurricanes, especially when accompanied by a tidal surge or flooding, can contaminate the public water supply. Drinking contaminated water may cause illness. You cannot assume that the water in the hurricane-affected area is safe to drink.

Listen for public announcements about the safety of the municipal water supply. Safe water for drinking, cooking and personal hygiene includes bottled, boiled or treated water. Your state or local health department can make specific recommendations for boiling or treating water in your area. Here are some general rules concerning water for drinking, cooking and personal hygiene. Remember:

- Do not use contaminated water to wash dishes, brush your teeth, wash and prepare food, wash your hands, make ice, or make baby formula. If possible, use baby formula that does not need to have water added. You can use an alcohol-based hand sanitizer to wash your hands.

- If you use bottled water, be sure it came from a safe source. If you do not know that the water came from a safe source, you should boil or treat it before you use it. Use only bottled, boiled or treated water until your supply is tested and found safe.

- Boiling water, when practical, is the preferred way to kill harmful bacteria and parasites. Bringing water to a rolling boil for 1 minute will kill most organisms.

- When boiling water is not practical, you can treat water with chlorine tablets, iodine tablets or unscented household chlorine bleach (5.25% sodium hypochlorite):

  - If you use chlorine tablets or iodine tablets, follow the directions that come with the tablets.

  - If you use household chlorine bleach, add 1/8 teaspoon (about 0.75 mL) of bleach per gallon of water if the water is clear. For cloudy water, add 1/4 teaspoon (about 1.50 mL) of bleach per gallon. Mix the solution thoroughly and let it stand for about 30 minutes before using it.

Note: Treating water with chlorine tablets, iodine tablets or liquid bleach will not kill parasitic organisms.

Use a bleach solution to rinse water containers before reusing them. Use water storage tanks and other types of containers with caution. For example, fire truck storage tanks and previously used cans or bottles may be contaminated with microbes or chemicals. Do not rely on untested devices for decontaminating water.

If there is flooding along with a hurricane, the waters may contain fecal material from overflowing sewage systems and agricultural and industrial waste. Although skin contact with floodwater does not, by itself, pose a serious health risk, there is risk of disease from eating or drinking anything contaminated with floodwater.

Do not allow children to play in floodwater areas. Wash children's hands frequently (always before meals) and do not allow children to play with floodwater-contaminated toys that have not been disinfected. You can disinfect toys using a solution of 1 cup of bleach in 5 gallons of water.

For more information about water purification after a hurricane or other weather emergency, please visit CDC's Web page on "Hurricanes and Your Health and Safety."

How to Prevent Injury after a Hurricane

When the wind and waters recede, people in the areas affected by a hurricane will continue to face a number of hazards associated with cleanup activities. The National Institute for Occupational Safety and Health (NIOSH) offers the following guidelines for preventing injury:

Wear Protective Gear

For most work in flooded areas, wear hard hats, goggles, heavy work gloves, and watertight boots with steel toe and insole (not just steel shank).

Wear earplugs or protective headphones to reduce risk from equipment noise. Equipment such as chainsaws, backhoes and dryers may cause ringing in the ears and subsequent hearing damage.

Beware of Electrical Hazards

- If water has been present anywhere near electrical circuits and electrical equipment, turn off the power at the main breaker or fuse on the service panel. Do not turn the power back on until electrical equipment has been inspected by a qualified electrician.

- Never enter flooded areas or touch electrical equipment if the ground is wet, unless you are certain that the power is off. Never handle a downed power line.

- When using gasoline and diesel generators to supply power to a building, switch the main breaker or fuse on the service panel to the Off position prior to starting the generator.

- If clearing or other work must be performed near a downed power line, contact the utility company to discuss de-energizing and grounding or shielding of power lines. Extreme caution is necessary when moving ladders and other equipment near overhead power lines to avoid inadvertent contact.

Avoid Carbon Monoxide

Carbon monoxide is an odorless, colorless gas that is poisonous to breathe. During flood cleanup, operate all gasoline-powered devices such as pumps, generators and pressure washers outdoors and never bring them indoors. This will help ensure your safety from carbon monoxide poisoning.

For additional information on carbon monoxide, see "Protecting Yourself from Carbon Monoxide Poisoning after an Emergency" and "Carbon Monoxide Poisoning" (from CDC's National Center for Environmental Health [NCEH]).

Prevent Musculoskeletal Injury

Special attention is needed to avoid back injuries associated with manual lifting and handling of debris and building materials.

To help prevent injury:

- Use teams of two or more to move bulky objects.

- Avoid lifting any material that weighs more than 50 pounds (per person).
- Use proper automated-assist lifting devices.

Beware of Structural Instability

Never assume that water-damaged structures or ground are stable. Buildings that have been submerged or have withstood rushing floodwaters may have suffered structural damage and could be dangerous.

- Do not work in or around any flood-damaged building until it has been examined and certified as safe for work by a registered professional engineer or architect.
- Assume all stairs, floors and roofs are unsafe until they are inspected.
- Leave immediately if shifting or unusual noises signal a possible collapse.

Avoid Hazardous Materials

Floodwaters can dislodge tanks, drums, pipes and equipment, which may contain hazardous materials such as pesticides or propane.

- Do not attempt to move unidentified dislodged containers without first contacting the local fire department or hazardous materials team.
- If you are working in potentially contaminated areas, avoid skin contact or inhalation of vapors by wearing appropriate protective clothing and respirators.
- Frequently and thoroughly wash skin areas that may have been exposed to pesticides and other hazardous chemicals.
- Contact NIOSH for more information on proper safety equipment.

Be Prepared for Fires

Fire can pose a major threat to an already badly damaged flood area for several reasons:

- Inoperative fire protection systems
- Hampered fire department response
- Inoperable firefighting water supplies
- Flood-damaged fire protection systems. At least two fire extinguishers, each with a UL rating of at least 10A, should be provided at every cleanup job.

Prevent Drowning

When entering moving water, you are at risk for drowning, regardless of your ability to swim. Because people in vehicles are at greatest risk of drowning, it is important to comply with all hazard warnings on roadways and to avoid driving vehicles or heavy equipment into water of unknown depth. NIOSH recommends that you avoid working alone and wear a Coast Guard-approved life jacket when working in or near floodwaters.

Reduce Risk of Thermal Stress

While cleaning up after the hurricane, you are at risk for developing health problems from working in hot or cold environments.

To reduce heat-related risks:

- Drink a glass of fluid every 15 to 20 minutes.
- Wear light-colored, loose-fitting clothing.
- Work during the cooler hours of the day.

To reduce cold-related risks when standing or working in water that is cooler than 75° F (24° C):

- Wear rubber boots.
- Ensure that clothing and boots have adequate insulation.
- Take frequent breaks out of the water.
- Change into dry clothing when possible.

Prevent Fatigue-Related Injuries

Continued long hours of work, combined with exhaustion, can create a highly stressful situation during cleanup. People working on hurricane and flood cleanup can reduce their risks of injury and illness in several ways:

- Set priorities for cleanup tasks and pace the work. Avoid physical exhaustion.

- Resume a normal sleep schedule as quickly as possible.

- Be alert to emotional exhaustion or strain. Consult family members, friends or professionals for emotional support.

How to Cope with Stress after a Hurricane

The days and weeks after a hurricane are rough. In addition to your physical health, you need to take some time to consider your mental health. Remember that some sleeplessness, anxiety, anger, hyperactivity, mild depression or lethargy are normal and may go away with time. If you feel any of these symptoms acutely, seek counseling.

Your state and local health departments will help you to find the local resources, including hospitals or health care providers, that you may need.

Individual responses to a threatening or potentially traumatic event may vary. Emotional reactions may include feelings of fear, grief and depression. Physical and behavioral responses might include nausea, dizziness and changes in appetite and sleep pattern, as well as withdrawal from daily activities. Responses to trauma can last for weeks to months before people start to feel normal again.

Seek medical care if you become injured, feel sick, or experience stress and anxiety.

You can do many things to cope with traumatic events, including:

- Keep as many elements of your normal routine incorporated into the disaster plans as possible, including activities to allay children's fears.

- Be aware that you may have fewer resources with which to attend to your day-to-day conflicts, so it is best to resolve what you can ahead of time.

- Turn to family, friends and important social or religious contacts to set up support networks to help you to deal with the potential stressors.

- Let your children know that it is okay to feel upset when something bad or scary happens.

- Encourage your children to express feelings and thoughts, without making judgments.

Dealing With Wild and Domestic Animals in a Disaster

Be cautious if you encounter wild or stray animals. They may be disoriented and dangerous following a hurricane or flood. Try to confine the animal without putting yourself at risk of being bitten. Call the animal control agency in your county.

Wild and domestic animals may escape or be killed in disasters. Escaped animals may wander onto land where they can:

- contaminate water supplies.

- cause a buildup of manure.

- overgraze sensitive ecosystems.

- cause damage to crops.

Decaying carcasses create biologic waste and attract flies and rodents, which can spread disease. They may also contaminate groundwater and cause bad odors. Animal carcasses should be disposed of as soon as possible to avoid creating a health hazard to animals or humans. Contact your local animal control department or local health department for specific disposal guidance.

Hand Washing in Emergency Situations

After an emergency, it can be difficult to find running water. However, it is still important to wash your hands to avoid illness. It is best to wash your hands with soap and water, but when water is not available, you can use alcohol-based products made for washing hands.

Preventing West Nile Virus (WNV)

After a hurricane, mosquitoes may breed in standing water during the summer and autumn months. The easiest and best way to avoid West Nile Virus is to prevent mosquito bites.

- When you are outdoors, use insect repellents containing DEET (N, N-diethyl-meta-toluamide). Follow the directions on the package.

- Many mosquitoes are most active at dusk and dawn. Be sure to use insect repellent and wear long sleeves and pants at these times or consider staying indoors during these hours.

Light-colored clothing can help you to see mosquitoes that land on you.

- Make sure you have good screens on your windows and doors to keep mosquitoes out.

- Get rid of mosquito breeding sites by emptying standing water from flowerpots, buckets and barrels. Change the water in pet dishes and replace the water in bird baths weekly. Drill holes in tire swings so that water drains out. Keep children's wading pools empty and on their sides when they are not being used.

Appendix F • Natural Disasters: Tornadoes

Knowing what to do when you see a tornado or when you hear a tornado warning can help protect you and your family. During a tornado, people face hazards from extremely high winds and risk being struck by flying and falling objects. After a tornado, the wreckage left behind poses additional injury risks. Although nothing can be done to prevent tornadoes, there are actions you can take for your health and safety.

Being Prepared

Stay Tuned for Storm Watches and Warnings

When thunderstorms are in your area, turn on your radio or TV to get the latest emergency information from local authorities. Listen for announcements of a tornado watch or tornado warning.

Local Warning System

Learn about the tornado warning system in your county or locality. Most tornado-prone areas have a siren system. Know how to distinguish between the siren's warnings for a tornado watch and a tornado warning.

A tornado watch is issued when weather conditions favor the formation of tornadoes – for example, during a severe thunderstorm.

During a tornado watch:

- Stay tuned to local radio and TV stations or a National Oceanographic and Atmospheric Administration (NOAA) weather radio for further weather information.

- Watch the weather and be prepared to take shelter immediately if conditions worsen.

A tornado warning is issued when a funnel cloud is sighted or indicated by weather radar. *You should take shelter immediately.*

Thunderstorms

Because tornadoes often accompany thunderstorms, pay close attention to changing weather conditions when there is a severe thunderstorm watch or warning. A severe thunderstorm *watch* means severe thunderstorms are possible in your area. A severe thunderstorm *warning* means severe thunderstorms are occurring in your area.

Keep fresh batteries and a battery-powered radio or TV on hand. Electrical power is often interrupted during thunderstorms – just when information about weather warnings is most needed.

Important Measures to Take

- Take a few minutes with your family to develop a tornado emergency plan. Sketch a floor plan of where you live, and walk through each room and discuss where and how to seek shelter.

- Show a second way to exit from each room or area. If you need special equipment, such as a rope ladder, mark where it is located.

- Make sure everyone understands the siren warning system, if such a system exists in your area.

- Mark where your first aid kit and fire extinguishers are located.

- Mark where the utility switches or valves are located so they can be turned off – if time permits – in an emergency.

- Teach your family how to administer basic first aid; how to use a fire extinguisher; and how and when to turn off water, gas and electricity in your home.

Source: Centers for Disease Control and Prevention (http://www.bt.cdc.gov/disasters) Accessed March 2, 2011.

F • Natural Disasters: Tornadoes

- Learn the emergency dismissal policy for your child's school.

- Make sure your children know –

  - what a tornado is.

  - what tornado watches and warnings are.

  - what county or parish they live in (warnings are issued by county or parish).

  - how to take shelter, whether at home or at school.

Extra Measures for People with Special Needs

- Write down your specific needs, limitations, capabilities and medications. Keep this list near you always – perhaps in your purse or wallet.

- Find someone nearby (a spouse, roommate, friend, neighbor, relative or co-worker) who will agree to assist you in case of an emergency. Give him or her a copy of your list. You may also want to provide a spare key to your home or directions to find a key.

- Keep aware of weather conditions through whatever means are accessible to you. Some options are closed captioning or scrolled warnings on TV, radio bulletins or call-in weather information lines.

Practicing Your Emergency Plan

Conduct drills and ask questions to make sure your family remembers information on tornado safety, particularly how to recognize hazardous weather conditions and how to take shelter.

Write Down Important Information

Make a list of important information. Include on your list –

- important telephone numbers, such as emergency (police and fire), paramedics and medical centers

- names, addresses and telephone numbers of your insurance agents, including policy types and numbers

- telephone numbers of the electric, gas and water companies

- names and telephone numbers of neighbors

- name and telephone number of your landlord or property manager

- important medical information (for example, allergies, regular medications and brief medical history)

- year, model, license and identification numbers of your vehicles (automobiles, boats and RVs)

- your financial institution's telephone number, and your account types and numbers

- radio and television broadcast stations to tune to for emergency broadcast information

Storing Important Documents

Store the following documents in a fire- and waterproof safe:

- Birth certificates

- Ownership certificates (autos, boats, etc.)

- Social security cards

- Insurance policies

- Wills

- Household inventory

  - List of contents of household; include serial numbers, if applicable

  - Photographs or videotape of contents of every room

  - Photographs of items of high value, such as jewelry, paintings, collection items

Reducing Household Hazards

The following suggestions will help reduce the risk for injury during or after a tornado.

Possible Hazards

Inspect your home for possible hazards, including the following:

- Are walls securely bolted to the foundation?

- Are wall studs attached to the roof rafters with metal hurricane clips, not nails?

Utilities

- Do you know where and how to shut off utilities at the main switches or valves?

Home Contents

- Are chairs or beds near windows, mirrors or large pictures?

- Are heavy items stored on shelves more than 30 inches high?

- Are there large, unsecured items that might topple over or fall?

- Are poisons, solvents or toxic materials stored safely?

Securing Your Home's Structure

No home is completely safe in a tornado. However, attention to construction details can reduce damage and provide better protection for you and your family if a tornado should strike your house. If an inspection reveals a possible hazard in the way your home is built, contact your local city or county building inspectors for more information about structural safety. They may also offer suggestions on finding a qualified contractor to do any needed work for you.

Walls and Roof Rafters

Strengthen the areas of connection between the wall studs and roof rafters with hurricane clips.

Shutting Off Utilities

Gas

After a tornado, *do not* use matches, lighters or appliances or operate light switches until you are sure no gas leaks are present. Sparks from electrical switches could ignite gas and cause an explosion.

If you smell the odor of gas or if you notice a large consumption of gas being registered on the gas meter, shut off the gas immediately. First, find the main shut-off valve located on a pipe next to the gas meter. Use an adjustable wrench to turn the valve to the "off" position.

Electricity

After a major disaster, shut off the electricity. Sparks from electrical switches could ignite leaking gas and cause an explosion.

Water

- Water may be turned off at either of two locations:

  1. At the main meter, which controls the water flow to the entire property.

  2. At the water main leading into the home. If you may need an emergency source of fresh water, it is better to shut off your water here because it will conserve the water in your water heater.

- Attach a valve wrench to the water line. (This tool can be purchased at most hardware stores.)

- Label the water mains for quick identification.

Arranging and Securing Household Items

- Arrange furniture so chairs and beds are away from windows, mirrors and picture frames.

- Place heavy or large items on lower shelves.

- Secure your large appliances, especially your water heater, with flexible cable, braided wire or metal strapping.

- Identify top-heavy, freestanding furniture, such as bookcases and china cabinets that could topple over.

- Secure your furniture by using one of two methods.

  1. L brackets, corner brackets or aluminum molding, to attach tall or top-heavy furniture to the wall.

  2. Eyebolts, to secure items located a short distance from the wall.

- Install sliding bolts or childproof latches on all cabinet doors.

- Store all hazardous materials such as poisons and solvents –

  - in a sturdy, latched or locked cabinet.

  - in a well-ventilated area.

  - away from emergency food or water supplies.

During a Tornado

Signs of an Approaching Storm

Some tornadoes strike rapidly, without time for a tornado warning and sometimes without a thunderstorm in the vicinity. When you are watching for rapidly emerging tornadoes, it is important to know that you cannot depend on seeing the funnel cloud – clouds or rain may block your view. The following weather signs may mean that a tornado is approaching:

- A dark or green-colored sky

- A large, dark, low-lying cloud

- Large hail

- A loud roar that sounds like a freight train

If you notice any of these weather conditions, take cover immediately and keep tuned to local radio and TV stations or to an NOAA weather radio.

NOAA Weather Radios

NOAA weather radios are the best way to receive warnings from the National Weather Service. By using an NOAA weather radio, you can receive continuous updates on all the weather conditions in your area. The range of these radios depends on where you live, but the average range is 40 miles. The radios are sold in many stores. The National Weather Service recommends buying a radio with a battery backup (in case the power goes off) and a tone-alert feature that automatically sounds when a weather watch or warning is issued.

Sighting a Funnel Cloud

If you see a funnel cloud nearby, take shelter immediately (see the following section for instructions on shelter). However, if you spot a tornado that is far away, help alert others to the hazard by reporting it to the newsroom of a local radio or TV station before taking shelter as described later. Use common sense and exercise caution: If you believe that you might be in danger, seek shelter immediately.

Taking Shelter

Your family could be anywhere when a tornado strikes – at home, at work, at school or in the car. Discuss with your family where the best tornado shelters are and how family members can protect themselves from flying and falling debris.

The key to surviving a tornado and reducing the risk of injury lies in planning, preparing and practicing what you and your family will do if a tornado strikes. Flying debris causes most deaths and injuries during a tornado. Although there is no completely safe place during a tornado, some locations are much safer than others.

At Home

Pick a place in the home where family members can gather if a tornado is headed your way. One basic rule is to *avoid windows*. An exploding window can injure or kill.

The safest place in the home is the interior part of a basement. If the home has no basement, go to an inside room, without windows, on the lowest floor. This could be a center hallway, bathroom or closet.

For added protection, get under something sturdy such as a heavy table or workbench. If possible, cover your body with a blanket, sleeping bag or mattress and protect your head with anything available – even your hands. Avoid taking shelter where heavy objects, such as pianos or refrigerators, are on the area of floor that is directly above you. They could fall though the floor if the tornado strikes your house.

In a Mobile Home

Do not stay in a mobile home during a tornado. Mobile homes can turn over during strong winds. Even mobile homes with a tie-down system cannot withstand the force of tornado winds.

Plan ahead. If you live in a mobile home, go to a nearby building, preferably one with a basement. If there is no shelter nearby, lie flat in the nearest ditch, ravine or culvert and shield your head with your hands.

If you live in a tornado-prone area, encourage your mobile home community to build a tornado shelter.

On the Road

The least desirable place to be during a tornado is in a motor vehicle. Cars, buses and trucks are easily tossed by tornado winds.

Do not try to outrun a tornado in your car. If you see a tornado, stop your vehicle and get out. Do not get under your vehicle. Follow the directions for seeking shelter outdoors (see next section).

Outdoors

If you are caught outside during a tornado and adequate shelter is not immediately available:

- Avoid areas with many trees.
- Avoid vehicles.
- Lie down flat in a gully, ditch or low spot on the ground.
- Protect your head with an object or with your arms.

Long-Span Buildings

A long-span building, such as a shopping mall, theater or gymnasium, is especially dangerous because the roof structure is usually supported solely by the outside walls. Most such buildings hit by tornadoes cannot withstand the enormous pressure. They simply collapse.

If you are in a long-span building during a tornado, stay away from windows. Get to the lowest level of the building – the basement if possible – and away from the windows.

If there is no time to get to a tornado shelter or to a lower level, try to get under a door frame or up against something that will support or deflect falling debris. For instance, in a department store, get up against heavy shelving or counters. In a theater, get under the seats. Remember to protect your head.

Office Buildings, Schools, Hospitals, Churches and Other Public Buildings

Extra care is required in offices, schools, hospitals or any building where a large group of people is concentrated in a small area. The exterior walls of such buildings often have large windows.

If you are in any of these buildings:

- Move away from windows and glass doorways.
- Go to the innermost part of the building on the lowest possible floor.
- Do not use elevators because the power may fail, leaving you trapped.
- Protect your head and make yourself as small a target as possible by crouching down.

Shelter for People With Special Needs

Advance planning is especially important if you require assistance to reach shelter from an approaching storm.

- If you are in a wheelchair, get away from windows and go to an interior room of the house. If possible, seek shelter under a sturdy table or desk. Cover your head with anything available, even your hands.
- If you are unable to move from a bed or a chair and assistance is not available, protect yourself from falling objects by covering up with blankets and pillows.
- If you are outside and a tornado is approaching, get into a ditch or gully. If possible, lie flat and cover your head with your arms.

After a Tornado

Injury may result from the direct impact of a tornado, or it may occur afterward when people walk among debris and enter damaged buildings. A study of injuries after a tornado in Marion, IL, showed that 50% of the tornado-related injuries were related to rescue attempts, cleanup and other post-tornado activities. Nearly one-third of the injuries resulted from stepping on nails. Other common causes of injury included falling objects and heavy, rolling objects. Because tornadoes often damage power lines, gas lines or electrical systems, there is a risk of fire, electrocution or an explosion. Protecting yourself and your family requires promptly treating any injuries received during the storm and using extreme care to avoid further hazards.

Injuries

Check for injuries. Do not try to move seriously injured people unless they are in immediate danger of further injury. Get medical assistance immediately. If someone has stopped breathing, begin CPR if you are trained to do so. Stop a bleeding injury by applying direct pressure to the wound. Have any puncture wound evaluated by a physician. If you are trapped, try to attract attention to your location.

General Safety Precautions

Here are some safety precautions that could help you to avoid injury after a tornado:

- Continue to monitor your battery-powered radio or television for emergency information.

- Be careful when entering any structure that has been damaged.

- Wear sturdy shoes or boots, long sleeves, and gloves when handling or walking on or near debris.

- Be aware of hazards from exposed nails and broken glass.

- Do not touch downed power lines or objects in contact with downed lines. Report electrical hazards to the police and the utility company.

- Use battery-powered lanterns, if possible, rather than candles to light homes without electrical power. If you use candles, make sure they are in safe holders away from curtains, paper, wood or other flammable items. Never leave a candle burning when you are out of the room.

- Hang up displaced telephone receivers that may have been knocked off by the tornado, but stay off the telephone, except to report an emergency.

- Cooperate fully with public safety officials.

- Respond to requests for volunteer assistance from police, firefighters, emergency management and relief organizations, but do not go into damaged areas unless assistance has been requested. Your presence could hamper relief efforts and you could endanger yourself.

Inspecting the Damage

- After a tornado, be aware of possible structural, electrical or gas-leak hazards in your home. Contact your local city or county building inspectors for information on structural safety codes and standards. They may also offer suggestions on finding a qualified contractor to do work for you.

- In general, if you suspect any damage to your home, shut off electrical power, natural gas and propane tanks to avoid fire, electrocution or explosions.

- If it is dark when you are inspecting your home, use a flashlight rather than a candle or torch to avoid the risk of fire or explosion in a damaged home.

- If you see frayed wiring or sparks, or if there is an odor of something burning, you should immediately shut off the electrical system at the main circuit breaker if you have not done so already.

- If you smell gas or suspect a leak, turn off the main gas valve, open all windows and leave the house immediately. Notify the gas company, the police or fire departments or the state fire marshal's office and do not turn on the lights, light matches, smoke or do anything that could cause a spark. Do not return to your house until you are told it is safe to do so.

Safety During Cleanup

- Wear sturdy shoes or boots, long sleeves and gloves.

- Learn proper safety procedures and operating instructions before operating any gas-powered or electric-powered saws or tools.

- Clean up spilled medicines, drugs, liquids and other materials.

Children's Needs

After a tornado, children may be afraid the storm will come back again and they will be injured or left alone. Children may even interpret disasters as punishment for real or imagined misdeeds. Explain that a tornado is a natural event.

Children will be less likely to experience prolonged fear or anxiety if they know what to expect after a tornado. Here are some suggestions:

- Talk about your own experiences with severe storms or read aloud a book about tornadoes.

- Encourage your child to express feelings of fear. Listen carefully and show understanding.

- Offer reassurance. Tell your child that the situation is not permanent and provide physical reassurance through time spent together and displays of affection.

- Include your child in cleanup activities. It is comforting to children to watch the household begin to return to normal and to have a job to do.

Note: Symptoms of anxiety may not appear for weeks or even months after a tornado. They can affect people of any age. If anxiety disrupts daily activities for any member of your family, seek professional assistance through a school counselor, community religious organization, your physician or a licensed mental health professional.

Appendix G • Answers to Learning Checkpoints and Review Questions

Chapter 1

Learning Checkpoint 1

1. False. First aid usually does not replace the need for medical care (calling 9-1-1 or the victim seeing a health care provider). First aid is intended to help the victim until professional help can be given. With minor injuries, however, the victim sometimes does not need to see a health care provider.

2. True. First aid such as giving CPR or stopping bleeding can make the difference between the victim living or dying. In other cases, an injury or illness could become worse if first aid is not given before the victim gets professional help.

Learning Checkpoint 2

1. d. All of the above. These are all important aspects of first aid training.

2. d. All of the above. You should have a first aid kit available wherever an injury may occur.

Learning Checkpoint 3

1. d

2. d

3. Usually first at the scene is an emergency medical responder, who may be a law enforcement officer, firefighter, ski patroller or other official with more advanced training.

4. When you call 9-1-1, be ready to give the following information:
   • Your name
   • The phone number you are using
   • The location and number of victims
   • What happened to the victim(s) and any special circumstances
   • The victim's condition
   • The victim's approximate age and sex
   • What is being done for the victim(s)

Learning Checkpoint 4

1. False. Never move a victim unless faced with a life-threatening situation such as fire. Moving a victim is likely to make an injury worse.

2. d. If your job description requires you to provide first aid, then you have a duty to act.

3. You have consent for an unresponsive adult victim, a child without a guardian present, a victim who nods consent, and a child whose parent or guardian consents. All of these are expressed or implied consent. You do not have consent of all victims all the time.

4. You should always do what you are trained to do, ask for consent, and stay with the victim until another trained person takes over. Do not try techniques you have not been trained to perform, and do not move most victims by trying to transport them yourself, which may lead to further injury.

Review Questions

1. d
2. b
3. b
4. a
5. d
6. d
7. c
8. c
9. d
10. a

Chapter 2

Learning Checkpoint 1

1. False. Bloodborne diseases may be transmitted through contact with several different body fluids, or by objects contaminated with any of those body fluids.

2. True. You can almost always avoid getting an infectious disease if you use precautions such as protective equipment and follow standard precautions.

3. d. All of the above. These are basic precautions based on the assumption that any person's body fluids may carry pathogens and any contact with these fluids may lead to infectious disease.

4. a (there may be pathogens in the blood on that bandage) and d (a cut on the finger could easily let pathogens enter your body). Shaking hands does not transmit HIV; being vaccinated for HBV prevents infection and does not cause it; coughing does not transmit hepatitis C; and urine does not normally transmit pathogens (unless it contains blood), although to be safe you should wear gloves when possibly contacting a victim's urine.

5. Signs and symptoms of latex allergy may include skin rashes, hives, itching eyes or skin, flushing, watery or swollen eyes, runny nose, or an asthmatic reaction.

Learning Checkpoint 2

1. False. The first thing to do is check the scene for safety. If you enter an unsafe scene to help a victim, you could become a second victim for EMS professionals to have to care for.

2. d. All of the above. These are all general principles for giving first aid.

3. All four of these are dangerous scenes you should not enter. Stay at a safe distance and call 9-1-1.

Review Questions

1. a
2. d
3. b
4. c
5. b
6. d
7. a
8. d

Chapter 3

Learning Checkpoint 1

1. heart, lungs
2. d
3. pharynx (throat)
4. a
5. These are cardiac problems that can affect tissue oxygenation: cardiac arrest, myocardial infarction and dysrhythmia. Asthma is a respiratory problem, not a cardiac problem, although it, too, can affect tissue oxygenation.

Learning Checkpoint 2

1. All eight listed injuries and illnesses may result in altered mental status.
2. c
3. A dislocation is the movement of one or more bones out of their normal position in a joint.
4. b. A femur fracture can cause severe bleeding, which may be life-threatening; the fracture may also cause soft tissue damage in the leg, but this is unlikely to be a life-threatening injury.
5. Even a small break in the skin can be very serious if a pathogen can enter the body, such as those pathogens causing serious illnesses (e.g., HIV).

Learning Checkpoint 3

1. d
2. People need a tetanus vaccine booster at least every 10 years to ensure immunity against tetanus infection, which may occur after any break in the skin.
3. a
4. c. Blood in urine may result from different injuries or illnesses but should always be investigated by a health care professional.

Review Questions

1. d
2. a
3. b
4. c
5. b
6. a

7. a

8. d

9. c

10. c

Chapter 4

Learning Checkpoint 1

1. b (check for responsiveness), c (look for normal breathing), a (check for severe bleeding).

2. Do not proceed to the secondary assessment if you find any life-threatening condition in your initial assessment. Instead, care for the life-threatening problem.

3. True. A victim who is coughing is breathing.

Learning Checkpoint 2

1. d. The secondary assessment is performed after the initial assessment and only if the victim has no life-threatening conditions requiring care.

2. S = signs and symptoms, A = allergies, M = medications, P = previous problems, L = last food or drink, and E = events leading to current situation.

3. As you examine each part of a victim's body you are looking for anything out of the ordinary, such as pain, bleeding, a swollen or deformed area, unusual skin color, temperature or moisture, or abnormal movement or sensation in an area. (Alternative answer: DOTS – deformities, open injuries. tenderness (pain), and swelling.)

Review Questions

1. b

2. a

3. c

4. a

5. b

6. a

7. d

Chapter 5

Learning Checkpoint 1

1. normal breathing, the heart. Basic life support keeps victims who are not breathing normally (and whose hearts have stopped) alive until they receive advanced medical care.

2. 1 to 8 years: This is the definition of a child for using an AED. For CPR, a child is 1 year up to the onset of adolescence or puberty.

Learning Checkpoint 2

1. b. Cardiopulmonary resuscitation. "Cardio" refers to the heart (chest compressions) and "pulmonary" means the lungs (rescue breathing).

2. Risk factors for cardiovascular disease include:
   • Smoking
   • High cholesterol levels
   • Inactivity
   • High blood pressure
   • Family history of heart disease
   • Growing older

3. The first crucial link in the Cardiac Chain of Survival is immediate recognition of cardiac arrest and activation of the emergency response system – calling 9-1-1 to access EMS.

4. Call first for any unresponsive adult not breathing normally. Give 2 minutes of CPR first for an unresponsive infant or child not breathing normally.

Learning Checkpoint 3

1. a. Rescue breaths move oxygen into the victim's lungs to be transferred into the blood. (Chest compressions move that blood to vital organs.)

2. False. Blowing too hard can put air in the victim's stomach and cause vomiting. Blow only hard enough to make the chest rise.

3. c. Watch the victim's chest rise and fall. This is the best way to confirm that your breaths are going into the victim's lungs.

4. Give each breath over 1 second.

Learning Checkpoint 4

1. c. Start CPR as soon as you determine the victim is unresponsive and not breathing (unless an AED is present and ready to be used).
2. In an adult or child, the correct position for chest compressions is on the lower half of the breastbone (sternum) in the middle of the chest.
3. Chest compression depth for adults: at least 2 inches. For an infant or child: at least $\frac{1}{3}$ the depth of the chest in an infant (about 1½ inches) or child (about 2 inches).
4. d. 30 to 2 (in all victims regardless of age).
5. a. Use the AED as soon as it is set up and ready. The AED unit will analyze the heart rhythm and determine whether the victim needs a shock to restore regular rhythm or needs CPR.

Review Questions

1. d
2. b
3. a
4. c
5. b
6. c
7. d
8. d
9. a
10. a

Chapter 6

Learning Checkpoint 1

1. True. The shock from the AED can restore a normal heart rhythm when the heart is fibrillating.
2. False. There is almost no risk in using an AED because the unit will not advise a shock unless it determines that the victim's heart is fibrillating; in this case the shock is appropriate and can restore a normal heartbeat.
3. About half of cardiac arrest victims are in fibrillation and require a shock to restore the heart to a normal rhythm.

Learning Checkpoint 2

1. a. The two pads of the AED must be correctly positioned on the victim.
2. c. Give the shock when the unit indicates it, after first making sure no one is in contact with the victim.
3. Resume CPR beginning with chest compressions.

Learning Checkpoint 3

1. A situation such as drowning or poisoning may cause cardiac arrest in a child, in which case the AED may restore a normal rhythm.
2. Do not put the pad on or very near to an implanted pacemaker or defibrillator; place it several inches away.
3. Remove any medication patches with a gloved hand before applying the AED pads.

Review Questions

1. c
2. c
3. d
4. a
5. b
6. b
7. a
8. b

Chapter 7

Learning Checkpoint 1

1. Trying to swallow large pieces of food, eating too quickly, eating while engaged in other activities, eating under the influence of alcohol or drugs or eating with dentures.
2. These items on the list should not be given to a child younger than 3:
   • Popcorn
   • Grapes
   • Marshmallows
   • Gum

Learning Checkpoint 2

1. c. Give abdominal thrusts to a choking adult unless he or she is coughing or able to speak.

2. True. A forcefully coughing victim is getting at least some air, and the coughing may dislodge the obstructing object.

3. True. Without air a victim will become unresponsive and the heart will stop; the victim then needs CPR.

4. d. All of the above.

5. The chest compressions of CPR may dislodge the obstructing object. Even if not, the chest compressions will circulate blood to vital organs.

Review Questions

1. d
2. a
3. b
4. a

Chapter 8

Learning Checkpoint 1

1. True. The body can quickly lose much blood from arterial bleeding.

2. False. The first thing to do always is to stop the bleeding.

3. A victim who has been bleeding severely may show the signs of shock, including cool, clammy skin.

4. Many different materials can form a barrier between you and the victim's blood, including bulky clothing or a plastic bag. (This topic is more fully discussed in Chapter 2.)

Learning Checkpoint 2

1. False. Internal bleeding can be life-threatening because significant blood may be lost from internal organs or blood vessels. The blood is lost from circulation even if it remains within a body cavity – the fact that it is still inside the body does not mean it reaches vital organs through circulation.

2. All of these are signs or symptoms of internal bleeding. Significant blood loss may cause shock, resulting in cool, clammy skin and confusion or lightheadedness.

3. d

Review Questions

1. b
2. a
3. d
4. b
5. c
6. c
7. a
8. d

Chapter 9

Learning Checkpoint 1

1. False. Never give fluids to a shock victim. The victim is likely to vomit.

2. True. A spinal injury can cause shock if it causes nervous system damage.

3. a. Stop the bleeding. Severe bleeding is life-threatening and must be managed before you do anything else.

4. b. Nausea, thirst and clammy skin. These are common signs and symptoms of shock.

5. Calling 9-1-1 is the most important action (after treating any life-threatening injuries) because the victim may need advanced medical care very soon to survive.

Learning Checkpoint 2

1. True. A victim who has experienced an allergic reaction in the past may have an emergency epinephrine auto-injector you can help them use. (Also tell the arriving EMS crew about the allergy.)

2. True. Allergic reactions to bee and wasp stings are common – and can be severe.

3. d. Breathing problems. These are caused by swelling of the airway and are most serious because they can be life-threatening.

4. Help the victim into whatever position is easiest for breathing, which is often sitting part-way up.

Review Questions

1. a
2. c
3. d
4. b
5. d
6. a
7. b
8. a
9. a
10. c

Chapter 10

Learning Checkpoint 1

1. Include these actions in wound care: Irrigate minor wounds with running water. Cover any wound with a sterile dressing and bandage. See a health care provider for a deep or puncture wound.
2. Soak a dressing in water if it sticks to the wound.
3. False. Puncture wounds have a greater risk of infection because germs may be trapped inside.
4. False. With all victims, assume there may be pathogens in the blood; follow standard precautions.
5. Use an antibiotic ointment only on abrasions and only if the victim is not allergic to the antibiotic
6. Signs of wound infection include a red, swollen area; warmth in the area; fever; and pus draining from the wound.
7. These victims need to seek medical attention: Jose, because his wound is deep (regardless of the fact that you stopped the bleeding). Rebecca, because any animal bite should be examined by a health care provider. Kim, because significant face wounds should be examined by a health care provider.
8. False. The bandage should be tight enough to put pressure on the wound to control bleeding, but if it is too tight it may cut off circulation.

9. In this situation the bandage is too tight and is cutting off her circulation. Unwrap the bandage and reapply it less tightly.
10. c. The bandage should cover the entire dressing to secure it in place. It should be dry and should not be able to be slid to one side because a bandage that loose will not adequately protect the wound.

Learning Checkpoint 2

1. Promote some bleeding of a shallow puncture wound to "wash out" any germs that may be deep inside.
2. False. Leave an impaled object in a wound because removing it could worsen the injury.
3. True. Keep an amputated part cold to help preserve it, but do not put it in direct contact with ice (which could freeze tissue).
4. For an eye injury you should cover the uninjured eye also, because movement of the uninjured eye will also cause the injured eye to move, which could worsen the injury.
5. Three ways to remove a small particle from the eye are: Pull the upper eyelid out and down over the lower eyelid. Flush the eye with water. Try to brush it out with a dampened cotton-tip swab or sterile dressing.
6. False. Let blood or fluid drain out.
7. 10 minutes. During this time, do not tilt the victim's head backward, do not have the victim lie down, and do not let the victim speak, swallow, cough, or sniff.
8. True. A dentist can usually reimplant a knocked-out tooth if it is kept in milk (or clean water if milk is not available) and the victim reaches the dentist soon.
9. False. Rinsing the mouth with cool water will not stop bleeding but will keep the blood from clotting in the wound.

Review Questions

1. b
2. a
3. c
4. a

5. a

6. b

7. d

8. b

9. c

10. b

Chapter 11

Learning Checkpoint 1

1. Following are the most common causes of fires leading to injury or death (list any three):
   - Smoking
   - Heating
   - Cooking
   - Playing with fire
   - Electrical wiring
   - Open flames
   - Appliances or other equipment

2. Specific actions to prevent fires in the kitchen:
   - Keep a fire extinguisher in the kitchen and know how to use it.
   - Tie back long hair or loose clothing when cooking or working around flames.
   - If food catches on fire in a microwave or toaster oven, leave the food there and turn the appliance off; keep other objects away until the flames go out.
   - Keep electrical cords away from counter edges where children may pull on them.

   In addition, other general measures such as these can help prevent fires in the kitchen or elsewhere in the home or workplace:
   - Make sure enough smoke detectors are installed and change batteries twice a year when you change clocks for daylight saving time.
   - Do not allow smoking, or ensure that it is done safely and materials safely extinguished. Never allow smoking in bed.
   - Keep curtains and other flammable objects away from fireplaces and stoves; use fireplace screens.
   - Have chimneys regularly inspected and cleaned to prevent chimney fires.
   - Never store gasoline or other highly flammable liquids indoors.
   - Prevent fires caused by electricity.
   - Keep power cords safely out of the way and away from children.
   - Check appliance cords for damaged areas or fraying.
   - Do not overload electrical outlets or use multiple extension cords.
   - Unplug appliances and extension cords when not in use.
   - Keep children from playing with fire.

3. False. The first thing to do is to make sure everyone is evacuated from the building.

4. Four factors that affect how serious a burn may be:
   - The type of burn (first-, second-, or third-degree)
   - How extensive the burn is (how much body area)
   - The specific body area burned
   - Special circumstances such as the victim's age and health status

Learning Checkpoint 2

1. False. Never break blisters on a burn, which could cause infection.

2. Small (less than 20% of the body – or 10% in a child).

3. First, stop the fire (have him stop, drop, and roll to put out the flames, or cover him with a coat or blanket).

   Cool the area with cold running water immediately to stop the burning (but not more than 20% of his body).

   Remove any tight clothing or jewelry.

   Call 9-1-1. Then treat for shock and cover the burned area with a dressing.

Learning Checkpoint 3

1. c. Immediately flush the eye with running water to stop the burning.

2. First, brush the chemical off the skin to stop the burning. (Wear gloves or otherwise protect yourself.) Remove clothing and jewelry from

the area and flush the entire area as quickly as possible with large amounts of running water until EMS personnel arrive. Have someone check the MSDS for the chemical involved.

3. False. The signs and symptoms of an injury caused by smoke inhalation may not become manifest for up to 48 hours. Any victim of smoke inhalation should receive medical attention.

Learning Checkpoint 4

1. False. The first thing to do is to unplug or turn off the electrical power.
2. Unplug the appliance or shut off the circuit breaker. Do not try to pull the victim away from the appliance or the appliance from the victim, because you, too, could be shocked.
3. a. Call 9-1-1 first. You cannot safely reach the victim or move the high-voltage wires yourself – you could make the situation worse.

Review Questions

1. a
2. b
3. d
4. c
5. d
6. a
7. a
8. b
9. c
10. d

Chapter 12

Learning Checkpoint 1

1. Signs of a possible skull fracture include a deformed area of skull, a depressed area felt during your examination, blood or fluid loss from the ears or nose, and an object impaling the skull. Do not put pressure on a bleeding wound with skull fracture.
2. False. Symptoms of brain injuries including concussion, bleeding, or swelling can be variable and may be confusing. Call 9-1-1 with any suspected brain injury.

3. Headache, memory loss, dizziness or confusion, and nausea and vomiting.
4. d. None of the above. No one assessment can always determine the presence of a spinal injury. Do not assume a victim without specific symptoms does not have a possible spinal injury.
5. Signs and symptoms of a serious brain injury may occur as late as 48 hours after a blow to the head.

Learning Checkpoint 2

1. True. Suspect a spinal injury in a victim with a head injury because head trauma may also injure the spine.
2. b. Check for breathing without moving the victim, if you suspect a spinal injury. Move the victim only if necessary.
3. Always suspect a spinal injury in these situations: fall from a roof, motor vehicle crash and a blow to the head.
4. Signs and symptoms of a spinal injury include tingling in the hands, breathing problems and a twisted neck.
5. a. Call 9-1-1 for all victims who may have a spinal injury.
6. Stabilize the head of a victim with a suspected spinal injury in the position in which you find the victim, because movement could worsen the injury.
7. Vomits. The victim could choke on the vomit and therefore must be rolled onto his side, while still supported at the head. Otherwise there is no reason to move the victim and risk further injury.
8. Stabilize the victim's head by holding it still with the victim staying in the driver's seat. Call for someone to call for 9-1-1. Monitor the victim's breathing.

Review Questions

1. a
2. b
3. c
4. d

5. d
6. a
7. b
8. d
9. c

Chapter 13

Learning Checkpoint 1

1. False. Loosely bandage a pillow or other support over the ribs. A tight bandage could cause further injury or breathing problems.
2. d. All of the above: Preventing movement of the arm helps prevent movement of that side of the chest. Preventing movement will also ease pain. A sling and binder may be used to immobilize the arm.
3. Do not remove the impaled screwdriver, which could worsen the injury. Instead, use bulky dressings to stabilize it, and bandage around it. Then call 9-1-1.
4. Treat a sucking chest wound by covering the wound dressing with a piece of plastic taped on three sides; this prevents air from being sucked in but allows air to escape. Then keep the victim lying down and call 9-1-1.

Learning Checkpoint 2

1. The signs and symptoms of a closed abdominal injury include bruising and a swollen abdomen.
2. A victim with an open or closed abdominal wound should lie on his or her back (or in the position found if unresponsive and breathing normally).
3. True. Keep a victim in shock from becoming cold. If necessary, cover him with a coat or blanket, and place something between him and the cold ground.
4. d. Cover organs protruding from a wound with a nonadherent dressing and plastic wrap to keep the organs from drying out.
5. Call 9-1-1 for any victim with an open or closed abdominal wound.

Learning Checkpoint 3

1. Movement. Movement of a fractured pelvis could increase the bleeding and worsen the injury.
2. True. Pelvic bones themselves may bleed heavily, or internal organs may be damaged and bleed profusely.
3. False. With a pelvis fracture, do not move the affected leg.

Review Questions

1. a
2. b
3. d
4. a
5. c
6. b
7. b
8. d

Chapter 14

Learning Checkpoint 1

1. a. Most musculoskeletal injuries. You do not need to know the exact nature of the injury before using RICE.
2. False. Do not put a cold pack directly on the skin because tissue damage could occur. Place a pad or cloth between the cold pack and the skin.
3. d. All of the above.
4. Rest the ankle.
   Put an ice or cold pack on the injured area (observe time limits).
   Compress the ankle with a roller bandage (over the cold pack).
   Elevate the ankle.

Learning Checkpoint 2

1. True. Call 9-1-1 for any serious fractures or fractures of large bones.
2. c. Immobilize the joints above and below a fracture area to keep the fractured bone from moving.
3. True. Shock may result in a fracture from blood loss or pain.

4. The signs and symptoms of a bone or joint injury include a deformed area, pain, swelling, and an inability to use the body part.

5. False. Moving or exerting a sprained joint will only make the injury worse.

Learning Checkpoint 3

1. False. Use ice or a cold pack, but remove it after 20 minutes (or 10 minutes if it produces discomfort), and wait at least 30 minutes before reapplying it.

2. False. Treat a muscle contusion with a cold pack, compression bandage, and elevation of the limb.

3. False. An area of skin discoloration can be caused by a fracture, dislocation, or sprain as well as by a contusion.

4. Gently stretch the muscle, apply a cold pack, and massage the muscle.

Review Questions

1. d
2. a
3. a
4. b
5. c
6. d
7. b
8. a
9. c
10. b

Chapter 15

Learning Checkpoint 1

1. You can make a rigid splint from many different materials, including a board, a piece of plastic or metal, a rolled newspaper or magazine, or thick cardboard.

2. Following are all actions to take when using a splint:
   • Pad the splint.
   • Put a cold pack around the splint.
   • Dress an open wound before splinting.
   • Splint in the position found.

3. Signs that circulation has been cut off in an extremity below the splint include swelling, skin cold and pale or discolored, and tingling or numbness.

4. Two things you should not do when contemplating putting a victim's arm in a sling are:
   • Do not move the arm into position for a sling if this causes more pain.
   • Do not cover the fingers inside the sling, because you need to check circulation.

Learning Checkpoint 2

1. Soft
2. Elbow, hand
3. a. A binder provides additional support and helps prevent movement of the arm.

Learning Checkpoint 3

1. You do not need to know for certain if the bone is broken, as there are signs and symptoms of a fracture (pain, inability to move the leg). Take these actions:
   • Have the victim stay lying down and immobilize the leg.
   • Call 9-1-1.
   • Put ice or a cold pack on the area.
   • Splint the leg if help may be delayed, using either an anatomic splint or a rigid splint from the upper leg to the foot.

2. d. A victim with a fracture of the femur may experience severe bleeding that can cause shock. The injury may be either open or closed.

3. With any fracture of an extremity, ideally the fracture should be splinted on both sides, using two rigid splints.

Review Questions

1. d
2. d
3. a
4. c
5. c
6. a
7. d
8. d

Chapter 16

Learning Checkpoint 1

1. True. With an unknown sudden illness, the victim should not eat or drink.

2. The common signs and symptoms of a heart attack include shortness of breath, chest discomfort, pain or pressure, sweating, indigestion, pale skin, and dizziness.

3. The chest pain of angina usually lasts only a few minutes and is recognized as angina by the person experiencing it. If it persists 10 minutes or more after taking prescribed medication, or the victim has other signs and symptoms of a heart attack, give first aid as for a heart attack.

4. Call 9-1-1. Do not delay, because the victim needs advanced medical care immediately.

5. a. Fluids drain from the mouth. A stroke victim may vomit or drool, possibly causing choking if the fluid does not drain out.

Learning Checkpoint 2

1. False. You do not need to know the specific cause of the breathing difficulty but can care for the victim anyway: call 9-1-1, help the victim to rest in the position for easiest breathing, assist with any prescribed medications, and be prepared to give basic life support.

2. d. Let the victim find the position for easiest breathing.

3. The best thing an asthma victim can do during an attack is to use his or her prescribed inhaler; the medication should control the attack.

4. False.

5. Call 9-1-1 for a hyperventilating victim if breathing does not return to normal within a few minutes.

Learning Checkpoint 3

1. Call 9-1-1 for a victim who faints if the victim does not regain responsiveness soon or faints repeatedly.

2. False. Lay the victim down and raise his or her legs, not the head, 6 to 12 inches.

3. c. Place something flat and soft under the victim's head. Do not try to hold the victim still, and do not put anything between the teeth.

4. Call 9-1-1 for a seizure victim –
   • if the seizure lasts more than 5 minutes.
   • if the victim is not known to have epilepsy.
   • if the victim recovers very slowly or has trouble breathing.
   • if the victim has another seizure.
   • if the victim is pregnant.
   • if the victim is wearing another medical ID.
   • if the victim is injured.

5. Seek urgent medical care for a young child whose abdomen is swollen and feels hard.

6. Common signs and symptoms of a low blood sugar diabetic emergency include dizziness, hunger, clumsiness, sweating, and confusion.

7. If you cannot judge whether the victim has low or high blood sugar, give sugar to the victim as for low blood sugar. Seek medical attention if the victim does not improve within 15 minutes or symptoms become worse.

Review Questions

1. d
2. a
3. c
4. a
5. b
6. d
7. c
8. a
9. d
10. b

Chapter 17

Learning Checkpoint 1

1. The common signs and symptoms of a swallowed poison include nausea, dizziness, drowsiness, vomiting and unresponsiveness.

2. Give the victim lots of fluids to drink.

3. c. Move the victim to fresh air.

4. This is likely a poisoning situation. Call 9-1-1 and give basic life support as needed. Put the

child in the recovery position. Tell the 9-1-1 dispatcher and the arriving crew about the open cleaning product.

Learning Checkpoint 2

1. False. Use soap and water to wash the area to minimize the reaction.
2. See a health care provider for severe reactions or swelling of the face or genitals, or signs of infection (fever, pus).
3. a. Hydrocortisone cream. (Also colloid oatmeal, baking soda paste or calamine lotion.)

Review Questions

1. b
2. a
3. d
4. c
5. a
6. d
7. d
8. c
9. b
10. b

Chapter 18

Learning Checkpoint 1

1. a. Remember: Alcohol is still a drug even though legal for those of age.
2. Because alcohol and other drug abuse typically begin at young ages, prevention efforts focus on children and adolescents.
3. The following are appropriate actions to help prevent misuse of prescribed drugs:
   - Read product information that comes with prescription medications.
   - Keep medications in their original labeled containers.
   - Ensure that a person with diminished judgment cannot unintentionally take too much medication. In addition:
   - Always take medications as prescribed – not only when feeling symptoms. Many medical conditions requiring drug treatment do not cause noticeable symptoms.

- Never use medications prescribed for someone else – even when you are certain you have the same condition as the person with the medication. People vary in their responses to medications, and only a health care provider can know what medication is appropriate for you.

Learning Checkpoint 2

1. For an intoxicated person who apparently has passed out, take these actions:
   - Check the person for responsiveness and normal breathing.
   - Position an unresponsive victim who is breathing normally in the recovery position; be prepared for vomiting.
   - Monitor the victim and provide BLS if necessary.
   - Check for injuries or illness.
   - Call 9-1-1 if the victim's breathing is irregular, if seizures occur or if the victim cannot be roused (coma).
   - In a cold environment, protect the person from hypothermia.
2. b
3. The following are appropriate actions to take for a person with a drug or medication overdose:
   - Call 9-1-1 or the Poison Control Center.
   - Check for injuries that may require first aid.
   - Try to keep the person awake and talking.
   - Try to find out what the person took.
   In addition:
   - Position an unresponsive victim in the recovery position because vomiting is likely – not on his or her back.
   - Because of the risk of being injured, never try to restrain a potentially violent person – leave this to law enforcement personnel.
   - Do not try to induce vomiting in any victim at any time unless so instructed by the Poison Control Center.

Review Questions

1. a
2. d

3. b
4. a
5. c
6. c
7. a
8. d

Chapter 19

Learning Checkpoint 1

1. a. See a health care provider immediately. Do not wait until you develop symptoms, and do not try to capture the animal. You cannot kill the rabies germs by treating the wound site.
2. Human bites can be serious because human mouths usually contain many germs.

Learning Checkpoint 2

1. Have the victim stay calm and lie down with the bitten area below the level of the heart. Call 9-1-1. Wash the bite wound with soap and water. For a poisonous snakebite on an extremity, wrap the limb with an elastic bandage.
2. Call 9-1-1 for a spider bite if the victim has trouble breathing or the bite is from a brown recluse spider.
3. Tweezers.
4. b. "Bull's-eye" rash is a common early sign of Lyme disease. A tick bite does not usually cause pain or burning at the site. Fever may occur with Lyme disease but usually not until much later.

Learning Checkpoint 3

1. A credit card or piece of rigid plastic.
2. Because she seems to be having an allergic reaction to the bee sting, you should first call 9-1-1, ask if she has an epinephrine auto-injector, monitor breathing and treat for shock.
3. c. Vinegar (or baking soda paste if vinegar is not available) can help stop the stinging. Boiling water would cause a burn. Ketchup and mayonnaise are not treatments.

Review Questions

1. d
2. d
3. a
4. c
5. b
6. a
7. c
8. c
9. b
10. d

Chapter 20

Learning Checkpoint 1

1. False. Rubbing frostbitten skin can cause damage. Instead, warm it against warm skin or in warm water.
2. Waxy white, gray, yellow or bluish.
3. Warm his ears with your warm hands (gently). Protect the ears from being rubbed on clothing or other objects. The victim needs immediate medical care.

Learning Checkpoint 2

1. False. Hypothermia can occur any time the climate is cool enough to feel cold.
2. True. Shivering does produce body heat but is not always enough. If the victim has signs and symptoms of hypothermia, help warm his body even if he is shivering.
3. d. Remove damp clothing and warm a hypothermic person with a blanket. Do not let him drink alcohol, and do not warm him too quickly with a heat source such as a fire or a hot shower.
4. Answers may vary depending on equipment the first aider is thought to have. Ideally, get the hypothermic victim out of the cold environment into a tent. Remove his cold, damp clothing and get him into dry clothing and a sleeping bag. If there is a stove, heat water to make him a warm drink.

Learning Checkpoint 3

1. False. Have the victim rest comfortably and drink a sports drink.
2. b. Give a sports drink or water to drink because the body needs fluids.
3. False. Do not give salt tablets. Give a sports drink if the victim is awake and alert.
4. Fluids.
5. Three ways to cool a heat exhaustion victim:
   - Put wet cloths on the forehead and body.
   - Sponge the skin with cool water.
   - Spray the skin with water from a spray bottle and fan the area.
6. First, get him out of the sun and into a cool place. Loosen or remove unnecessary clothing. Give a sports drink or water. Have him lie down and rest. Cool his body with one of the methods previously described.

Learning Checkpoint 4

1. False. Heatstroke is a medical emergency, and the victim may still be at risk. Call 9-1-1.
2. Call 9-1-1 for all instances of heatstroke.
3. A heatstroke victim may be acting very confused or disoriented, dizzy, and irrational; the victim may become unresponsive.
4. a. Have plenty of nonalcoholic fluids present. Be sure there is a shady spot for resting.
   b. Tell everyone to avoid too much exertion (especially those who are older or overweight). Make sure you keep drinking enough fluids. Stop and rest in the shade if you start feeling overheated. Tell everyone to watch for signs and symptoms of heat exhaustion in others: heavy sweating, thirst, fatigue, heat cramps, headache or dizziness, or nausea and vomiting. (Also be alert for the signs and symptoms of heatstroke – but it is better to stop and treat the person in the earlier stages of heat exhaustion.)
   c. Call 9-1-1 for a heatstroke victim.

Review Questions

1. a
2. d
3. b
4. c
5. a
6. c
7. b
8. b
9. a
10. d

Chapter 21

Learning Checkpoint 1

1. d
2. All of the conditions listed may cause altered mental status.
3. Following are guidelines to help calm an emotional victim:
   - Tell the victim who you are and say you are there to help. Avoid seeming judgmental.
   - Do not assume the victim is intoxicated, using drugs or otherwise impaired.
   - Reassure the victim that help is on the way (after 9-1-1 has been called).
   - Ask the victim for his or her name, and use it when speaking to him or her.
   - If possible, try to involve the victim's friend or family member present at the scene.
   - Let the victim tell you what he or she thinks is wrong.
   - Let the victim know you understand his or her concerns.
   - Make eye contact with the victim.
   - Speak in a caring, reassuring voice, but do not give false reassurances or lie about the victim's condition.
   - Do not argue with the victim. Show that you understand the victim's concerns by repeating or rephrasing what the victim tells you.
   - If the victim seems irrational or delusional, do not make statements that support his or her false beliefs, but do not challenge them, either.
   - Stay a safe distance away from the victim until your help is accepted. If the victim does not accept your help, do not attempt to restrain or force care on him or her.

- Tell the victim what you plan to do before doing it.
- Move calmly and slowly, touching the victim only as necessary.

4. False. It is better to encourage the victim to talk. Acknowledge that the person seems sad and ask why.

5. False. This is a common myth. Talking about suicide is a warning sign that the person is contemplating suicide.

6. To ensure your own safety and get help fast, take these steps in this order:
   a. Do not enter the scene if there is a risk to your safety. Encourage others present at the scene to withdraw.
   b. Call 9-1-1.
   c. Talk to the person calmly and quietly, and try to divert the person from any violent action by keeping him or her talking.

Learning Checkpoint 2

1. c
2. Following are common characteristics of victims of domestic violence:
   - They love their partners.
   - They feel guilty and may blame themselves for the violence.
   - They often have low self-esteem.
   - They depend emotionally and/or financially on their partners.

   In addition:
   - They are afraid of their partners.
   - They are often isolated from family and friends.

3. d
4. Important first aid actions for a victim injured in a rape include:
   - Be sensitive to the victim's psychological trauma and provide emotional support.
   - Ensure that 9-1-1 has been called.
   - Ensure privacy for the victim.
   - Try to involve a friend or family member of the victim or at least a first aider of the same sex.
   - Give needed first aid and stay with the victim until help arrives.
   - Preserve evidence of the rape.

Review Questions

1. b
2. a
3. d
4. b
5. c
6. d
7. a
8. b
9. a
10. a

Chapter 22

Learning Checkpoint 1

1. Following are generally accepted guidelines for a healthy pregnancy:
   - Minimize caffeine and alcohol consumption.
   - Take dietary supplements as recommended.

   In addition:
   - Eat a healthy diet.
   - Accept normal weight gain.
   - Stop smoking.
   - Do not use illicit drugs.
   - Get exercise.
   - Rest sufficiently.
   - Prevent injury.

2. b
3. b

Learning Checkpoint 2

1. Call 9-1-1 for heavy vaginal bleeding. Calm the woman and help her into a comfortable position. Give the woman a towel or sanitary napkins to absorb the blood, but do not try to pack the vagina.

2. a

3. All six of the signs and symptoms listed could indicate a possible problem with the pregnancy; the woman should see her health care provider for any of these.

Learning Checkpoint 3

1. False. Childbirth is a natural process that seldom involves complications or requires elaborate medical care.

2. Signs and symptoms that childbirth may occur soon include:
   - Woman feels urge to push.
   - Amniotic sac has ruptured.
   - Infant's head is crowning.

   In addition:
   - Contractions are less than 5 minutes apart.
   - Childbirth may occur sooner in a woman who has given birth before.

3. d
4. When assisting with childbirth, follow these guidelines for things not to do:
   - Do not try to delay the birth by having the woman hold her legs together or any other maneuver.
   - Do not place your hands or anything else in the woman's vagina.
   - Do not interfere with the childbirth or touch the infant until the head is completely out.
   - Do not pull on the head or shoulders.
   - Do not try to wash the infant's skin, eyes or ears.
   - Do not pull on the umbilical cord in an effort to pull out the afterbirth.

5. c
6. True. Some bleeding does normally occur with childbirth and delivery of the placenta. If bleeding does not stop soon after delivery of the placenta, massaging the abdomen may help the uterus to contract and stop bleeding.

Review Questions

1. b
2. b
3. a
4. d
5. c
6. d
7. b
8. c
9. c
10. d

Chapter 23

Learning Checkpoint 1

1. Rescue or medical help may be delayed in emergencies in situations such as this:
   - Rural areas
   - When hiking or camping in wilderness areas
   - When boating
   - During or after a natural disaster

2. d

Learning Checkpoint 2

1. The following are important principles for planning a trip into a wilderness location:
   - Do not go alone.
   - Tell someone where you are going and when you will return.
   - Take more food and water than you expect to need.

   In addition:
   - Take a first aid kit equipped for the location.
   - Be prepared for weather emergencies.
   - Know where you are at all times.
   - Do not use alcohol or other drugs.
   - Study the location in advance.

2. False. When dealing with a complex emergency in a remote location, the leader should be flexible, continually reassess the situation and change the plan as needed.
3. A cell phone may have a dead battery, may not have a signal or may stop working because of temperature extremes, moisture or other problems.
4. c

Learning Checkpoint 3

1. d
2. False. If you suspect a victim in a remote location may have a spinal injury, if it is unlikely that help will arrive soon you should assess the victim more carefully to see if a spinal injury can be ruled out so that the victim can move.

3. False. The condition of a victim with a brain injury will not improve by itself. This is a medical emergency – call for a helicopter if possible, or if you cannot communicate the need for rescue, consider evacuating the victim if it can be done safely.

4. b. It will be difficult to warm the victim and keep him warm while walking or being carried through a cold environment for three hours; with severe hypothermia he would probably not be able to walk, and three people generally cannot effectively carry someone. It is better to build an emergency shelter and warm the victim with dry clothing, extra clothing from others, warm fluids and even the body warmth of the other hikers.

5. 30 minutes

Learning Checkpoint 4

1. 3 to 5 gallons
2. The typical signs and symptoms of acute mountain sickness include:
   - Headache
   - Dizziness
   - Fatigue
   - Nausea

Review Questions

1. d
2. b
3. b
4. d
5. a
6. c
7. a
8. b
9. d
10. c

Chapter 24

Learning Checkpoint 1

1. a. Get everyone out. Any delay spent calling 9-1-1, using a fire extinguisher or taking other actions could result in someone being harmed by the fire.

2. d. All of the above. Stay low because there will be more oxygen near the floor, feel doors before opening them to avoid entering a fiery area, and use the stairs because a power outage caused by the fire could stall the elevator.

3. True. OSHA guidelines for fire prevention and safety apply in most workplaces.

4. False. Stay away from potentially hazardous materials; call 9-1-1 and let the professionals clean up the spill.

5. True. But because you cannot usually know if fumes from a spilled liquid are poisonous, act as if they are.

6. Support the victim's head and neck but do not move the victim unless there is an immediate threat. Give basic life support as needed.

7. c. The safest order in which to attempt a water rescue is reach-throw-go.

Learning Checkpoint 2

1. False. A victim with only a broken arm is considered stable and can walk, and is therefore a third priority.

2. True. Victims with life-threatening injuries are the first priority.

3. Following are the ranked priorities for these four victims:
   First – b. A man on the ground with no apparent external injuries but who is unresponsive
   Second – d. A man leaning against the rubble, looking very pale, who says he feels nauseous
   Third – a. A woman with a bruised face and abrasions on her arms, who is walking around holding her bleeding forehead
   Fourth – c. A man who is not breathing, whose chest has caved in under a steel beam and who is surrounded by a pool of blood

Learning Checkpoint 3

1. Consider moving a victim in these situations:
   - Fire is present.

- There is a strong smell of natural gas in the room.
- One victim is lying on top of another.

2. d. The blanket drag is an effective way to move a victim by yourself and provide some support for the victim's head.

Review Questions

1. c
2. d
3. d
4. a
5. b
6. c
7. c
8. b
9. a
10. d

Chapter 25
Review Questions

1. a
2. c
3. a
4. d
5. b

Chapter 26
Review Questions

1. c
2. b
3. d
4. a
5. b

Glossary

A

Abandonment: a type of negligence that occurs if someone who has begun to provide first aid stops, and the injury or illness becomes worse.

Abdomen: the area below the ribs and above the hips.

Abrasion: a wound in which the top layer of skin is scraped off.

Abuse: an intentional inflicting of injury or suffering on someone under the abuser's power, such as a child, spouse or elderly parent.

Acquired immunodeficiency syndrome (AIDS): a sometimes fatal disease caused by the human immunodeficiency virus (HIV).

Acute mountain sickness: a severe form of altitude sickness.

Acute myocardial infarction (AMI): a condition involving a sudden reduced blood flow to the heart muscle; heart attack.

Advanced cardiac life support (ACLS): medical procedures needed to restore a heartbeat beyond the procedures of basic life support.

Airborne transmission: a process by which a pathogen existing in an infected person is transmitted into a different person through the air, usually via small fluid droplets the infected person coughs or sneezes out.

Airway: the path air takes from the nose and mouth to the lungs.

Airway adjunct: a shaped tube-like device inserted into the mouth or nose that helps keep a victim's airway open during resuscitation or until the victim receives advanced medical attention.

Airway obstruction: a condition in which the victim's airway is partially or completely obstructed by the tongue, vomit or other body tissue or fluids, or a foreign object, preventing the flow of air to the lungs; choking.

Allergen: a substance that causes an allergic reaction in a person.

Allergic contact dermatitis: an allergic skin reaction.

Aloe vera: a type of plant; usually refers to a lotion or gel made with the plant's extract, which may be soothing for first-degree burns.

Altered mental status: a phrase used to describe a change from a person's normal responsiveness and awareness, including confusion, disorientation, dizziness, drowsiness, or partial or complete unresponsiveness.

Altitude sickness: a syndrome caused by low oxygen levels at high altitudes, causing headache, dizziness, fatigue, shortness of breath, nausea and other symptoms.

Alveoli: tiny air sacs in the lungs where oxygen and carbon dioxide pass into and out of small blood vessels.

Amniotic fluid: the fluid surrounding the embryo and fetus within the amniotic sac; often called "water."

Amniotic sac: a membrane surrounding the embryo and fetus in the uterus, containing amniotic fluid.

Amputation: the complete cutting or tearing off of all or part of an extremity: a finger or toe, hand or foot, arm or leg.

Anaphylactic shock: shock resulting from an extreme allergic reaction, typically to an insect sting, a particular food, medication or some other substance; also called anaphylaxis.

Anaphylaxis: another term for anaphylactic shock.

Anatomic splint: splinting one part of the body to another part.

Angina pectoris: chest pain caused by heart disease, usually occurring after intense activity or exertion; often simply called angina.

Ankle drag: an emergency move for an unresponsive victim or one who cannot walk, but which provides no head support for a potential spinal injury.

Antibiotic: a medication that kills bacteria.

Antivenin: an antidote to the poisonous venom of a particular species, administered to counteract the effects of a bite or sting.

Anxiety: fear or apprehension of impending danger usually producing physical signs and symptoms.

Arteries: blood vessels that carry oxygenated blood from the heart to body tissues.

Aspiration: the movement of vomit or other fluids or solids into the lungs.

Assessment: the process of checking a victim for conditions requiring treatment or first aid, divided into an initial assessment for life-threatening conditions and a secondary assessment for other problems.

Asthma: a chronic disease in which at times the airway becomes narrow and the person has difficulty breathing.

Atherosclerosis: a narrowing and "hardening" of the arteries caused by plaque.

Aura: a generalized sensation or a hallucinated sensation involving any of the senses that occurs before a seizure.

Automated external defibrillator (AED): a device used to shock a fibrillating heart to return it to a regular rhythm.

Avulsion: an open wound in which an area of skin or other soft tissue is torn partially from the body.

B

Bag mask or **bag-valve-mask (BVM):** a resuscitation mask unit connected to an airbag that is squeezed to provide air to a non-breathing victim.

Barrier device: a device such as a pocket mask or face shield used to provide a barrier between a victim and first aider when giving rescue breathing to reduce the risk of disease transmission.

Basic life support (BLS): first aid given to a victim with a life-threatening problem of the airway or circulation; refers to rescue breathing, CPR and use of AED.

Beach drag: a method for removing an unresponsive victim from shallow water that provides some head support for a potential spinal injury.

Behavioral emergency: a situation in which the victim's behavior, whether caused by injury or illness or by personality or mental health factors, results in an emergency situation such as potential suicide or violence.

Bladder: the organ that stores urine until it is passed to the outside.

Blanket drag: an emergency move for an unresponsive victim or one who cannot walk, providing some support for the victim's head as the rescuer pulls the blanket.

Blood pressure: the pressure of blood on the walls of blood vessels.

Bloodborne disease: a disease that can be transmitted from one person to another through contact with the infected person's blood or certain other body fluids.

Bloodborne transmission: a process by which a pathogen existing in an infected person's blood or other body fluid is transmitted into a different person through contact with that body fluid.

Body mass index (BMI): a measure of weight in relation to a person's height, used to determine overweight and obesity.

Body substance isolation (BSI): an infection-control concept, used primarily in health care facilities, that assumes that any body fluid or moist body tissue is potentially infectious.

Body system: a group of organs that work together to perform a major body function.

Brachial pulse: the pulse felt over the brachial artery in an infant's upper arm on the inside, about midway between the shoulder and elbow.

Breech presentation: the position in which the infant's buttocks or feet move first into the birth canal rather than the head; also called breech birth.

Bronchi (singular: bronchus): the passageways from the trachea to the lungs.

Bronchodilator: a drug that relaxes the muscles of the airway, often used in an inhaler by people with asthma.

Burn: damage caused to skin and other tissue by heat, chemicals or electricity.

C

Capillaries: tiny blood vessels between the arteries and veins where oxygen and nutrients in the blood pass into tissues and carbon dioxide passes into the blood.

Carbon monoxide: an invisible, odorless, tasteless and highly lethal gas resulting from fires, gasoline engines, furnaces and other causes.

Cardiac: refers to the heart.

Cardiac arrest: the condition in which the heart stops beating effectively.

Cardiogenic shock: shock resulting when any condition, such as heart attack, causes the heart function to be reduced to the point that blood is not circulating sufficiently.

Cardiopulmonary resuscitation (CPR): a basic life support procedure for a victim who is not breathing and has no heartbeat, consisting of chest compressions combined with rescue breathing.

Cardiovascular system: the body system that moves the blood, which transports both oxygen and nutrients, throughout the body to supply cells and remove wastes.

Carotid pulse: the pulse felt over the carotid artery in a neck of an adult or child.

Central nervous system: the part of the nervous system formed by the brain and spinal cord.

Cervix: the lower part of the uterus, opening into the vagina.

Cardiac chain of survival: a concept emphasizing five steps needed for cardiac arrest victims: immediate recognition of cardiac arrest and activation of the emergency response system, early CPR that emphasizes chest compressions, rapid defibrillation if indicated, effective advanced life support, and integrated post-cardiac arrest care.

Chest compressions: a technique used in CPR to circulate the blood or, with a choking victim, to expel an object.

Choking: a physical obstruction of the airway, such as by food or the tongue in an unresponsive person.

Cholesterol: a fatty substance the body needs to carry out important functions but that in high levels is a risk factor for cardiovascular disease.

Chronic: refers to an illness or health condition, often incurable, that the person has had for some time; chronic conditions often make the individual more susceptible to the effects of injuries or sudden illnesses.

Chronic obstructive pulmonary diseases (COPD): a group of respiratory diseases, including emphysema and chronic bronchitis, in which breathing can become difficult.

Cincinnati Prehospital Stroke Scale (CPSS): a screening process for rapid identification of a stroke outside the hospital.

Closed injury: an injury in which the skin is not broken.

Clothes drag: an emergency move for an unresponsive victim or one who cannot walk, providing some support for the victim's head against the pulled clothing and rescuer's hands.

Clotting: the process in which fibrin and platelets clump together with other blood cells to seal a leak in a blood vessel.

Competent: the victim is able to understand what is happening and the implications of his or her decision to receive or refuse first aid.

Concussion: a type of brain injury resulting from a blow to the head, involving a temporary impairment of brain function but usually not permanent damage.

Confidentiality: the general principle that one should not give out private information about a victim to anyone except for those caring for the victim.

Consent: the victim's permission for you to provide first aid.

Contraction: one of a series of rhythmic tightening actions of the uterine muscles during labor.

Contusion: a bruised muscle.

Coronary heart disease: blockage of vessels supplying heart muscle with blood, often leading to heart attack.

Cradle carry: an emergency move for a light, unresponsive victim or one who cannot walk, in which the rescuer carries the victim in his or her arms.

Cramp: a tightening of a muscle that usually results from prolonged use.

Cravats: strips of cloth used to tie a splint.

Crepitus: a grating sensation felt or heard when fractured bone ends rub against each other.

Crowning: the stage of childbirth when the infant's head is passing into the birth canal and is visible.

D

Defibrillation: the process of administering an electric shock to a fibrillating heart to restore a normal heart rhythm.

Dependence: a pattern of physical and behavioral changes resulting from frequent use of a substance, including tolerance to its effects and the occurrence of withdrawal symptoms after cessation.

Depressant: a drug that slows certain central nervous system functions and produces dulled feelings.

Depression: a temporary state or a chronic psychological illness involving feelings of sadness, hopelessness and worthlessness, often along with physical symptoms.

Dermis: the middle layer of skin, damaged in second-and third-degree burns.

Diabetes: a metabolic disorder in which not enough insulin is produced or the body has developed resistance in the use of insulin, resulting in blood sugar (glucose) levels not being well regulated by the body.

Diaphragm: a muscle between the abdomen and lungs that moves with breathing.

Direct contact: disease transmission that occurs when someone directly contacts an infected person, or fluids or substances from that person.

Disinfectant: a substance, such as a bleach solution, that kills most pathogens on contaminated surfaces.

Dislocation: movement of one or more bones out of their normal position in a joint, usually with ligament damage.

Dispatcher: an EMS professional who answers 9-1-1 calls, determines the nature of the emergency and sends the appropriate emergency personnel to the scene.

Duty to act: a legal obligation to provide first aid as trained, obligated by one's job requirements or role as a child's parent or guardian.

Dysrhythmia: an irregular heartbeat; sometimes called arrhythmia.

E

Elder abuse: physical, emotional or financial abuse or neglect inflicted on someone older than 60, often by someone else in the home.

Electrodes: the pads of an automated external defibrillator (AED), which attach to the main unit with cables and deliver the shock to a victim's chest when indicated.

Embryo: a developing human from the time of implantation in the uterus through the first 8 weeks.

Emergency medical responder: formerly called a first responder, a professional with BLS training who often arrives first at the scene of a medical emergency, such as a police officer, fire fighter, industrial safety officer, ski patroller or similar professional who is often close to the scene.

Emergency Medical Services (EMS): a comprehensive network of professionals linked together to provide appropriate levels of medical care for victims of injury or sudden illness.

Emergency medical technician (EMT): emergency personnel trained to give prehospital medical treatment to injured or ill victims and to transport victims to advanced care facilities.

Emergency position indicating radio beacon (EPIRB): an emergency device for marine uses that emits a signal that is picked up by satellites and relayed to rescue personnel.

Endocrine system: the body system that produces hormones that help regulate many body functions.

Enhanced 911: an EMS system that automatically provides the dispatcher with the caller's phone number and the location of a land telephone line being used.

Entrance/exit wounds: terms referring to two related wounds such as burned areas on the body where electricity entered and left the body or wounds caused by a bullet entering and exiting the body.

Epidermis: the outer layer of skin, damaged in first-degree burns.

Epiglottis: a tissue flap that prevents solids and liquids from entering the trachea.

Epi-Pen: a commercial emergency epinephrine auto-injector used for anaphylactic reactions.

Esophagus: the tube that carries food to the stomach from the throat.

Evacuation: the process of removing a victim from a remote location that cannot be reached by ambulance, including carrying the victim out and helicopter rescue.

Evisceration: protrusion of abdominal organs through an open wound in the abdominal wall.

Expressed consent: consent explicitly given by the victim for first aid.

External respiration: the process by which oxygen enters the blood from air that is inhaled and carbon dioxide exits the blood into air that is breathed out.

Extremities: the arms and legs.

F

Family radio service (FRS): small short-distance radios (often called walkie-talkies) that do not require a special license.

Febrile seizure: a seizure caused by high fever.

Femoral pulse: the pulse felt in the center of the groin crease.

Femur: the long bone of the upper leg.

Fetal alcohol syndrome: a pattern of growth and development problems found in infants whose mothers drank significant amounts of alcohol during pregnancy.

Fetus: a developing human in the uterus from the age of 8 weeks until birth.

Fibrillation: an abnormal heart rhythm, common after a heart attack, in which muscles of the heart are quivering instead of beating rhythmically; see Ventricular fibrillation.

Fibrin: a protein substance in blood that, with platelets, forms blood clots to prevent bleeding.

First-degree burn: a minor burn that damages only the skin's outer layer.

Flail chest: a fracture of two or more ribs in two or more places, allowing a segment of chest wall to move apart from rest of the chest.

Flowmeter: a piece of oxygen equipment that is used to adjust the rate of oxygen delivery to the victim.

Food poisoning: a type of poisoning that occurs after eating food that is contaminated with microorganisms, usually bacteria, or their toxins.

Fracture: a broken bone.

Frostbite: a condition in which localized skin and other tissue freezes and dies, as a result of exposure to freezing temperatures.

Full-thickness burn: another term for a third-degree burn.

G

Gastrointestinal system: the body system that extracts nutrients from food to meet the body's needs for energy.

Genitals: the male and female sex organs.

Good Samaritan law: a state law designed to protect people who give first aid in an emergency from lawsuits.

GPS: a small device, named for the global positioning system, that reads satellite signals to inform the user of location in longitude and latitude.

Ground fault circuit interrupter (GFCI): a shock-preventing device that can be added to electrical circuits near water sources, such as in bathrooms and kitchens, that immediately interrupts the flow of electricity if an electrical appliance contacts water.

H

Hammock carry: an emergency move with which three to six rescuers carry the victim in a "hammock" made with their arms.

Hazmat: an abbreviation for "hazardous materials," often used to refer to a hazmat incident or a hazmat team of professional rescuers.

Heat cramps: muscle cramps, often in the lower legs or abdominal muscles, that result from activity in a hot environment when sweating lowers the body's sodium levels.

Heat exhaustion: a condition of dehydration and depletion of salt and electrolytes in the body caused by heavy sweating if the person does not get enough fluids when active in a hot environment.

Heatstroke: a life-threatening condition in which the body's core temperature rises abnormally high when heat-loss mechanisms fail to maintain a normal body temperature in a hot environment.

Heimlich maneuver: another term for abdominal thrusts given to a responsive choking victim to expel the obstructing object.

Hemorrhage: bleeding, usually significant.

Hemorrhagic shock: shock caused by severe external or internal bleeding.

Hepatitis: the various forms of liver disease caused by the bloodborne hepatitis B virus (HBV), hepatitis C virus (HCV) or other hepatitis viruses.

High altitude cerebral edema (HACE): a rare but serious type of altitude sickness involving a life-threatening fluid buildup in the brain.

High altitude pulmonary edema (HAPE): a rare but serious type of altitude sickness involving a life-threatening fluid buildup in the lungs.

History: information about what happened with an injury or illness and other relevant facts about the victim and the condition.

Homeostasis: a balanced state within the body necessary for effective functioning.

Hormone: a chemical messenger carried in the blood that affects the functioning of one or more organs.

Human immunodeficiency virus (HIV): the bloodborne virus that causes acquired immunodeficiency syndrome (AIDS).

Humerus: the bone of the upper arm.

Hyperglycemia: high blood sugar.

Hypertension: high blood pressure.

Hyperventilation: fast, deep breathing usually caused by anxiety or stress.

Hypoglycemia: low blood sugar.

Hypothermia: lowering of the body's core temperature, a life-threatening emergency caused when the body cannot produce enough heat to compensate for heat loss in a cold environment.

Hypovolemic shock: shock that occurs when blood volume drops.

I

Immune system: the body system that helps fight disease.

Immunity: the state of being protected against an infectious disease.

Implied consent: consent for first aid for an unresponsive victim or a child without a parent or guardian present.

Indirect contact: disease transmission that occurs when someone contacts contaminated objects, food or drink, droplets in the air, or vectors such as insects.

Infection: an invasion of the body by a pathogen that may potentially cause disease.

Initial assessment: a quick first check of the victim for life-threatening problems, involving a check for responsiveness and breathing.

Inline stabilization: see Spinal motion restriction.

Insulin: a hormone secreted by the pancreas that helps regulate blood sugar levels.

Integumentary system: the body system that protects the body from the environment and germs and helps regulate body temperature; the skin, hair and nails.

Internal respiration: the process of oxygen and carbon dioxide moving into and out of the blood within internal body tissues.

Irrigation: the process of washing out a wound under running water or saline solution.

J

Joint: the point where two bones meet; most joints are capable of movement.

K

Kidneys: organs that filter wastes from the blood and produce urine.

L

Laceration: a cut in the skin that may penetrate and also damage underlying tissue.

Latex: a rubber material, commonly used in medical examination gloves, to which some people are allergic.

Ligament: a tough, fibrous band that holds bones together in a joint.

Log roll: a technique in which several rescuers turn a victim with a suspected spinal injury either onto the back or side while keeping the head supported in line with the body.

Lyme disease: a potentially serious bacterial infection that may result from the bite of a tick carrying the bacteria.

M

Medical direction: the process by which EMS personnel are guided in certain medical interventions in the field by a physician.

Miscarriage: spontaneous death of an embryo or fetus before the middle of the second trimester.

Morning sickness: nausea and vomiting common in early pregnancy.

Musculoskeletal system: the body system that gives the body shape and strength and makes movement possible.

Myocardial infarction: see Acute myocardial infarction (AMI).

Myocardium: heart muscle.

N

Nasal cannula: an oxygen delivery device usually used on a breathing victim who does not require a high concentration of oxygen; also called nasal prongs.

Nasopharyngeal airway: a nasal airway inserted through the nose and into the pharynx.

Needlestick: an unintentional puncture of the skin with a used medical (syringe) needle, that may be contaminated with pathogens.

Negligence: a breach of duty, when one has a duty to act, that results in injury or damages to a victim.

Nervous system: the body system that controls all body functions and movement and allows for sensory perception and consciousness.

Neurogenic shock: shock that occurs when a nervous system problem allows vessels to dilate to the point that blood volume is not sufficient to fill blood vessels and be pumped to vital organs.

Nitroglycerin: prescription medication for angina and heart attack that increases blood flow through partially restricted coronary arteries.

Nonrebreathing mask: an oxygen delivery device composed of a mask and a reservoir bag, used on a breathing victim.

O

Occlusive dressing: an air- and water-tight dressing used to seal a wound.

Open wound: an injury in which the skin is torn or cut open, often leading to bleeding.

Organ: a body part that accomplishes one or more specific functions.

Oropharyngeal airway: an oral airway inserted through the mouth and into the pharynx.

Osteoporosis: a bone condition involving a loss of calcium, common in old age.

Overdose: taking too much of a drug or substance, causing detrimental or life-threatening effects.

P

Pacemaker: a small electronic device implanted under the skin in some patients with heart disease, that helps the heart maintain a regular rhythm.

Packstrap carry: an emergency move for an unresponsive victim or one who cannot walk, in which the rescuer carries the victim over the rescuers' shoulders.

Panic attack: a sudden, overwhelming fear that is excessive for the situation.

Paradoxical movement: the movement of a segment of the chest in a patient with flail chest, in which the flail segment moves in the opposite direction of the rest of the chest wall.

Paralysis: an inability to move a body part, such as the arms or legs, caused by nerve damage.

Paraphernalia: things used in the preparation or taking of drugs, such as needles and syringes, eye droppers, straws used for snorting, pipes, razor blades, plastic bags, and pill bottles.

Partial-thickness burn: another term for a second-degree burn.

Pathogen: a microorganism, such as bacteria and viruses, that can cause infectious disease.

Pelvis: refers generally to the area below the abdomen and specifically to the pelvic bones between the hip and the lower spine.

Personal locator beacon (PLB): a type of emergency position indicating radio beacon intended to be used by individuals in emergencies in remote land locations.

Personal protective equipment (PPE): any equipment used to protect against contact with blood or other body fluids, including gloves, barrier devices and other devices.

Pharynx: the throat.

Physical abuse: a physical injury (ranging from minor bruises to severe fractures or death) as a result of punching, beating, kicking, biting, shaking, throwing, stabbing, choking, hitting (with a hand, stick, strap or other object), burning or otherwise harming a person.

Physical examination: the process of examining an injured or ill victim head to toe to find conditions requiring first aid or medical attention.

Piggyback carry: an emergency move for a light responsive victim, in which the rescuer carries the victim on his or her back with arms under the victim's legs.

Placenta: an organ that develops in pregnancy to supply the embryo and fetus with oxygen and nutrients from the mother by means of the umbilical cord.

Plaque: a buildup of cholesterol and other substances inside arteries, eventually causing atherosclerosis and potentially blocked arteries.

Platelet plug: platelets sticking together at the site of an injury in a blood vessel, which may reduce or stop minor bleeding.

Platelets: structures in blood that assist in clotting at the site of an injured blood vessel to prevent bleeding.

Poison Control Center (PCC): one of a national network of centers designed to provide information about specific poisons in an emergency.

Poison: any substance that enters or touches the body with effects that are injurious to health or life-threatening.

Prenatal: before birth.

Presentation: the position of the infant in the uterus and vagina at the time of birth.

Pressure bandage: a bandage applied over a wound to maintain pressure to control bleeding.

Pressure regulator: a piece of oxygen equipment that connects to the oxygen tank to reduce the pressure of oxygen leaving the tank to a safe level.

Prolapsed cord: a situation in which a segment of the umbilical cord protrudes through the birth canal before childbirth.

Pulse: rhythmic changes in blood pressure in arteries caused by the heartbeat, which can be felt in certain body locations.

Puncture: a hole into the skin caused by a sharp penetrating object that may also damage deeper tissues.

R

Rabies: a viral disease, fatal if not treated in time, that is transmitted by the bite of an infected animal.

Rape: forced sexual intercourse, including vaginal, anal or oral penetration by the offender, including with a foreign object.

Recovery position: a position used for breathing unresponsive victims while waiting for help to arrive; the victim is positioned on the side to keep the airway open and allow fluids to drain from the mouth; also called the HAINES recovery position (High Arm IN Endangered Spine).

Reproductive system: the body system that makes human reproduction possible.

Rescue breathing: a BLS technique to get needed oxygen into the lungs of a non-breathing victim.

Respiratory arrest: the condition in which breathing has completely stopped.

Respiratory distress: the condition in which the victim's breathing is ineffective or difficult.

Respiratory system: the body system that provides the oxygen needed by body cells and removes the waste product carbon dioxide.

Resuscitation: the alternate term for basic life support skills for a victim in cardiac or respiratory arrest.

RICE: an acronym standing for rest, ice, compression and elevation; a procedure used with most musculoskeletal injuries.

Rigid splint: a splint made from something unbendable, such as a board.

Risk factor: anything that makes it more likely that a person will develop a particular disease.

Rule of nines: a method for calculating the percentage of body surface area of a burn.

S

SAMPLE: an acronym referring to the history of an ill or injured victim, standing for Signs and symptoms, Allergies, Medications, Previous problems, Last food or drink, and Events leading up to the injury or illness.

Scope of care: actions one is qualified to perform, such as specific first aid techniques one learns in a first aid course.

Secondary assessment: an assessment performed after determining the victim does not have life-threatening problems, including obtaining a history and performing a physical examination.

Second-degree burn: a burn that damages the skin's deeper layers but does not penetrate to tissues beneath the skin.

Sedative: a drug that calms and sedates certain nervous system responses; a type of depressant.

Seizure: a brain disturbance caused by many different conditions, including epilepsy and high fever in infants and children; may produce convulsions.

Sexual abuse: any kind of sexual activity with a minor – including fondling, rape, sodomy, indecent exposure, or exploitation through prostitution or the production of pornographic materials – or with an adult without consent.

Suction device: a device used to clear blood, vomit or other substance from a person's airway; could he manually powered or powered by battery or pressurized oxygen.

Sexual assault: a wide range of victimizations, generally involving unwanted sexual contact, with or without force, including grabbing or fondling as well as verbal threats.

Sharps: a general term referring to medical needles and other sharp objects that may be contaminated with an infected person's blood and that could easily penetrate another person's skin to spread the infection, therefore requiring safe disposal.

Shepherd's crook: a rescue pole with a hook at the end to reach a victim from the edge of a swimming pool.

Shock: a life-threatening condition that occurs when vital body organs are not receiving enough oxygenated blood; usually results from bleeding.

Shoulder drag: an emergency move for an unresponsive victim or one who cannot walk, providing some support for the victim's head as the rescuer pulls the victim by the shoulders.

Skeletal muscles: muscles that attach to bones and create body movements.

Sling: a device used to support and immobilize the arm, made of a wide bandage or cloth tied around the neck.

Soft splint: a non-rigid splint made from a pillow or folded blanket.

Spinal column: refers generally to the vertebrae, extending from the base of the brain to the "tailbone," as well as to the nerves, or spinal cord, running through the vertebrae.

Spinal cord: the nerves running through the vertebrae.

Spinal motion restriction: supporting the head in line with the body to prevent movement in a victim thought to have a spinal injury.

Splint: a device for immobilizing a part of the body.

Sprain: damage to ligaments and other structures in a joint.

Standard precautions: infectious disease prevention behaviors combining the major features of universal precautions and BSI precautions.

Standard of care: refers generally to how first aid should be performed; what others with the same training would do in a similar situation.

Sternum: the breastbone.

Stimulant: a drug that stimulates the central nervous system and produces feelings of energy and well being.

Stoma: a hole in the neck used for breathing that was surgically created as a result of an injury or illness.

Strain: a tearing of muscle or tendon tissue.

Stroke: a sudden impairment of blood circulation to a part of the brain; also called a cerebrovascular accident (CVA) or brain attack.

Subcutaneous layer: the deepest layer of skin, damaged in third-degree burns.

Substance abuse: the intentional and often frequent non-medical use of a substance for its effects, typically without regard for potential negative health effects.

Substance misuse: using a drug for an unintended purpose or using in larger amounts than prescribed, perhaps unintentionally.

Sucking chest wound: an open wound in the chest caused by a penetrating injury that lets air move in and out of the chest during breathing.

Sudden illness: any medical condition that occurs suddenly and requires first aid until the person can be seen by a medical professional.

Sudden infant death syndrome (SIDS): a condition, the exact cause of which is poorly understood, that results in an apparently otherwise healthy infant dying suddenly in its sleep.

Sun protection factor (SPF): a numerical rating of sunblock and sunscreen products, indicating how well the skin is protected; with an SPF of 20, for example, 20 hours of sun exposure to skin covered with the sunblock is the equivalent of 1 hour of exposure of unprotected skin.

Superficial burn: another term for a first-degree burn.

Supplemental oxygen: oxygen in a tank administered to ill or injured victims.

T

Tendon: a fibrous band of tissue that attaches muscle to bone.

Tetanus: a serious infection caused by common bacteria, also called lockjaw.

Third-degree burn: a burn that damages the skin all the way through and may burn muscle or other tissues; a medical emergency.

Thorax: the chest area enclosed by the ribs (including the back of the body).

Tourniquet: a band, such as a rope or belt, tightened around a limb above a wound to stop bleeding by cutting off circulation to the limb below the band; used only as an extreme last resort because usually the limb has to be amputated.

Toxemia: a hypertensive problem of pregnancy.

Trachea: the tube carrying air from the larynx to the bronchi.

Tranquilizer: a drug with calming, anxiety-reducing effects.

Transient ischemic attack (TIA): a temporary interruption to blood flow in an artery in the brain; sometimes called a mini-stroke.

Trauma dressings: thick, bulky dressings used with large or irregular wounds or dressings used to stabilize an impaled object.

Triage: a process of setting priorities for the care of multiple victims.

Tripod position: a position often taken by a person in respiratory distress: sitting and leaning forward, with hands on knees.

Two-handed seat carry: an emergency move for a responsive victim, in which two rescuers carry the victim in a "seat" made with their arms.

U

Umbilical cord: an organ containing an artery and vein that connects the embryo and fetus to the mother.

Universal precautions: a set of preventive behaviors, used with all victims, all the time, always assuming that blood and other body fluids may be infected; includes hand washing, using gloves and other personal protective equipment, and other actions to prevent transmission of bloodborne diseases.

Urinary system: the body system that removes liquid wastes from the body and helps maintain the body's water balance.

V

Vaccine: a form of a dead or weakened pathogen that triggers the body's immune response, creating immunity.

Vascular spasm: a mechanism in which the damaged blood vessel constricts to slow the bleeding and allow clotting to occur.

Vasoconstriction: contraction of blood vessels.

Vasodilation: dilation of blood vessels.

Vector transmission: the process by which a bloodborne pathogen is transmitted from an infected person or animal through the bite of a tick, mosquito or other insect.

Veins: blood vessels that carry deoxygenated blood back to the heart from body tissues.

Ventricles: two of the heart's four chambers that pump blood to the body and lungs

Ventricular fibrillation (V-fib): an abnormal heart rhythm, that commonly occurs with heart attacks, in which the ventricles of the heart are quivering instead of beating rhythmically

Vertebrae: the bones the back and neck.

VHF radio: very-high frequency radios typically used on boats, typically for distances of less than 30 miles.

W

Walking assist: a method to help a victim walk by supporting part of the victim's weight with your arm around the victim.

West Nile virus (WNV): a bloodborne disease spread mostly by the bite of infected mosquitoes.

Withdrawal: a physical or psychological reaction caused by abrupt cessation of a drug in someone who has become dependent on it.

Index

— ❖ —

Why a Revised Edition?

We first published *The Creative Curriculum for Infants & Toddlers* in 1997. Our decision to write a curriculum for programs serving very young children was not made lightly. For years, we had resisted the idea, telling colleagues who asked that we felt it wasn't necessary: "Caring for infants and toddlers is about building relationships and making the most of everyday experiences and routines," we said. "You don't need a curriculum to tell you how to do this."

While building relationships must be at the core of any infant and toddler program, we came to believe that a comprehensive curriculum is as vital to serving this age group as it is for any other. Knowing what we do about the critical importance of the first few years of life and the long-term benefits of quality programs on children's healthy development, we also recognized how difficult it is for programs to achieve quality when they lack the resources to train and retain staff. We tried to address this need by developing a practical yet comprehensive approach for staff development that applies the latest research to everyday programming. We chose the format of a curriculum because we wanted to offer an alternative to resources that emphasize only activities without providing a comprehensive framework for making decisions.

Curriculum development is not a finite task that can be completed and set aside. Over the past two years, we have had the opportunity to talk with colleagues, to evaluate how our materials are interpreted, and to assess how effectively the approach is being implemented. We decided to publish a revised edition in order to incorporate suggestions we received and modifications in our own thinking about how to best explain developmentally appropriate practice for infants and toddlers.

Our goal in this revision has been to make absolutely certain that we effectively convey the concept that curriculum for infants and toddlers is primarily about building responsive relationships. We wanted to clarify how adults create environments and offer a variety of experiences in response to children's growing abilities, personalities, interests, and needs. By taking time to observe and get to know children as individuals, caregivers/teachers can respond in ways that nurture each child's curiosity about the world and self-confidence. In this revised edition, we have also modified the individualizing and planning forms, and updated the information and checklists on health and safety, as well as the resources. Programs using both editions will find the content and format completely compatible.

It is our hope that *The Creative Curriculum for Infants & Toddlers* will help those who work with infants and toddlers and their families to visualize and implement a high-quality program that is developmentally, individually, and culturally appropriate.

Acknowledgments

Many individuals helped us to shape *The Creative Curriculum for Infants & Toddlers* into a product that conveys our best thinking on how to create and maintain a high-quality program for very young children and their families. We would like to begin by thanking the four Early Head Start programs who contracted with us for staff development support and served on a Design Team to assist us in conceptualizing our approach: Brattleboro Town School District, Brattleboro, Vermont; Project Chance, Brooklyn, New York; Sacramento Employment and Training Agency, Sacramento, California; and United Cerebral Palsy of Washington and Northern Virginia.

A very special acknowledgment goes to our editor, Emily Kohn, who was always supportive, but also willing to challenge our thinking and patiently helped us re-work many drafts of the book. The chapters on routines are based extensively on Amy's experiences as head of the Bank Street Infant and Family Center. These experiences were also the basis of a book for parents that Amy wrote with Leah Wallach (*The Ordinary is Extraordinary: How Children Under Three Learn*, New York: Simon & Schuster, 1988). The first draft of *The Creative Curriculum* was reviewed by a group of experts who gave us extremely constructive comments. We are very grateful for the feedback and recommendations we received from Cathy Gutierrez-Gomez, Dorothy Hartigan, Dianne Itterly, Trudi Norman-Murch, Bart O'Connor, Peter Pizzolongo, Michele Plutro, Valerie Rhomberg, Sherrie Rudick, Sarah Minteer Semlak, Janice Stockman, Rachel Theilheimer, Ruth Uhlmann, and Jean Racine.

Once the book was in print, we received recommendations for strengthening our approach from several infant/toddler specialists. Ron Lally advised us to more explicitly emphasize how the child initiates actions on the environment, what caregivers/teachers learn from observing each child, and to include more on young infants. Abbey Griffin and Sarah Minteer Semlak reviewed the entire manuscript, concurred with these recommendations, and gave us specific changes to many of the chapters. We also wish to thank Karen Sokal-Gutierrez, M.D. for helping us update the information on health and safety.

Our words came to life during the production process when Jennifer Barrett O'Connell "introduced" us to our children, families, and caregivers/teachers through her illustrations. We felt we were truly meeting in person the people we had only known in our minds! And we are grateful for the expert support of Debra Al-Salam, who was part of this project from the beginning—organizing the process, inputting our changes to countless drafts, managing the review process, and collaborating with Maggie Pallas to produce the first edition, and Cindy Shaw for this revised edition.

Finally, we want to thank the entire staff at Teaching Strategies for their support and encouragement during the development of both editions. We are especially grateful for the invaluable assistance we received from Toni Bickart, Larry Bram, Caitlin Pike, and Sharon Yandian.

Table of Contents

Why a Curriculum?

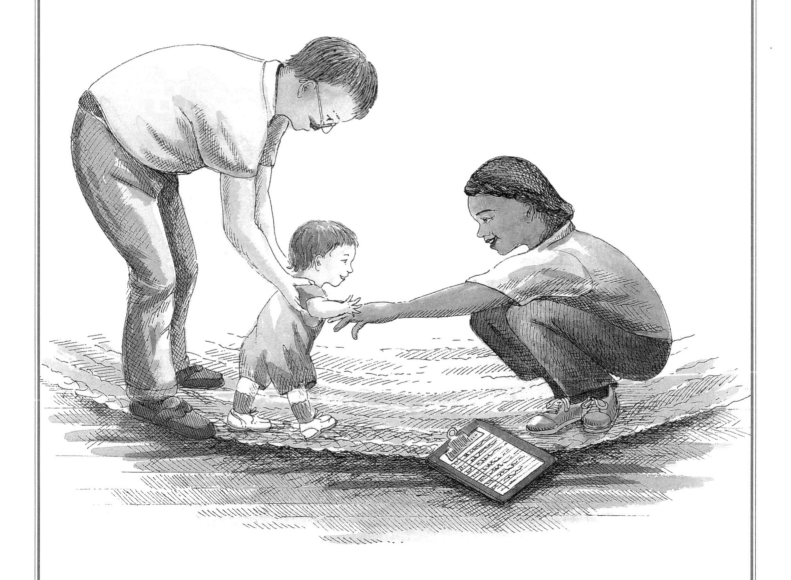

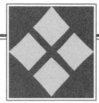

Why a Curriculum for Infants and Toddlers?

As someone who cares for infants and toddlers in center-based programs and family child care settings, you have an awesome responsibility. We now know that the first three years of life are more critical to a child's development than we ever imagined. Research tells us that more rapid brain development takes place during these years than at any other time of life. During this period, children are discovering who they are, how others respond to them, and if they are competent. They are also learning how to relate to others, what it means to express their feelings, and whether they are loved. Their brains are being "wired" into patterns for emotional, social, physical, and cognitive development.

Your work is extremely important, for you are helping to build both a foundation and a future for each child and each family. Whether you call yourself a caregiver, teacher, provider, early childhood educator, "educarer," nanny, or child development specialist, we see your role as blending the abilities and ideals represented by all of these titles. In this *Curriculum*, we have chosen to use the title caregiver/teacher, because we feel that it comes closest to representing the full spectrum of what you do. Our *Curriculum* is addressed to you—the center–based staff and family child care providers who are committed to offering a high-quality program for infants and toddlers and their families.

What Is a High-Quality Program for Infants and Toddlers?

Every high-quality program whose mission is care and education shares certain characteristics. First and foremost, it meets the standards of the profession. These standards describe seven key indicators that identify an early childhood program of high quality.[1] As you read through this list of indicators, think of the role that you play to ensure that your program is a standard bearer for quality. Notice also that a developmentally appropriate program

---

[1] Based on Derry G. Koralek, Laura J. Colker, and Diane Trister Dodge, *The What, Why, and How of High-Quality Early Childhood Programs: A Guide for On-Site Supervision,* Revised Edition. Washington, DC: National Association for the Education of Young Children, 1995, Ch. 1.

contains three interwoven elements: age appropriateness, individual appropriateness, and cultural/social appropriateness.[2]

(1) The program is based on accepted theories of child development. We know that at each stage of life, children take on special developmental tasks and challenges related to their social, emotional, physical, and cognitive development. For infants and toddlers, development occurs in all of these areas as they use their senses to gain a sense of security and identity and to explore the people and objects in their world.

The key to meeting the developmental needs of infants and toddlers can be found in the responsive relationships children build with the important adults in their lives— including you. This is why it is so important to have small-sized groups and low adult-to-child ratios. For the same reason, it is also important for each child to have a primary caregiver, and, whenever possible, for that person to remain paired with the child throughout the first three years.

(2) The program is individualized to meet the needs of every child. A knowledge of child development tells you what is age appropriate—that is, what children, in general, are like at a given age. For example, most two-year-olds are energy in motion, testing limits as well as patience. However, what you don't know from child development theory, but learn through interactions and observations, is that a particular infant with colic can be soothed by laying him across your knees and gently rocking him from side to side, and that a certain toddler, who has limited manual dexterity but loves to paint, can do so with a special headband that holds a paint brush.

The information you gather from working with children and talking with their families enables you to make the program individually appropriate for each child. You do this by making changes to the environment, planning activities, and developing strategies that build on your intimate knowledge of each child's temperament, interests, culture, emerging capabilities, and preferred learning styles.

(3) Each family's culture is respected and family members are encouraged to participate in the program. Since the 1960s and the first days of Head Start, there has been a recognition that parents and early childhood professionals are natural partners in promoting children's growth and development. In programs for infants and toddlers, it is almost impossible to serve children without also serving their families.

(4) The physical environment is safe, healthy, and contains a variety of toys and materials that are both stimulating and familiar. Every high-quality early childhood program provides an environment where children can be safe and healthy, yet free to move around, explore, and experiment. Infant and toddler environments also need to be warm and engaging so that children and families feel welcome and comfortable. A soft, stuffed chair where you can curl up with a baby and read a book, or a covered fish tank at floor level are places that stir children's imaginations and are conducive to building trusting relationships.

---

[2] Sue Bredekamp and Carol Copple, Eds. *Developmentally Appropriate Practice in Early Childhood Programs*, Revised Edition. Washington, DC: National Association for the Education of Young Children, 1997.

To create this type of environment, you continually check indoors and out to remove hazards and prevent children from injuring themselves and others. You follow hygienic procedures for diapering, toileting, hand washing, food service, and management of illness. In addition, you arrange the indoor and outdoor environments to promote active exploration, and you include attractively displayed and accessible play materials and toys that reflect the children's culture, interests, and skill levels.

(5) Children select activities and materials that interest them, and they learn by being actively involved. During their earliest years, children are learning to trust the world, to actively explore their environment, and to do things for themselves. When an infant stares with delight at a colorful scarf and you bring it within her reach, you are following her interests. Likewise, when you place a wedge-shaped pillow on the floor near the open shelf on which dolls are displayed, you enable a child with cerebral palsy, who lacks upper body strength, to reach for the dolls on her own, when she wishes. The more you provide opportunities for children to follow their own interests, the more they learn from experience, and the greater the chances that they will continue to be successful learners throughout their lives.

(6) Adults show respect for children and interact with them in caring ways. We know from research that if any single factor defines quality in an early childhood education program, it is the caring nature of adult-child interactions. Children's healthy development depends on being cared for by adults who will respond immediately and appropriately to their needs and communications. This means not just talking with children in a soothing voice, but responding to a child's needs to be held, rocked, and comforted. It also means being a sensitive and responsive communicator, both verbally and non-verbally. Even children who are not yet able to talk need you to engage in meaningful conversations with them. Infants and toddlers are most likely to thrive when they have a primary caregiver who reflects their emotions, who is there to share the highs and lows of each and every day, and who experiences with them the excitement of new discoveries.[3]

(7) Staff and providers have specialized training in child development and appropriate programming. High-quality programs are planned, implemented, and continually revised by trained professionals who have the knowledge and skills to oversee a program that is developmentally appropriate. This training comes in many forms: through college courses, by obtaining a Child Development Associate (CDA) credential, by attending workshops and seminars, by being part of a network of colleagues such as a family child care providers' association, and from using a developmentally appropriate curriculum.

Where your program is located isn't as important as what you do in the program. If yours is a quality program, the seven characteristics highlighted above will be in evidence. What, why, and how you do things are far more important than anything else. High quality is high quality, and it takes many forms.

---

[3] This type of caregiving is described in the literature as "involved teaching." See Helen Raikes, "A Secure Base for Babies: Applying Attachment Concepts to the Infant Care Setting," *Young Children,* July 1996, pp. 59–67.

The Relationship of Curriculum to High-Quality Programming

How do we move from these seven indicators of high-quality to everyday practices? ZERO TO THREE: The National Center for Infants and Toddlers provides us with a clear definition of the components of a quality program and the roles of the key players who interact in ways that promote children's growth and development.[4] Their publication, *Caring for Infants and Toddlers in Groups*, is filled with abundant examples of practices that are developmentally appropriate contrasted with practices that are not appropriate. There can be no question about what a quality program should provide.

Why then do you need a curriculum? We believe that the guidelines alone are not enough to help you plan and implement a program for infants and toddlers. While a clear definition of developmentally appropriate practice is a vital part of quality programming, it is not a substitute for curriculum. Curriculum provides a framework for pulling all the pieces of developmentally appropriate practice together—the what, why, and how you do things. It provides a vision of where developmentally appropriate practice will take you and guides you through the processes of planning, implementing, and evaluating the program.

At the same time, a curriculum helps you to individualize your program. It gives you a framework for learning about each child and shows you how to respond to each child's special circumstances, abilities, and learning style, and to each family. A curriculum based on developmentally appropriate practice offers you the "big picture" of where you want to lead each child and family—and how you can grow as a professional. It is your blueprint for action.

The Creative Curriculum for Infants & Toddlers

Like all formal curriculum models, *The Creative Curriculum for Infants & Toddlers* outlines what children learn during the first three years, the experiences through which children achieve these learning goals, what staff and parents do to help children reach these goals, and the materials needed to support the implementation of the curriculum.[5]

The National Association for the Education of Young Children (NAEYC) identifies three key components of a curriculum:[6]

❖ **Content**—what emerges from the goals and objectives. The focus is on helping children to learn about themselves, about their feelings, about others, about communicating, about moving and doing, and to acquire thinking skills. In addition to goals for children, *The Creative Curriculum for Infants & Toddlers* includes goals and objectives for the other key players in the learning process: the children's families and you, yourself.

---

[4] J. Ronald Lally, Abbey Griffin, Emily Fenichel, Marilyn Segal, Eleanor Szanton, and Bernice Weissbourd. *Caring for Infants and Toddlers in Groups: Developmentally Appropriate Practice.* Arlington, VA: ZERO TO THREE/The National Center, 1995.

[5] Note that this definition of curriculum reflects the Revised Head Start Program Performance Standards (Federal Register, Vol. 61, No. 215, Tuesday, November 5, 1996, Rules and Regulations).

[6] Sue Bredekamp and Teresa Rosegrant, Eds. *Reaching Potentials: Appropriate Curriculum and Assessment for Young Children*, Vol. I. Washington, DC: National Association for the Education of Young Children, 1992, p. 10.

❖ **Processes**—what you do to help children learn. They include strategies for setting up the environment, selecting toys and materials, interacting with children, and planning activities. Most importantly, processes focus on decision making. All day, every day, you use routines and provide activities to respond to children's growing abilities, interests, and needs. *The Creative Curriculum for Infants & Toddlers* provides a framework for making decisions that are developmentally, individually, and culturally appropriate for each child.

❖ **Context**—the setting in which learning takes place. For children under age three, relationships are the context. By building strong bonds with children and their families, you create a climate where learning flourishes. Using *The Creative Curriculum for Infants & Toddlers* to design and implement your program enables you to lay the groundwork for a lifetime of learning.

Here is how these components of our curriculum fit together.

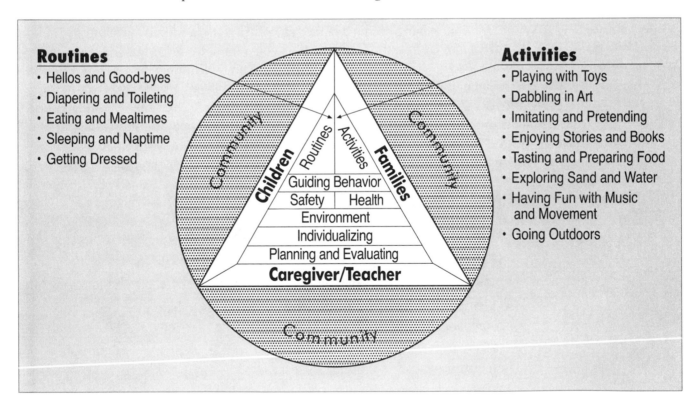

As you can see, you are at the foundation of the curriculum. The children and families in your program are the focal points of your work. As shown in the graphic, they are also your equal partners. Your relationship with them is central to all that happens in your program.

Surrounding all of you is the community in which you live. The values and culture of your community are a constant influence on your program. The community also symbolizes the interaction between your program and the larger society in which it exists: services are received from the community, but something is also given back.

By implementing *The Creative Curriculum for Infants & Toddlers,* you set the stage for children's learning. You do this by planning and continually evaluating your program. You individualize the program based on what you learn about each child and family from your observations and daily interactions. You create a warm, inviting environment, ensure that children are safe, and follow practices that promote children's health. You guide children's behavior in positive ways.

You use daily routines as opportunities to build relationships with children and promote learning. And you plan activities that respond to the growing interests and abilities of the children in your care.

Using This *Curriculum* to Make Decisions Each Day

While decision making occurs whether or not you have a formal curriculum, *The Creative Curriculum for Infants & Toddlers* gives you a framework for making decisions based on knowledge, your observations, and thoughtful reflection. How does this framework translate into practice? The best way to illustrate this process is to go back to the concept of decision making. Each day you make hundreds of decisions—both large and small—in your work with children and families. You think about questions such as the following:

❖ Should I hand the teething ring to the baby or let her reach for it?

❖ How can I personally greet each child and family if I'm in the middle of changing a diaper?

❖ How many books should I leave out for my toddlers to look at?

❖ Do the pretend play props reflect the children's home cultures?

❖ How can I be sure that the outdoor equipment is safe for the children to use?

❖ What is the best way for me to work with parents to help their child use more language?

❖ How can I help a new colleague to get to know the children and our curriculum?

To illustrate how you might use the *Curriculum* in your work, we take you through a typical day caring for infants and toddlers. On the following pages, we highlight some of the major responsibilities you have to juggle each day, and identify the chapters where they are addressed.

A Typical Day Caring for Infants and Toddlers

Review your plans for the day. As you walk into your center or make a cup of coffee before the first family arrives on your doorstep, think about the day ahead.

- ❖ Collect all the ingredients for playdough.
- ❖ Take a mental scan of all your children. Who needs a new challenge? Who is ready for more cooperative play?
- ❖ Plan how you will give special attention to a child who has seemed especially quiet and withdrawn for the past two days. Make a point to talk with her grandmother.

> **Planning** ahead for an **art activity** gives you a mental picture of what to expect and frees you to be responsive to the individual needs of children and families. *(Chapters 5 and 17)*

> Knowing **infants and toddlers** and consulting with **family members** allows you to meet **individual needs.** *(Chapters 2, 3, and 6)*

Check over the environment. In the quiet of the morning, take a good look at the space.

- ❖ Hang a mobile over the changing table to give infants something interesting to see that they can touch or kick and make move.
- ❖ Note any toys that need to be repaired or replaced. Remove the broken fire truck with the sharp edge from the shelf.
- ❖ Replace a missing outlet cover immediately.
- ❖ Put a new picture book on the shelf to catch toddlers' interest. Remind yourself to sit down and read with children.

> Creating a **safe, welcoming environment** with interesting things to see and do encourages children to explore and learn. *(Chapters 7, 8, and 16)*

> **Reading** with children each day is critical to their development. *(Chapter 19)*

Greet children and their families. Do a quick health check as you welcome each child and family.

- ❖ Smile hello and explain you will be with an arriving family as soon as you finish changing a diaper.
- ❖ Ask parents questions about what has happened since you last saw their child. "When did she last eat?" "How did she sleep last night?"
- ❖ Share some of your plans for the day. "We will walk to the park later."
- ❖ Encourage a father to have a cup of juice or to read a book with his daughter as she settles in for the day.

> **Building relationships** with children's families forms a bridge for the child between home and child care. *(Chapter 1)*

> **Knowing families** helps you to better understand their needs and concerns. *(Chapter 3)*

Help children and families say good-bye to one another. Be there to assist with separations.

- ❖ Encourage parents to say good-bye, no matter how tempting it is to sneak out while their child is occupied.
- ❖ Suggest a good-bye ritual, such as walking with you to the door.
- ❖ Invite a child's grandmother to call later in the day to see how the child is doing.
- ❖ Reassure a toddler that mommy will come back just like she always does. Help him join in an activity you know he will like.

> Helping parents say **good-bye** instead of sneaking out promotes trust and strengthens the relationship between parents and their children. *(Chapter 11)*

> Listening to children and responding to their feelings helps you build **relationships.** *(Chapter 1)*

Change diapers and help toddlers learn to use the toilet. Changing a diaper or helping a child use the toilet can be much more than a simple mechanical task.

> *Diapering and toileting provide excellent opportunities for one-on-one time with children. (Chapter 12)*

> *Making daily **safety** and **health** checks and taking precautions reduces the chances of injury and guards against the spread of disease.*

> *You **individualize** by observing so you know when a child is ready to begin working on a new skill, such as using the toilet. (Chapter 6)*

- ❖ Talk to an alert young infant before lifting her. "Let's change your diaper so you'll be comfortable."
- ❖ Observe safety practices, such as never leaving a child on the changing table unattended and wiping up spills to avoid falls.
- ❖ Wash your hands—and children's—and disinfect the changing table after each diaper change.
- ❖ Play "Where Is Your Tummy?" as you change a child's diaper.
- ❖ Look for signs that indicate a toddler is getting ready to be a toilet-user—staying dry for long periods, saying when she has to urinate, or showing a real interest in sitting on the potty.
- ❖ Encourage perseverance and self-confidence. "Accidents happen. Let's find a pair of dry pants."

Encourage children to explore and play. Through their senses and actions, infants and toddlers learn about objects, what they can do, and what to expect.

> *Offering children a range of appropriate **activities** helps them feel competent as learners. (Chapters 16 through 23)*

> *Making changes to the **environment** keeps it stimulating and challenging. (Chapter 7)*

- ❖ Provide materials that encourage infants and toddlers to use all their senses—rattles, unbreakable mirrors, squeeze toys, texture balls, finger foods to taste and smell, fill and dump toys, simple rhythm instruments, playdough, books, and simple puzzles.
- ❖ Give the mobile a push as you change an infant's diaper.
- ❖ Surprise children—cover a table with a blanket to create a tent.
- ❖ Give a child with a disability who uses a walker the extra time needed to move to and explore different areas of the room.
- ❖ Share your enthusiasm and pleasure in children's discoveries. "You found our new puzzle!"

Observe children. Watch carefully and ask yourself, "What is this child doing?" "What does it tell me?"

> *Observing helps you get to know each child so that you can **individualize** your program. Being aware of your own cultural beliefs helps assure that your observations are as objective as possible. (Chapter 6)*

> *Making daily observations allows you to **evaluate** the program and make needed changes. (Chapter 5)*

> *Observing children gives you insight on their **health** and development and indicates whether screening for special needs is indicated. (Chapter 9)*

- ❖ Note differences in temperament—who is more reticent and cautious, who is more active and quick to engage, who is more laid back and less demanding.
- ❖ Look for why a certain child seems to get upset so easily, why another bites, why another seems to disappear and get little attention.
- ❖ Use a system for recording your observations, such as jotting notes in a notebook or on index cards.
- ❖ Talk with your director or colleagues about an infant who doesn't respond to loud noises.
- ❖ Be aware that your beliefs may interfere with objective observations.

Respond to children as individuals. Your challenge is to provide enough variety to meet the needs, interests, and abilities of each child.

❖ Give children choices by setting out a variety of materials each day.

❖ Share a book about dogs with a child who is fearful of real dogs.

❖ Continually observe and ask yourself, "What is this child interested in?" "What kind of experience is she having?"

❖ Use your observations and what you have learned from talking with parents to help you better understand each child's needs, interests, temperament, and learning style.

❖ Be sensitive to each child's individual temperament and preferences. For example, a child who is tactily sensitive (highly sensitive to touching or being touched) will be reluctant to fingerpaint.

> Children learn best when they are given the opportunity to select their own play **activities.** (*Chapters 16 through 23*)

> Using observations gives you objective insights about a child's development, interests, and needs, which are the basis for **individualizing** your program. (*Chapter 6*)

> Sharing **stories and books** is important for children's language and literacy skills and is pleasurable as well. (*Chapter 19*)

Prepare and serve snacks and meals. Appreciate the many learning opportunities and nurturing feelings that are associated with food.

❖ Serve a variety of healthy foods.

❖ Talk with families about cultural or dietary considerations. Learn about children's allergies, their special nutritional requirements, and food preferences. Post menus so parents know what their children eat each day.

❖ Hold an infant on your lap during snack so he can enjoy all the activity. Invite toddlers to help put out plates and napkins, spread apple butter on their crackers, and pour their own juice from small plastic pitchers.

❖ Feed babies when they are hungry, not according to a preplanned schedule, and hold them on your lap when feeding them a bottle.

❖ Sit and talk with older infants and toddlers while they eat.

❖ Separate wash cloths, toothbrushes, and placemats for each child.

> Serving nutritious foods helps assure children's good **health** today—and tomorrow. Food habits begin at birth. (*Chapter 9*)

> Communicating with **families** about **mealtimes** helps you work together to build bridges between children's worlds of home and child care. (*Chapters 3 and 20*)

> **Tasting and preparing food** and **mealtimes** are wonderful learning opportunities for infants and toddlers. (*Chapters 13 and 20*)

Encourage children to sleep and take naps. The younger the child, the more individualized the schedule for sleeping and naptime.

❖ Allow children to nap when they feel the need, while you play with those who are awake.

❖ For toddlers, play quiet music or dim the lights to signal naptime.

❖ Base rituals to encourage sleep on each child's temperament and preferences. Sit with one child in a rocking chair; place another in his crib and talk quietly to him for a few minutes.

❖ Observe health and safety precautions. Be sure each child has his or her own space for sleeping and that pillows, heavy blankets, and large stuffed animals are not placed in cribs.

> Allowing children to **sleep and nap** as needed ensures they get enough rest. (*Chapter 14*)

> **Music** can be used as a transition from one activity to another. (*Chapter 22*)

> Creating a **safe, healthy** environment allows children to thrive. (*Chapters 8 and 9*)

Individualizing activities ensures that children get the most out of them. *(Chapter 6)*	**Offer a variety of activity choices.** Note what toys and materials children have been most interested in and place them where they will be accessible.

Offer a variety of activity choices. Note what toys and materials children have been most interested in and place them where they will be accessible.

> ❖ Take the time to watch what children do and ask yourself, "What is the child experiencing? What am I learning about him? What's my role?"
>
> ❖ Talk to children as they explore and play to describe what they are doing, looking at, and experiencing.
>
> ❖ Bring out hats and pocketbooks for the toddlers who are playing with doll babies.
>
> ❖ Be aware that what children take from an experience may be different from what you had planned. Don't be disappointed if a walk to the corner turns into watching an earthworm right outside your door.
>
> ❖ Share ideas for activities and tips for doing them with families, so they can try planned activities at home. "This is the playdough recipe we made today. Your child loved it"

Side notes (left column):

Individualizing activities ensures that children get the most out of them. *(Chapter 6)*

Art, pretend play, sand and water, and **music and movement** can be particularly soothing activities. *(Chapters 17, 18, 21, and 22)*

Sharing activities with **families** enables them to extend children's learning at home. *(Letters to Families)*

Clean up. Children learn from being involved in cleaning up.

> ❖ Be sure shelves and containers have picture labels so mobile infants and toddlers can help put their toys away.
>
> ❖ Encourage older infants and toddlers to join you as you put things away and wipe the tables.

Side notes (left column):

Clearing away the clutter in the **environment** helps children see what is there so they can make choices. It also makes your job easier. *(Chapter 7)*

Low, open shelves that are labeled allow children to use and return **toys** on their own. *(Chapter 16)*

Take children outdoors. Take children—even young infants—outdoors every day, when weather allows.

> ❖ Set aside a shaded soft area for young infants and quiet activities, an area with a small climber and swings, and an area for riding toys and for sand and water play in your play yard.
>
> ❖ Offer infants the opportunity to sleep, watch what other children are doing, and enjoy the fresh air—in a carriage, on a blanket, or in a baby carrier.
>
> ❖ Create safe places where mobile infants can crawl, cruise, climb, run, ride wheel toys, kick and throw balls, garden, and play with sand and water.
>
> ❖ Secure the straps on a stroller and insist that toddlers hold your hand when crossing the street during a neighborhood walk.

Side notes (left column):

Going outdoors allows children to use their rapidly developing motor skills and explore a new environment. *(Chapter 23)*

Encouraging children's explorations, while at the same time ensuring children's **safety** outdoors, requires your ongoing attention. *(Chapter 8)*

Guide children's behavior. By helping children learn how to control their behavior, you encourage inner control and the beginning of self-discipline.

- ❖ Redirect the mobile infant who is interested in objects, but not aware of those in her path.

- ❖ Help a child who is out of control: "I am going to help you stop kicking. We'll find something else for you to do."

- ❖ Have realistic expectations of children's behavior. An infant is not misbehaving when he cries—he is communicating with you. Toddlers are not being selfish when they fight over the ball—they are not yet ready to share.

- ❖ Consult with families about challenging behaviors, and together develop an approach to handling the problem.

- ❖ Take time to carefully observe when, where, and under what circumstances a child hits and bites. With the information you gain, you can successfully help him to express his feelings in acceptable ways.

- ❖ Use the environment to promote positive behavior: provide duplicates of popular toys; put quiet activities away from those that are active, noisy, or messy; store pencils and other sharp objects up high and out of children's reach; use pillows to create a safe space for infants that keeps them out of toddler traffic; use trays, placemats, and carpet squares to help mobile infants and toddlers define their space.

> Developing positive relationships with children allows you to **guide their behavior** and helps them take their first steps toward self-discipline. *(Chapter 10)*

> Understanding child development enables you to have realistic expectations for **children's behavior** that can be shared with families. *(Chapters 2 and 3)*

> Reorganizing the **environment** can help address and prevent potential problems. *(Chapter 7)*

Help children and families reunite and head for home at the end of the day. Parents and children may need you to help them say hello to one another and good-bye to you.

- ❖ Invite family members to come a few minutes early and spend some time playing with their child before they have to leave.

- ❖ Help parents understand their son's confusing end-of-the-day behavior. When he has a tantrum about putting on his coat, explain he may have saved his deepest feelings for them—the people he loves and trusts most of all.

- ❖ Share news of the day with each child's family: "She finished her whole bottle at 3:30." "He helped feed the fish today." "She made it all the way to the top of the climber outside."

- ❖ Be available to help children gather their belongings, put on their coats, and say good-bye as they leave.

> Helping families look at **hellos and good-byes** through their children's eyes can be very reassuring. Departures are also an important time for building a bond with families. *(Chapter 11)*

> How you say good-bye to children and families is key to a strong **relationship**. *(Chapter 1)*

> **Dressing** children can be a time to build relationships and promote learning. *(Chapter 15)*

Reflect on your day. Take a moment to think about your day and what you learned, so that you can note any changes for the future.

- ❖ Identify an activity that went well and note who participated.

- ❖ Make notes about why the fingerpainting activity got out of control.

- ❖ Review your notes on individual children and think about new experiences you can plan for them.

> Reviewing your day enables you to **evaluate** what worked well and what aspects of your program need to be changed. *(Chapter 5)*

> Observation is the basis for **individualizing** your program goals and objectives. *(Chapter 6)*

| Taking good care of yourself enables you to do your job. **You are your most important resource.** *(Chapter 1)* |

| When you model **healthy** behaviors, you teach children to value them, too. *(Chapter 9)* |

Take care of yourself. Only by taking care of yourself will you have the resources and energy to care for the children and families in your program.

❖ Learn to lift children by bending your knees to protect your back.

❖ Display artwork or a special poster where you can see and enjoy it.

❖ Eat a nutritious breakfast and get a good night's sleep each day.

❖ Invite toddlers to join you in a few exercises each afternoon.

❖ Talk with a friend when something is bothering you.

| Being aware of and using **community** resources helps to strengthen families and enhances the quality of your program. *(Chapters 4 and 9)* |

| Being a **professional** means respecting the privacy of children and families and treating them honestly and ethically. *(Chapter 1)* |

Meet and talk regularly with colleagues in child care and your community. Remind yourself that caring for infants and toddlers and working with families is both rewarding and demanding work. This work is easier and better done with the support of colleagues.

❖ Think about all the people who could help you with the daily questions and concerns about children and their families. This list might include your director, co-workers, members of your provider association, someone from the Child and Adult Care Food Program, and people from various social service agencies in your community.

❖ Call on community resources as issues arise. Discuss your concerns about typically developing children and those with special needs, always maintaining the confidentiality of individual children and families.

❖ Talk with colleagues regularly—at staff meetings, family child care association meetings, or even monthly pot-luck dinners.

❖ Meet with the case manager from the county early intervention program.

The order and types of activities described in "A Typical Day" may vary from those in your program. There is, however, one important constant: being aware of *why* you do *what* you do will help ensure that your daily decisions add up to a high-quality program. Throughout this book, we will explore the ideas, strategies, and practices introduced in "A Typical Day."

Your Journey Through This Book

Depending on your experience and needs, you can use this book in different ways. You can read it chapter by chapter. You may choose to select chapters according to a prioritized need—health and safety first, for example. Or, you may wish to begin by consulting the routines and activities chapters first. However you begin, it is important to keep in mind that creating and maintaining a quality program is an ongoing journey, not a task that one can accomplish and cross off as "done."

For many of you, *The Creative Curriculum for Infants & Toddlers* will confirm the excellent practices you already have in place. For some, this will be your first introduction to caring for infants and toddlers. For all readers, we hope that the *Curriculum* will enhance what you do well and give you new ideas for improving your program.

Goals and Objectives for Caregivers/Teachers

To help you keep track of where you have been and where you are going as you journey through this book, we begin the *Curriculum* with goals and objectives for you, the caregiver/teacher.

Goal 1: To build responsive relationships

- To form positive, trusting relationships with each child over time
- To form positive relationships with families to support children's growth and development
- To work with colleagues and community representatives to support children and families

Goal 2: To plan and manage a developmentally appropriate program

- To plan and evaluate a program that meets the needs of the children and families served
- To observe children regularly and individualize the program based on these observations
- To create a warm and welcoming environment that supports children's growth and development
- To ensure the safety of children in the program
- To promote the health of children in the program
- To guide children's behavior in positive ways

Goal 3: To promote children's development and learning

- To use routines as opportunities for growth and learning
- To provide activities that will facilitate children's growth and development

Goal 4: To continue learning about children, families, and the field of early childhood education

- To participate in training to expand skills and knowledge
- To participate in professional early childhood education organizations
- To observe colleagues to learn new successful techniques and approaches

Goal 5: To maintain professional standards

- To be ethical in all dealings with children, families, and community representatives
- To respect the privacy and confidentiality of children and parents
- To demonstrate respect for all children and families

Goal 6: To be an advocate in support of children and families

- To educate others about the need for high standards and quality programs
- To work with community agencies in support of children and families

The *Goals and Objectives for Caregivers/Teachers* are presented in the form of a self-assessment tool in Appendix A. You can use this form to help you track your own professional development, to indicate those parts of your job you do well, and to identify areas you want to work on.

Goals and Objectives for Children and Families

As you begin reading through *The Creative Curriculum for Infants & Toddlers* and applying it to your own program, you will note that we have grouped children into three categories to highlight developmental differences that will influence the decisions you make. These categories are:

- ❖ young infants (birth through 8 months);
- ❖ mobile infants (8 to 18 months); and
- ❖ toddlers (18 to 36 months).

A listing of goals and objectives for each of the age groups can be found in Chapter 5, Planning and Evaluating Your Program. Forms to help you individualize your program are based on these goals and objectives. These forms, entitled *Individualizing Goals and Objectives for Young Infants, Individualizing Goals and Objectives for Mobile Infants, and Individualizing Goals and Objectives for Toddlers* can be found in Appendix B. In Chapter 6, Individualizing for Children and Families, we have modeled the process of individualizing by using the forms for toddlers to plan for 35-month-old Valisha Curtis.

Because families are your partners in creating a quality program, Chapter 5 also includes a list of goals and objectives for your work in building relationships with families. A form, entitled *Goals for Working with Families* can also be found in Appendix B. You can use it to plan and track your work with each family in your program.

Introducing Our Children, Families, and Caregivers/Teachers

We would like to introduce our cast of characters—the infants and toddlers, families, and caregivers/teachers you will meet as you journey through *The Creative Curriculum for Infants & Toddlers*. Though each child and family is distinct in culture, interests, temperament, and background, as a group they typify all of the children and families you serve. The programs described highlight the range of settings in which infants and toddlers can receive quality care, and the varied backgrounds of the caregivers/teachers who ensure that the care is of the highest quality.

Julio Gonzales, 4 months, lives in Florida with his parents Marta and José, and his 15-month-old sister, Maria. His parents speak Spanish at home.

Linda Marquez has a two-year degree in early childhood education. She is bilingual and works at a center that serves a migrant community.

Jasmine Jones, 8 months, lives on a U.S. military base in Germany with her mother, Charmaine, a Master Sergeant in the Air Force. Jasmine sometimes spends nights with her caregiver/teacher's family when her mother has to work.
Janet Walker became a family child care provider so she could stay at home with her own five children.

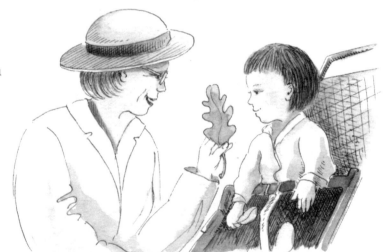

Willard O'Keith, 11 months, is the only child of Kevin and Monica who are graduate students in Iowa. **Grace Lincoln,** his caregiver/teacher, works at the university-sponsored child care center.

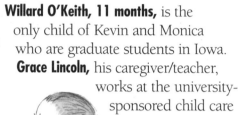

Abby Kennedy, 16 months, was adopted from Korea when she was one week old. She lives with her parents, Robin and Edward, and her older sister, Talia, age nine.
Dr. Brooks Peterson, a family child care provider, is a retired psychologist who provides child care for two or three children at a time.

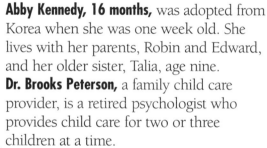

Leo New, 20 months, lives on a reservation in Arizona with his parents, Virginia and Elmer. **Barbara Yellowcloud,** a center-based teacher, earned her CDA credential and is currently taking distance learning courses by satellite.

Matthew Gerry, 26 months, lives with his parents, Nancy and Pete, and a newborn sister, Kara, in a Chicago suburb. **Mercedes de Jesus** takes care of both Matthew and Kara in her family child care home. She works weekends as a caterer.

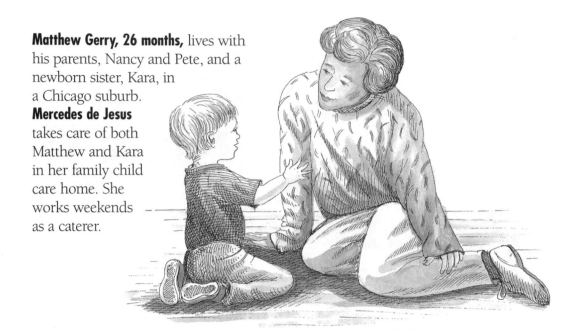

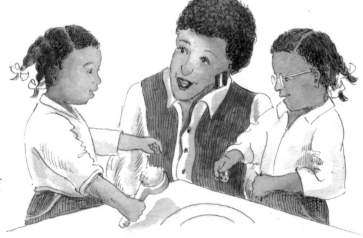

Gena Domenica, 30 months, lives in Rhode Island with her parents, Neal and Rebecca, and eight siblings ranging in age from 11 months to 21 years. Born with cerebral palsy, Gena has limited mobility.

Ivan Powell, a center-based teacher, is very comfortable working with children who have special needs. He is taking courses towards an AA degree.

Valisha and Jonisha Curtis, identical twins, 35 months, live in Los Angeles with their parents, Yvonne and Johnny, and their brother Patrice, age 5. Jonisha wears eye glasses as the result of an injury.
La Toya Thompkins cares for six children in her home.

Part
I Who's Who

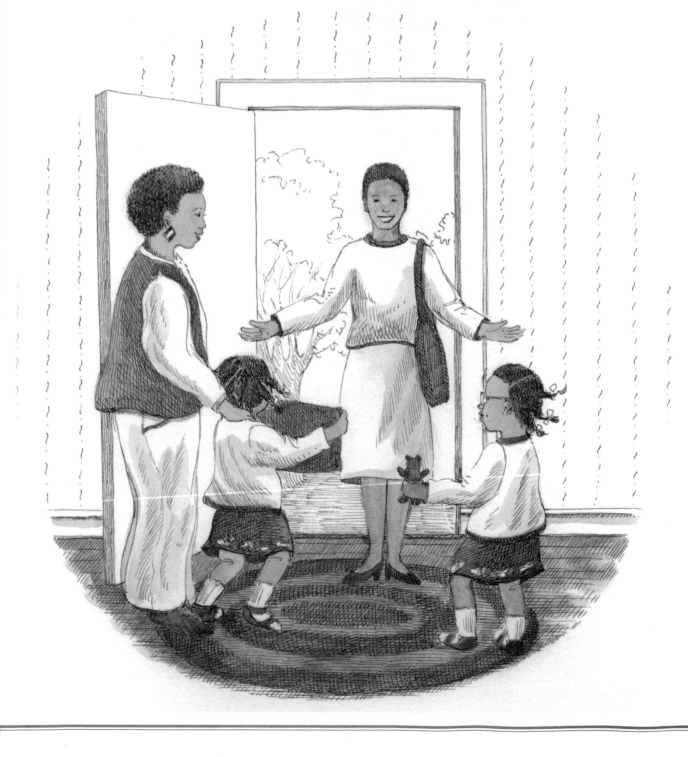

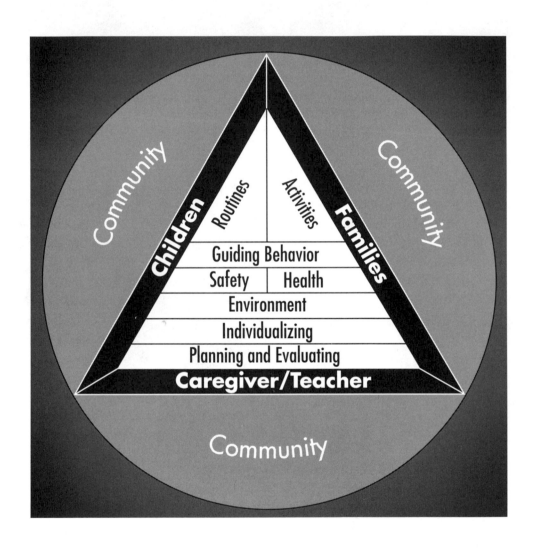

Who's Who in a Quality Program

A quality program begins with the key players—caregivers/teachers, the children, their families, the community—and the trusting, responsive relationships that exist among them. The program evolves and changes as a result of the interactions between these key players as illustrated by the picture of our curriculum framework on the preceding page.

As a caregiver/teacher, you play a central role in nurturing these relationships. The infants and toddlers you care for are learning who they are as people. By observing, you get to know and appreciate each child as an individual. As you respond to their cues, you help children feel good about who they are and you encourage them to want to engage with other people and objects in their world. As the children grow and change, you respond in ways that promote greater independence, more complex use of their skills, and further learning. Knowledge of child development and the individual characteristics of each child with whom you work forms the basis for the many decisions you make each day.

Children are part of families, and you interact daily with family members. Because research shows that effective programs require the joint efforts of families and teachers, good relationships with families are critical to the success of your program. Equally important, they help build strong families. You build relationships with parents as you establish an atmosphere of trust and respect. In this kind of atmosphere, you and family members each can contribute your own expertise to benefit and support the children in your lives.

Because families may look to you to guide them to other resources in the community, you need to be familiar with the services your community provides. To increase your awareness of available resources, you begin to build relationships with colleagues, professional groups, and the people who work in various community agencies. As you reach out, you'll discover how much you have to offer your community, based on your commitment to and knowledge of children and families. Building community relationships takes time, but once built, they can enrich your program, your community, and you, yourself.

No one can tell you that creating and maintaining a quality program for infants and toddlers is easy. It's not. And as valuable and important as your work is to children and families, many people do not appreciate the critical role you play. But the more you learn and grow professionally, the more effectively you can speak about the value of your work as an essential support for families. The relationship focus of your work makes it special and gives it a unique place in the lives and future of the children you care for and the families you support. As society comes to appreciate the value of your chosen profession, you will be more likely to earn the recognition, income, and benefits you deserve.

❖   ❖   ❖

Building Relationships: The Focus of Your Work

Whether you work in your home or a center, building relationships with infants, toddlers, and their families is the focus of your work. You are the one who can make sure that your program meets the needs of the children and families you serve. For this reason, we place you at the foundation of our curriculum.

People who work with infants and toddlers don't always appreciate the critical importance of their work as they face the fourteenth diaper change of the day. Or reach for the tissue box once again. Or explain to an upset mother why one of her child's socks is missing. While these tasks may at times seem unimportant or dull, it's important to keep in mind that every interaction is an opportunity to build the relationships that allow children to thrive. Children who receive responsive care in the first three years of life learn how to care for others.

Building Relationships with Children

During the first three years of life, infants and toddlers are learning who they are. Through their interactions with you and their families, they gain answers to questions such as:

❖ Do people respond to me?

❖ Who are the people I can depend on?

❖ Am I important to others?

❖ Am I competent?

❖ How should I behave?

❖ Do people enjoy being with me?

❖ What should I be afraid of?

❖ Is it safe for me to show how I feel?

❖ What things interest me?

The daily interactions you have with children help shape their sense of themselves and how they will relate to other people. When you respond to infants' needs consistently, promptly, and lovingly, you help them learn to trust and show them what it means to be in a caring relationship with another person. When you guide toddlers' behavior in respectful, positive ways, you promote self-discipline and help children learn to express their feelings in acceptable ways. As you listen to children, create a safe environment filled with interesting things to do and opportunities to be competent, and share your pleasure in their discoveries, you help children feel good about themselves and their growing skills.

Each child in your program will benefit from a relationship with a **primary caregiver.** This person builds close bonds with a small number of children and families. Having a primary caregiver gives children a secure base. They learn to trust someone familiar who will care for them as they explore and who will be there to comfort them when they are tired, upset, or frightened. Their relationship with a primary caregiver helps children feel secure enough to relate to other adults in the child care setting. In a family child care home you are likely to be each child's primary caregiver. In larger child care homes and center-based programs, primary caregivers may be assigned or self-selected to form these all-important relationships.

Strategies for Building Relationships with Children

How do you build relationships with children? As in all aspects of your work, knowing yourself is a good place to start. The more aware you are of your own feelings, attitudes, and values, the more aware you can be of those of others. To be self-aware requires a willingness to ask questions such as, "Why am I acting this way?" as you find yourself, for example, becoming overly involved with one child, or shying away from another. Recognizing that your feelings shape your interactions will help you form relationships and respond to children individually. Here are some ways to build relationships with children as you care for them each day.

Allow time. Often, the demands of caring for a group of children can keep you so busy that you feel you have no time simply to be with an individual child and get to know one another. To help you slow down, remind yourself that building relationships is a central part of your work.

Be dependable. Let children know they can count on you. Be there to greet them at the door each morning. Respond promptly to a child who is crying. Keep your promises: "Yesterday I said you could help make playdough today. Are you ready?"

Handle children's bodies with respect. Explain to an infant, "I'm going to pick you up now so I can change your diaper." Ask a toddler, "Could you please help me take off your wet shirt?"

Look, listen, and respond to children. Give a child your full attention. Observe the child's facial expressions and body language. Learn to distinguish an infant's cries, so you'll know whether to offer him something to eat or comfort him. Sit down and listen to a toddler's story about helping to make pancakes at home.

Use caring words to let children know they are respected and understood.
Think about what you say and also how you say it. Even infants who
can't talk yet and don't know the meaning of the words you say are
sensitive to the sound of your voice. Use the child's home
language whenever possible. Practice using
caring words and a caring tone. For example, when comforting an upset child, you
might say, "You are having a hard time. I
can tell by your tears you're feeling sad.
Let's sit here in the rocking chair together
and see how we can help you feel better."

**Adapt daily routines to meet individ-
ual needs.** Offer an infant a bottle when
she is hungry, regardless of whether it is
snacktime or mealtime. Give a
toddler time to finish his puzzle
before you change his diaper.

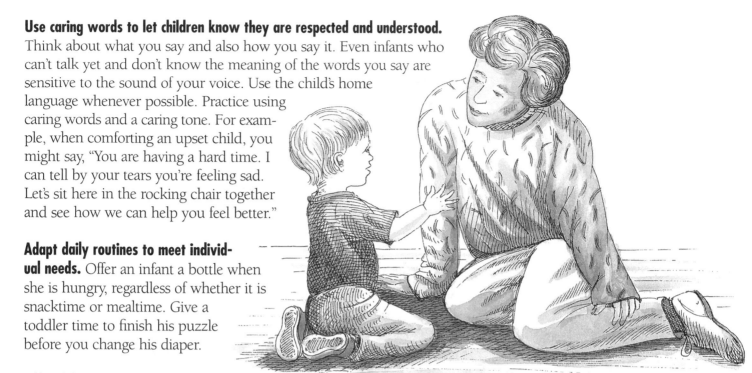

**Offer children opportunities to make
decisions, whenever possible.** Give children clear alternatives when the choice is theirs to
make. At snacktime, asking children to choose among slices of banana, peach, or pear
shows you respect their tastes and their growing decision-making skills.

Have realistic expectations of children's behavior. Knowing about child development means
you won't be surprised, for example, if two toddlers fight over the same toy. Instead of
getting upset or blaming the children, you'll know to provide duplicates of favorite items,
and also to show children how they can use a toy together.

Tell children when you leave the room. Let children know that you are going into the
kitchen or upstairs to a meeting. This tells them you won't suddenly disappear. Rather
than keeping tabs on you, they can focus on what they are doing.

Attend to your own needs. To build and maintain relationships, you need to focus on
children and not be distracted by your own concerns. Take a few minutes each day
to take care of yourself so that you will have the energy you need for the children.

What If You Don't Like a Child

Have you ever worked with a child you didn't really like? If so, you are not alone. Though
it can be a hard thing to admit, especially when talking about an infant or toddler, owning
up to your feelings is part of being a professional. In rare cases, you may decide that things
are not going to work out and that it is time to part ways with a child and family. More
often, acknowledging your negative feelings is a signal to call on your professional self
to figure out why you and this child don't seem to "fit." Often it is because you have
very different temperaments and personalities. It may help to share your feelings with a

colleague, or even to ask a colleague to observe you and this child together. Consider this story, shared by Barbara.

> "When I first cared for Leo, I found myself reacting negatively to what I saw as his passivity and unresponsiveness. As I observed him, however, what I learned about temperament came alive. I realized that because I'm active—you could say 'feisty'—I was judging his very different way of being. Leo, in fact, is very attentive. He watches carefully and approaches when he is ready. He will not just respond to my tendency to sweep little ones up in my arms. I have to slow down for him until he gives me the signal. Now I love everything he does and how he does it."

All relationships have their ups and downs. Some are clearly easier than others. We believe, however, that the extra effort you put into building positive relationships with every child will be repaid many times over.

Building Relationships with Families

Children need you and their families to work together. By working together, you can both get to know a child better than either of you could on your own. Your relationship builds a bridge between a child's two worlds: home and child care.

Parents are specialists about their child. For example, Jasmine's mother, Charmaine, is able to share with Janet, Jasmine's family child care provider, that Jasmine cries for a bottle as soon as she wakes up from her morning nap, and that lately she has been afraid of dogs. Janet is a specialist, too. From her training and experience, she knows that babies' needs should be met quickly, so she makes sure to have a bottle ready when Jasmine wakes. She also knows that when Charmaine travels, Jasmine is likely to have more frequent episodes of fearfulness. Sharing knowledge with one another helps both gain a more complete picture of Jasmine and how to respond to her needs.

Beginning a Relationship

When a family member comes to visit your program, take time to share a little about yourself—your background, training, and why you have chosen to work with infants and toddlers. Take them on a tour of your space. Describe your program and curriculum. Most important, assure families of your belief that they are—and will remain—the most important people in their children's lives. Let them know that your goal is to work with them to help their children grow and thrive.

Listen to parents. Ask them about their hopes and dreams for their child. What concerns do they have? What do they want from you and from your program for their child? If you listen carefully enough, you will begin learning about a family's culture and values. Continue to set the stage for a good working partnership by clarifying responsibilities you and the family have to one another. You'll probably want to provide printed copies of policies and procedures including information about fees, the program's hours, a yearly calendar, and what happens in case of illness (children's and yours).

We strongly recommend making home visits as a way to get to know and build relationships with families. A home visit provides a unique opportunity to see a child and his or her family in their natural environment, which builds mutual understanding. Your willingness to visit families at home sends a strong message that you want to reach out to them. But be aware that not all families feel comfortable about inviting you into their homes. For this reason, we suggest that you first visit those families with whom you feel welcome. It may take a little selling on your part to help other families understand that your purpose is to reinforce the connection between home and child care for their child.

Sharing Information Daily

Sharing information about the basics of daily living—sleeping, eating, and toileting—can help everyone be more responsive to children's needs. For example, when a parent tells you that his child was up most of the night, you'll know that the child might need a nap earlier than usual. If you tell a child's grandmother that her grandchild didn't eat lunch, she may decide to offer him a snack before going home. Telling a father how his toddler poured her own juice from a small pitcher, may lead him to allow extra time for waterplay in the bathtub at home.

Sharing information about events in a child's life can also help you understand a child's feelings. For example, knowing that a child's grandfather is very ill may explain why she has been more clingy and whiny than usual. With this information in mind, you may decide to spend extra one-on-one time with her and to talk about her grandfather.

Communication can take many forms. Little conversations at the beginning and end of the day are good ways to share news of a child's day and to tell families what will be happening at the program in the near future. Some programs use a clipboard with a standard form on which they jot down notes about each child's day.

Occasional social events are another way to communicate with children's families. A pot-luck supper or a weekend picnic can give families an opportunity to know you better and to meet and talk with other families. Conversations that start with sharing a recipe or during a game in the park can continue long after the event is over.

Sometimes, sharing information can bring up feelings of self-doubt and worry. For example, a mother may be afraid to tell you that her child doesn't sleep through the night. Perhaps she fears this information makes her seem incompetent. You may worry about admitting that you haven't been successful in stopping a child in your program from biting. When these kinds of feelings arise, remember that no one knows all the answers when it comes to caring for children. Only by sharing your questions can you and a child's family pool your ideas, seek information on ways to handle a situation, and build the kind of working relationship that benefits children.

While sharing information with families is very important, always be careful to respect confidentiality. Letting families know that your conversations will go no farther will help them feel more comfortable about sharing their concerns.

Holding Conferences with Parents

Conferences are another way to build relationships with families. These conferences can serve many purposes. They can help you and parents feel more comfortable working together. They can give you all a chance to learn more about a child. They can also provide an uninterrupted time to talk about the child's development, set new goals, and discuss how you might deal with a particular issue a child or family may be facing.

Planning in advance helps to ensure a successful conference.

- ❖ **Arrange a time that is convenient for families**. Make a special effort to invite fathers and other males who are important in a child's life.

- ❖ **Let families know what to expect.** When you set up the conference, explain that conferences are formal times to communicate and plan for their child. Ask what other topics families want to talk about.

- ❖ **Think carefully about the points you want to cover.** Review your observation records and ask co-workers if they have any information or insights to contribute. Sharing stories and observations will help families get a clear picture of their child and of your program as well.

- ❖ **If language differences are a barrier, invite someone to help interpret.** Many families have someone they know who can serve as an interpreter. If this is not an option, try to make other arrangements.

- ❖ **Give some thought to where you will meet.** Find a comfortable place with adult-size furniture. Be sure the area is private and separate from the children.

Because conferences are not everyday events, think about ways to put everyone at ease. Here are some suggestions for making everyone comfortable during a conference.

- ❖ **Begin by welcoming parents.** Like Ivan, offer an observation that says you know and enjoy their child: "Gena is trying so many new things. You should have seen the delight on her face as she tasted kiwi today."

- ❖ **Discuss the purpose of your time together.** Follow Mercedes's example: "Today we have the chance to think about how Matthew is doing. You said you wanted to know more about how he spends his days here. I thought we could begin there, then talk about the new skills he is learning. Are there some other topics you wish to discuss?"

- ❖ **Be sure there are many opportunities for parents to make comments and ask questions.** Grace does this by being sensitive to nonverbal cues: "Kevin, you have a puzzled look on your face. Did you want to ask me something else about Willard's progress?"

- ❖ **If a family speaks a language you are not familiar with, ask for some help.** Learn some basic words in their language.

- ❖ **At the end of the conference, summarize the main ideas you've talked about.** Review any actions you've all agreed to take. Here's how Ivan does this: "Why don't we go over to the library right now. I can recommend some books that Gena might enjoy having you read to her."

Resolving Differences

There will be times you and the children's families will disagree about something. Many of the differences come from the fact that you both care deeply about a child and want the best for him or her. However, you each may have different ideas about what is "the best." Sometimes these conflicts are due to differences in your cultural backgrounds and beliefs about how to promote children's development and learning.

When you and parents disagree, there are usually three courses of action you can take. You can let an issue go—that is, ignore it. You can choose to face the problem and work it out. Or, you can decide things are unworkable and end your relationship.

Let an issue go. Sometimes an issue really isn't all that important. If you decide on this option, however, be sure your reason is not merely to avoid a conflict. The example below shows how this option can be effective if, like Barbara, you really let the issue go.

> Barbara felt annoyed when Leo's parents kept forgetting to bring a blanket for him to use at nap time. Yet, when she considered all the problems and stresses in their lives, she realized it was quite amazing they even got Leo to child care. Barbara decided to let the issue go. She used one of her blankets for Leo. For everyone, the situation was resolved.

Work together to find a solution. If an issue is bothering you and you don't try to resolve it, you will probably become annoyed and children will sense that something is not quite right. It's worth taking time to find a resolution, as Linda did in the following example.

> Julio had been at the Shane Center for just one month, but each week his parents had been coming later and later to pick him up. The Center closed at 6:00 P.M., and Linda had to leave on time to attend a class. Linda was annoyed at Julio's parents because her reminders had not made a difference. Finally, she arranged a conference to explain to them how difficult it was for her when they were late. Julio's father said they didn't know they were causing a problem. If they had to be late from now on, the parents agreed to have a cousin pick up Julio.

Here are some steps you might try to resolve a difference:
- ❖ Identify the problem or issue.
- ❖ Work together to make a plan for dealing with the issue.
- ❖ Try your plan for a particular length of time.
- ❖ Check in with each other to see how things are going.
- ❖ Make changes as needed.

End your relationship. Sometimes, it's impossible to resolve a difference in a way that will allow you to continue working comfortably. Under these conditions, your decision may be to part ways. The following example shows how Mercedes made this difficult choice.

Sarah's parents insisted that she was toilet trained. Although she had several accidents each day and showed no interest in using the potty, her parents refused to let Mercedes put her in diapers. Mercedes and the family had many discussions about toilet training but these only led to arguments and Sarah was showing signs of increasing tension. For these reasons, Mercedes decided it was best to part ways.

Remember, this decision should only be considered as a last resort. When following this course of action, try to help families find alternative child care arrangements, for example, by suggesting they contact a child care resource and referral agency.

Differences can often stir up feelings of frustration and anger. These feelings can make it difficult to resolve problems. Try to be aware of issues that are "hot-spots" for you. Recognizing what they are may help you deal with them before they become a problem. Sometimes, talking with co-workers who have had similar experiences can help you understand a situation and may give you ideas of how to work with families toward a resolution. Here are some principles that may help guide you through the process of attempting to resolve conflicts.

Keep the children's best interests in mind. Children need you and their families to deal with your differences in ways that don't interfere with their care.

Let parents know you understand their feelings. Often the issues that come up generate strong feelings. Just acknowledging that you understand can put parents at ease.

Build on your history together. A disagreement doesn't have to mean that one of you is doing something wrong. Instead, a disagreement can be a point from which both you and families can learn and grow.

Have realistic expectations. Resolving differences often takes much time and discussion. Some differences may never be resolved. However, as long as you both are willing to discuss an issue, your relationship with families and your support of the child can continue.

When you know that conflicts are a normal part of sharing the care of a young child, you can look at them as opportunities to better understand a family's point of view. The more you know about children and families, the more likely you will be able to determine the best approach to handling conflicts. The next two chapters discuss getting to know children and families.

❖   ❖   ❖

Knowing Infants and Toddlers

All curriculum planning begins with knowing the children—how they grow and develop; what makes each child unique; and the cultural context or family environment in which a child develops. The more you know about children, the more effectively you can meet their needs.

Generally, all infants and toddlers in your program follow a similar path of development, though in their own ways and at their own pace. In less than 36 months, the children in your program will change from being totally dependent on others to care for them to being able to choose which shirt they want to wear and proudly pouring their own juice.

This chapter provides information on child development—how children three and younger grow and develop and learn. We discuss how infants and toddlers learn:

- ❖ about themselves—self-concept development;
- ❖ about their feelings—emotional development;
- ❖ about other people—social development;
- ❖ to communicate—language development;
- ❖ to move and do—physical development; and
- ❖ to think—cognitive development.

This chapter, also explores how children differ in terms of individual temperaments and special needs. (In the chapter, Knowing Families, we discuss the influence of culture.)

Learning About Themselves

In the first three years of life, infants and toddlers begin creating a picture of who they are, what they can do, and what they think and feel. It is a picture that will affect every area of their development. How you respond to children helps shape this picture. When you are respectful, share your pleasure in children's accomplishments and discoveries, and create an environment in which they can participate in daily routines and activities, you show children they are important, interesting, and competent. Your attitudes and actions help give children a good beginning during these important early years.

Building a Sense of Self

According to child psychiatrist Margaret Mahler, children go through a process that she calls a psychological birth.[1] Separated from their mother physically at birth, they spend the next three years developing a sense of themselves as individuals who are attached to, but separate from their parents. This is the journey of separation-individuation.

Around the age of four to five months, babies "hatch." They have a look of new alertness and almost overnight seem more persistent and goal-directed. We can see them beginning to understand that their parents or primary caregivers are separate from them as they pull at familiar adults' hair, study their face, and reach to explore a piece of jewelry or pair of glasses. Before long, infants discover that they can lose sight of important adults—a frightening discovery. More intensified clinging behavior and stranger and separation anxiety are evidence of children's growing attachment to their parents and primary caregivers. Jasmine, for example, may use a blanket, a piece of cloth from her mother's clothing, or a stuffed toy as a "transitional item." Holding onto the object, or smelling or feeling the piece of cloth, helps Jasmine hold a mental picture of her mother until she returns.

By the time infants are 10 to 16 months old, they act like explorers in love with the world. They are often so busy walking and practicing other new skills that their parents sometimes have to literally stand in front of them and wave good-bye to catch their attention. At this stage, parents sometimes worry their children don't care if they stay or go. This is not the case at all. If you observe carefully, you'll notice that children often seem a bit subdued or quiet when members of their family are not present. Quite the reverse is true at the end of the day. When a family member walks in the door, it's as if the child's emotional temperature rises. Games that involve going away and being found—peek-a-boo, putting things into boxes or cabinets, closing them in, then opening them and pouring them on the floor—are favorites of mobile infants and help them to deal with these issues of separation.

Toddlers are testing where their power to hold onto those they love ends and also learning how to comfort themselves. They may become upset and cling when it's time to say good-bye. Having "seen the world," it's as if they have gained a new awareness of how small and vulnerable they are. Their developing ability to use language, such as "mommy coming back" or "mommy at work," is one way toddlers reassure themselves. Dramatic play also helps them to understand and gain control of their world. Put out props that remind children of mommy, daddy, or grandma going to work and coming back and you might see a toddler like Matthew marching around with a briefcase and a jacket repeating, "Matt go to work."

By the end of the toddler years, most children are "psychologically born." They are able to hold the memory that their parents will return, but separations can still be difficult at times.

---

[1] Margaret S. Mahler, Fred Pine, and Anni Bergman. *The Psychological Birth of the Human Infant: Symbiosis and Individuation*. New York: Basic Books, 1975.

Building Trust and Autonomy

How children feel about themselves as they relate to others and learn who they are affects every area of their development. The psychologist Erik Erikson has identified eight stages through which each person passes in the lifelong process of developing a sense of self. Infants and toddlers are working on the first two stages.[2]

Infants are at the first stage: developing trust. Young infants have physical needs: to be fed when they are hungry; changed when soiled or wet; and allowed to sleep when they are tired. They also have emotional needs: to be comforted when upset; to have someone to talk with and interesting things to explore; and to be held and loved. When you meet their needs consistently, promptly, and lovingly, you help infants learn to trust themselves and their world.

Sometimes adults worry they will spoil infants by always responding to their needs. The reality is that infants need what they need when they need it. When you hold an infant securely in your arms and take time to sing a song or play "Where is your nose?" when you change a child's diaper, you are helping to build a sense of trust.

Toddlers are at the second stage: developing autonomy. According to Erikson, toddlers need to stretch their wings and assert themselves. At the same time, though, they need you to set clear and firm limits.

The world can be an exciting place to toddlers. Sometimes, it can feel so big that it's overwhelming. As a result, toddlers typically find themselves wanting the impossible: to be big and to stay little at the same time. As toddlers struggle with these feelings, you may find it difficult to know how best to respond to them. The most caring and knowledgeable adult can find herself at wit's end when a two year old screams, "No!" as she tries to help him put on his coat. Then she finds the same child five minutes later, dissolved in tears of frustration and wanting to be cuddled like a baby.

For toddlers, *no* is a favorite word. Saying *no* plays an important role in developing a sense of self. This powerful word helps children block out the often overpowering voice of adults and assert, "This is me."

You can help the toddlers in your program develop their independence and a positive sense of themselves. One way is to look at the world through their eyes so you can better understand what they may be experiencing. Using this approach can help you recognize that they aren't out to "get you"—even though it may feel that way sometimes. Rather, they are grappling with growing up. This understanding can help you respond to their often challenging behaviors with respect, appreciation, and with much needed humor.

Learning About Their Feelings

Day after day, your interactions with infants and toddlers help shape their emotional life. According to psychiatrist Daniel Stern, when there is **attunement,** a child learns that other

---

[2] Erik Erikson. *Childhood and Society.* New York: W.W. Norton & Company, Inc., 1950.

people can understand and share his feelings.[3] For instance, Linda is attuned to Julio when she smiles and mirrors his pleasure in making a sound with his rattle. As she does this, she is reinforcing the pathways in his brain that create emotions. When an attuned adult such as Linda mirrors back an emotion and an infant responds, the adult is helping to reinforce the signals in the child's brain that produced that emotion.

However, when an infant and adult are not in emotional "sync" with one another most of the time, the child's brain circuits and emotions may become confused. Examples of being emotionally "out-of-sync" would be the adult who usually responds angrily when an infant feels sad, or responds to a toddler's joy with a resigned sigh.

Milestones of Emotional Development

Stanley Greenspan, a psychiatrist and pioneer in the field of emotional development, has charted milestones in children's emotional growth.[4] The following paragraphs describe each milestone briefly.

Self regulation and interest in the world (birth+). During this first stage, young infants have their own ways of dealing with sensations, taking in and acting on information, and finding ways to calm and soothe themselves. They need you and their parents to take note of these individual differences and respond to them in appropriate ways.

Falling in love (4 months+). By four months, some infants eagerly reach out for relationships. Others need to be gently sold on them. More hesitant infants need you and their parents to continue to woo them, even when some of your attempts to engage them are ignored or rejected.

Developing intentional communication (8 months+). By this stage, infants need to know that their families and caregivers can understand and respond appropriately to the signals they communicate. For example, they need adults to read their cues that signal the need for calm and when they are ready for more active play.

Emergence of an organized sense of self (10 months+). By 10–18 months, infants and toddlers need adults to recognize and show appreciation of all the new abilities they have mastered. When you follow a child's lead during play, help her shift from one activity to another, and extend her play, you help her see herself as a complex, organized individual.

Creating emotional ideas (18 months+). By 18–24 months, children use pretend play to act out their feelings and to put into words their curiosity about sexuality, aggression, rejection, and separation. When you help children express their feelings through words and gestures, you promote their emotional development. If children's emotions make you uncomfortable, you may find yourself cutting off play that includes anger and aggression. Rather than limit children's exploration of these emotions, acknowledge their feelings and model or suggest an appropriate way to express them.

---

[3]Based on Daniel Stern, *The Interpersonal World of the Infant.* New York: Basic Books, 1987.
[4]Based on Stanley Greenspan and Nancy Thorndike Greenspan. *First Feelings: Milestones in The Emotional Development of Your Baby and Child From Birth to Age 4.* New York: Viking Penguin, 1985.

Emotional thinking: the basis for fantasy, reality, and self-esteem (30 months+). By about 30 months, children begin to move from acting out their emotions to using reasoning. For example, rather than simply hugging a doll, a child might explain that the doll is sad because she fell down and hurt her knee. During this stage, children need you to set limits and guide their behavior in positive ways that take their feelings into account.

Learning About Other People

A child's social development begins at birth. Infants and toddlers learn about how to relate to other people through daily interactions with their families and other important adults. They learn how to treat others by experiencing how they are treated. Developing a supportive, loving relationship with each infant and toddler in your care is the most important way for you to promote positive social development.

Typically, during the third month of life, a special moment occurs: an infant smiles directly and purposefully at an important adult. Over the next month or two, there are further signs of recognition: infants respond more strongly by kicking or cooing and by protesting when an important adult moves out of sight. This is the time when, according to Greenspan, infants first "fall in love" with another person. It is also the time when, as Mahler noted, they begin to recognize that they are separate people and that being with other people is an enjoyable experience.

Mobile infants enjoy watching other children and may imitate what they see others do. They can crawl or walk to you and climb on your lap for a hug or a story. By noticing infants' cues, playing peek-a-boo, and rolling a ball back and forth, you help infants learn the give and take of responding to others. They discover that relating to another person is interesting, fun, and rewarding.

Toddlers, too, are naturally curious and interested in other people. By providing simple props and encouraging pretend play, you invite children to explore the roles and activities of the important people in their lives and, as a result, to feel closer to them. Toddlers are also very observant of one another. In a group setting, they quickly learn whose mommy and daddy, bottle, and shoes belong to whom. Have you ever been amazed at the ways toddlers can attend to and care for each other? They may, for example, hold a cup to a child's mouth who cannot do this independently, or gently pat another child who is crying.

At the same time, the reverse of this caring attention is equally common. You may have observed how often biting, hitting, and pinching occur, and how difficult it is for toddlers to share. Toddlers tend to have strong feelings and often don't know how to express them. Sharing is a developmental task that develops over time and requires considerable practice. As you set behavioral limits and respond to toddlers with respect and understanding, you lay the groundwork for their future relationships with others.

Learning About Communicating

Language development is one of the major accomplishments that occurs during the first three years of life. In this brief time, a child moves from communicating needs nonverbally through facial expressions, gestures, body movements, and crying to communicating through words or sign language. During these years, children learn they are communicators. They acquire a vocabulary of hundreds of words and learn the rules for using them. They learn all this simply by being around adults who communicate with them and encourage their efforts to communicate.

The Development of Language in Infants

Infants are born with a unique ability to relate to other human beings. They come into the world ready to communicate and connect with their caregivers. A newborn turns her head to the sound of her mother's voice. When their eyes meet, the baby's face brightens and quiets. Infants cry to communicate needs. During the first few months, infants begin making other sounds. They gurgle, coo, and squeal, using sounds to establish contact with adults. By about six to nine months, infants begin to babble sounds in their home language. In addition to making sounds, infants also listen and respond. Observers have videotaped infants as young as 12 hours making tiny movements in sync with someone's voice.

As they get older, infants may respond by smiling, kicking, and turning their heads to look at someone talking. They may also cry, turn away, or withdraw, should their surroundings become too noisy. Children this age understand more than they can say. Before they are able to talk, they look at objects we name and make gestures such as waving good-bye during leave-taking, or blowing on their carrots when you caution they are hot.

At about one year, some infants say a few recognizable words, usually the names of people and things that are important to them. In English-speaking families, favorite words often include *mama, dada, bottle, cat*, or *ball*. Soon, children start to use a mix of words and babble, forming sentences spoken with great expression. The language an infant hears determines the "language connections" that are formed in her brain as well as the sounds she makes and can distinguish. This is why children exposed to two languages from infancy can become truly bilingual.

The Development of Language in Toddlers

By the time they are about eighteen months old, many toddlers have at least 20 words in their oral vocabulary and continue to understand much more than they can say. They can use language to express a need, for they have learned that words can help them "get" something. They may begin putting words together to express a thought such as "Daddy go" or "me do." By the age of two, many children's vocabularies have expanded to as many as 50 to 60 words. Between the ages of two and three, they may be able to say anywhere from 200 to 1,000 words or more and use simple sentences.

As in all aspects of development, young children develop language at their own rates. Some say their first words at eight months. Others hardly speak at all until they are almost two. Many factors influence how and when language develops. Some are individual differences present from birth. Others depend on a child's experiences with communication. One of your important tasks is to respect individual differences in language development.

Remember that learning to talk takes much practice. By sharing your pleasure in children's communication rather than correcting their mistakes, and talking with them even when they don't have words to respond, you help children build on their natural desire to communicate.

Learning to Move and Do

Physical development refers to gradually gaining control over gross (large) and fine (small) muscles. It includes acquiring gross motor skills that, over time, allow a child to roll over, sit, crawl, walk, run, and throw a ball. It also includes developing fine motor skills such as holding, pinching, and flexing fingers. As children develop these skills, they can use them to draw, write, eat with a spoon, and cut with scissors.

The exciting result of developing new motor skills is that it leads infants and toddlers to make other new discoveries. As they explore, they begin to make sense of their environment. For example, as Julio gains control of his head, he can use his eyes and ears to locate a sound. As Jasmine learns to use her fingers, hands, and wrists, she can touch, taste, and smell the slice of pear on her high chair tray. And as Jonisha turns the pages of her book one at a time, she is able to identify pictures of familiar objects and animals and recall a familiar story.

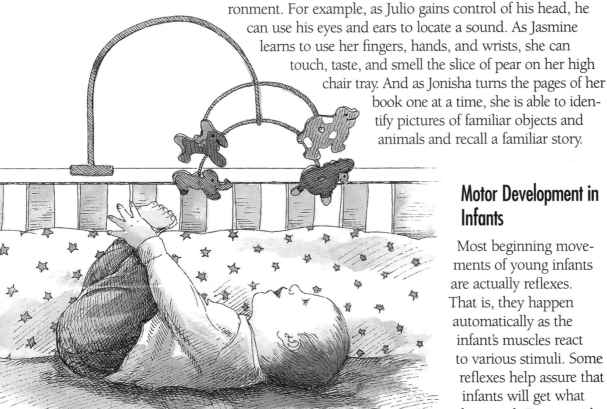

Motor Development in Infants

Most beginning movements of young infants are actually reflexes. That is, they happen automatically as the infant's muscles react to various stimuli. Some reflexes help assure that infants will get what they need. For example, when you touch the cheek of a newborn, she starts moving her mouth in search of a nipple. When you touch her mouth, or when her mouth touches the nipple of a breast or bottle, she begins sucking. Young infants have other reflexes, too.

For example, one—called **reciprocal kicking**—occurs when an infant kicks first one foot, then the other. This reflex suggests skills yet to be developed, such as walking.

Over time and bit by bit, infants gain control of their muscles. Although they develop at different rates, infants learn to control their bodies in the same general way—from head to toe and from the center of their bodies out through their arms and legs to their fingers and toes. You can see this as you watch a child learn to lift his head, then sit, crawl, and walk.

During their first 18 months, infants make a remarkable journey. They change from having little control over their muscles to developing distinctive motor skills such as sitting, walking, and eye-hand coordination. These skills form the foundation of moving and doing throughout their lives.

Motor Development of Toddlers

Toddlers have a wide range of gross and fine motor skills. They can walk and run well and are developing new skills such as throwing and catching a ball and hopping. They can use their fingers and hands to turn the pages of a book, make strokes with a crayon, roll, pound and squeeze playdough, paint, and begin to cut with scissors. They need many opportunities and a safe environment to practice, refine, and build on these skills. You can promote motor development by encouraging children to try new skills, or by helping them to slow down a little so they can gain more control.

Using the toilet—an achievement welcomed by caregivers and parents alike—requires that children be aware of and able to control their bladder and bowel muscles. Every child develops at his or her own pace, but typically children are physically mature enough to begin using the toilet between 24 and 30 months.

Learning to Think

The psychologist Jean Piaget spent more than 60 years observing, studying, and writing about how children think. According to his ideas, children actively construct their own understanding of the world by interacting with people and objects. They use all their senses and motor skills to explore actively. Children learn when they roll over, crawl around and over everything in their path, run, jump, knock things over, and lift them up. They learn as they grasp a rattle, pound playdough, and smell the grilled cheese sandwiches you make for lunch. They learn as they live their everyday lives with their parents and with you. As they eat, get dressed, have their diapers changed, sit on a potty, or move a chair across the room, they collect information about how things work. They also learn as they play. When Jasmine pulls herself up on the sofa and discovers a new way to play peek-a-boo with you, and when Willard crawls around pretending to be a tiger, they increase their understanding of the world and their place in it.

Piaget also found that children approach learning very differently than adults do. It is not just that they have less information, it's that they experience the world differently. He noticed that at different ages, children answer questions in certain special ways. Piaget found that toddlers would usually explain things in terms of their appearance. For example, they describe a cracker broken into many pieces as more food than the same cracker when it is whole. Piaget also noted that toddlers seem to believe that everyone sees things from the same viewpoint they do, and that they alone are the cause of events: "I fell down because I made a big noise."

Stages of Intellectual Development

According to Piaget, children pass through four stages of intellectual development. Infants and toddlers go through the first stage and into the beginning of the second.[5]

The first stage, which Piaget calls the **sensorimotor stage,** begins at birth. It lasts until a child is about one-and-a-half or two years old. At this stage, infants and toddlers learn as they move and use their senses of touch, taste, hearing, sight, and smell. For example, when Julio sucks on a toy, Jasmine squeezes, smells, and tastes the slice of banana, or Abby notices the sounds of birds and airplanes, they are using their senses to learn about their world. They are beginning to understand **object permanence**—that something or someone continues to exist even when out of sight. When a child who used to forget the spoon that she dropped from her highchair tray now drops the spoon and signals with a smile that she expects you to pick it up, you know she has learned about object permanence. Peek-a-boo, a favorite game of most young children, reinforces this concept.

During this stage, children learn how to use tools and begin to understand cause and effect. When Abby wants the pull toy on the other side of the table, she gets it by pulling the string. She has learned that certain actions (pulling the string) have certain results (the toy attached to the string will move). Jasmine, on the other hand, might whine to let Janet know she needs help, not realizing she could pull on the string to get the toy herself.

Piaget calls the second stage the **preoperational period.** The preoperational period begins at about age two and lasts until about age seven. During this stage, children learn to use language and mental images in their thinking. For example, toddlers can separate from their families more easily because they can create mental images of family members to hold onto throughout the day. They do lots

---

[5] Jean Piaget. *The Origins of Intelligence.* New York: International Universities Press, 1952.

of make-believe play, exploring daily events and activities, roles, and feelings. They begin to understand that time exists and to recognize that there is order to the day. Toddlers, for example, may begin looking for their parents after story time, knowing that is when they usually begin arriving.

Children in the preoperational stage tend to be egocentric. This means they believe everyone thinks like they do and that they have the power to control the world. A toddler, for example, may believe he can make the traffic on a busy street come to a standstill simply by yelling, "Stop!" And they believe things that move are alive which helps us understand why a flushing toilet or a vacuum cleaner can be so scary.

Little by little, as they explore and play, children collect new information to add to what they already know. The way they think begins to change as they realize that the moon does not follow them and that a broken cracker is actually the same amount as an unbroken one.

Recognizing a Child's Individuality

Knowledge of child development helps us to predict how children—in general—will behave at different stages of development. However, each child is an individual with particular characteristics. In addition to a general understanding of child development, you must take the time to learn about the special characteristics of each child.

Think of two infants you know well. What are they like? From the minute they are born, infants differ in terms of:

- their activity level;
- the regularity of when they eat, sleep or toilet;
- how they approach (or withdraw) from people and things;
- how often they display happy or sad moods and how frequently their moods shift;
- the intensity of their reactions;
- their sensitivity to stimuli such as bright lights, loud noises, and touch;
- whether or not they like to be cuddled;
- the amount of time it takes them to adapt to a new situation or routine;
- how easily they can be distracted from activities; and
- their persistence.

Yet because infants are so small and appealing, people often make assumptions about what they need, how they should be treated, and how they will respond. Do you?

Imagine an infant crying in his crib. How would you comfort him? Most adults would naturally pick him up and hold him closely. Yet, some infants don't enjoy being cuddled. They find it uncomfortable—even painful. They are better comforted by being placed on their stomach over your knees and gently rocked.

Try to understand what each child needs. For example, an infant who tenses in your arms isn't rejecting you. She may be asking you to try a different way of comforting her.

She may respond better if you start by massaging and rubbing her back. Ask family members how they comfort the child. A toddler who tests limits isn't out to test your patience. He may be simply trying to figure out who he is. Looking through a child's eyes can help you get to know a child and appreciate his or her special characteristics.

Understanding Different Temperaments

Children are born with unique temperaments—inborn characteristics that tend to shape emotional responses.[6] When you are aware of a child's temperament, you can sometimes predict how that child may react and behave in certain types of situations. You may also be able to do a better job of understanding and interpreting particular behavior. When your predictions are correct, you can respond appropriately. Yet, it's always important to remember that children don't fall into neat categories. While you may see general patterns in their behavior and your responses, you'll need to keep on your toes and be ready to respond to them in different ways at different times.

Abby may be described as a *flexible* child. She eats and naps regularly, is typically cheerful, and adapts easily to changes. When she is upset, she usually cries quietly and looks at her parents or Brooks for support. Abby is generally an easy child to live with, but she does have her challenging moments; last week she had a tantrum in the super-market. Although she tends to be less demanding than other children, she needs the adults in her life to observe her regularly, read her signals, and offer support, encouragement, or comfort when necessary.

Gena can be described as generally *cautious* or *fearful*. She often needs time to warm up to new situations or new people—though she took a liking to Ivan within a few days of starting at the Crane School. Gena tends to watch things from the sidelines. Ivan has learned that his presence and encouragement can sometimes help draw Gena into activities. He has learned to respect Gena's style and give her the time she needs to open up to new experiences.

Willard could be described as *feisty, active,* or *intense*—take your pick. When he is happy or needs something, he lets his parents and Grace know. When he wants a toy another child is playing with, he may yell or cry loudly, even hit or push. Grace—who used to think Willard was a real handful, and even looked forward to the occasional days he wasn't at the Kendrick Center—has been surprised lately at how much she enjoys his spirited style. She has also discovered that Willard loves looking at pictures of children and their families in the program's photo album. Grace and Willard spend some quiet time doing this together each day.

Understanding children means appreciating their unique ways of interacting with the world and with people. It means taking time to learn about children's strengths, interests, challenges they like, challenges that frustrate them, and ways they are comforted. With this knowledge, you can respond in ways that address each child's needs.

---

[6] Infant researchers Alexander Thomas and Stella Chess have identified three basic types of temperaments. *The Program for Infant/Toddler Caregivers,* developed by West Ed/Far West Laboratory for Educational Research and Development, in collaboration with the California Department of Education, has named these *flexible, fearful,* and *feisty.*

Children with Special Needs

All infants and toddlers have needs to be met. Some needs are probably more familiar to you than others. You may have several suggestions for helping a child who has difficulty saying good-bye to his parents in the morning, or for another who has temper tantrums. At the same time, you may feel hesitant about working with a child who has cerebral palsy or who is visually impaired. You may wonder, "How can I ever meet the needs of these children?" It can be challenging to help young children with disabilities see themselves as competent, valuable, independent individuals.

Experts believe that all children can benefit when children with disabilities are included in early childhood programs. *The Creative Curriculum for Infants & Toddlers* can help you in your work with all children, including those with disabilities. It provides a framework for assessing where each child is developmentally. It also gives you ideas of how children with very different interests and abilities can be included and feel successful in open-ended activities and daily routines. Experts believe that children with disabilities should have the same experiences as all children. You are in a position to bring this idea to life for the children and families in your program.

The Creative Curriculum's emphasis on building relationships is extremely important for young children with disabilities—who may be isolated—and for their families—who may fear bringing their child out into the real world. Some of the children may receive special services, such as occupational, physical, or speech/language therapy. It is helpful and important to invite specialists in these fields to your program to share ideas about common goals and strategies.

In 1975, federal legislation mandated a free, appropriate public education for all children with disabilities and special needs. Since 1986, states have offered services to three- to five-year-old children.[7] Beginning in 1990, states have been able to use federal funds to offer **early intervention services** for infants and toddlers with disabilities and their families. These services are designed to minimize the effects of developmental delays or diagnosed disabilities. The important provision in the law which applies to children from birth to age three is called Part C (formerly known as Part H).

Understanding Part C

Children are identified and become part of the program in many ways. Each state is required to have a "child find system" which identifies children in need of services and makes referrals to service providers. A child may be identified at birth as having a disability, during a check-up at the pediatrician's office, by a specialist such as a physical therapist, or by someone providing care and education, such as yourself.

Under Part C, state or community teams—which may include speech and physical therapists, physicians, social workers, public health nurses, and educators—work with

---

[7] *Education for All Handicapped Children Act,* P.L. 94-142, 1975. *Early Intervention Amendments,* P.L. 99-457, 1986. Part H is part of this legislation. *The Individuals with Disabilities Education Act,* P.L. 101-476, 1990. P.L. 102-119, Reauthorized Part H, 1991. The 1997 reauthorization reclassified it as Part C. P.L. 105-17.

family members to create an individualized family service plan (IFSP). IFSPs contain the following information:

❖ current developmental information, including a detailed picture of a child's abilities and emerging skills;

❖ desired developmental outcomes for the child and family on which team members agree; and

❖ specific developmental objectives that allow team members to see what progress is being made.

Your involvement with your local early intervention program may come about in a variety of ways. You may be the person who suspected a developmental delay and got the whole process started by suggesting to the family that they call the state's Part C Coordinator, who helped them make a local contact. You may know about a family's IFSP because you were contacted as the family's primary entry point into the system and have been involved from the beginning. Alternately, you may have been overlooked. If this is the case, talk with the child's family about requesting a review of their IFSP and adding your name to the team. In any case, you are an important member of the early intervention team, as you have the opportunity to work with the child each day to achieve developmental goals.

The new legislation requires each state to have one agency with central responsibility and a central directory of services. To help you learn more about Part C and how it can support the children and families in your program, there is a directory of Part C Coordinators and Lead Agencies in each state in Appendix E. You can also research the topic directly on the Internet through the ERIC (Educational Resources Information Center) Clearinghouse on Disabilities and Gifted Education (http://www.cec.sped.org/ericec.htm) or by contacting the ERIC web site (http://www.ericeece.org). Your local school district office is another good resource.

The Americans with Disabilities Act

Another law that applies is the Americans with Disabilities Act, which requires child care providers to make "reasonable accommodations" to care for children with disabilities. This includes children who have chronic medical conditions, such as asthma, seizures, and sickle cell disease. It's important to work with the family and health care provider to develop a detailed Individualized Health Plan for the child. This plan details all the accommodations needed for feeding and activities, routine medications and health procedures, measures to prevent medical crisis, and how to recognize and respond to medical emergencies. You will also need to have on-hand the medication and supplies needed, participate in training in the necessary health procedures, and have an emergency back-up plan.

Strategies for Addressing Special Needs

The suggestions that follow apply to all infants and toddlers. You'll find them particularly useful in your work with children who have diagnosed disabilities or other special needs.

See children as children first. Learn about each child's strengths and interests first, then consider the child's special needs. Indeed, this attitude can be, in the words of Gena's father, Neal, "the greatest gift anyone could have given us." He explains, "Sometimes as a parent of a child with a disability, you struggle so hard to overcome problems that you forget to enjoy your child. The first day we took Gena to the Crane School, we didn't know what to expect. When Ivan asked Gena about her stuffed lamb, Franklin—before talking with us about her impaired speech and dexterity—we knew we were in the right place."

The goal for all children is to feel included and successful. For this to happen, you must look beyond the specific diagnosis to see what effects it has on a particular child. You must be careful not to generalize about children on the basis of their diagnoses.

Learn about the effects of a specific disability. Consider how a specific disability may or may not affect the child's daily life in your program. Use this information to help you decide what, if any, adjustments you need to make. For example, you may need another adult to help you during certain parts of the day. Or you may need to move furniture so a child's wheelchair can fit into every part of the room.

Work closely with children's families. Parents of a child with a disability are your greatest sources of support and information. Ask them to share what they know about their child's condition. Invite them also to share tips and strategies they use at home. For example, Gena's parents, Neal and Rebecca, helped Ivan learn to position Gena in ways that give her the best possible control over her body. Also, ask parents about their involvement with the local early intervention program. If they are unaware of local services, give them the necessary information.

Set goals and work with a specialist. Use the goals and objectives from a child's IFSP to guide your work with that child. Many objectives will be the same as those you've set for all children and will fit easily into your regular planning and daily schedule. Others may mean adding special toys, adapting equipment, or changing routines (such as blinking lights to catch the attention of a deaf child). These strategies should be included in the child's plan. As with all children, you should observe continually and assess the goals you have set, adapting them as necessary. With parental permission, work with the child's therapist(s) to come up with strategies that will work in your program.

Encourage, but do not force independence. Some children may need extra support to develop skills as well as self-confidence. Feeling competent is important for all children. Recognize, however, that children may have needs beyond your experience and expertise. If this is the case, seek the help of specialists in your community. Your openness to learn about various disabilities and reach out to experts will set a good model for the children—and adults—in your program.

Getting to know infants and toddlers can sometimes be challenging—and is always interesting and exciting. In the next chapter, we focus on families—your partners in getting to know children.

Knowing Families

The families you work with each day are at a very exciting but vulnerable stage in their lives. Parenting an infant or toddler can be wonderful. It is a chance to watch a brand new human being unfold. So much change takes place in the first three years that parents constantly marvel as their child explores and joyfully discovers new things about himself and his world. But parenting can also be demanding and overwhelming. As one parent put it, "I love my baby. But taking care of him is harder than I ever imagined. I feel so lost."

When you made the decision to work with infants and toddlers, you may not have considered how much you would also be working with children's families. It probably wasn't long before you realized, however, that to help children develop, you must also create a partnership with their families. Therefore, the more you know about families, the more responsive and supportive you can be of their needs. In turn, families who feel you understand and respect the central role they play in their child's life will be your greatest supporters.

This chapter can help you to get to know families by recognizing:

❖ the stages of parenthood that apply to families with children younger than three;
❖ the special concerns of families with children under three;
❖ the influence of culture in children's lives and the need to appreciate cultural differences; and
❖ the importance of involving the men in children's lives in your program.

Stages of Parenthood

The birth of a new baby means not only the birth of a new person, but also the birth of parents in a newly arranged family. According to pediatrician T. Berry Brazelton, "Falling in love with a baby may well happen at birth, but staying in love is a learning process—learning to love oneself as well as the baby."[1]

---

[1] T. Berry Brazelton. *On Becoming A Family: The Growth of Attachment.* New York: Delacorte Press, 1981, p. xiv.

Just as children follow certain stages in their development, so do parents. According to Ellen Galinsky, parents pass through six stages, each based on children's development. In each stage, parents reorganize the ways they think about themselves and their world and the way they respond to the child's changing behavior.[2]

Parents of infants and toddlers pass through three of these stages of parenthood: image-making (the way they think their new life with a child will be), nurturing (the way they care for and protect their children), and authority (the way they place limits on their children's behavior).

Recognizing these stages can help you understand what parents may experience as they learn about themselves and their children. This can help you decide how best to respond. As you read about each of these stages, keep in mind that your task is not to move parents from one stage to another. This will happen naturally as their children grow. Rather, it is to be aware of their interests and needs at certain stages so that you can support them as necessary. Your support can help them feel competent as they face new challenges.

If you are a parent yourself, you may find it helpful to reflect on your own feelings and experiences to better understand the parents with whom you work. If you are not a parent, observe and try to look through the eyes of parents. Ask yourself, "What are they experiencing?" Regardless of your background, remember that parents are often glad to share their feelings and stories with someone they trust—someone they can count on to listen carefully and respectfully.

The Image-Making Stage

This first stage of parenthood begins before a child is born. Parents-to-be start preparing and rehearsing for the great change that is about to take place in their lives—even if it is with a second or third child. Part of how they do this is to imagine their new life.

At this stage, expectant parents spend much time dreaming about what their child will be like. They also think about what kind of parents they will be and how being a parent will change their relationships with each other and their own parents. This is a time of roller coaster feelings. Parents may often feel "ready" and then "not ready" to deal with these changes in their lives.

Expectant parents (regardless of whether they have other children) will often appreciate your listening to their hopes, dreams, and fears—if and when they want to share them with you. They may also welcome your introducing them to other parents in your program who are awaiting the birth or adoption of a child.

The Nurturing Stage

The next stage begins with the birth of the infant. During this stage, parents bring together the picture of the child they imagined with the real child they hold in their arms. Many new parents report feeling a deep love and caring for their infant, while others experience this bonding as a more gradual process. They also report the challenge that occurs when

---

[2] Ellen Galinsky. *The Six Stages of Parenthood.* Reading, MA: Addison-Wesley Publishing Company, 1987.

the imagined picture of joyful parents and a smiling infant does not always match the reality. In fact, accepting these differences causes growth in parenthood. As Leo's mother said, "I thought my baby would be a smiler. Instead, he cried a lot. So did I during those first months!" Particularly when an infant is born with a disability, parents may feel as if their entire world has come apart.

In addition to getting to know a new infant, parents are redefining their relationship to each other, to their other children (if they have them), and to their own parents. At the same time, their immediate task is to become attached to their new infant, just as the infant's task is to become attached to them. Attachment creates possessive feelings in everyone who cares for a child—parents, grandparents, and child care providers alike. As a result, one of your jobs is to recognize these possessive and competitive feelings. You can turn them into cooperative feelings by supporting the parents in their primary roles.

It's easy to understand why parents with a new infant often feel overwhelmed. Everything they thought they knew and felt gets called into question: Am I feeding too much or too little? Is the baby sleeping enough? For employed mothers—should I really be working? It's a big relief when they can depend on you to keep their child (the new infant or an older brother or sister) safe in a quality program. You can help parents by listening to them and reminding them they are handling a great deal. A supportive word can sometimes make a world of difference to an unsure parent.

The Authority Stage

The third stage sets in slowly and gradually as children become more mobile and begin exploring the larger world around them. Parents who put aside many of their own needs during the Nurturing Stage now realize that there are times when they must say "No" to their children. What parents should control and what can be left up to the child become important decisions that must be resolved almost every day.

During this stage, both parents and children face the challenge of limits. As children explore, test, and accept limits, parents also explore and struggle with establishing and enforcing these limits. While it may appear that parents are often ambivalent or wishy-washy, this is the normal fumbling state that parents go through as they learn to be authorities.

Because setting limits is difficult and complicated, parents may look to you for direction. There are two things you can do. First, you can model or demonstrate how you set clear, realistic limits with their child and the other children in your program. Second, you can share your knowledge about infant and child development with parents. For example, understanding that Matthew is declaring his independence when he protests, "No!" as his parents try to put on his boots at the end of the day can help lessen the stress that often occurs when adults feel tested and not in control.

Parents also often look to other parents as they move from trying to be perfect to being "good enough." When you help parents of toddlers connect with one another, you open the way for them to encourage and learn from one another. They can also share the delights of watching their children develop.

Special Concerns of Families with Children Younger Than Three

Although each family has its own culture, values, strengths, and needs, most families of young children share some characteristics. These include:

- ❖ the stress of parenting an infant, including lack of sleep;
- ❖ conflicting feelings about how to share the care of the baby;
- ❖ confusion over who is who in their child's life; and
- ❖ the need to feel that they are part of their child's day, even when they are not physically with their child.

The Stress of Parenting an Infant

Being the parent of an infant takes a great deal of energy. It can be very demanding and stressful at times. Not only are new parents often confused by a child's behavior and unsure of what to do, but they are also very, very tired. Lack of sleep makes it easy for new parents to lose perspective and to despair that they will never learn as much as they need to know. When a parent is very young, single, or worried about having enough money to buy food or medical services, the stress is even greater.

What's more, many parents find child care centers or homes to be scary, no matter how welcoming your setting is or how warm and friendly you are. Are you surprised? Many caregivers who feel nervous around parents are often amazed to learn that parents see them as "all-knowing professionals." Kevin tells about being afraid to pick up Willard that first day: "I'd never been in a child care setting before. I didn't know who was in charge or what was allowed."

Why is this information important to you? It's because some families will feel comfortable asking you for the support they need. Others will not. They may be too overwhelmed with the changes in their lives. They may not yet trust you or they may view asking for help as a sign of failure. But you are in a good position to be helpful because you see parents every day. It's up to you to listen carefully and figure out how best to offer help. Sometimes that help can be a cup of juice or the way you assure a hassled parent that, based on your experience, a child's behavior is absolutely typical and nothing to worry about.

Conflicting Feelings About Sharing Care

Sharing the care of young children by placing them in a child care program often may stir up conflicting feelings. Some parents may feel sorrow, guilt, or some fear about leaving their child with you, no matter how professional you are and how highly rated your program.

Once a child is enrolled in the program, parents want you to be competent and want their child to like you. They may worry, however, that their child will like you better than he or she likes them. These feelings can be stressful for parents. Sometimes the stress is reflected in their children.

You also might have feelings about sharing care. As you become attached to a child, you may feel a bit competitive with a parent. You may resent having to work with parents when you really want to work with children. You may also have feelings about parents who choose to work instead of staying home to care for a very young infant.

How can you deal with these conflicting feelings? First, be aware that parents' feelings —and yours—go hand-in-hand with sharing care. Help parents see that their mixed feelings are normal and should not be cause for embarrassment. Raising and caring for infants and toddlers is passionate work. As for you, it is natural to feel deeply protective and attached to young children. You'll need to recognize these feelings for what they are, so they won't get in the way of working together with parents in the best interests of the child.

Confusion Over Who Is Who

Parents and caregivers each play an important but different role in a child's life. Infants and toddlers know who is who. Yet the adults in their lives sometimes don't feel so sure.

The difference, though, should be very clear. Parents are the most important people in their child's life. Their relationship is forever. It is built upon a deep trust and a love unlike any other. No matter how skilled and experienced you are, you can never take a parent's place.

However, the emotional bond you build with each child is also important, even though your relationship is temporary. As you develop these relationships, you show children that they can trust people outside their families. Because you are more objective than parents, you can more easily give children the time and space they need to get through a bumpy stage of development or to master a new skill.

With these differences in mind, you can understand how helpful it is to reassure parents who have young children in child care that they are the most important people in their child's life. You may also want to remind parents that you are aware of who is who, too.

Wanting to Feel a Part of Their Child's Day

Parents depend on you to fill them in on what has happened in their children's lives during the hours when they are apart. You may do this in many ways. For example, when parents come to pick up their children in the evening, you may share stories of the day. You may take photos of the children, write notes to send home, or hang a calendar of the day's highlights on the wall. In general, families will be very glad to hear the news you share.

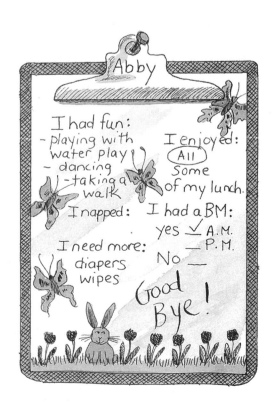

There is one major exception, however. No one wants to miss one of their child's "firsts." For example, if you see the first time a child sits up or takes first steps, you may not want to share this information fully. Instead, consider saying something like this: "Willard's been pulling himself up a lot today! I'll be curious to know what his evening is like. I'm going to remember to ask you tomorrow morning."

Understanding the Influence of Culture

All people learn about their own culture simply by living it. Families have beliefs and practices associated with every aspect of life that they pass on to their children. Like the children with whom you are now working, your belief system was influenced by your family, specifically by your parents or whoever was directly responsible for raising you. As a caregiver, it is important that you have a clear understanding about your culture and how its influences affect your work.

For example, most people and many cultures have strong beliefs about names and how names should be treated. Being aware of these beliefs allows you to honor them as much as possible. Avoid changing or shortening a child's name because you feel it is hard to pronounce or is difficult to spell. If necessary, ask someone for a correct pronunciation and to help you practice saying it.

Learning from Families

It is easy to misinterpret what families do or say if you do not understand something about their culture. However, you also must avoid assigning cultural labels to families. Rather than making assumptions about cultural influences, it is better to ask questions and consider the values behind each family's beliefs.

Children's families can teach you a great deal about their cultural beliefs and traditions. Invite parents to spend time in your program whenever possible. Observe how they interact with their children. Arrange for a home visit. As your relationship grows, talk about culture. Ask questions. Think together about how your culture(s) shape each of you and how you respond to children.

Use these questions and any others you want to add to guide your efforts to understand families whose cultures are different from yours.

- How does the family define who is in their family? What gives them a sense of family?
- How do families select a child's name?
- How does the family balance children's independence with doing things for them?
- When should toilet training begin and how should it be handled?
- What, when, and how are children fed?
- How is discipline handled?
- Do family members have different and distinct roles in raising children?
- Are boys and girls treated differently?
- Is it acceptable for children to be noisy and to get dirty?
- What kinds of questions are children asked?
- How do people interact with one another? Do they look each other in the eye? Are they taught to pause and think carefully about a response before giving it? Do they touch each other as they communicate?
- How do families show respect for elders?

Incorporating Children's Cultures Into Your Program

By including experiences that are consistent with those the children have at home, you provide children with cultural continuity. This is especially important for infants and toddlers, because they are developing a sense of identity. Here are several ways you can achieve cultural continuity, even if your cultural background is different from that of the families in your program.

Use children's home language(s) as much as possible. In the best of all worlds, there would be an adult from the same culture(s) who spoke the same language(s) as the children in your program to build a bridge for children between home and child care. Because this is often not the case, you'll need to think creatively about how to bring children's language(s) into your setting. For example, encourage family members to speak in their home language when they visit and to teach you some important words. Ask families to make tapes of stories and music their children know from home. Get help, as necessary, to translate written communications. Identify someone a family trusts who would be willing to serve as a language resource, especially for conferences, home visits, and in emergency situations.

Reflect children's cultures in daily routines. Knowing how daily routines are handled at home can help you make children feel at home in child care. For example, a child who is expected to eat neatly at home may need extra reassurance when she spills her juice at lunch.

Reflect children's families in the environment. Display photographs of children's families which they have chosen to share. Incorporate foods, activities, toys, and songs that children know from home into their daily lives in child care.

Working Towards Understanding

When the adults in their lives share a consistent approach, children gain a sense of continuity that helps them feel safe and secure in child care. This doesn't mean you have to agree about everything. More likely, there will be times when you and a child's parents will have different points of view about caring for their child. The question is, "How can you achieve mutual understanding?"

> Gena's parents often sent her to child care in her best clothes. They became upset when the clothes were soiled with dirt and paint at the end of the day. Ivan felt it was very important for Gena to have many hands-on experiences. He explained this to the Domenicas and found they agreed. Together they worked out a solution. Ivan would keep a set of "play clothes" that Gena could change into on the days her parents dressed her in good clothes. That way she could participate in all activities without fear of getting dirty. At the same time, she could protect her good clothes.

When there are differences, a good policy is to problem-solve together and work at a compromise, as long as you feel the compromise will not harm the child. (See Chapter 1 for a discussion on resolving conflicts.)

Involving the Men in Children's Lives[3]

A quality program needs to involve everyone who is important in a child's life. Too often, however, men in children's lives are overlooked. Why is this? Primarily it's because our culture defines caring for children—in our homes and in child care programs—as "women's work." Perhaps it is also because most people who work with infants and toddlers are women who may feel more comfortable with other women. And some may not want to share child care with men, preferring to hold onto raising children as their special area of expertise. In addition, some people may think men are not good caregivers, especially for infants and toddlers.

Men themselves may be uncomfortable walking into a setting that is largely female. A society that values toughness for males rather than gentleness and caring doesn't encourage comfort in a child care setting. If a man has grown up without a caring father or other man in his own life, he may find it even more difficult to become involved with his own young children.

At the same time, more and more men are seeing how much their fathers missed and are taking a more active parenting role. Our culture increasingly supports men as nurturing influences in children's lives. Courts, too, are more willing to grant fathers custody of children. The number of single fathers is increasing. If men aren't involved in your program, you need to think about reversing the situation. Here are some suggestions to help you get started.

Examine your attitudes about men (even if you are a man). You may especially want to think about these questions.

> ❖ What kinds of experiences have you had with the men in your life—your father, brother, husband, or partner?
> ❖ Do you think men really care about children as much as women do? Why?
> ❖ Do you think men can contribute to your program? How?

Expect that men will participate. Ask for the name and address of a child's father if he doesn't live with the child. If possible, try to arrange for home visits when fathers will be there. It's helpful to assume that men are interested, that they care and want to do their best for their children.

Create a welcoming environment. First of all, let fathers (and other men who come to the program) know that you recognize that being in a child care setting can be a somewhat uncomfortable experience. Offer suggestions of things that men can do, as Barbara does

---

[3] Based on James A. Levine, Dennis T. Murphy, and Sherill Wilson. *Getting Men Involved: Strategies for Early Childhood Programs.* New York: Scholastic, 1993.

when she says to Elmer, "Do you want to go over and read with Leo? I'm sure he would love it." Other ways to make men feel at home at the program may include:

- ❖ sharing an observation that shows how well the child is doing;
- ❖ adding selections such as *The Father's Almanac* to your parent library; and
- ❖ including men in the photographs you display.

Provide meaningful ways for men to be involved. Men can do many different things in your program. They can nurture and play with children. They can help with routines, such as serving meals and snacks. They can help with maintenance and repair work. But even more important, having men involved in your program helps everyone. Children benefit by seeing male role models. Fathers and other men in children's lives benefit by developing stronger relationships with children. You and your program benefit as men bring new kinds of knowledge and interests that enrich children's lives.

As you think about the families in your program and get to know them better, you will learn about their many strengths and want to give them all the support they need. As much as you want to help, you are only one person and you represent only one program. However, you all—families, children, and programs—exist within a community that not only benefits from the services you offer, but can provide needed services. This is the topic of the next chapter.

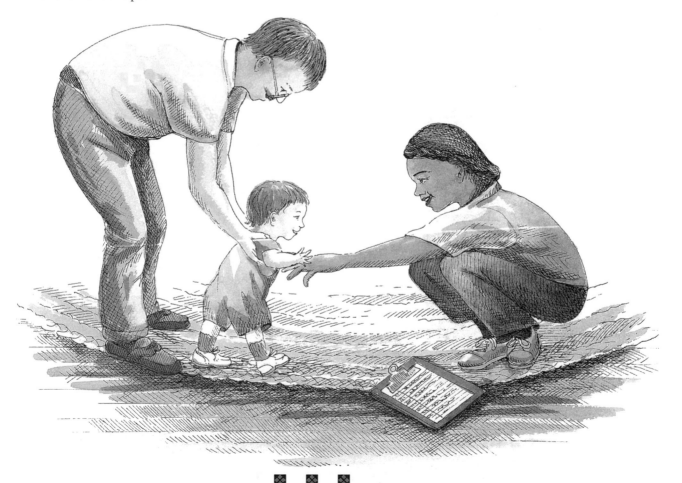

Community: Building a Network of Support

Your program is a part of your larger community. On the one hand, you give your community or neighborhood a valuable service that helps make it a better place for all families and children. On the other hand, your community gives you and the families you serve resources, including libraries, well-baby clinics, parks, and the support of neighbors and colleagues that can enrich your program. As a result, the relationship between your program and your community is a two-way street.

This chapter focuses on the community's role in your program. We discuss how you can work within the community to build a network of support for children and families by:

- ❖ recognizing why your program needs support;
- ❖ being aware of what other communities are doing;
- ❖ appreciating what you have to contribute to the community; and
- ❖ becoming involved in efforts to make your community a better place for children and families.

The Need for Support

Clearly, families today are under tremendous stress for a wide variety of reasons. These reasons include poverty; the break-up of the basic family unit; lack of affordable, quality health care; and widespread violence. Indeed, we need to redefine the term *family* in light of the current realities. Today, half of America's children live with only one parent at some point in their lives. In the past, more parents were part of an extended family in which elders helped out and provided advice. Today, families are often isolated. One significant result of these and other complications is that infants and toddlers—and their families—are at risk. In *The State of America's Children Yearbook 1999,* the Children's Defense Fund alerts us to the problems that face American children and families every day.[1]

---

[1] *The State of America's Children Yearbook 1999.* Washington, DC: Children's Defense Fund, 1999, p. xii.

Risks Facing American Children and Families

Every 25 seconds	a baby is born to an unmarried mother.
Every 40 seconds	a baby is born into poverty.
Every 1 minute	a baby is born to a teen mother.
Every 2 minutes	a baby is born at low birthweight.
Every 3 minutes	a baby is born to a mother who had late or no prenatal care.
Every 18 minutes	a baby dies.
Every 2 hours	a child is a homicide victim.
Every 4 hours	a child commits suicide.

In view of these sobering statistics, families may need many different kinds of support —including dental and medical services, family counseling, public housing, special education services, assistance in paying for food and eye glasses—and not know where to turn for help. You may be the first support person who really gets to know a family— their strengths as well as their needs. As a result, many families may look to you not only to provide quality child care, but also to guide them to other resources in the community.

Why You Need Support

As families' needs become more complex, so do the demands on you. Everyone working with infants and toddlers can benefit from the ongoing support of others who do the same kind of work. Whether you work with colleagues every day or see each other regularly at association meetings or training sessions, you'll find that ongoing professional connections can help you in many ways. You can share experiences and challenges and brainstorm solutions. When you feel supported, you can be more open to exploring new ideas. You will probably enjoy your work more, and as a result, you will be more likely to do a better job.

It is very likely you will also need to call on other people to help families address issues outside your area of expertise, such as physical or mental health concerns, or the need for job training. The better you know your community, the more likely it is you will know who offers which services and how to help families connect with the resources they need. How to provide this help depends largely on your community. In some communities, services for families are well coordinated. In other communities, service providers and services are fragmented.

If the latter is the case in your community, be persistent. Talk with everyone you know. Call your mayor's office. Contact organizations such as your city's health department and your local child care resource and referral agency. Only by persisting will you be able to find the services needed by the children and families in your care.

What Communities Are Doing

People all across the country are working together to make their communities more family-friendly. Generally, since funding for social services is often the first budget item to be cut, communities must find new and creative ways to make the most out of available resources. As communities recognize the need for coordinated, accessible services that build on families' strengths and focus on prevention, groups of people are coming together to try to meet this need.

Professionals in a wide variety of fields—education, health and mental health, social services, and business—are joining with parents to identify services that already exist and those that families still want and need. Knowing what others are doing can allow your community to build on their successes and lessons learned. Here are some examples of what communities are doing.[2]

❖ In Hampton, Virginia, a group of community partners launched the Healthy Families Partnership (formerly known as the Hampton Family Resource Project). Its goal is to ensure that every child in Hampton is born healthy and enters school ready to learn. The Partnership offers the following services: home visiting, parent education, young family centers in libraries, *The Healthy Stages* newsletter available to all families with children under 18, and Healthy Teen, a pregnancy prevention program.

❖ The KCMC Child Development Corporation in Kansas City is combining its Head Start funds with resources of other non-profit agencies and businesses. The Corporation aims to provide all children with comprehensive services that meet the Head Start Program Performance Standards.

❖ In Dover, New Hampshire, a community survey identified the needs of parents with young children. Results revealed that new mothers wanted a place that offered child care and other services, to which they could go at least weekly. The community responded by opening a center staffed by early childhood professionals. The Center is now open daily and provides information that parents say they need.

❖ In North Carolina, Family Ties is a state-wide community-based outreach initiative designed to identify low-income families with children under six who need child care or child development services. Its aim is to share information with families about existing community resources and programs, to obtain information about families' needs, and to build local leadership.

❖ In Indiana, Step Ahead Councils in 92 counties have completed needs assessments and are working to create plans of action for addressing families' needs.

---

[2] Based on Amy Laura Dombro, Nina Sazer O'Donnell, Ellen Galinsky, Sarah Gilkeson Melcher, and Abby Farber. *Community Mobilization: Strategies to Support Young Children and Their Families.* New York: Families and Work Institute, 1996.

❖ The Parent Voices Project, conceived by the California Child Care Resource and Referral Network, is currently working with local child care resource and referral agencies to examine how to identify and support parent advocates for child care.

❖ In West Virginia, Family Resource Networks (FRNs) in local communities are bringing together major parties that have an interest in children and families, including families themselves. These groups assess and determine the priority of community needs and create strategies to address those needs. For example, the Cabell-Wayne FRN found that families wanted more accessible services and a more helpful, respectful attitude from service providers. In response, the FRN is working to create services that are family-friendly, community based, and that focus on preventing problems—such as violence in the schools—before they occur.

❖ In Hawaii, Healthy Start, a home-based intervention program targeted to pregnant women and mothers with children up to the age of three months, attempts to provide support to families that may be at risk for child abuse. The participants are identified by screening hospital birth records, interviewing new mothers, and following up on referrals from physicians and public health agencies. The program has been so successful that today there are more than 100 Healthy Families America programs in 20 states, all based on Hawaii's Healthy Start model.

What You Have to Offer

You offer your community a valuable service. You have an in-depth view of the strengths and needs of its children and families, based on your knowledge of child development and your daily experiences running a program. Your insights, combined with your commitment to support families, can contribute to the well-being of your community, as well as to its individual members. You can also contribute by sharing your interests and skills from the "personal" side of your life, be they writing, illustrating, home repair, or speaking another language.

In addition, you can help parents become lifetime advocates for their children, working with other support people in their lives as well as on a community-wide level. When you work with families, you help them feel competent and fully involved in their children's child care experience. A positive experience with you can lead family members to feel more empowered in their relationship with, for example, their child's health care provider, and eventually, with their child's school. Such experiences often lead to participation in other community efforts to improve children's lives.

Getting Involved

Your community may be at the forefront in addressing the needs of children and families. Alternatively, it may not put a high priority on these issues and activities. If this alternative is the case, you will need to lobby for changes. Either way, getting involved is a positive step. Here are some suggestions to help you build relationships with community partners and to become involved in efforts that will benefit children and families in your program.

Identify community partners. A community partner can be just about anyone: the family child caregiver down the street; your physician or pediatrician; your local Part C coordinator, a teacher, principal, or guidance counselor at your local school; the priest, minister, or rabbi where you worship; a business owner; a librarian; or your neighbor who volunteers at the food bank. Some of these people may have information or offer services that families in your program can use. Each of them can probably introduce you to other people and programs.

Reach out. Each week, talk with one new person who shares your commitment to improving the lives of children and families.

Introduce yourself and your program. Let people know what you do and the types of things you know about. Describe your program. Share your goals for children and families. Invite new partners to come and visit.

Learn about what your new partners do. Find out about any special terms they may use in talking about their work. Ask questions. Read the literature from partners' organizations. Try to visit when possible. Learn to speak their "language."

Figure out ways to begin working together. For example, if you care for a child with a disability, invite specialists working with that child to participate in your program. Attend therapy (occupational, physical, speech/language) with a child and family to see what kinds of goals and strategies are addressed and to offer your perspective.

Stay in touch. Keep up to date on the services your community offers. Put your name on their mailing lists. Mark a time on your calendar to call community partners each month.

Find out about ongoing efforts—big and small—in your community. You may hear about a project or meeting from a neighbor, co-worker or community partner, or on the radio or TV. You may see a notice in the newspaper or find one posted on the bulletin board of a community center, school, or place of worship. You may even call the local paper, your local resource and referral agency, or the mayor's office.

Learn more. Attend a meeting. Join a community work group. Talk with people who are already involved. Try to get a picture of what is happening.

Think realistically about *when* to get involved and *how*. You may decide that for the time being, your focus needs to be on your program. However, if you want to become involved in a community effort and aren't sure how to go about it, explore various options for your involvement until you find one that fits.

Be patient. Remember, and remind others if necessary, that creating change takes time. Acknowledge accomplishments and celebrate small successes. This will help you keep going when the going is slow.

Because all these suggestions sound very time consuming, you may think you can't possibly handle more than your day-to-day work. Why not try just one suggestion as a start? Who knows? You may end up being president of your local professional organization, or a member of your city council!

Part
II The Big Picture

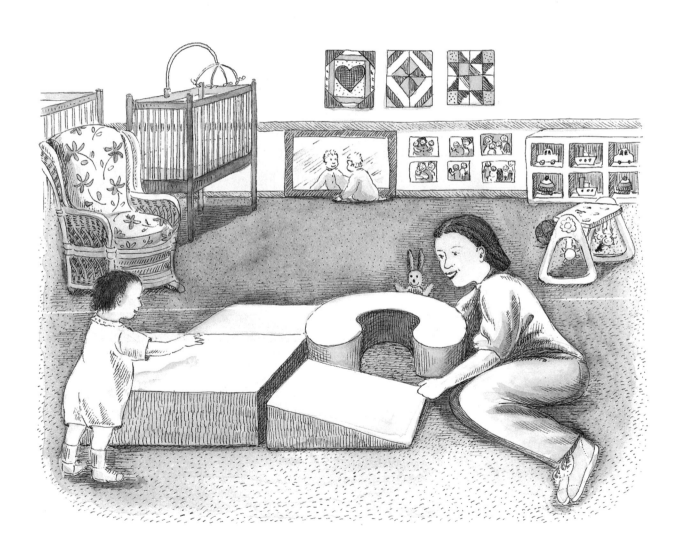

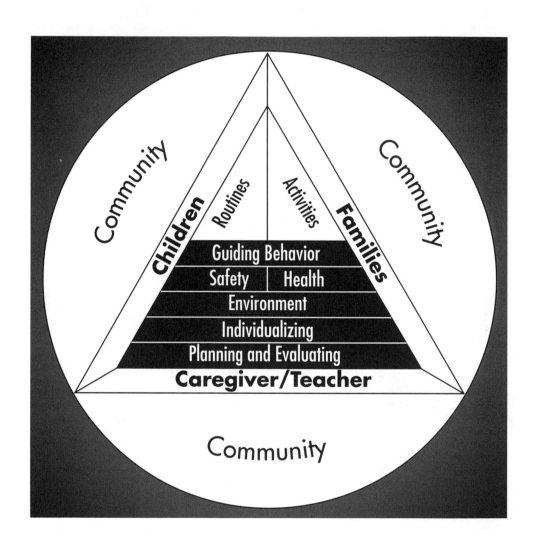

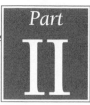
Putting Quality
Into Action:
The Big Picture

O ften when people think about curriculum, they focus on the routines and activities that consume a child's day. But before any routine or activity takes place, you must set the stage and provide a context for learning. In Part II we discuss six components of quality—what we call "The Big Picture."

Planning and evaluating. Quality programs are well thought out. You define program goals and objectives for your work with children and families. Long-term and short-term plans follow taking into consideration the changing needs, interests, and special characteristics of the children and families you serve. Then you develop a schedule that is adaptable and responsive to children's changing needs. As you continually assess what is working and what isn't, you use what you learn from evaluation to guide your decisions and take steps that improve your program.

Individualizing. The more organized you are, the more time you have to observe children regularly. Observation enables you to learn about each child and individualize your program. It also helps you to follow their growth and development—one of the most interesting and rewarding aspects of working with young children. Using specific strategies for observing, you will be able to set goals for each child and plan your work with families.

Creating a welcoming environment. To implement the program you have planned, you begin by creating a welcoming and warm environment. Such an environment can help children feel more comfortable in child care and can also put parents more at ease about leaving their children. Equally important, a well-designed environment enables you to work efficiently so you have the time and energy you need to care for infants and toddlers in an unhurried and nurturing way.

Ensuring children's safety. Safety is a number one priority for parents and for anyone working with infants and toddlers. You ensure children's safety by routinely checking your indoor and outdoor environments for potential problems. You prepare yourself for possible emergencies and practice safety habits yourself to provide a model for children. And day in and day out, you work to balance your concerns for children's safety with children's need to take "reasonable risks" as they explore.

Promoting children's health. Healthy children are ready to learn. You promote children's health by informing yourself of health requirements, taking preventive measures, and constantly checking your program for practices that promote and maintain good health. Each day you model health practices that children can make part of their own lives. In addition, knowing you may be the first to recognize and report suspected cases, you learn the signs of child abuse and neglect and your legal responsibilities.

Guiding children's behavior. Young children learn from adults what behavior is acceptable and what is not. When adults take a positive approach to guiding behavior, they help children learn how to relate positively to others. Then children can develop self-discipline and learn to make good decisions for themselves. Working with infants and toddlers also means knowing how to handle the challenging behaviors—such as biting and temper tantrums—that are sure to come up.

When all of these elements are in place, you will have created an appropriate setting in which infants and toddlers feel secure enough to explore and learn through daily routines and activities.

❖   ❖   ❖

Planning and Evaluating Your Program

Many people believe that caring for children younger than three means simply following the children's lead each day. While this is certainly a central focus of responsive caregiving, it is not the whole story. To make sure the setting and the experiences you provide are appropriate and engaging, you must have plans in place.

A plan shows you where you are going. Even when you change your plans to respond to children's needs, you will still have an overall picture of what you hope to accomplish. Because planning gives you a sense of what to expect, it actually enables you to be more flexible and responsive in your daily work.

To illustrate, think about what's different when you plan ahead to offer fingerpainting as a play choice versus what happens when you spontaneously decide to let children fingerpaint. When you plan, you can select a time of day when children can paint without interruption, you can assemble the materials ahead of time, and you can prepare the environment to reduce messes. As a result, you can focus your attention on the children rather than the activity. Not only does the fingerpainting itself become more manageable, but your time and energy are now devoted to making the experience meaningful for the children.

Evaluation goes hand in hand with good planning. To continue with the fingerpainting example, your observations tell you if the activity is successful. When this is the case, you may decide to prepare for and carry out fingerpainting again in much the same way. If you observe problems, you consider whether your plans were appropriate or whether they need adjustment.

This chapter focuses on two aspects of creating a quality program: planning and evaluation. You will learn about:

- ❖ making evaluation a regular part of the planning process;
- ❖ defining your program's goals for children and families;
- ❖ long-term planning and evaluation;
- ❖ short-term planning and evaluation; and
- ❖ creating a daily schedule.

Making Evaluation a Regular Part of the Planning Process

The needs, interests, and special characteristics of the children and families you serve are continually changing. As a result, your response to these needs, interests, and characteristics must continually change, too.

Evaluation allows you to judge how successfully you have targeted goals and strategies and implemented your plans. When you informally observe children at play, you are evaluating. When you administer a standardized observational instrument, you are also evaluating. So too, when you consult your colleagues and the children's families for their opinions, you are evaluating. Through these different types of evaluation, you gather the information you need to make informed decisions to answer questions, such as the following:

❖ Are all of the children engaged?

❖ Are the materials appropriate for and interesting to the children?

❖ Is each child getting individual attention?

Evaluation, as defined here, is a process that helps you in your work. It is not the threatening concept so many of us tend to fear. Evaluation helps you determine if you're "on target"—and if not, how to get there. It is the flip side of the planning process. If you believe in planning, then you are already a believer in evaluation.

Here is what the planning and evaluation process looks like in action.

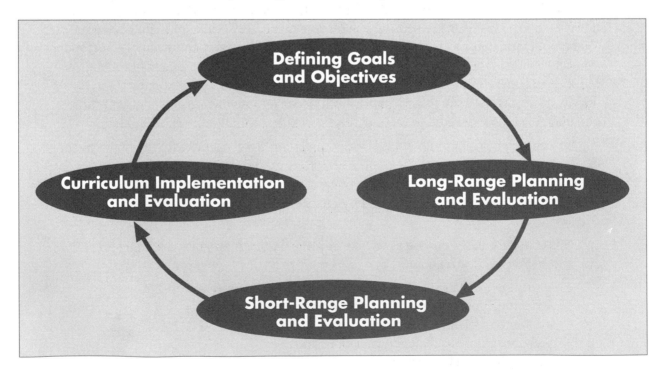

The remainder of this chapter explores how you can plan and evaluate your program to achieve your desired goals.

Defining Program Goals and Objectives

The ultimate goal of planning and evaluation is to achieve a high-quality program. As discussed in the Introduction, leading organizations, such as ZERO TO THREE/The National Center and the National Association for the Education of Young Children, have identified standards of quality for programs serving infants and toddlers.[1] These standards are reflected in the two sets of goals which form the framework for this *Creative Curriculum*: (1) Goals and Objectives for Children; and (2) Goals and Objectives for Working with Families.

Goals and Objectives for Children

Goal 1: To learn about themselves

* To feel valued and secure in their relationships
* To feel competent and proud about what they can do
* To feel supported as they express their independence

Goal 2: To learn about their feelings

* To communicate a broad range of emotions through gestures, sounds, and—over time—words
* To express their feelings in appropriate ways

Goal 3: To learn about others

* To develop trusting relationships with nurturing adults
* To show interest in peers
* To demonstrate caring and cooperation
* To try roles and relationships through imitation and pretend play

Goal 4: To learn about communicating

* To express needs and thoughts without using words
* To identify with a home language
* To respond to verbal and nonverbal commands
* To communicate through language

Goal 5: To learn about moving and doing

* To develop gross motor skills
* To develop fine motor skills
* To coordinate eye and hand movements
* To develop self-help skills

Goal 6: To acquire thinking skills

* To gain an understanding of basic concepts and relationships
* To apply knowledge to new situations
* To develop strategies for solving problems

---

[1] J. Ronald Lally, Abbey Griffin, et al. *Caring for Infants and Toddlers in Groups: Developmentally Appropriate Practice*. Washington, DC: ZERO TO THREE/The National Center, 1995.

Sue Bredekamp and Carol Copple, Eds. *Developmentally Appropriate Practice in Early Childhood Programs*, Revised Edition. Washington, DC: National Association for the Education of Young Children, 1997.

Goals and Objectives for Working with Families

Goal 1: To build a partnership with families

- ❖ To involve families in the program's planning and evaluation process
- ❖ To listen to and discuss families' questions, concerns, observations, and insights about their children
- ❖ To communicate regularly with families at arrival and departure times about how things are going for their child at home and at the program
- ❖ To schedule regular conferences and/or home visits
- ❖ To discuss with families ways to handle children's challenging behaviors
- ❖ To resolve differences with families in a respectful way
- ❖ To help families gain access to community resources

Goal 2: To support families in their parenting role

- ❖ To demonstrate respect for a family's approach to childrearing and their feelings about sharing the care of their child
- ❖ To celebrate with families each new milestone in their child's development
- ❖ To incorporate family rituals and preferences into the daily life of the program
- ❖ To offer workshops/training on child development and other topics of interest to families
- ❖ To help families network with one another for information and support

Goal 3: To support families in their role as primary educators of their child

- ❖ To encourage family involvement and participation in program activities
- ❖ To provide families with strategies to support children's learning at home

Goal 4: To ensure that the home cultures of the children's families are reflected in the program

- ❖ To support children's use of their home language
- ❖ To encourage children's awareness of and interest in home languages spoken at the program
- ❖ To seek families' assistance in learning about the children's home culture
- ❖ To include objects and customs from the children's home cultures in the program's environment, routines, and activities
- ❖ To interact with children in a style that is respectful of their home culture

Choosing Your Target Goals and Objectives

Taken together, these two sets of goals and objectives may be viewed as a master list. Your ultimate aim is, of course, to realize all of these goals. In reality though, achieving desired results occurs in small steps rather than leaps. For most programs, it is helpful to start out by pinpointing goals and objectives that most need your attention and to add other goals and objectives over time.

Therefore, to implement *The Creative Curriculum,* your first step is to review these two sets of goals and objectives. Consider how they relate to your program by responding to these questions:

❖ Are there certain goals you've already achieved and need only to continue doing what you're doing to maintain them?

❖ Are there other goals you haven't been as successful in reaching as you'd like to be?

❖ Are there goals you haven't focused on but think you should?

❖ Are there goals that need your attention as a result of special circumstances?

There are several informal methods you can use to determine your focus. First of all, your own observations (see Chapter 6), will give you a firm idea of what children need, which parts of *The Creative Curriculum* work well, and which parts of your program need strengthening. You can also interview colleagues, families, and consultants, to ask their opinions about your program's needs. Then, as a team, you can decide which goals need your attention.

Alternatively, you can conduct a more formal standardized evaluation of your program. Instruments, such as *The Assessment Profile—Infant/Toddler Version* or *Family Day Care Version* (Abbott-Shim & Sibley) and the *Infant/Toddler Environmental Rating Scale* (ITERS) or *Family Day Care Rating Scale* (FDCRS) (Harms & Clifford), can help you determine how well your program meets recognized standards for environment, scheduling, health, safety, programming, and adult-child interactions.[2] With the information collected, you can decide on which goals to focus your energies.

At the same time that you decide to concentrate your energies on specific goals, it's important to remember two things:

❖ **If you use** *The Creative Curriculum for Infants &Toddlers,* **you won't be neglecting other goals while you concentrate on those you've selected**. This is especially true of the goals for children, since the areas of child development are so interrelated. For example, suppose you target the goal of helping children learn about themselves. As you help a child develop a sense of self, you also help the child develop social, emotional, physical, and thinking skills.

❖ **Although you may have chosen goals with specific children or families in mind, your efforts benefit all the children and/or families in the program.** Suppose, for example, you want to address some parents' unrealistic expectations about their children's development. You offer a workshop, and in so doing, all families benefit.

Thus, you can recognize that the purpose of targeting two or three specific goals is to give them the extra attention they need. It does not mean neglecting other goals.

---

[2] Both versions of *The Assessment Profile* can be obtained by contacting Quality Assist, 368 Moreland Avenue, Atlanta, GA 30307. Copies of the *ITERS* and *FDCRS* can be ordered from Teacher's College Press, Columbia University, New York, NY 10027-6694.

Long-Range Planning and Evaluation

Once you and your colleagues have identified specific goals and objectives, you've begun the long-range planning and evaluation process. Long-range planning requires thinking ahead—typically for a month or more—about how to meet these targeted goals and objectives. There are five steps to follow when planning for the long term.

1. Identify the targeted goals and objectives for children and families.
2. Identify specific strategies to reach each goal and objective. Develop a plan.
3. Implement your plan.
4. Evaluate your plan. How is it working?
5. Based on your findings, make a plan for the following month. It may focus on the same goal(s) and objective(s) or new ones.

To give you an idea of how to apply these steps, here are two examples that demonstrate how La Toya and Grace developed long-range plans for their programs.

La Toya's Long-Range Planning Process

Step 1: Identify Target Goals and Objectives

I feel good about all the interesting activities I offer children in my family child care program. I also feel good about how much children help with daily routines, such as setting the table. One thing I don't feel good about is that there's a great deal of hitting among the children. The children's parents are concerned that they've been hitting and having tantrums at home, too. I reviewed the goals and objectives for children in the Curriculum and I've decided to spend extra time to help the children learn about their feelings and how to express them in appropriate ways.

Step 2: Identify Strategies and Develop a Plan

I know toddlers have a wide range of feelings and that their feelings can be very intense. I plan to introduce a variety of activities which let children express their feelings in positive ways.

Step 3: Implement the Plan

I am talking more with the children about their feelings and reactions. I offer activities such as playing with dough and dancing to music, which let them express their emotions in positive ways. And today the children and I made up a song about things to do when they are happy, sad, and angry.

Step 4: Evaluate the Plan

The children were very interested in all these activities. On Tuesday I heard Valisha say, "I'm mad at you, Eddie!" She stomped her foot—a big improvement over smacking him the way she used to! I think children want and need more chances to talk about feelings and express themselves in positive ways.

Step 5: Review and Revise Plan

Because this is such an important topic and because we've had some obvious improvements, I plan to continue focusing on feelings as one of my target goals for children. Next month I'll ask colleagues at our provider association meeting to share their ideas for dealing with children's hitting and for helping children express feelings positively. I'll also pay more attention to ways I guide children's behavior.

Grace's Long-Range Planning Process

Step 1: Identify Target Goals and Objectives

I feel good about the way I relate to the children, but it bothers me that I don't know much about their families' backgrounds. Since our center serves the whole university community, there are many different cultures represented. To be perfectly honest, I sometimes feel uncomfortable working with families that are so different from mine. I've decided to make a real effort to focus on the goal of helping to reflect the children's home cultures into our program.

Step 2: Identify Strategies and Develop a Plan

As a first step, I plan to explore how my own background influences my views on child rearing and how I might learn more about the children's families' backgrounds.

Step 3: Implement the Plan

Last week, I attended a workshop on culture and child rearing. I've also talked with some of the professors at the university about the subject. Most importantly, I have been talking with my own parents and siblings about our family beliefs. I'm starting to talk openly with the families in my program about their beliefs and values.

Step 4: Evaluate the Plan

To my surprise, I discovered how much my past influences my work. I realize now that growing up in a home where we were encouraged to be quiet makes it particularly challenging for me to deal with children like Willard, who are very active and noisy.

Step 5: Review and Revise Plan

Next month, I am going to invite members of the children's families to tape songs they sing at home with the children. I also plan to continue our discussions about what we want for the infants and toddlers in our lives. This is a goal I think I should continue to focus on for some time.

Short-Range Planning and Evaluation

Short range planning is a way to make long-range plans materialize. It gives you an overall sense of direction for the week and a list of the materials you will want to have readily available. Making a commitment to do weekly planning encourages you to reflect on what you know about each of the children in your care. Based on your observations, you can evaluate and make changes to the environment that will take advantage of each child's interests and growing abilities.

Think about weekly planning as "planning for possibilities." You set the stage and then follow a child's lead, taking time to enjoy the experience together. Infants and toddlers often respond in unexpected ways to new materials in their environment and to planned activities. Your ability to watch and respond to what children do each day is one of the joys of working with infants and toddlers. If you view planning in this way, you are more likely to watch what happens and take advantage of opportunities that emerge.

The *Weekly Planning Form* we designed for this *Curriculum* asks you to consider six aspects of weekly planning.

Target goals/objectives. Which goal(s) and objective(s) are you going to focus on this week with children? How do you plan to work with their families? For example, if you are focusing on helping children learn to express their feelings in appropriate ways, you may note that you will offer comforting and expressive activities, such as water play, pretend play, and playdough, and that you will plan to sing songs about feelings, and consult with parents.

Changes to the environment. Are there changes to make? Do you need duplicates of materials to keep children from fighting over toys? Do materials reflect the children's cultural backgrounds? Does the fact that puzzle pieces end up scattered on the floor mean that the puzzles are too difficult and should be put away for now? That they aren't stored so that children can use them independently? That children aren't encouraged to clean up after themselves?

Special activities I plan to offer this week: What activities would extend opportunities for children to explore and make discoveries. Think about what experiences you can provide indoors and outdoors. Consult chapters 16–22 for ideas about activities, but don't feel pressured to plan a special activity every day.

Changes to daily routines. How are daily routines and transitions going? Are children getting cranky because they are spending too much time waiting? Or do they feel proud as they help with "real work," such as feeding the fish or wiping the table after snack? Are any changes needed?

Family involvement. What are some different ways to involve parents in implementing *The Creative Curriculum*? These may include discussing a concern, asking for their help in making materials, inviting them to participate in an activity or in daily routines.

To do. What will your need to do to carry out your plans.

Adapting Your Plans

When you work with infants and toddlers, the one thing you can expect is the unexpected. Each infant has a uniquely personal schedule. As you zip up the last jacket and head for the door, an infant may begin crying to tell you he is tired or hungry or needs his diaper changed. Toddlers, too, have an amazing ability to capsize the best laid plans. You can't predict when a toddler may decide to flush her socks down the toilet or try out a balancing act on the back of the sofa.

You'll need to be able to adapt your plans if you're to respond to the children's changing needs and interests. Here are some steps you can follow.

Review your weekly planning form. Visualize your day first thing in the morning. Try to imagine how all the parts of the day will fit together.

Assess the realities of the day. Is there an infant who is going to need extra time and attention because she is teething? Did a family bring in a bag of freshly picked apples tempting you to replace your plans to make French toast for snack with making applesauce? Are you feeling a little worn down and not up to taking the walk you planned?

Adapt your plans as necessary. No matter how carefully you plan, you must always be ready to adapt. Therefore, throughout the day, keep these two points in mind.

❖ **Remain flexible.** There is no way to predict that a toddler will throw a tantrum and require some extra attention. As a result, you won't be able to introduce the large chalk activity you had planned. Nor can you foresee that a bulldozer will begin working at the end of your road, giving you a new destination for neighborhood walks.

❖ **Be responsive to individual children's needs and interests.** If you know a child needs you to be ready to step in and keep her from biting another child, you may decide to postpone your plans for making playdough with the children. Instead, you might bring out the playdough you made a few days ago or spend extra time singing and reading with the children. You can make playdough tomorrow or next week.

After reviewing how La Toya filled out the *Weekly Planning Form* (see the example on the following page), try using this form to plan your program over the next week or two. Then evaluate how it works for you and change it to suit your needs. (See Appendix B for a blank form.)

Weekly Planning Form

Target goals/objectives: *To learn about their feelings/To be able to express their feelings in appropriate ways*

Week of: *10/18*

Changes to the Environment

Create a reading nook with soft pillows and a hanging book pocket so child can sit and look at books.

Add more blocks so several children can build together.

Add doctor props to pretend play area because Eddie has a series of doctor appointments coming up.

Rotate and clean toys.

Special Activities I Plan to Offer This Week

	Monday	Tuesday	Wednesday	Thursday	Friday
Indoor Opportunities to Explore and Discover	Serve apple butter—children spread it on crackers	Make playdough	Playdough	Fingerpainting Sing songs about feelings	Fingerpainting
Outdoor Opportunities to Explore and Discover	Paint with water	Blow bubbles	Blow bubbles		Walk to Library for Story Time

Changes to Daily Routines *Make a point of inviting children to help me prepare snacks and lunches and to set the table. See if this helps lunch time go smoother.*

Family Involvement *Talk with the Curtises who are concerned about Valisha hitting other children. Ask them what they do to help Jonisha when her sister hurts her. Share the new article about positive guidance with all families.*

To Do *Borrow a set of blocks from provider association's toy lending library. Copy article on guiding behavior for all families.*

Creating a Daily Schedule

Infants and toddlers need a schedule that is regular enough to be predictable, yet flexible enough to meet their individual needs and to take advantage of learning opportunities that continually emerge in everyday experiences. In general, the younger the children, the more flexible and individualized the schedule must be. Yet even babies gain a sense of security when the schedule is somewhat regular. Responsive care respects an infant's biological rhythms as well as the interests of toddlers.

When an infant like Julio falls asleep soon after arriving at child care, he needs a nap even though the other children are awake and playing. When the wind begins swirling leaves in the backyard, toddlers like Jonisha and Valisha need some time to dance with the leaves, even though the schedule says it is time to come inside and get ready for lunch.

A daily schedule is important for children, families, and you. A schedule offers infants and toddlers a feeling of predictability that helps them develop a sense of trust about the world. It offers parents a sense of what their child is doing during the day. Finally, a schedule gives you a picture of the day that can be adapted as necessary to meet the needs of individual children.

Components of a Daily Schedule

A good daily schedule contains the same basic components day after day. Depending on the length of your program day and the ages of the children you serve, your daily schedule will probably include time for the following:

- ❖ arrivals and departures;
- ❖ feeding/preparing and eating snacks and meals;
- ❖ diaper changing/toileting;
- ❖ dressing;
- ❖ indoor and outdoor play (including clean-up and transitions for older children); and
- ❖ sleeping/naptime.

A good schedule offers children a balance between the following types of activities:

- ❖ time with others, time alone, and one-on-one time with a "special" adult;
- ❖ quiet times and active times; and
- ❖ activities children choose and those offered by adults.

The chart on the next page shows how you can adapt your daily schedule to meet the needs of children as they grow.

Adapting the Schedule to Meet Children's Needs

Young Infants	How You Can Adapt Your Daily Schedule
They depend on you to meet their basic needs—to be fed, kept dry and comfortable, and picked up and held.	Create a daily schedule that is flexible so you can respond to individual biological needs.
They like to spend time with familiar adults seeing and doing interesting things.	Allow plenty of unhurried time throughout the day to spend with individual children.
They are learning to trust themselves and other people.	Respond to children when they need you, regardless of your scheduled plans.

Mobile Infants	How You Can Adapt Your Daily Schedule
They begin to remember more from one day to the next.	Follow your schedule consistently so that children will learn to predict what happens next.
They sense how you feel about them.	Organize your plans so that you'll have time to enjoy children and demonstrate your pleasure in what they do.
They like doing things for themselves.	Allow enough time for children to participate as fully as possible at mealtimes and in other daily routines.

Toddlers	How You Can Adapt Your Daily Schedule
They rely on familiar routines to organize their picture of the world.	Follow your daily schedule consistently, but allow for flexibility.
They can often become overwhelmed if things get too hectic.	Plan the day to eliminate unnecessary confusion. Use transitions to help children move from one part of the day to another.
They can concentrate for longer periods of time.	Allow time for children to play and pursue their interests unhurriedly.

Individualizing the Schedule for Infants

You will discover, if you haven't already, that each child in your care has a unique schedule for eating, diapering and toileting, playing, and sleeping. The younger the children in your care, the more likely you'll need to juggle your schedule to meet these individual needs. Just as one child finishes a bottle and falls asleep, another may wake up hungry.

Here's how one particular day went for two infants, Julio and Abby. Notice that although they do many of the same kinds of activities, the timing and specific content of what they do differs. The difference results, in large part, because of their different ages, abilities, and temperaments.

Julio's Day (4 months old)	Abby's Day (16 months old)
Morning	**Morning**
Arrival: Julio arrives at the Shane Center with his mother, Marta. Marta says a long good-bye and hands Julio to Linda.	**Arrival:** Abby arrives at Brooks's home with her father, Edward. She cries as he says good-bye. Brooks comforts her by reading a book to her.
Mealtime: Julio sits in a rocking chair with Linda. She cradles him in her arm as she gives him a bottle.	**Handwashing:** Abby and Mollie wash their hands so they can help Brooks prepare their breakfast.
Diaper change: Julio gazes at Linda as she changes his diaper and talks to him. He begins rubbing his eyes.	**Food preparation/Mealtime:** Abby helps Brooks and Mollie set the table and make scrambled eggs. They eat breakfast together, then clean up and wash their hands.
Naptime: Julio falls asleep in his crib as Linda pats him gently and sings a lullaby.	**Indoor play:** Abby squeezes, pounds, pokes, and rolls playdough. She notices new photos hanging on the wall and looks at them with Brooks.
Diaper change: Julio's diaper is dry when Linda checks it.	**Diaper change:** Abby plays a game touching her nose, tummy, and so forth with Brooks.
Indoor play: Julio lies on a mat with two other babies near a low, shatterproof mirror. Linda sits at the edge of the mat and talks with the children about what they are doing and seeing.	**Indoor play:** She sings songs with Brooks and Mollie. Mollie and Abby pretend to feed their babies a bottle.
Mealtime: Julio drinks part of a bottle sitting in Linda's lap, then burps as Linda pats him on the back.	**Clean up:** Abby and Mollie help put the blocks away and fold up the tunnel.
Diaper change: Julio kicks his legs as Linda changes his diaper. She pushes the overhead mobile. He tracks it with his eyes as it turns.	**Diaper change:** Abby protests as Brooks picks her up to change her diaper. Brooks assures her it will only take a minute and then she can get down and go outdoors.
Dressing: Linda puts on Julio's jacket. She sings to him as she dresses him.	**Dressing:** Abby takes her jacket off her hook. Brooks helps her put it on. Mollie proudly helps with the Velcro™ tab.
Outdoor play: Julio goes outdoors in a Snugli™ Linda is wearing. He closes his eyes when a gust of wind blows across his face. Linda describes what it might feel like.	**Outdoor play:** Abby takes a walk around the block with Brooks and Mollie. She notices sounds of birds and cars. She points out three different dogs.
Midday	**Midday**
Diaper change: Linda changes Julio gently but quickly, knowing the other children need her attention.	**Diaper change/Handwashing:** Abby's diaper is dry when Brooks checks it. She washes her hands for lunch, taking time to splash a bit.
Mealtime: Julio refuses the bottle Linda offers. He sits in an infant seat and watches the children eat. Linda tries again in 10 minutes, and he's hungry.	**Mealtime:** Abby carries napkins and paper cups to the table. She eats most of her grilled cheese sandwich and several carrot sticks. She uses a spoon and her fingers to eat and drinks some milk from a cup. Then she cleans up and washes her hands.
Naptime: Julio begins dozing off. Linda rocks him, puts him in his crib on his back, and gently pats his tummy.	

continued on next page

Julio's Day (4 months old)	Abby's Day (16 months old)
Diaper change: Linda talks quietly to Julio as she changes his diaper and plays a peek-a-boo type game with him. **Mealtime:** Julio drinks part of a bottle sitting in Linda's lap.	**Brushing teeth:** Brooks finishes drying Abby's hands with a towel and gets down the toothbrushes. Abby and Mollie brush their teeth. **Transition:** Brooks reads the girls a story and plays some quiet music to set the mood for naptime. **Diaper change:** Abby yawns and lies quietly as Brooks changes her diaper. **Naptime:** Abby falls asleep on her cot in the living room as Brooks sits nearby. **Diaper change:** Brooks changes Abby's diaper and sings her favorite song. **Snacktime:** Abby and Mollie spoon some cottage cheese on crackers and eat them. Abby also scoops some of the cottage cheese onto the table. They each drink a cup of milk and wash their hands when done.
## Afternoon **Indoor play:** Julio sits in Linda's lap as she sings with older infants. **Diaper change:** Linda notices Julio is wet and changes his diaper. He squirms and she finishes promptly. **Indoor play:** Linda places Julio on a mat on the floor under a low hanging mobile. Julio can bat the mobile with his fists. **Departure:** Julio sits in a rocking chair with his mother, Marta, while she relaxes and talks with Linda. After about 20 minutes, Marta puts on Julio's jacket, says good-bye, and they leave for home.	## Afternoon **Indoor play:** Abby carries five large cardboard blocks, one by one, into the middle of the living room. She carefully places each one on the floor. When Brooks brings over a bin of rubber farm animals, Abby puts some animals on top of the blocks. **Clean up:** Abby watches as Mollie and Brooks start to put away the blocks. When Brooks hands Abby a block and asks her to help, Abby puts it on the shelf. **Diaper change:** Abby and Brooks talk about farm animals. They "moo" together as Brooks changes Abby's diaper. **Dressing:** Abby gets her jacket and takes it over to Mollie, who is busy putting on her own jacket. Brooks helps Abby and explains that Mollie can help her tomorrow. **Outdoor play:** Abby and Mollie play in the sandbox in Brooks's backyard. Abby watches the sand fall through a sieve. **Departure:** Robin picks up Abby. She explains they have to hurry to go pick up Talia at a friend's. Brooks helps Abby put on her coat as Robin gathers her things. Robin and Abby say good-bye and leave.

A Schedule for Toddlers

By the time children are toddlers, their day is more consistent and predictable. For example, toddlers typically eat and sleep as a group and have a designated time for play. A consistent daily schedule helps toddlers feel more in control, and thus more competent and secure. Of course, it is still important to be flexible about responding to individual children's needs.

Here is a sample schedule for toddlers.[1] Notice that frequently several activities take place at the same time.

Sample Toddler Schedule	
Early Morning	Greet parents and children. Help children and parents say good-bye. Encourage children to explore the environment and materials in their own way. Set up and invite children to participate in adult-directed activity, such as playing a simple lotto game. Clean up and wash hands. Prepare and eat snack. Discuss plans and news of the day. Clean up and wash hands.
Late Morning	Change diapers and use toilet, wash hands. Help children get ready to go outside. Take small group walks (to the park, to mail a letter, to the playground). Come inside, take off coats, and hang on hooks. Wash hands, read stories.
Midday	Help prepare and eat lunch. Clean up and wash hands. Change diapers and use toilet, wash hands. Brush teeth. Read stories, play music. Help children prepare for naps. Wake up and cuddle time. Change diapers and use toilet, wash hands. Prepare and eat snack, wash hands.
Late Afternoon	Play indoors and outside. Read stories or do quiet play, such as table art or toys. Help parents and children reunite and leave for home.

The schedule you develop for your program may vary from the ones we have oulined. However, they will give you a starting point for planning a schedule that meets the needs of your children and your program.

---

[1] K. Modigliani, M. Reiff, and S. Jones. *Opening Your Door to Children*. Washington, DC: National Association for the Education of Young Children, 1986.

Planning for Transitions

Every day is filled with transitions—the periods of time between one activity and the next. With toddlers, who have a more structured schedule, transitions are more apparent. The most important transitions, and often most difficult, are at the beginning and end of the day. These are the times when infants and toddlers say good-bye and then hello to their families. (This will be discussed in detail in Chapter 11.) However, any transition can become a problem if children don't know what to do or if they are required to wait for long periods of time. Young children can't wait. When they are made to do so while adults get organized, disruptions (restlessness, pushing, hitting) are bound to occur.

Here are some suggestions of ways you can avoid making infants and toddlers wait by preparing for transitions and involving children in the process.

Plan ahead. Then you'll know what you'll be doing and can feel prepared for each new activity.

Be organized. Have the supplies for the next activity ready so you don't have to search for them while the children wait.

Give children a warning. Before a change takes place, say something like, "It's almost time to clean up. Think about finishing what you are doing."

Divide the group so children won't have to wait. For example, while some toddlers are brushing their teeth, the others might be listening to a story or helping you set up cots.

Guide children through a transition. You can do this by describing what you are doing or singing songs or chants. For example, you can have a special song for clean up time or for getting ready for lunch.

Planned transitions help children build a sense of order about their world. They feel competent when they know what is expected and are engaged. From your point of view, a well-organized day means that you feel more calm and can take the time you need to observe children and enjoy their development. In the next chapter, we will explore in detail how you can go about doing this.

Individualizing for Children and Families

I n the last chapter, we discussed planning and evaluating your program. In this chapter, we look at how you can plan and adapt your program's goals and objectives for each individual child and family. Because children and families come to your program with distinct needs, strengths, and values, your challenge is to customize the program's goals to fit the *particular* circumstances of *each* child. One of the hallmarks of a high quality program is this ability to individualize.

To individualize for children, you begin by identifying goals and objectives on which to focus, then determine with the children's families how you can best support children's mastery of them. In addition, you can customize your work with families to meet their individual needs and interests.

As you read through this chapter, you will learn about:

❖ using the forms for *Individualizing Goals and Objectives for Children;*
❖ observing children systematically to get to know them as individuals;
❖ organizing your observations;
❖ putting it all together into the *Summary of Development* and the *Planning Form for Individualizing;* and
❖ using the *Goals for Working with Families* form.

Individualizing Goals and Objectives for Children

The goals and objectives for children listed in Chapter 5 identify social, emotional, physical, and cognitive skills for all children. However, as everyone who works with infants and toddlers knows, no two children are alike in their development. One nine-month-old may be crawling while another is already starting to walk. One 18-month-old may be expressing her thoughts in words, while another relies on grunts and gestures. Development in all areas follows its own timetable.

To truly meet the needs of every child in your care, you'll need to find out where each one is in terms of development. Then you can meet that child at a wholly appropriate level and help him or her to reach the next step.

To do this in a systematic way, we have created forms for *Individualizing Goals and Objectives*. There are three versions of the form: one each for young infants, mobile infants, and toddlers. Each version lists the six goals, identifies the objectives within each goal, and provides three examples of behaviors that indicate mastery of the objective. There is space for you to record your notes right on the form.

Objectives. The examples for illustrating mastery of an objective are age-specific and are based on child growth and development over time. For this reason, Linda would select the checklist for young infants when observing Julio, Brooks would use the mobile infant checklist with Abby, and La Toya would use the toddler checklist for Valisha and Jonisha. The examples only suggest some of the behaviors reflecting a child's mastery of the given objective. They are not intended to be a complete list, but rather to give you an idea of types of behaviors to look for.

Notes (Date each entry). For each objective, you have space to record examples of behaviors that illustrate mastery. While your examples may be similar to the ones listed on the form, they do not have to be. Your examples may also be conclusions you've drawn from your observations. To illustrate, La Toya might chose to note "Valisha proudly told me her name" (9/23/98) as an example of Valisha's mastery of the objective, "To feel valued and secure in their relationships."

We recommend that you use the *Individualizing Goals and Objectives* forms in an ongoing way. Each time you enter a note, be sure to date it so that you will have a record of the child's progress over time.

Every three months, summarize the notes section onto the *Summary of Development* form. You can then use the information you've collected as a planning tool. This form can also serve as a basis for your parent conferences.

A reminder, however: these forms are meant to serve as planning tools for individualizing your program. They are *not* intended to be a list of skills or milestones children should acquire by a certain age. Most certainly, they should not be used to compare the progress of one child with that of another.

Here is a sample form that La Toya has been using with Valisha. She is now at the point where she is ready to summarize the information onto the *Summary of Development* form and share it with the Curtises.

Individualizing Goals and Objectives for Toddlers
(18–36 months)

Name of child: _Valisha Curtis_   **Caregiver/Teacher:** _La Toya Thompkins_

Date of birth: _1/2/96_

Goal 1: To learn about themselves	
Objectives	**Notes (Date each entry)**
To feel valued and secure in their relationships Examples: ❖ points out family picture in a scrapbook ❖ knows which child is out for the day after seeing who is there ❖ looks to caregivers for comfort and at times may comfort caregiver	- V sat on my lap after her parents left and snuggled close to me (9/1/98) - She proudly tells me her name is Valisha Renée Curtis and that she is a twin (9/26/98) - V comforted her sister who was crying after naptime (10/1/98)
To feel competent and proud about what they can do Examples: ❖ pours own juice at snack time and says, "I did it!" ❖ helps another child find the crayons ❖ stands on one foot and calls, "Look at me!"	- V called me over to see her painting of a giant red cat (9/30/98) - V told me girls can play the steel drums (10/5/98) - V started setting the table for our snack before I asked (10/19/98)
To express their independence Examples: ❖ insists on putting on own jacket ❖ willingly joins in a new activity ❖ cheerfully says "good-bye" to parents and goes to play	- V insisted on putting all the prunes and raisins to be soaked for a holiday black cake into the bowl by herself (11/2/98) - V insisted on zipping her jacket herself even though she was having difficulty doing so (11/9/98)

Goal 2: To learn about their feelings	
To communicate a broad range of emotions through gestures, sounds, and—eventually—words Examples: ❖ says, "I did it!" after using the potty successfully ❖ hugs a doll and lovingly feeds it a bottle ❖ raises hand to make a "high five"	- V made Fluffy a pretend breakfast, then gave Fluffy a hug and told her, "You're a good cat." (10/12/98) - V's face mirrors Jonisha's moods, especially when she's sulking (10/5/98, 10/20/98)
To express their feelings in appropriate ways Examples: ❖ roars like a lion when angry instead of biting ❖ recognizes feelings in others (e.g., "Camilo sad") ❖ bites on a bagel when has urge to bite	- V began to bite on a bagel when she was mad, but changed her mind and threw it on the floor (11/6/98)

Goal 3: To learn about others

Objectives	Notes (Date each entry)
To develop trusting relationships with nurturing adults Examples: ❖ imitates adult activities (e.g., reading a newspaper, setting the table) ❖ eager to help with chores (e.g., preparing meals, feeding the fish) ❖ calls adult over to show an accomplishment (e.g., a painting, block structure)	- V told me, "I can help" as she came into the kitchen, climbed up on the chair, and reached for a spoon to help me make French toast for breakfast (10/5/98) - V called me over to show me how she had braided her doll's hair (10/10/98)
To show interest in peers Examples: ❖ enjoys including other children in pretend play (e.g., driving in a car or going food shopping) ❖ refers to other children by name ❖ comments on who is a girl and who is a boy	- V likes to play with toys Jonisha is interested in (10/6/98, 10/15/98, 11/2/98)
To demonstrate caring and cooperation Examples: ❖ responds to emotions of other children (e.g., helps adult pat a crying child) ❖ works with another child to complete a task (e.g., putting away a puzzle) ❖ feeds and puts doll to bed	- V gave Jonisha a hug when she fell and scraped her knee (10/30/98)
To try out roles and relationships through imitation and pretend play Examples: ❖ acts out simple life scenes (e.g., making dinner, going to the doctor) ❖ puts hat on and says, "I'm going to work" ❖ uses object to represent something else (e.g., box as car, block as phone)	- V played "going to the doctor" with Jonisha and Eddie (11/16/98)

Goal 4: To learn about communicating

Objectives	Notes (Date each entry)
To express needs and thoughts without using words Examples: ❖ uses facial expressions to show excitement ❖ catches adult's eye for attention and reassurance when needed ❖ tugs on pants to indicate need to go to bathroom	- V brought her <u>Millions of Cats</u> book over and held it out to me to read (9/26/98)
To identify with a home language Examples: ❖ speaks in home language with family members and others ❖ uses main language spoken in child care with those who don't speak home language ❖ recognizes tapes of stories and songs from home culture	- V uses West Indian phrases with her family and me— "When will Johisha and they have a turn?" (10/14/98)

Goal 4: To learn about communicating (continued)

Objectives	Notes (Date each entry)
To respond to verbal and nonverbal commands Examples: ❖ follows directions such as, "Will you carry these napkins to the table, please?" ❖ responds to adult's facial expression (e.g., stops throwing blocks after a stern look) ❖ goes over to cot when lights are dimmed for naptime	- V followed my directions about how to whisk an egg when we made French toast (10/26/98)
To communicate through language Examples: ❖ tells a story ❖ tells about what happened over the weekend ❖ talks with other children while playing together	- V told me in vivid detail about going to a street fair over the weekend and playing steel drums (10/15/98) - She engages adults and children in conversation (10/20/98) - She can recite nursery rhymes by heart (11/2/98)

Goal 5: To learn about moving and doing

Objectives	Notes
To develop gross motor skills Examples: ❖ walks up stairs ❖ throws a ball ❖ runs	- V is very comfortable climbing stairs holding onto the railing (9/18/98) - She can balance on one foot (11/2/98)
To develop fine motor skills Examples: ❖ threads large beads ❖ scribbles with marker or crayons ❖ pastes papers together	- V tries to use scissors but ends up frustrated and tearing the paper because cutting is so hard for her (9/8/98) - She draws with crayons and uses fingerpaints (10/28/98)
To coordinate eye and hand movements Examples: ❖ places pieces in a simple puzzle ❖ closes Velcro™ fasteners on shoes ❖ pours juice into a cup	- V can do the cat puzzle that has six pieces (9/30/98) - She mixes paints together to form new colors (11/1/98)
To develop self-help skills Examples: ❖ uses the potty and washes hands ❖ pours own milk and juice from small plastic pitcher ❖ puts on own jacket and hat when going outside	- V can button her sweater with help (9/30/98) - She uses the toilet by herself though I have to remind her to wash her hands (10/3/98) - She helps me set and clean the table (10/5/98, 10/11/98, 10/15/98, 10/19/98)

Goal 6: To acquire thinking skills

Objectives	Notes (Date each entry)
To gain an understanding of basic concepts and relationships Examples: ❖ experiments with mixing colors when painting ❖ tells another child, "Your mommy comes back after nap" ❖ runs to the tree and says, "I run fast"	- V wants to explore everything (9/18/98) - She asked if she will be bigger when she turns three (10/20/98) - She told me how her socks turned purple in the wash (11/3/98)
To apply knowledge to new situations Examples: ❖ sees a picture of a zebra and calls it a horse ❖ paints on side of building with water after painting at easel ❖ completes new puzzle using familiar strategy of turning pieces until they fit	- When V's cat puppet was torn, she suggested we use tape to fix it like we do with our books (10/16/98) - She identifies pictures of objects when we read books (10/21/98)
To develop strategies for solving problems Examples: ❖ cooperates with others in implementing a plan (e.g., carries a large pillow across the room for a jumping game) ❖ asks "Why?" questions ❖ dips paintbrush in water to clean it	- When V wanted more potatoes at lunch, she asked Eddie to pass them to her (9/22/98) - V held the bag upside down and shook it to get the raisins out (11/2/98)

Systematically Observing Children to Get to Know Them as Individuals

In addition to identifying the content goals and objectives for individual children, you also need to know how to best help children acquire these targeted objectives. When you understand what motivates a child, how the child approaches new tasks, and what his or her preferred learning style is, you can plan for that child.

You can gather this type of information in many ways. One of the most effective is to use systematic, focused observations, as Brooks did with Abby.

> Several months ago Brooks first observed Abby reaching for the spoon with which she was being fed. Brooks then decided to give Abby her own spoon to hold. A few days later, knowing that things would get messy but deciding it was worth it, Brooks gave Abby a small bowl of applesauce to eat with her spoon. Since then, Abby has become quite skilled at using a spoon to feed herself. She has also moved on to other self-help skills, such as wiping up spills and throwing away her napkin.

When Brooks observes, she uses a two-step process: she describes what she sees, then asks herself what it means. This type of careful observation is like watching children from the outside to understand what they are experiencing on the inside. Brooks figured out that in grabbing the spoon, Abby was asserting her independence and her desire to be in charge of feeding herself.

Through focused observations, you can gather information about children's

- ❖ family, culture, and home life;
- ❖ temperament;
- ❖ special interests;
- ❖ likes and dislikes;
- ❖ behavioral challenges; and
- ❖ learning styles.

Making a Commitment to Observe

There's no doubt that you already know a great deal about the children in your program. Why, then, are we now asking you to devote time regularly to observing in a focused way? Aren't informal observations—that one child has a cold, another isn't being very social, and that a third is spending most of the day playing dress-up—enough?

While informal observations certainly have their place, they don't provide enough information to make informed decisions about children. For this you need observations that are typical of the child, objectively reported, and accurately recorded. You'll need to plan and make a commitment to observe children routinely.

Although you may appreciate the value of observing, you may still wonder how you will fit observation time into your routine and activity-packed day. With only so many minutes in the day, something has to give. All too often that something is the time for focused observation.

The chart that follows identifies some of the main reasons people give to explain why they don't observe regularly and suggests strategies to overcome these obstacles.

Obstacles to Observing	Strategies to Overcome Them
"I don't have time in my schedule for observing."	Make observation a priority. Be aware that you are always observing as you care for children. However, when you observe in a purposeful way, you gain additional and valuable insights.
"I don't speak a child's home language."	Even a child who is not yet talking will have body language unique to a culture you might not understand. Consider asking someone who does speak the child's home language to observe with you.
"I can't observe and adequately supervise other children at the same time."	Schedule planned observations at times when children won't need constant supervision. If your program allows, you might make arrangements to have substitute staff, parent volunteers, or back-up providers on hand during scheduled observation times. Figure out a place where you can observe from the sidelines but still see and hear everything.
"There are too many things that need to be observed. I don't know where to begin."	Begin slowly. Choose one or two children to observe. Then, over time, gradually widen the scope until you are observing all children regularly.
"I miss what is happening when I have to go get a pen and paper."	Keep a pad of paper, notebook, index cards, and a pen in your pocket or in a convenient place. That way, you will always be ready to note something of interest.
"I'm afraid of breaching children's (and families') confidentiality."	You'll want to keep all your written observations in a secure place, such as filing cabinet you can lock.
"I don't know how to be objective."	Practice writing only what you see and hear. Keep a list of "red-flag" terms to avoid (such as active, quiet, bright, good, fussy, or happy) as a reminder. Request that your program provide training and assistance on becoming a better observer.

Recording Your Observations

Doing a focused observation implies having a purpose in mind. It also implies that you are systematic and use specific skills to make observations that are both accurate and objective. Focused observations can take many forms.

Anecdotal observations are recorded information about one specific event or behavior. They range from notations of developmental milestones (Jasmine pulled herself up on the sofa) to descriptions of children's behavior (Jonisha asked Eddie to join her at the sand box). Anecdotal records are often jotted down on index cards, large-sized adhesive labels, or Post-its™, and can be as rich in detail as you want.

Running records are a narrative sample of what you see and hear during a specified period of time—usually between 2 and 20 minutes. How long you spend doing a running record depends on the time available, the presence of another adult who can watch the children while you observe, and the purpose of the observation. (Remember, lots can happen in even 2 to 3 minutes.) For example, seeing how children build with blocks might require more time than observing the effectiveness of your morning drop-off procedures.

Checklists are observations of a specific list of items, skills, or behaviors. Checking off an item indicates that the observed child performed the skill or behavior.

Rating scales require you to use a scale to judge the degree to which a child exhibits a specific behavior. Rating scales usually are numerical (on a scale of 1 to 5) or use descriptive phrases to cover a range of behaviors.

Sampling observations record behavior over a period of time or during a particular event. In time sampling, you record what children are doing at set intervals, such as every 10 or 15 minutes. In event sampling, you add up the number of times that children engage in a specific behavior, such as using the outdoor play equipment.

Videotaped observations allow you to study children in their natural setting with no exaggeration or distortion. Because videotapes are capable of instant replay and freeze framing, you can use them for in-depth investigation.

As you become a more skilled observer, you will probably make use of all these forms. However, you may want to begin with only one or two types of observations, and then progress to other approaches. We suggest that a good way to begin is by keeping anecdotal and running records. These methods are straightforward, do not require use of any standardized forms, and provide rich data.

On the following pages are sample anecdotal and running records that La Toya recorded as she observed Valisha. As you read through them, think about how this information can help La Toya in planning for Valisha.

Sample Anecdotal Records

Date	Observations
9/12/98	I spent 20 minutes with Valisha today reading every book I have about cats! She must have asked me to read Millions of Cats a million times. She held onto the books and pointed to the pictures when I asked questions. She's got most of our cat books memorized.
9/23/98	Valisha got very angry when I wouldn't let her bring Iris, the cat from next door, into the house. Nothing I said to her made any difference. When I firmly said "No," she had a real temper tantrum.
10/2/98	Valisha spent almost 30 minutes today stacking blocks. This caught my attention, because she usually gets angry and quits if she encounters any problems. I noticed that she watched Eddie making a tower and then went over to build next to him.
10/7/98	Valisha asked if I would help her write a letter to her brother Patrice, who is in Port-of-Spain visiting their Granny and aunts and uncles. I suggested we do a tape recording so that she could send him a letter he could hear. Valisha's face lit up at the suggestion, and she immediately went to fetch Jonisha to join in. She then suggested we tape her and Jonisha playing the steel drums.
10/8/98	Valisha napped for two full hours today. This seems to have become her pattern.

Sample Running Records

Child: Valisha Curtis

Age: 33 months

Date: 10/15/98

Observer: La Toya Thompkins

Time: Began: 10:10 AM Ended: 10:20 AM

Setting: Kitchen. Mrs. Cruickshank (Eddie's mother) is helping Valisha, Jonisha, and Eddie soak fruit for a holiday black cake

Mrs. C. entered the kitchen. V. ran to her, and hugged her. Mrs. C. greeted each child by name and turned toward Valisha, who was pulling at her pant leg. "Mrs. C., Mrs. C.," said Valisha, "did you see my Granny when you went home? Did you see Auntie Janice and Uncle Vic? Did Granny send anything for me?"

Mrs. C. stooped over to hug Valisha and told her that she didn't get to see her relatives because she had been in San Fernando where her own relatives lived, not Port-of-Spain. Valisha nodded. Mrs. C. started explaining how they were going to make the black cake.

"Can I help? Can I help?" asked Valisha, flashing a big smile to Mrs. C. Mrs.C. said she could help by soaking the prunes and the raisins. "Let's go," said Valisha, leading Mrs. C. to the table where the fruit was sitting in bags.

Child: Valisha Curtis

Age: 33 months

Date: 10/24/98

Observer: La Toya Thompkins (tape recorded)

Time: Began: 4:15 PM Ended: 4:20 PM

Setting: Outdoors

"Please, please," Valisha kept repeating. "I want to play ball with the boys." "I know you do Valisha. But you're just getting over bronchitis, and you shouldn't be running around. Why don't you take this book over to the picnic table instead?" Valisha grabbed the book out of my hand, yelled "No," and threw the book on the ground. "That's not how we treat our books," I said. "Please pick it up." Scowling all the while, Valisha picked up the book and handed it to me. "I'm sorry, Valisha," I said. "I know you'd like to play with the boys, but it's not a good idea until you're feeling better. Can you think of something more quiet you'd like to do?" Valisha took a moment and then her face lit up as she said, "Fluffy." "That'd be fine," I said. "Why don't you get Fluffy and some of the other stuffed animals and bring them outside to play with us."

Organizing Your Observations

To make use of your observations, you need to have some method of organizing the information you've collected. One way is to keep a portfolio—samples of children's actual work (artwork or tape recordings of their singing); photos of their work (making playdough, building with blocks, preparing snack); written records (logs of books children have had read to them, comments by children on their work); and systematic observations.

La Toya keeps portfolios to plan and individualize, to track children's progress, and to share information with families. Here's a sampling of what's inside Valisha's portfolio:

- ❖ background information
- ❖ injury/incident reports
- ❖ dated artwork (fingerpainting, drawings, paintings, collage)
- ❖ photographs of Valisha cooking peas and rice, playing dress-up
- ❖ log of books that La Toya has read one-on-one with Valisha
- ❖ audiotape of Valisha and Jonisha singing a calypso song
- ❖ anecdotal records
- ❖ running records
- ❖ event sampling
- ❖ the *Individualizing Goals and Objectives for Toddlers* form

Samples of background information and event sampling are shown below.

Background Information

Child: Valisha Curtis

Home Language: English

Parent(s)/Guardian(s): Yvonne and Johnny Curtis

Date: 9/7/98

Family History: Valisha and her sister Jonisha are identical twins, age 32 months when they entered the program. (Jonisha, unlike Valisha, wears eyeglasses due to a car accident when she was 21 months old.) The twins live with their parents and a brother Patrice (age 5) in an apartment complex in central Los Angeles, in a largely West Indian community. Valisha's mother is from Trinidad. She has a large, extended family living in Port-of-Spain. Valisha's father is originally from Oakland, California. Johnny and Yvonne have been married for four years. Johnny is a mechanic, taking courses to become an airline mechanic. Yvonne is a receptionist at Virgin Records. With her boss's encouragement, she recently enrolled at a local community college.

Johnny drops off the girls in the morning at 7:45 AM. Yvonne picks the children up at 6:30 PM.

Event Sampling:
Number of times Valisha offered to be a helper (assisted me or another child) on October 2nd:
Total—4 times

Putting It All Together: Using the Planning Form for Individualizing

Once you have observed and documented children's progress, you have a wealth of information you can use to individualize your program. The next step is to turn this information into a plan for action. This can best be done in two steps.

First, as noted at the beginning of this chapter, you'll want to summarize the information you've been collecting about a child's development onto the *Summary of Development* form every three months or so. This information can then be shared with the child's family.

The second step in the process is to put all of the information you now have at your fingertips into a usable format. For this, we suggest that you use the *Planning Form for Individualizing*. It is our thought that this can best be completed during a parent conference so that you and the child's family can together develop joint goals for their child's continued development.

To illustrate how these forms help in planning for a specific child, see the two sample forms on the next pages. The first one shows how LaToya summarized the information she had collected on Valisha using the *Summary of Development* form. The second one shows how LaToya and Valisha's parents together completed the *Planning Form for Individualizing*.

As you read the forms, remember that every child in your program should receive the same attention given Valisha. And each child will benefit from the knowledge you gain through careful observations and planning.

Summary of Development

Name of child: _Valisha Curtis_

Date: _11/20/98_

Comment on what you learned about this child in any of the following areas of development.

What is the child learning about:

Self:

Valisha has a strong self-concept. She is proud of her family and her heritage. She is independent, self-confident, and likes to be a helper to me and others. She is very "twin conscious."

Feelings:

Valisha is brimming with emotions—that she doesn't always know how to handle. She is beginning to redirect her anger, but she still needs to work on this. Valisha takes her emotional cues from her sister. For example, when Jonisha sulks, Valisha mimics her.

Others:

While Valisha shows occasional interest in her peers, her sister remains her main play interest. She is happy to be a helper on her own, though.

Communicating:

Valisha is extremely verbal and enjoys telling stories, reciting rhymes, singing songs, and acting out dramatic stories. She adores books—especially <u>Millions of Cats</u>.

Moving and Doing:

Valisha is quite proficient in the gross motor area. She runs, climbs, and balances herself on one foot with ease. Her self-help skills are also excellent. She has mastered toileting. Valisha's fine motor skills pose some problems for her. She can't yet use scissors without becoming frustrated and angry.

Thinking:

Valisha is skilled at problem solving, doing simple puzzles, and figuring things out for herself.

Planning Form for Individualizing

Name of child: _Valisha Curtis_   **Parent(s)/Guardian(s):** _Yvonne & Johnny Curtis_

Date of birth: _1/2/96_   **Caregiver/Teacher:** _La Toya Thompkins_

Date completed: _12/2/98 (35 months)_

This child likes

Anything having to do with cats, including her favorite book <u>Millions of Cats</u> (by Wanda Gag); being a helper; West Indian culture; soft, cuddly toys; and being a twin.

This child's temperament is

Outgoing, active, and lively. She is very verbal and engages everyone in conversation; she is usually ready to join in new activities. She is quick to anger, though—especially when frustrated or not allowed to have her way. She echos Jonisha's moods and facial expressions.

This child learns best by

Observing and then doing things for herself. She follows verbal directions well. She likes to practice skills on her own.

This child's special needs are

Needs help to deal with her emotions when she begins feeling out of contro. She is dependent upon her sister for emotional cues. Needs longer naps than other children her age.

To individualize for this child, I intend to make these changes:

To the environment (including equipment & materials):

Ask Reggie to build a climbing structure to go with the outdoor playhouse he built. Provide more soft toys for Valisha to cuddle during dramatic play. Encourage Valisha to do sensory activities, such as sand and water play, art, or dramatic play. These activities will provide outlets for expressing her emotions in safe, appropriate ways.

To routines, transitions, and planned activities:

Give Valisha lots of opportunities to help do "real work." Encourage her mastery of the self-help skills she is working on now. Avoid focusing too much on the helper role—she's still a little girl and needs lots of opportunities to just have fun. However, since this is an area where Valisha thrives independently of Jonisha, I want to encourage her talents.

To the daily schedule:

Allow Valisha to nap as long as she needs to—even if the other children are up and ready for their snack. Valisha can have her snack when she gets up—it's more important for her to get the sleep she needs to function well.

To interactions:

Help Valisha to express her strong feelings in appropriate ways—take deep breaths, count to 10, and express her anger or frustration by stomping her foot rather than hitting.

When I work with Valisha on new skills such as using a scissors, I should give her lots of opportunities to do these things herself as that's how she learns best.

Using the Goals for Working with Families Form

Throughout this curriculum, we have emphasized the importance of family in a young child's life. It is for this reason that in Chapter 5 we included goals and objectives for your work with families in addition to goals and objectives for children.

We believe that to serve a child well, you must also individualize your program to serve that child's family. For this reason, we have developed the *Goals for Working with Families* form. You can use this form, which appears in Appendix B, to document your work with each family and to evaluate your progress in achieving each goal and objective. There are two different sections to complete.

Documentation of what was done. In this section, you record what you've done to meet a particular objective and indicate when that activity took place. You'll find that by implementing *The Creative Curriculum for Infants & Toddlers,* you will be addressing many of the objectives for working with families in the course of your everyday activities. For example, if you have sent home copies of the letters to families that are included in chapters 7–23 of the *Curriculum,* you can list this activity under the Objective, "To provide families with strategies for supporting children's learning at home," which comes under Goal 3: To support families in their role as primary educators of their child. (You'll note in the example below that La Toya has done this.)

Next steps. This section asks you to reflect on what else you might do to further a particular objective. Your responses to this section should fit what you already know about this family's make-up and needs.

Again, using La Toya as an example, the following pages show what a completed form might look like. With this information, La Toya can make the accommodations to her program she's listed under "Next Steps." This will enable her to serve the Curtis family even more successfully. Like La Toya, when you individualize your program for children and families, you plan for high quality.

Goals for Working with Families

Parent(s)/Guardian(s): _Yvonne and Johnny Curtis_   **Child:** _Valisha Curtis_

Completed by: _La Toya Thompkins_

Goal 1: To build a partnership with families	
Objectives	**Notes (Date each entry)**
To involve families in the program's planning and evaluation process	During our initial meeting, I asked Yvonne and Johnny what their goals are for Valisha while she's in my care. (8/30/98)
To listen to and discuss families' questions, concerns, observations, and insights about their children	Yvonne and I had tea together. She asked my advice about a number of topics—hitting, biting, if the twins should be separated, etc. (9/12/98)
To communicate regularly with families at arrival and departure times about how things are going for their child at home and at the program	I talk with Johnny every morning and Yvonne every evening about how the twins' day went. (daily)
To schedule regular conferences and/or home visits	First conference. (12/2/98)
To discuss with families ways to handle children's challenging behaviors	Valisha has hit Jonisha both here and at home. We're all working on ways to redirect her anger. We've seen some progress.
To resolve differences with families in a respectful way	So far we haven't had any differences that need to be resolved. We've been a good team!
To help families gain access to community resources	I do know that Yvonne's taking night school classes that her job is paying for.

Next steps:

I intend to meet with the children's parents formally once a month — not just in the informal ways I do now. I'll inquire if Yvonne needs any further support, now that she's going to school at night.

Goal 2: To support families in their parenting role

Objectives	Notes (Date each entry)
To demonstrate respect for a family's approach to childrearing and their feelings about sharing the care of their child	I always talk with the Curtises about discipline matters. We think together about how best to handle things. I want to make sure Valisha gets consistent messages from me and her parents. (9/22/98)
To celebrate with families each new milestone in their child's development	When Valisha became toilet trained (without accidents after naps), I bought her some "big girl" panties to wear at home. (9/20/98) I always send home artwork and creations—such as her first sculpture. (10/6/98)
To incorporate family rituals and preferences into the daily life of the program	Before naptime, I sing the children a Trinidadian lullaby Yvonne taught me. It's quite similar to the ones we sing in Jamaica.
To offer workshops/training on child development and other topics of interest to families	
To help families network with one another for information and support	I sponsored a potluck supper so all the families could get to know one another. It was very successful. (10/3/98)

Next steps:

I need to ask parents if they'd like to have a workshop on any particular topics. If so, I'll coordinate with my providers' association. It might be fun to have an expert on twins come speak—since 2 other providers I know care for twins and one has a set of triplets!

Goal 3: To support families in their role as primary educators of their child

Objectives	Notes (Date each entry)
To encourage family involvement and participation in program activities	I've asked the Curtises to join us on field trips, but so far they haven't been able to because of their jobs. (9/27/98)
To provide families with strategies to support children's learning at home	I've given the Curtises the Letters for Families on Health, Safety, Hellos and Good-byes, Art, and Books. We've discussed them and they've given me feedback on what they've tried. (a letter a week in September & October)

Next steps:

Find a way for the Curtises to become involved in the program that won't interfere with their jobs. Continue giving out Letters to Families and discussing them with the Curtises.

Goal 4: To ensure that the home cultures of the children's families are reflected in the program

Objectives	Notes (Date each entry)
To support children's use of their home language	English is the first language for all of us. We all use West Indian sayings when we speak.
To encourage children's awareness of and interest in home languages spoken at the program	Not applicable.
To seek the families' assistance in learning about the children's home culture	When Valisha's Uncle Ronnie was visiting, he came over to show the children how to play classical music on the steel drums. Ronnie's a semi-professional musician (he plays with the Amoco Renegades) and it was super. (9/6/98)
To include objects and customs from the children's home culture in the program's environment, routines, and activities	We have a pan (steel drums) in the music area along with Carnival costumes. The children love to dance to calypso and soca. (I can occasionally get them to hear some reggae.) We prepare lots of West Indian foods at mealtimes and snack (e.g., caloloo, pelau, peas and rice, macaroni pie). (daily)
To interact with children in a style that is respectful of their home culture	Being West Indian myself, this is no problem for me. I place great value on family and try never to undermine any relative. (daily)

Next steps:

Continue doing the same types of activities. I'll ask the parents for any suggestions.

Creating a Welcoming Environment

One of the first steps in implementing the program you've planned is to set up your home or center. It should be both a welcoming place for children and families and a pleasant and efficient place in which you can work. The environment you create has a profound effect on the feelings and actions of the children in your care, their families, and on you, yourself.

Children will spend most of their waking hours in your program. A new environment, no matter how welcoming, can be unsettling for them. They will probably be most comfortable when they are in a place that feels "homelike." A familiar environment produces the same feelings of safety and security they experience when they are with their own families. Thus, the trust children have built at home needs to be transferred to this new environment.

A warm and friendly environment can also be very reassuring to families. Areas specifically designed with families in mind send the message that they, as well as children, are always welcome. Environments that reflect children's backgrounds and special needs offer further security to children and families. You want to be sure that your program's environment communicates a sense of trust and security to all children and families.

Finally, because you also spend most of your work time in this environment, it should be a place where you enjoy spending time. If you design your environment so that you can work efficiently, you will have the time and energy you need to relate to each child in a caring, unhurried, and nurturing way.

In this chapter you will learn about:

- ❖ planning a responsive environment for infants and toddlers;
- ❖ arranging the environment to convey positive messages;
- ❖ creating appropriate indoor spaces;
- ❖ defining play areas outdoors;
- ❖ selecting and organizing materials;
- ❖ adapting the environment for children with special needs; and
- ❖ including children's families and cultures in the environment.

Planning a Responsive Environment

Because infants and toddlers grow and change so quickly, the environment must be changed continually to provide new challenges and inspire new interests, as shown on the chart below.

Planning a Responsive Environment		
What Children Can Do	**Ways You Can Arrange the Environment**	**How This Supports Development**
Young Infants Notice and watch what goes on around them.	Place pictures on the wall at child's eye level.	Encourages infants to focus and attend to objects.
Reach for, bat, and poke at objects.	Hang mobiles where infants can see and kick them.	Teaches infants they can have an impact on the world.
Respond to being held and rocked.	Have comfortable places for holding infants, such as soft chairs and hammocks.	Builds relationships and a sense of trust.
Developing the ability to sit and crawl.	Install soft carpet so infants can crawl comfortably.	Promotes physical development.
Mobile Infants Pull themselves up to a standing position.	Be sure furniture is sturdy, with protected edges. Use mats with a variety of surfaces.	Allows mobile infants to explore in safety and builds large muscles.
Push, pull, fill, and dump objects.	Offer a variety of playthings, including household objects.	Builds motor skills as well as coordination.
Take comfort from familiar objects and reminders of home.	Display pictures of family members and invite families to make audiotapes.	Helps children feel safe and secure. Reduces separation anxiety.
Sometimes need to be alone.	Create private spaces.	Helps children develop a sense of self.
Toddlers Walk, run, climb, and play with objects and toys.	Arrange the space so toddlers can move around safely.	Allows toddlers to explore freely and independently.
	Organize toys on low shelves and label them with pictures.	Promotes independence because toddler can find and return toys on their own.
Sometimes want to do more than they can do.	Offer materials and activities that meet children's level of development.	Provides a variety of appropriate challenges so toddlers experience a sense of their own competence.
Play alongside and also with others.	Define areas where two or three children can play. Provide duplicates of toys.	Promotes the ability to engage in sustained and purposeful play.

Arranging the Environment to Convey Positive Messages

Have you ever watched children when they first enter a new environment? They look around and try to decide what kind of place it is. If you could read their minds, they might be asking themselves:

- ❖ Do I feel comfortable here?
- ❖ Do people know who I am and do they like me?
- ❖ Is this a place I can trust and where I can feel safe?
- ❖ Can I explore and go wherever I want?
- ❖ Can I count on people to take care of me?

Your daily interactions with infants and toddlers—the caring way in which you hold them, meet their needs, and encourage them to explore their world—are the most important way you answer these very typical questions and concerns. However, how you organize the physical environment also sends powerful messages to children and their families. Listed below are five positive messages you can send children and examples of how the environment can convey these messages.

"This place is comfortable."

- ❖ Special blankets and toys from home are in each child's crib or cubby.
- ❖ Familiar household objects—aluminum pots and pans, utensils, plastic containers—are available as play materials.
- ❖ There are home-like touches—plants, curtains, pillows covered in attractive fabrics, a fish tank.
- ❖ Cuddling places are available—stuffed chairs, couches, rocking chairs, and hammocks.
- ❖ There are "nooks and crannies" in which children can snuggle and feel protected.

"We know who you are and we like you. You belong here."

- ❖ Pictures of children and their families are displayed at a child's eye level and are laminated so children can touch them.
- ❖ There are places for each child to store belongings from home.
- ❖ Pictures and materials reflect the ethnic and individual characteristics of children and families.
- ❖ A message board tells parents about each child's day.

"This is a place you can trust."

- ❖ Furniture is arranged so children can explore freely and not get hurt.
- ❖ Toys and books are consistently displayed in the same places so children know where to find them.
- ❖ There are soft places where children can crawl and walk without fear of being hurt if they fall.
- ❖ Sick children have a comfortable place where they can rest or wait until their parents come.

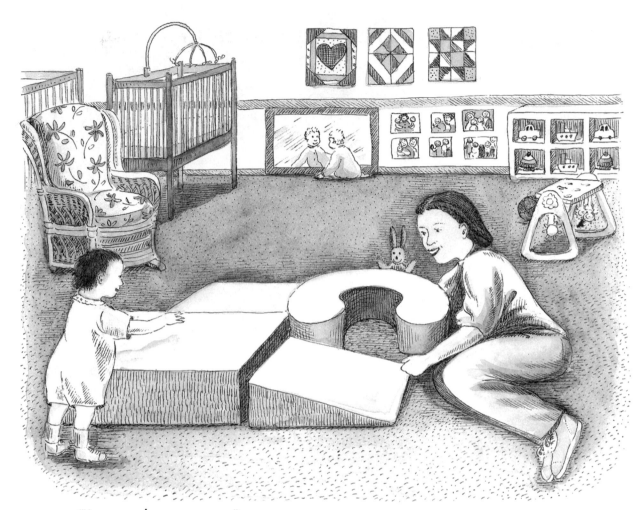

"You can explore on your own."

❖ Areas that are off limits are blocked so children can't get there.

❖ Walls are decorated with interesting pictures and textures children can touch.

❖ Electrical outlets are covered and the rooms have been "child-proofed."

❖ Toys are on low shelves with picture labels so children know where to find and return them.

"We will take care of you."

❖ Child-adult ratios are low, group sizes are small, and each child has a primary caregiver.

❖ Changing tables are comfortable and safe; everything needed is within reach.

❖ Each child has his or her own crib or cot for resting.

❖ Food preparation is efficient so children can be fed on their individual schedules.

Take a look around your program setting. What messages do children receive? Consider the examples listed above and think about whether there are any changes you want to make.

Creating Indoor Spaces

Most of your day with infants and toddlers is spent in routines and activities. The daily routines of saying hello and good-bye, preparing and eating food, napping, diapering and toileting, and dressing occupy much of a young child's day—and therefore much of yours. As infants become more mobile, they need places to explore safely. They are ready for activities such as playing with toys and blocks, exploring sand and water and art materials, cooking, music and movement, and exploring books. These routines and activities translate into the following types of spaces you may want for your indoor environment:

- ❖ a greeting area;
- ❖ a food preparation and eating area;
- ❖ a sleeping area;
- ❖ a changing area and bathroom; and
- ❖ play areas with spaces for both active and quiet play; individual and group play.

If you work in a center-based program, you will need to create the areas described above. A counter-top with a bottle warmer and small refrigerator may serve as your kitchen, and you may define a play area with movable, low shelves or furniture. In a family child care home, these places exist naturally. Your own family members may feel less intruded upon if you ask them to help you figure out how to arrange your home for child care—and still preserve their sense of privacy. In either setting, arrange the indoor space to be inviting to children and an easy place to work. Here are some guidelines to keep in mind.

Include special touches. Think about places you enjoy. What makes them special? Is it the decorative touches, such as plants and pictures? Is it the soft furniture and reading materials that invite you to sit down and relax? These same features can make a family child care home or center just as welcoming to children and families.

Avoid overstimulating children. Even if you have all the toys and materials anyone could want, resist the temptation to put everything out. Think how overwhelming a warehouse store filled with merchandise can be. Displaying a few carefully selected toys on low shelves is more likely to lead to purposeful play than shelves with many playthings.

Allow for movement. Movement, as we discussed in Chapter 2, is essential for a child's healthy development. Children who are in an environment where they are free to move safely will develop the physical skills that help them feel competent.

Be aware of how space affects behavior. Large open spaces encourage mobile infants and toddlers to run and use their large muscles. Small, enclosed areas promote social interaction and make it easier to concentrate. Your environment should offer both types of spaces.

Make each space easy-to-maintain. Ideally, you'll use washable area rugs to cover areas where children will crawl or move. You'll have children eat and do messy activities in spaces with washable flooring. If your environment includes spaces that aren't washable, you can use an old shower curtain to cover the floor during messy activities.

Organize and label storage space. Take the time to assess what you need so you'll know where to put things. Place shelves, bins, and hooks where you can reach them easily. Make picture labels to show where children's toys and belongings belong. Good storage allows you full use of your resources, and makes it easy for a substitute caregiver/teacher.

Minimize the physical strain on your body. Take care to avoid back problems that may result from lifting and holding infants and toddlers. Be sure there are comfortable places with good support for you to sit with children. Install sturdy steps so toddlers can climb up to a changing area.

Continually evaluate how the environment is working. Observe how children use the space and how they react to changes you make. Be prepared to make adjustments to meet the changing needs and growing abilities of infants and toddlers.

The chart on the facing page shows how indoor areas can meet the needs of infants, toddlers, and adults. In addition to the spaces identified on the chart, mobile infants and toddlers will benefit from defined spaces for a variety of play activities.

❖ **Imitating and pretending.** Items such as simple dress-up clothes (hats, assorted bags), a toddler-sized table, chairs, cooking utensils, and dolls inspire dramatic play. Prop boxes can be used anywhere.

❖ **Playing with toys.** This area might have a carpeted platform, rug, or low table. You can store small toys such as pop beads, puzzles, sorting games, and small blocks in labeled dishpans. Cardboard or plastic blocks, and a few props are all toddlers need for construction and building activities.

❖ **Enjoying stories and books.** You can display books in see-through holders hung on the wall, or stand the books on a low shelf. Soft places to sit, such as a covered mattress or a pillow invite children to settle in with a book.

❖ **Dabbling in art.** This area should be set up on washable floors and located near a sink. It might include a table, low easels, and shelves with paper, colored markers, crayons, and playdough.

❖ **Tasting and preparing food.** Utensils and ingredients for a cooking activity can be brought out and used on a low table so that mobile infants and toddlers can easily participate.

❖ **Exploring sand and water.** Outdoors, sand and water play can take place in tubs, sand boxes, or wading pools. Indoors, children can use a low sink, shallow dish pans placed on low tables, or a sand and water table. Props may include basters, plastic containers, rubber animals, funnels, and scoops.

❖ **Having fun with music and movement.** You'll probably want to locate a tape player and tapes in a place that is convenient for you. Musical instruments might be stored in a box and brought out when needed.

How Indoor Areas Can Meet the Needs of Infants, Toddlers, and Adults

Area	Infants	Toddlers	Adults
Greeting Area	Bulletin board for parent notices; cubbies or individual storage tubs; photos of children at play and with their families; children's artwork; bench or adult-height counter to make dressing and undressing children easier; comfortable seating for adults.		
Sleeping Area	Cribs, bassinets, or cradles set apart to accommodate different sleep schedules; mobiles to look at; restful colors	Mats/cots; special toys and blankets from home; restful colors	Chairs/hammocks to sit in and cuddle children or to watch them nap or play quietly
Eating Area	Infant seats, high chairs, and tables with support chairs in an area with a washable floor; supply of bottles and child-size eating utensils	Low tables and chairs in an area with a washable floor; plastic dishes and cups; child-sized utensils; small pitchers; paper towels for spills	Sink and counter storage for food, trays, and utensils; serving and clean-up equipment; some places to sit and feed babies, such as rocking chairs
Diapering/ Toileting	Wall-mounted, large unbreakable mirror; soft toys to hold and watch; changing table with raised lip	Changing table with steps; potty chairs or low toilets; steps up to a sink to wash hands; soap and paper towels where children can reach them; waste baskets conveniently placed	Convenient location near sink or bathrooms; covered diaper pail; changing tables at 36"; shelves with supplies easily accessible; spray bottle with bleach solution
Gross Motor Play	Mats and protected areas in which to roll over, crawl, sit, and pull up; shatterproof mirrors; pictures of babies, families, and animals to look at	Open spaces for active play; furniture for climbing, sliding, and stepping up and down; large cubes/blocks; riding toys; tumble mats; tunnels; large cardboard boxes to crawl into	Movable, low dividers to define spaces
Quiet Play	Infant seating with grasping toys within reach where infants can watch the action; backpacks	Lofts/platforms on which to sit; soft chairs; a stocked aquarium with cover on a bottom shelf; tape player and tapes	Comfortable places to sit, cuddle, and read

Learning from Others

Many people find it helpful to visit other programs to see different ways of organizing space. You can join a tour of homes run by your local family child care association, or exchange visits with another provider or with the staff from a nearby center. During your visit, ask yourself questions such as the following.

- ❖ What areas can I identify?

- ❖ Is each area inviting for children and adults? In what ways could each space be made more inviting?

- ❖ Can adults easily reach the materials they need to carry out routines and activities efficiently?

- ❖ Are there clear pathways so children and adults can get to and around the various areas?

- ❖ How does the space make it easy for adults to supervise and take care of children? Are any improvements needed?

- ❖ Are there places for children to be alone—away from the "crowd"—when they desire?

When you return, ask yourself the same questions about your environment. A few changes can really make a difference to you and to the children.

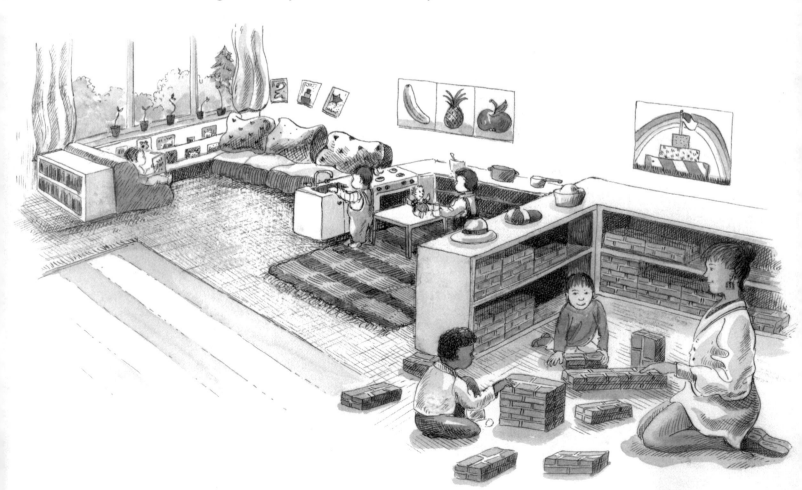

Defining Play Areas Outdoors

Time outdoors each day is important for children's physical health and emotional well-being. Children love to be outdoors, even when the weather isn't perfect. A change of scenery and fresh air is also beneficial for you.

Think about what you enjoyed doing most outdoors when you were a child. Do you recall rolling down a grassy hill? Looking up at the sky and watching the clouds change shape? Jumping from curbs and low walls? Running as fast as you could? Picking bouquets of flowers? Collecting leaves? Watching bugs? The outdoor environment offers many different kinds of experiences for children—it truly doubles the learning environment.

Going Outdoors Must Be Manageable

To make the time spent outdoors fun for the children and enjoyable for you takes some planning. As always, children's developmental abilities can guide your decisions.

Young infants want to look around and take in the action. To spend time outdoors with young infants, you need:

- a way to transport them outside;
- enclosed spaces where infants can reach, grasp, roll, and kick freely;
- soft places such as grass, colorful blankets, or mats;
- elevated swings in which infants can safely take in the sights; and
- shade or covered areas.

Mobile infants are going to crawl and cruise as they explore the outdoors. Think about these additions to your outdoor space:

- mats, cardboard boxes, and tunnels;
- plastic railings children can hold onto;
- logs and tree stumps children can pull up on and straddle;
- containers children can fill and dump;
- seat swings, low to the ground; and
- tires embedded in the sand.

Toddlers will run, climb, jump, push, pull, haul, and dump when they get outside. An outdoor space for toddlers should include a variety of surfaces (soft and hard) and a range of equipment. Here are some ideas that will delight most toddlers:

- balls of all sizes and textures;
- wagons, buckets, and baskets that children can fill, haul, and dump;
- riding toys, carts, and push and pull toys;
- hollow blocks, plastic crates, ladders, and planks for creating new structures;
- low easels with chalk, paint, or colored markers;
- brushes and buckets for painting with water;
- sand boxes (covered when not in use) and props for digging and pouring;
- sling swings, hung low so children can swing on their tummies;
- small slides and rocking toys children can use on their own;

❖ water play containers and materials, finger paints, and playdough; and

❖ musical instruments.

Don't forget to consider your own comfort outdoors. Benches, a porch swing, soft mats, or logs can be good perches from which to keep a watchful eye on the children and engage them in activities as you cuddle others on your lap.

Evaluate your outdoor space and think about whether it offers children age-appropriate challenges and experiences. Consider activities you offer children indoors that they could do outdoors equally well. You will find many suggestions of indoor activities you can take outside in the activity chapters.

Selecting and Organizing Materials

The materials you select make your environment an interesting place for infants and toddlers to investigate and explore. Safety—which is addressed in detail in the next chapter—is always the first concern. Check every day to be sure that toys and play equipment are in good condition—that is, they have no broken parts, chipping paint, or splinters. Remove anything with parts that are small enough for a child to swallow. (If an object can fit into an empty film container, it is too small for infants and toddlers.)

Materials Should Reflect Children's Interests and Abilities

For very **young infants,** you are by far the most interesting part of the environment. An adult who responds to their sounds, expressions, and actions is better than any "busy box." Infants are attracted to variations in color, contrast, design, and texture in materials, toys, and carpets. An uncluttered background makes it easier for them to focus on interesting objects and shapes. They will track and respond to the movements of a mobile, particularly if it makes noise. Once infants begin to hold on to objects and explore more actively, their toys and materials must be chewable, washable, and easy to grasp. Anything that responds to their actions by making a noise or moving will encourage infants to continue exploring —and learning.

Mobile infants who can crawl, climb, or walk to get what they want will be attracted to toys and materials that are displayed at their eye level. Everyday objects such as wooden spoons, buckets, pots and pans, hats, and telephones are as fascinating as anything you can purchase in a toy store. Mobile infants are ready for new challenges that allow them to test out their new skills: stacking, filling and dumping, pushing and pulling, and fitting objects together. As they get older and more mobile, they will enjoy ride-on toys, low climbing structures, and materials that promote pretend play. Dolls, cars and trucks, balls, and push and pull toys are very popular with this age group.

Toddlers, with their strong drive to be independent and increasing gross and fine motor skills, benefit from an environment that offers them opportunities to manipulate and explore objects for a purpose. Toddlers especially like materials they can sort, match, fit together, or arrange in an interesting way. Providing duplicates of popular materials minimizes the need to share and makes it easier for toddlers to relate in positive ways to one another. With their increased fine motor skills, toddlers enjoy exploring and creating with art materials such as playdough, paint, and crayons. They increasingly engage in pretend play: a block can become a car; a toy telephone can inspire a lengthy phone conversation; a variety of hats, props, and dolls can lead to dramatic play.

In deciding which toys and materials to put out and when, ask yourself the following questions.

❖ Will the toy interest infants and toddlers?

❖ Will they be able to use these materials safely?

❖ Do children have the skills to handle the toy?

❖ Will this toy help children learn?

The list that follows offers some suggested toys and materials. You will find more detailed lists for young infants, mobile infants, and toddlers in each of the activity chapters in Part IV.

To promote fine motor skills:

Rattles	Clutch balls	Containers to fill and dump
Bean bags	Busy boxes	Cardboard boxes with lids
Stacking rings	Interlocking blocks	Large wooden beads and shoelaces
Nesting cups	Shape sorting boxes	Wooden and rubber puzzles (3 to 8 pieces)

To promote gross motor skills:

Riding toys	Large cardboard boxes	Balls of all sizes
Climber and slide	Push and pull toys	Low steps covered with carpet
Wagons	Tumbling mats	Foam furniture covered with vinyl
Tractor tires	Cars and trucks	

To encourage children to use their senses:

Playdough	Large nontoxic crayons	Paper for coloring and tearing
Finger paint	Sand and water table with containers and scoops	Ribbons, scarves, and fabrics

To inspire dramatic play:

Dolls	Suitcases	Doll beds or shoe-box beds
Telephones	Plastic dishes	Full length mirrors
Dress-up clothes	Pots and pans	Hats and simple dress-up clothes

To encourage children to explore shape, size, and balance:

Sponge blocks	Hollow or unit blocks	Rubber animals
People props	Large cardboard blocks	Small cars and trucks

To invite quiet, peaceful play:

Tape recorder	Cardboard and cloth books	Picture books for toddlers
Bean bag chairs	Soft cushions	Music and story tapes

To engage children in cooking:

Potato mashers	Metal or plastic bowls	Utensils
Wooden spoons	Plastic knives	Plastic measuring cups and spoons

The Value of "Beautiful Junk"

How many times have you heard about a child ignoring a new toy and playing with a cardboard box instead? Toys don't have to be expensive and new to be good. With the help of children's parents, you can collect many materials—for example, an empty appliance box to crawl through and dramatic play props such as pots and pans, hats, and telephones. You can make toys, too. An oatmeal box and wooden spools make a great "drop-in and dump-out" toy. The lid of a used "wipes" box can be cut out to fit shape blocks. Magazine pictures can be mounted on cardboard, laminated, and cut into three pieces to make simple puzzles. Keep in mind, too, that garage sales or second-hand stores often have many inexpensive resources.

How You Display Materials Is Important

The way children use and care for materials may depend, in large part, on the way the materials are organized and displayed. Here are some suggestions for organizing and displaying toys and materials.

- ❖ **Display toys that children can safely play with on their own.** Arrange toys neatly on low shelves so children can reach them safely.

- ❖ **Remember that less can be more.** Young children are easily overwhelmed. Display a few carefully selected toys.

- ❖ **Display toys on a surface painted in a neutral color.** Leave space between materials so children can see what is available and choose exactly what they want.

- ❖ **Store toys with small pieces in clear plastic containers.** You may want to store some toys with many pieces on higher shelves to avoid chaos.

- ❖ **Place picture labels on containers and shelves.** This shows that everything has a place and helps children participate in cleaning up. Make labels from photographs, pictures in catalogs, or draw them on cardboard.

Adapting the Environment for Children with Special Needs

To fully include children with special needs in your program, you may need to make some changes to the physical environment. The changes or additions will depend on the type of disability and the severity. Your objective is to enable the child with special needs to participate and interact as fully as possible—to be part of the action!

Physical Challenges

Most of the furniture and equipment described in this chapter and in the activity chapters in Part IV is appropriate for children with physical disabilities. For example, a pool of balls, soft mats to crawl on, tumble forms to climb over are all usable. In some instances, though, you may need to modify the arrangement of furniture and obtain adaptive equipment.

If you have a child who is in a wheel chair or who uses a walker to get from one area to another, take a careful look at your space to see where barriers exist. You may need to increase the size of a doorway, rearrange tables or play areas, and install ramps and grab bars in the bathroom, so that a child (or family member) in a wheelchair can have access to the program environment.

Outdoor time is important for all children. Hammock swings can provide the support and stability a child needs to feel comfortable and view the changing scenes. A therapy ball is a large ball that can be used to sit or lie on to challenge a child's balancing skills or to provide various forms of sensorimotor experiences. It can be used to stimulate a child's motor reactions, or to relax a child with hypertonic reactions (spasms). Children who have seizure disorders or problems with balance may need to wear a helmet to protect their head in case they fall. These are just a few examples of ways you can ensure access to outdoor play for all children.

To participate fully in some activities and during small group times, children with physical disabilities may need assistance in order to sit. A beanbag chair or a large pillow can be molded to provide the support needed. In addition, there are a variety of specialized chairs available as described below.

- ❖ **Educube chair** is a hard chair with a raised back and sides that provides stability and support for a child who cannot maintain balance to sit.
- ❖ **Tumbleform chair** is a semi-hard foam chair that comes in various sizes and is used for children who cannot sit independently.
- ❖ **Pummel chair** is a hard chair designed for a child's specific needs and contains a pummel that is placed between the legs to separate the legs (typically seen with children who have cerebral palsy).

Children can learn to use materials and toys independently with the addition of bolsters and wedges. **Bolsters** are used to position a child either straddling or sitting to keep the child's legs apart, or, if the child lies prone across the bolster, to prop the arms forward and keep the head up. They come in various sizes to accommodate the size and special

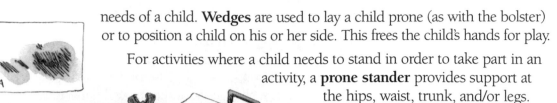

needs of a child. **Wedges** are used to lay a child prone (as with the bolster) or to position a child on his or her side. This frees the child's hands for play.

For activities where a child needs to stand in order to take part in an activity, a **prone stander** provides support at the hips, waist, trunk, and/or legs. This helps a toddler who cannot stand independently (such as a child with spina bifida) at a water table or easel.

Some simple adaptations can make it possible for a child with a disability to explore and learn from sensory activities such as art, cooking, and sand and water play. Some children are "tactily defensive"— they may not enjoy touching or using sensory materials such as paint, water, or playdough. Provide gloves, sticks, or paint brushes to allow these children to participate in the activity. Have on hand large markers and crayons for children who have a weak grasp, and attach Velcro™ straps to paint brushes or writing utensils to help a child who cannot maintain a grasp.

Sensory Impairments

If you have a child who is hearing impaired or who is blind, examine your environment from the child's perspective. Children with sensory impairments need clear sensory cues. An environment that has too many sights, sounds, smells, and textures can be overwhelming.

Children who are hearing impaired will use visual cues, touch, and vibration to interpret what is happening around them. Good room acoustics and a minimum of conflicting noises will help them to use what hearing they do have.

Children who are visually impaired learn to tune into the sounds and textures in their environment. The sounds of music, bubbles in a fish tank, and familiar voices are reassuring. A piece of felt or fur can help them identify their cubby. Clear pathways and well-defined areas, as well as textural cues, such as a defined line between the carpet and tile, help children know they have entered a new area.

Involving Specialists

It's important to keep in mind that you are not expected to be an expert. As in most situations, the best experts are the children's families. Additionally, there are resources to help you identify changes you can make so that your environment maximizes the opportunities for all children to participate as fully as possible.

If you have a child with a disability in your program, chances are he or she is receiving services from one or more specialists (for example, an occupational or physical therapist or an early childhood special educator). With parental permission, invite these individuals to come observe (and work with) the child in your environment. Specialists know a great deal about the particular challenges a child faces and how best to help that child meet those challenges. (See the discussion in Chapter 2 on Part C.) Ask for suggestions of ways to help the child be fully included and successful. Often the simplest suggestion can turn frustration and failure into an opportunity for success.

Including Children's Families and Cultures in the Environment

Family members are more likely to feel welcome if your environment conveys the message that you want and value their input and participation. Look around your home or center. In what ways does the physical environment suggest to families that they are welcome and considered important to your program?

During home visits, you can learn a great deal about how culture influences a family's environment. Think about what seems to be important to each family and find ways to incorporate some of these items into your environment. For example, a colored weaving from Bolivia might make a decorative wall hanging, and family photographs reinforce the connection between home and the program.

Listed below are messages that invite families to feel a part of the program, and some ways these messages can be conveyed by the environment.

"You are always welcome here."

❖ Make the entrance way attractive with decorative touches such as plants and pictures.

❖ Provide places for parents to hang their coats and safely store belongings.

❖ Hang a sign that conveys a welcoming message.

❖ Set up a schedule for parent volunteering and post a calendar.

"Transitions can be difficult; take your time."

❖ Allow space near children's cubbies where parents can linger with their children.

❖ Have adult-sized chairs for parents.

❖ Offer private spaces where mothers can nurse.

❖ Display photographs of children with their families in the entrance way.

"Make yourself at home; observe your child at play."

❖ Place a few adult-size chairs in the room where parents can sit and observe the program or join in a snack or meal.

❖ Display signs on room dividers or walls that explain what children are learning in each area of the room.

"Your interests, ideas, and help can enrich our program."

❖ Display and acknowledge examples of contributions families have made to the program.

❖ Create a suggestion box and invite parents to contribute ideas for the program.

❖ Select books and pictures that reflect the cultures of all families.

❖ Post a schedule of work days or "fix-it nights" to encourage family members to work together to improve the environment—such as building a sandbox for the outdoor play area, repairing toys, bringing fresh flowers, or painting a room.

"We are all learners."

❖ Create a bulletin board where you can display articles and information of interest to parents.

❖ Set aside a place where parents can sit and look through books and magazines on parenting and child development.

❖ Post information on adult education, GED classes, and conferences.

There are many ways to set up your environment so that it is warm and welcoming to children, family members, and to you. A primary consideration must be ensuring children's safety so that they are free to play and explore without fear of hurting themselves. This topic is covered in detail in the next chapter.

❖   ❖   ❖

— ❈ —

Sharing Thoughts About Our
Program Environment

Dear Families:

When you visit our program, the first thing you'll notice is how we've arranged our space. This is also what children notice. Therefore, we want our setting to be as welcoming, comfortable, and interesting as possible.

Our space for young infants (birth–8 months) has comfortable places where we can sit and hold them, soft carpet and mats for infants to lie on and crawl over, and places where they can safely watch the action. Because we know infants are learning all the time, we provide interesting objects for them to watch and to explore.

Our mobile infants (8–18 months) are eager to pull up on anything available, so we make sure all furniture is sturdy. Because they're interested in things that remind them of home, we've posted family pictures on the walls at their eye level.

Toddlers (18–36 months), as you well know, are constantly on the move. Therefore, we've arranged the space so they can explore freely and safely. You'll see lots of toys and materials that encourage toddlers to build, pretend, look at books, draw and mold, respond to and make music, and even cook.

How We Can Work Together

Your child will feel most comfortable if the program environment feels familiar. We need your help to build this connection between child care and home. Here are some suggestions to consider:

❖ *Bring us a few pictures of your child with family members.* After we cover them with clear Contact™ paper to protect them, we'll display them where your child can see them every day. Children love to have this connection with the most important people in their lives.
❖ *Make a tape for your child.* Record yourself reading your child's favorite stories or favorite songs that you sing together. We'll play these tapes during quiet periods of the day to remind children of their parents.
❖ *Tell us about your child's favorite things.* If you have some favorite books your child likes to read with you, or some music that you play on special holidays or events, we'd love to include it in our program, too. We believe it is very important for children to see aspects of their culture in the child care setting
❖ *Bring "loveys" from home.* If your child has a favorite toy or blanket that provides comfort for those times when he or she might miss family members, please feel free to bring it to the program.

We welcome your ideas and contributions to making our program a place where your child will be comfortable and happy.

Sincerely,

©1999, Teaching Strategies, Inc., Washington, DC. Permission granted to reprint, for non-commercial uses only, by programs implementing *The Creative Curriculum for Infants & Toddlers*.

Algunas ideas acerca del ambiente de aprendizaje de nuestro programa

Estimadas familias:

Cuando ustedes visiten nuestro programa, lo primero que notarán será cómo hemos organizado nuestro espacio. Para los niños más pequeños (recién nacidos – 8 meses) hay lugares cómodos en los que nos podemos sentar y sostenerlos, una alfombra suave y colchones para que los pequeños se acuesten o gateén, y lugares en los que pueden observar lo que ocurre sin ningún peligro. Porque sabemos que los infantes aprenden todo el tiempo, les ofrecemos objetos de su interés para observar y explorar.

Nuestros infantes ya se mueven por doquiera (8 – 18 meses) y están deseosos de asirse de lo que puedan. Además, como a ellos les interesan las cosas que les recuerdan su hogar, hemos pegado en las paredes a la altura de su vista, fotografías de sus familias.

Los mayorcitos (18 – 36 meses), como ustedes lo saben, se mueven constantemente. Por eso, hemos organizado el espacio de tal manera que puedan explorar libremente y sin peligro. En el mismo, hay una gran diversidad de juguetes y de materiales que los estimulan a construir, pretender, observar libros, dibujar y moldear, responder a la música y producirla, e incluso, a cocinar.

Cómo podemos trabajar juntos

Sus hijos se sentirán más a gusto si el ambiente del programa les resulta familiar. Pero, para lograr establecer el vínculo entre el hogar y el programa de cuidado infantil, necesitamos de su ayuda. Las siguientes son unas cuantas sugerencias:

❖ *Traigan al programa unas cuantas fotografías de sus hijos con miembros de su familia.* Después de recubrirlas, las colocaremos a la vista de los niños.

❖ *Graben una cinta para sus pequeños.* Grábense leyéndole a sus hijos sus historias preferidas o cantando juntos sus canciones favoritas.

❖ *Menciónennos cuáles son sus objetos preferidos.* Si sus hijos tienen libros preferidos, o alguna música que toquen en fechas o eventos especiales, nos encantaría incluirlas en nuestro programa. Estamos convencidos de que es muy importante que los niños vean aspectos de su propia cultura en el ambiente del programa de cuidado infantil.

❖ *Traigan algunos de los objetos preferidos de los niños.* Si su hijo(a) tiene algún juguete o una manta que le ofrezca seguridad en los momentos en que pudiera extrañar a los miembros de su familia, siéntanse en libertad de traerlos a nuestro programa.

Nosotros le damos la bienvenida a sus ideas y contribuciones para convertir nuestro programa en un espacio en el que sus hijos se sientan cómodos y felices.

Les saluda atentamente,

©1999, Teaching Strategies, Inc., Washington, DC. Se permite la reproducción, únicamente con fines no comerciales, a los programas que ponen en práctica *The Creative Curriculum for Infants & Toddlers.*

Ensuring Children's Safety

A sk parents to tell you their chief priority when looking for child care, and most will reply, "A place where my child is safe." No matter what else a program does, if it does not keep children safe from harm, it is not doing its job. Safety is a basic requirement of any quality program.

In this chapter you will learn about:

- ❖ carrying out safety procedures that meet the changing developmental needs of children;
- ❖ preventing injuries;
- ❖ planning for and responding to emergencies;
- ❖ helping children become aware of safety; and
- ❖ balancing concerns for children's safety with their need to explore and take risks.

Ensuring children's safety takes both commitment and knowledge. In this chapter, we provide information that will help you make decisions about how best to keep infants and toddlers safe.

Safety Procedures and the Developmental Needs of Children

As children grow, their needs change. For example, many of your safety concerns with infants involve the routines that take up so much of their everyday experience—sleeping, diapering, and feeding. As infants become more mobile, you must shift your attention to making the environment safe for them to explore. What was once of little concern may now pose a major safety hazard.

Because maintaining children's safety can be a huge job, taking a developmental approach helps you focus your energy and resources. Remember that you don't have to implement every safety procedure. You need only concern yourself with safety measures that make sense for the ages and stages of the children in your care. Suppose, for example, that all the children in your program rest on mats, cots, or beds. If this is the case, you don't need to deal with safety precautions about cribs.

The following chart offers guidelines to help you respond to infants and toddlers at different developmental stages. As you read through this chart, think about how this information applies to the children in your program.

Young Infants		
What Children Are Doing Developmentally	**What You Can Do to Keep Them Safe**	**How This Supports Their Development**
Put everything in their mouths.	Provide sanitized non-toxic toys that have no breakable parts and cannot be swallowed.	Providing infants with safe playthings allows them to use all their senses (including their mouths) to explore and learn.
Use their whole bodies to learn—they wiggle, squirm, and roll over.	Place infants in areas where they can safely view the world from different viewpoints. Be especially watchful when changing a baby.	Providing safe spaces encourages movement and exploration. Infants learn as they investigate their environment.
Learn to sit.	Make sure high chairs, strollers, and swings have safety buckles.	Sitting without fear of falling gives infants a new point of view for exploring the world.
Hold a bottle.	Give each child his own bottle. Hold infants while they feed themselves. Do not prop bottles for infants who can't yet feed themselves.	Holding infants provides security and encourages them to want to feed themselves. Propped bottles discourage learning this skill and are also a choking hazard.

Mobile Infants

What Children Are Doing Developmentally	What You Can Do to Keep Them Safe	How This Supports Their Development
Crawl and pull themselves up by grabbing onto furniture.	Provide protected areas for crawling. Make sure furniture won't tip over from an infant's weight or roll away.	Crawling and pulling themselves up encourages infants to explore their world.
Enjoy getting into things.	Provide safe playthings and play space. Cover outlets and hide electrical wires. Always keep children in sight.	Playing without always having to be told, "No," encourages exploration and learning and creates a positive bond with the caregiver/teacher.
Understand many words, but not rules.	Set boundaries with furniture. Explain rules but don't expect children to fully understand or obey them.	Reinforcing your words with actions ("We need to play in front of the bookcase, where your toys are.") helps children learn to understand language and to begin to understand what rules mean.
Begin walking.	Provide carpeted surfaces. Remove objects that might trip a child. Do not use walkers which give infants more mobility than is safe for their developmental level.	Practicing in a safe environment helps children master the skill.

Toddlers

Walk, run, climb, and get into things.	Provide open space for active play both indoors and outdoors.	Recognizing that they can fall without being injured encourages exploration and active learning.
Master self-help skills: toileting, dressing, nose blowing, teeth brushing, and hand washing.	Keep tissues, paper towels, and soap where children can reach them. Make sure faucet water is set below 120°F and that step stools for reaching the sink are steady.	Maintaining a safe environment encourages children to develop and use self-help skills. Mastering these skills makes children feel independent and competent.
Begin to understand rules but need to test limits.	Latch doors and gates to enclose play areas. Be ready to explain rules many times.	Using fences or furniture to enclose play areas helps children understand what rules and limits mean.

Preventing Injuries

Prevention aims to stop possible problems before they occur. By anticipating the causes of injuries, you can take measures to keep them from happening.

Probably the most important prevention measure you can take is to check indoor and outdoor environments routinely for potential problems. Begin by making sure that these *policy-related* measures are in place.

- ❖ A stocked first-aid kit is kept at the program, in any vehicles used for transporting children, and in a fanny pack or book bag that can be taken on walks and field trips.

- ❖ Smoke detectors are located outside all sleeping areas and at the top of any stairway.

- ❖ ABC-type fire extinguishers are located on every floor and near the kitchen stove.

- ❖ Evacuation plans are posted and up-to-date safety contingency plans are readily accessible.

- ❖ All paint is non-toxic and lead-free.

- ❖ Furniture is the appropriate size for the ages of the children.

- ❖ Cribs (if in use) have no more than 2⅜ inches of space between slats (to prevent head entrapment), and cornerposts that extend no more than 1⁄16 inch.

- ❖ Cribs (if in use) have mattresses that come within "two fingers" of the sides of the crib (to prevent suffocation).

- ❖ Furnishings, cloth toys and books, bedding, and carpeting are flame resistant.

- ❖ Stairs and hallways are well lighted.

- ❖ Stairs have child-height handrails; steps have non-slip treads; bathtubs (if used) contain skid-proof mats or stickers.

- ❖ Indoor and outdoor play equipment conforms to height standards for age of child (18 inch maximum for young infants, 2 feet for mobile infants, 3 feet for toddlers).

- ❖ Outdoor play areas are enclosed by fences or natural barriers at least 4 feet in height (the bottom edge of which is no more than 3½ inches above the ground).

- ❖ Outdoor play equipment is securely anchored with 9 feet of clearance space for the use of each item (15 feet for any equipment with moving parts, such as swings).

- ❖ All indoor and outdoor play equipment is surrounded by resilient surface material such as rubber matting specifically made to absorb shock. (Grass is not an appropriate outdoor surfacing.)

- ❖ Tool sheds, garages, workbenches, and balconies are locked and off-limits to children.

- ❖ Adult sporting and hobby equipment is stored out of children's reach.

❖ Any glass doors are made of safety glass and have decals at child's eye level (to alert child to their presence).

❖ All visitors are required to sign in.

❖ Children are released only to authorized individuals.

❖ Appropriate adult-to-child ratios are maintained.

You'll also need to check regularly to be sure that you're carrying out injury-prevention practices. To assist you in monitoring your program, Appendix C contains a safety checklist you can use to identify and address potential problems.

The following equipment, materials, and toys should <u>not</u> be used by your program.

- Walkers, unless indicated by a child's IFSP, Individual Family Service Plan (may cause falls and injuries)

- Trampolines (may cause falls and injuries)

- Toys or objects having a diameter of less than 1¼ inches (choking hazard)

- Toys or objects with detachable parts (choking hazard)

- Toys or objects with attached cords or strings longer than 12 inches (strangulation hazard)

- Unused refrigerators (suffocation hazard)

- Plastic bags (suffocation hazard)

- Styrofoam packing material (choking hazard)

- Uninflated or underinflated balloons (choking hazard)

- Marbles (choking hazard)

- Straight or safety pins (internal injuries)

- Talcum powder (gets in children's lungs)

- Foods such as whole grapes, cough drops, hot dogs (unless cut into cubes or strips), olives, hard candies, gum, and peanuts (choking hazards)

- Plants poisonous to children such as azaleas, daffodils, diffenbachia, ivy, and mistletoe (A complete listing is available from your Regional Poison Control Center or Cooperative Extension Service.)

- Art materials that are harmful if swallowed by young children: powdered clay, powdered paint, glazes with lead, oil-based paint, cold-water dyes, permanent markers, instant pâpier maché, epoxy, and instant glues

Planning for and Responding to Emergencies

Emergencies are facts of life. While prevention goes a long way to make your program safe, you can't eliminate every danger. At some time, a toddler may fall off a climber and hurt herself, or an infant may choke on a piece of fruit. You may smell gas in the kitchen or find yourself without electrical power during a sudden storm.

If you've ever experienced an emergency, you know just how difficult it is to think clearly. Even if you've had some prior training, it is not at all easy to remain calm and do what you are supposed to do. Things happen quickly. If others around you are upset, it's hard not to feel this way too.

Because many of us tend to panic or freeze up when an emergency arises, we need to prepare ourselves thoroughly ahead of time. When we're prepared, we don't have to worry about reacting properly, because we're on "automatic pilot."

Preparing Yourself

There are three basic steps to follow if you're to feel prepared for an emergency situation: participate in training; maintain a well-stocked first-aid kit; and have up-to-date emergency plans readily available.

Training

Everyone who works with infants and toddlers ought to be certified in pediatric first aid. Pediatric first aid, which includes first aid for choking and rescue breathing (blowing air from your lungs into a child's) are your first lines of defense in saving a child's life.

Knowing what to do immediately is the most important step you can take. In fact, a recent study of injuries at a child care center showed that 85% of the children needed no further treatment than first aid.

If you are not certified in pediatric first aid or need refresher training, call your local Red Cross chapter to find out where and when such courses are offered. You can get the same information by writing to:

American Red Cross
Attn: Public Inquiry Office
1621 N. Keat Street, 11th Floor
Arlington, VA 22209

Experts recommend that every adult who works with young children—whether in a family child care home or part of a center-based team—be trained in emergency management of the following conditions:[1]

---

[1]American Public Health Association and American Academy of Pediatrics. *National Health and Safety Performance Standards: Guidelines for Out-of-Home Child Care Programs.* Arlington, VA: National Center for Education in Maternal and Child Health, 1992, p. 23.

1. bleeding
2. burns
3. poisoning
4. choking
5. injuries, including insect, animal, and human bites
6. shock
7. convulsions or nonconvulsive seizures
8. musculoskeletal injury (such as sprains, fractures)
9. dental emergencies
10. head injuries
11. allergic reactions
12. eye injuries
13. loss of consciousness
14. electric shock
15. drowning

Although what you do for a child varies according to the type of injury, there are some basic common sense procedures that apply across the board.[2] Consider posting this *Emergency Procedures List.*

1. **Find out what happened.** Discover who was injured, if the scene is safe, and if there are bystanders who might be of assistance.

2. **Check for life-threatening problems.** These are known as the ABCs:
   A = open the airway;
   B = check for breathing;
   C = check for circulation (pulse and bleeding).

3. **Call your local emergency medical services—911 or an ambulance—if you have any doubts about the seriousness of the problem.** In situations that are life-threatening, it may be advisable to call the emergency medical service before administering any first aid, so that the ambulance can be dispatched and on its way while you are tending to the child. Use your judgment and good common sense to decide if the child has a better chance of survival if you call for an ambulance before or after you administer emergency first aid.

4. **Check for injuries, starting at the head and working down.** You will need to give this information to medical personnel.

5. **Regroup. Calm the other children.** If the injured child needs your attention, ask a co-worker or back-up provider for assistance.

6. **Contact the child's parents or guardian** as soon as possible.

7. **Follow local procedures for filing an injury/incident report.** Be sure families get a copy.

Above all, experts in safety recommend the following:

- **Do not move a child who may have a serious head, neck, or back injury,** unless it is to save the child's life. Movement may make injuries worse.

- **Do no harm.** *Harm* means failing to do anything or making things worse.

[2] Abby Shapiro Kendrick, Roxanne Kaufmann, and Katherine P. Messenger, Eds. *Healthy Young Children: A Manual for Programs.* Washington, DC: National Association for the Education of Young Children, 1995, pp. 93–102.

Maintaining a First-Aid Kit

Your first-aid kits ought to contain everything you need, should any type of safety-related emergency arise. Store kits where you can get at them easily, but the children cannot.

Make a point of checking your program's first-aid kits several times a year to ensure that they are always fully stocked. You will find a checklist in Appendix C to help you make sure your first-aid kit is fully equipped.

Sample Emergency Plan

Type of Emergency: FAINTING

What I Need To Do:
1. Place the child in a flat position.
2. Loosen clothing around the neck area.
3. Turn the child's head to one side.
4. Keep the child warm and the mouth clear.
5. Make sure the child has nothing to swallow.
6. Call for medical assistance **immediately.**
7. Notify the child's parent or guardian.
8. Complete an injury/incident report. Make sure parent/guardian has a copy.

Emergency Plans

As the name suggests, emergency plans tell you what to do in a crisis: who to call (parents, doctors); what to do for a child (administer first-aid, not move the child); and the order in which procedures should be followed. Plans also should include procedures to follow if you have to leave your home or center. Fires, gas leaks, and other natural disasters are the usual reasons to evacuate a building.

You should have on hand written plans to cover each type of medical emergency cited earlier. In developing plans, be aware that first-aid procedures for opening airways, rescue breathing, and treating choking require different responses for children younger than 12 months than they do for children older than 12 months. If you care for children with special needs, you may need to add special precautions.

Many people who work with children like to develop symptom-based plans. These plans describe, for example, what to do for a child who has convulsions, faints, or starts to vomit uncontrollably. To the left is one such plan for responding to a child who has fainted.

In developing your emergency plans, make sure that they include how you will supervise the group as you attend to an injured child. As part of your emergency planning, keep the telephone numbers posted for Emergency Medical Services, police, fire, poison control, and Child Protective Services. Also, keep directions posted on how to reach your program, so that you can give emergency staff this information at a time when you may not be able to think clearly. There are several resources you can consult. Chapter 8 of *Healthy Young Children: A Manual for Programs* (Kendrick, Kaufmann, and Messenger, Eds.) and *American Red Cross Child Care Course Health and Safety Units* (American Red Cross and American Academy of Pediatrics) are two excellent manuals that outline medically-approved procedures. Experts in your community are another resource. The Red Cross, hospitals, and military installations often have staff eager to help.

Evacuation Plans

Evacuation plans should state the procedures you will follow to get children out of your house or building and to a safe place. For example, you may need to have a special evacuation crib positioned near an exit door which could hold several infants in case of fire or smoke. Your first and only priority must be to save lives, not property. Evacuation plans should be approved by a fire marshal and shared with families. These plans also need to be posted as a reminder. When volunteers or other staff have a first language other than

English, it's a good idea to have plans translated into all applicable languages. During an emergency, quick comprehension may be vital.

Below is a sample evacuation plan Mercedes developed for Matthew and his seven-week-old sister, Kara. Mercedes' family child care home is housed on the ground floor of an apartment building.

Sample Evacuation Plan

1. Sound the alarm.
2. Grab the outdoors first-aid kit (black book bag), which contains list of emergency contacts. Place the kit over my left shoulder.
3. Brace Kara on my right hip.
4. Take hold of Matthew with my left hand.
5. If we need to exit from the front door, unlock the door and lead the children outside.
6. If we need to exit from the back door, unlock the sliding door, and lead the children to the picnic area.
7. If we need to exit by a window, open the window, climb out with Kara and then place her on the grass. Go back to window and help Matthew climb through.
8. When the children are in a safe area, double check they both are with me.
9. Take the children to a neighbor's apartment and notify the fire department.
10. Calm the children down, if need be.
11. Notify the children's parents to let them know what happened and that everyone is safe.

Practice evacuation procedures once a month so that they become automatic for both you and the children. Document your efforts.

In addition, you'll want to develop plans for any natural disasters likely to occur in your area. If you live in a hurricane, earthquake, or tornado zone, you'll need to know what to do if one strikes. If your home or program is in an area where flooding occurs, you should know how to manage during this type of disaster. The Federal Emergency Management Agency (202-646-4600) or your local Red Cross can give you guidance in developing an appropriate emergency plan. Your plans should also include caring for children up to three days, in case they are stranded at your program.

Once the plans are developed, review them with supervisors, colleagues, and volunteers. Keep these suggestions in mind.

❖ **Share your emergency plans with families.** Knowing your plans gives the children's parents peace of mind. In addition, parents often have information you can use as you develop these plans. For example, a child may have specific health concerns that would affect how you administer first aid. Or parents might wish to indicate which emergency contact to call first.

❖ **Make sure that you have all emergency-related forms on file.** These might include emergency transportation permission forms, permission to administer medication, and a Power of Attorney should hospitalization or surgery be immediately required. Together with the children's parents or guardians, you can decide which forms make sense for you to maintain. In addition, you will want to have updated emergency contact forms as well as injury/incident reports on hand. In family child care, you'll also want to have a designated back-up provider who has been pre-approved by the children's parents.

❖ **File your plans so that you can get at them as quickly as possible.** You need to be able to use your plans at a moment's notice.

❖ **Keep emergency supplies on hand.** Keep formula, food, water, clothing, diapers, and medication on hand to use when implementing your plans.

Helping Children to Become Aware of Safety

Throughout this chapter, we've underscored the idea that adults must take responsibility for young children's safety. Yet ultimately, children need to become responsible for their own safety. This transfer of responsibility is not something that happens overnight or occurs magically when children reach a certain age. Safe practices are learned gradually throughout life.

You may be surprised to know that a significant part of this process takes place without any concentrated effort on your part. By attending to children's safety needs in the ways we've discussed thus far, you create a "culture of safety." Children become aware of the importance that safety plays in their lives by spending day after day in a safe setting with you.

Infants learn about safety first hand. When you strap them into a stroller and check their toys for jagged edges, they learn that safety is important.

Toddlers, too, learn that safety is valued by watching you. When they observe you removing a nail that has started to work its way out of a toy shelf, they learn about safety measures. At the same time, they also begin to realize that they can do things to keep themselves and others safe. For example, when Barbara invites Leo to help pick up toys someone might trip over, she encourages him to take an active role in promoting his own safety. He also learns that safety is something over which he can have some control.

Here are some ways to encourage children to practice safety-related behaviors.

❖ **Model good safety practices.** This is probably the best way to help young children learn about safety. Young children are great imitators.

❖ **Make children informed partners in your safety routines.** As you practice good safety habits, let children know what you are doing and why. Explain why you are testing the batteries in the smoke alarms. Go over the procedures for using knives safely, and explain why they are stored in the kitchen.

❖ **Talk with children about safety rules.** Help them understand that there are things that they can do to keep themselves safe: "Chairs are for sitting. If you want to climb, use the climber."

❖ **Involve the children's families in your safety efforts.** Share the things you do with families, so that they can extend these activities at home. You can also learn about families' safety practices at home. When children observe both you and their families practicing safety measures, they recognize more strongly the importance of safety in their lives.

Of course, your use of these strategies will vary with the developmental level of each child. Very young infants won't be able to understand all of what you are telling them. But even the youngest children will get the message that safety is important, since you take the time to talk to them about it. Your interest and attention to safety are what is most important at the early ages.

Older toddlers can begin to understand safety messages and rules. However, they don't always grasp the consequences of a rule, because they are just beginning to understand cause and effect. That is why Matthew might one day proudly follow a "walk when inside" rule and another day stare at you in defiance when you remind him of the rule.

Try to remember that children Matthew's age are testing limits—not your patience. You may find it helps children to learn safety rules by stating them simply in positive language with a few short reasons. Then, by repeating these rules often and enforcing them with consistency, children gradually learn that "We throw balls. Blocks are for building."

By making children active partners in safety awareness, you set the stage for future self-responsibility.

Balancing Concerns for Children's Safety with Their Need for Exploration

Everyone agrees that safety plays an important role in a quality program. At the same time, everyone also agrees that children should have opportunities to experiment and take reasonable risks. Children need to be free to explore their surroundings. Learning can only take place when children use all of their senses to interact with the people and objects in their environment.

Can there be such a thing as too much attention to safety? Aren't cuts and scrapes an inevitable part of growing up? Where is the line between precaution and freedom? How do you balance your obligation to protect children with the need to let them "be children?" These are important questions. They deserve a thoughtful response.

Clearly, you don't want to be so cautious and watchful that you overprotect children. To make children fearful of their environment is to do them a disservice. Jim Greenman makes this observation in strong language: "Children are cheated if we sacrifice challenge and experience before the altar of ostensible safety."[3]

Children need to be able to take risks. For one thing, we know from research that if children are kept under too close supervision, they are likely to postpone their risk-taking

---

[3] Jim Greenman. *Caring Spaces, Learning Places: Children's Environments That Work.* Redmond, WA: Exchange Press, 1988, p. 78.

to another time and place—when things may not be as safe as they are at your program.

Risk-taking, too, is tied up with creativity. Creative people are those who are willing to risk failure. If we cut off children's risk-taking ability, we may very well eliminate creativity as well.

Your task is to somehow find a balance—to create a safe environment where children can explore and learn.

Making Decisions about Balancing Safety and Exploration

Take a few minutes to reflect on the following questions.

❖ Do children feel free to explore the indoor and outdoor environments
  in my program?
❖ Do children find the environment sufficiently challenging?
❖ Am I preoccupied with safety concerns?
❖ Am I always saying "No" to children in an effort to protect them?
❖ Do I encourage children to take reasonable risks?

Your answers to these questions should give you an idea of your thinking on this issue.

After asking himself these questions, Ivan felt confident that he had a good balance in his program at Crane School. While he did a daily safety check and closely supervised children, he did not feel he was overprotecting them. Rather, Ivan believed that he went out of his way to encourage children to solve problems, resolve conflicts, and be creative in their play. Because he was working with children with special needs like Gena, Ivan thought it was especially important to make sure they did not become fearful, but were encouraged to take reasonable risks.

La Toya, on the other hand, had to admit that she was somewhat obsessed with safety. She recognized she had become increasingly watchful ever since the time a toddler in her family child care program seriously injured himself trying to climb a jungle gym. While she is aware that she might be overprotecting all children as an overreaction to this one incident, she is afraid to let up on her caution.

If, like La Toya, you don't feel comfortable about the balance in your program, discuss the issue with the children's families and some colleagues whose teaching and advice you respect. Ask for their responses to these same questions. They may have observed these same things. You may, however, be surprised to learn that they view things differently.

After talking with families and colleagues, take a second look at your practices. Think about ways you can best find a balanced approach that serves your children and their families, as well as yourself. For example, would it be helpful to devote more attention to prevention so that you're not constantly saying "no" to protect them?

Periodically review your approach to safety. Always bear in mind, though, that freedom to explore does not mean that you should lower your standards. Children's safety should never be compromised.

❖ ❖ ❖

Sharing Thoughts About Children's Safety

Dear Families:

Your child's safety is just as important to us as it is to you. Preventing accidents and preparing for emergencies is basic to our program.

For children, a safe program meets many needs. First and foremost, a safe program keeps children free from harm. A safe program also makes children feel secure. When an infant picks up a rattle without fearing being cut or bruised, she learns to trust her world. When an older infant holds on to a steady shelf to pull himself up, he, too, gains confidence that he is in a safe place. Once he realizes that he won't be hurt, he doesn't mind pulling himself up and falling back down over and over again! It is through explorations such as these that children learn.

How We Can Work Together

Safety efforts will be most successful if we join forces to protect your child. Here are some thoughts.

❖ *Look at our evacuation and emergency plans.* Perhaps you'd like to take part in one of our monthly fire drills. This will give you a first-hand demonstration of our safety preparations.

❖ *Make it a point to review your child's records regularly.* Once a month or so we can look at your child's file together and see if anything needs to be added or changed. For example, has your child developed an allergic reaction to a particular food or medicine? In what order should we contact people in an emergency? Whatever works best for your family is what we should do.

❖ *Remember that you are a "safety role model" to your child.* When you arrive here in the morning and help your child wipe up mud that he brought in on his boots, you show him how to prevent injuries. We can plan ways together to present positive safety messages to your child.

❖ *Be a second pair of eyes and ears.* You can be a great help by looking out for safety details and sharing your observations. If you see an area that needs improvement, let's make sure it gets the attention it needs.

We welcome your suggestions of ways to keep your child safe. That way, we all gain peace of mind.

Sincerely,

©1999, Teaching Strategies, Inc., Washington, DC. Permission granted to reprint, for non-commercial uses only, by programs implementing *The Creative Curriculum for Infants & Toddlers.*

Algunas ideas acerca de la seguridad de sus hijos

Estimadas familias:

Para nosotros, la seguridad de sus hijos es tan importante como lo es para ustedes. Por consiguiente, prevenir los accidentes y estar preparados para las emergencias, es básico para nuestro programa.

Un programa seguro, satisface muchas de las necesidades de los niños. En primer lugar, lo más importante es que, con un programa seguro los niños viven libres de peligro. También, que ellos se sienten seguros. Cuando un(a) niño(a) agarra un sonajero sin temor a cortarse o a golpearse, aprende a confiar en su mundo. Cuando uno mayorcito se agarra de un anaquel para ponerse de pie, también adquiere confianza con respecto a encontrarse en un lugar seguro. Una vez que se dan cuenta de que no se harán daño, a los niños no les importa ponerse de pie y volver a tirarse al suelo, una y otra vez. Mediante esta clase de experiencias es que los niños aprenden.

Cómo podemos trabajar juntos

Nuestros esfuerzos en pro de la seguridad de sus hijos tendrán éxito si combinamos nuestras fuerzas. Las siguientes son unas cuantas sugerencias:

❖ *Observen nuestros planes de evacuación y emergencia.* Quizá ustedes deseen participar en alguno de nuestros simulacros mensuales. Así, presenciarían una demostración directa de nuestra preparación.

❖ *Háganse el propósito de revisar con regularidad los registros de sus hijos.* Por lo menos una vez al mes, podríamos revisar la carpeta de sus hijos y ver si es necesario cambiar o añadir algo. Por ejemplo, ¿su hijo(a) ha tenido alguna reacción alérgica a algún alimento o medicamento específico? En caso de emergencia, ¿en qué orden y a quién debemos contactar? Lo que sea que funcione mejor para su familia, es lo que debemos hacer.

❖ *Recuerden que ustedes son un "modelo de seguridad" para su hijo(a).* Al ustedes llegar en la mañana, y ayudarle a sus hijos a limpiar el lodo que pudieran traer en sus botas, les están demostrando cómo prevenir posibles lesiones. Juntos, podremos planear formas de presentarle mensajes positivos y seguros a sus hijos.

❖ *Sean un segundo par de ojos y de oídos.* Ustedes pueden ser de gran ayuda al notar detalles de la seguridad y al compartir con nosotros sus observaciones. Si ustedes notan que un área necesita mejoras, les garantizaremos darle la atención necesaria.

Les agradecemos sus sugerencias para mantener seguros a sus hijos. De esa forma, todos podremos estar tranquilos.

Les saluda atentamente,

©1999, Teaching Strategies, Inc., Washington, DC. Se permite la reproducción, únicamente con fines no comerciales, a los programas que ponen en práctica *The Creative Curriculum for Infants & Toddlers*.

Promoting Children's Health

To be healthy is to be more than disease-free. Good health is a state of well-being. It includes emotional and social wellness, as well as physical vigor. Children who get the sleep they need and who eat nutritious foods are ready for learning. A healthy child is a strong child, in every sense of the word.

This chapter focuses on ways to promote children's total well-being. As you read through the chapter, you will learn about:

- ❖ meeting children's health requirements from birth to age three;
- ❖ preventing health problems;
- ❖ responding to child abuse and neglect;
- ❖ responding to sick children;
- ❖ helping children develop good nutrition and other health habits; and
- ❖ using partnerships to promote children's health.

Meeting Children's Health Requirements from Birth to Age Three

At every stage of development, children have health needs common to all children and some that are particular to children at a given developmental stage. Young infants, for example, need to be fed and changed when they need it, not when some prearranged schedule permits it. Their health and well-being depend on your responsiveness to their biological needs. Mobile infants, who are hard at work exploring every aspect of their environment, need space and opportunities for active play. Your challenge is to create play spaces that are free of germs—but not sterile in warmth and charm. Toddlers are busy finding out who they are and what they can do. When you teach them self-help skills that will keep them healthy, they become confident of their own capabilities.

While your approach to children's health adjusts to each child's needs at a particular stage of development, all young children need an environment as germ free as possible. This is particularly important since young children tend to put everything in their mouths, regardless of where that object has been before.

Table tops should be cleaned/disinfected with a bleach solution before and after meals as should toys after being mouthed by a child and also on a weekly basis. Adults should remove their shoes or wear shoe coverings when walking in areas where infants crawl and play.

The National Health and Safety Standards: Guidelines for Out-Of-Home Child Care Programs, developed by the American Public Health Association and the American Academy of Pediatrics, provides detailed guidance on sanitizing and disinfecting infant and toddler environments in both center-based programs and family child care homes.[1] This reference book can help you to follow safe procedures. (See Resources in Appendix E for a list of some other useful references.)

As you reflect on the chart that follows, think about the children in your care and their stage of development.

Young Infants		
What Children Are Doing Developmentally	**What You Can Do to Keep Them Healthy**	**How This Supports Their Growth**
Put everything in their mouths.	Sanitize toys, diaper changing surfaces, table tops, and eating utensils with a solution of ¼ cup bleach to one gallon of water.	Children learn by using all of their senses. By making it safe to put objects in their mouths, they can learn without becoming sick.
Get hungry and thirsty according to their own individual time clocks.	Give infants expressed breast milk (if parents so desire and local health regulations permit), formula, or warmed milk in bottles on demand. Use water rather than milk or juice when giving infants a bottle before sleeping. Label bottles with children's names. Formula and expressed milk should be dated.	Help infants develop a sense of trust, feed them when they are hungry or thirsty. Juice or milk that stays in a baby's mouth during sleep can lead to tooth decay. Labeling bottles prevents the spread of germs. Dating milk guards against spoilage. Expressed milk can be kept safely for 48 hours in the refrigerator and for 5 weeks in the freezer at 0° F.

continued on next page

---

[1] American Public Health Association and the American Academy of Pediatrics. *National Health and Safety Standards: Guidelines for Out-Of-Home Child Care Programs.* Arlington, VA: National Center for Education in Maternal and Child Health, 1992.

Young Infants (continued)

What Children Are Doing Developmentally	What You Can Do to Keep Them Healthy	How This Supports Their Growth
Soil or wet their diapers and their clothes.	Change babies who are awake as soon as they have soiled themselves. Change diapers in an area removed from food preparation and eating. Place disposable diapers in covered, lined containers; soak soiled clothing and linens. Wash your hands and the child's hands when finished. Wash and disinfect the changing table after each use. Seal soiled clothes in plastic bags to be sent home daily. Record each diaper change.	Diapering children on demand meets their physical needs. Because germs are present, careful sanitation procedures need to be followed. Tracking the infant's bathroom habits (and noting anything unusual) provides a health record for each child.

Mobile Infants

What Children Are Doing Developmentally	What You Can Do to Keep Them Healthy	How This Supports Their Growth
Use their fingers to feed themselves.	Offer children a healthy range of foods, such as bananas, crackers, or cheese. Give them plastic drinking cups filled halfway with milk or juice.	When children try a variety of foods, they lay the groundwork for healthy nutrition practices. When they can feed themselves, the children feel competent.
Begin to undress themselves and often cooperate in letting you dress them.	Encourage children to let you know when their diapers need changing but discourage them from removing them themselves. Wash children's hands if they touch soiled clothing. Also, encourage children to keep coats and jackets on when playing outdoors in chilly weather.	Children can learn self-help skills, without exposing themselves to health dangers.
Crawl and pull themselves up with the aid of furniture.	Sanitize floors, table tops, and toys daily with bleach solution (¼ cup bleach to one gallon of water). Keep cleaning supplies in locked cupboards. Keep room temperature in the 65°–72°F range and be sure play areas are well ventilated.	Crawling and standing help children explore the world around them. Sanitizing surfaces reduces children's exposure to germs.

Toddlers		
What Children Are Doing Developmentally	**What You Can Do to Keep Them Healthy**	**How This Supports Their Growth**
Begin to understand rules, but need to test limits.	Be prepared to discuss health rules with toddlers many times. These rules may include wiping up spills, throwing dirty tissues in the trash, washing hands before touching food, and so forth.	Children need encouragement as well as positive feedback to follow rules.
Learn self-help skills such as toileting, dressing themselves, blowing their noses, brushing their teeth, and washing their hands.	Give children opportunities, time, and praise for mastering these skills. Keep tissues, paper towels, soap, and outdoor clothing where children can get at them on their own. Provide covered trash cans where children can throw away used tissues and paper towels.	Mastering these skills begins with teaching children to be responsible for their own health. Setting up experiences for success reinforces skill mastery.
Begin to learn about healthy foods from the foods you serve. Begin to associate food and nutrition with pleasant experiences by participating in mealtime conversations.	Serve toddlers family style lunches and snacks. Encourage children to serve themselves and to try a variety of foods. Discuss in simple terms how foods keep our bodies healthy.	Serving family style meals promotes self-help skills and encourages children to begin taking responsibility for their own nutrition. Offering children a wide variety of food sets a pattern for lifelong eating habits.

Preventing Health Problems

The best way to promote children's health is to prevent problems before they occur. Consider this example. Leo, who is highly allergic to citrus fruits, broke out in hives after a parent volunteer, unaware of his allergy, offered him some orange juice for snack. Both the parent volunteer and Leo panicked as welts began to appear all over his upper body. Luckily, Barbara was nearby and able to calm them both. She also knew what to do, because she had an emergency plan on file for responding to Leo's allergy.

Had better preventive steps been in place, however, the volunteer never would have offered Leo orange juice. From now on, Barbara will be sure to alert all staff—including classroom visitors—to any allergies the children have. Moreover, she will post this information in the eating area, where it will be a constant reminder.

In this section we describe three ways you can prevent health problems: checking children for potential health problems; observing children regularly for signs of child abuse or neglect; and checking daily to be sure that preventive health measures are in place.

Health Check-Ups

Prevention begins with regular check-ups so that problem areas can be identified at the earliest possible point. Some problems can be corrected on the spot. Others can be minimized through treatment and follow up, or at least can receive the attention they need. All children, including seemingly healthy ones, should be checked on a regular basis.

Examining children for health-related problems allows health professionals to determine whether a child is healthy and has no apparent problems, is possibly at risk and in need of further assessment, or is definitely at risk and in need of follow-up treatment.

Infants and toddlers, as a group, are potentially at risk for a number of health problems, including developmental delays and vision and hearing difficulties. Individual children may be at further risk of developing diseases based on heredity, family health habits, and environmental factors, such as the presence of lead paint in the home.

Every family should take their child to a health professional for regular check-ups, immunizations, developmental guidance, and when their child is ill. If your program does not conduct health check-ups, we urge you to work with families to obtain these services. This may mean reminding families when immunizations are due or helping them find assistance. (See the last section of this chapter for further guidance on this issue.)

The American Academy of Pediatrics recommends that infants and toddlers receive complete physical examinations when they are 1 month, 2 months, 4 months, 6 months, 9 months, 12 months, 15 months, 18 months, 24 months, and 36 months old.[2]

Each of these visits should include a family history, height and weight measurements, and a vision, hearing, and a developmental assessment. Head circumference measurements should be recorded during visits in the child's first year of life. In addition, the Academy recommends these tests/readings:

- hematocrit or hemoglobin tests at the 9-month examination;
- blood pressure readings at the 36-month check-up;
- tuberculin tests for children at risk; and
- an initial dental exam after 12 months and again at approximately 36 months when the child has all 20 baby teeth.

In addition to physical examinations, all children need to be immunized against preventable diseases such as measles, chicken pox, and pertussin (whooping cough). The Centers for Disease Control and the American Academy of Pediatrics set and regularly revise a schedule for what and when infants and toddlers should receive immunizations.[3] Be sure to check for updates, as recommendations are subject to change.

[2] American Academy of Pediatrics Committee on Practice and Ambulatory Care. *Recommendations for Preventive Health Care*, Elk Grove, IL: American Academy of Pediatrics, September 1995.

[3] *Recommended Childhood Immunization Schedule: United States January, 1995.* Approved by the Advisory Committee on Immunization Practices, the American Academy of Pediatrics, and the American Academy of Family Physicians.

Parents can request a free copy of the brochure *Immunization Protects Children*, which contains an immunization schedule for children birth through age 16. Parents should send a stamped, self-addressed envelope to:

The American Academy of Pediatrics
PO Box 747, 141 Northwest Point Blvd.
Elk Grove Village, IL 60007
Tel.: (847) 228-5005

It's important that you work with families whose children have not yet had immunizations and check-ups. For example, if a child comes into your care who did not receive the medical attention he should have, you can refer the family to the local department of public health or local chapter of the American Academy of Pediatrics.

In addition to medical examinations for health problems, children also need to be screened for developmental problems in any of these areas:

* gross and fine motor skills;
* perceptual discrimination;
* cognition;
* attention skills;
* self-help skills;
* social skills; and
* receptive and expressive language skills (for older children).

Although these screenings increase the chances of identifying and addressing problems, a word of caution is in order. There is always the danger of missing a problem or of diagnosing a problem that really isn't there. Diagnosing a disability when it is not there happens most frequently when the screening instruments used do not accurately reflect the development of children from certain cultural or linguistic backgrounds. Clearly, we don't want children to be considered at risk for a disability or developmental delay because they come from a cultural or linguistic background different from the mainstream. We also don't want their disabilities or delays to go undetected for the very same reason.

The best way to deal with this issue is to become **culturally responsive**. In theory, to be culturally responsive is to honor the beliefs, interpersonal styles, attitudes, and behaviors of the multicultural families you serve.[4] In practice, it means working with health professionals to ensure that the screening instruments and practices used are accurate and culturally appropriate.

If you have concerns about a child's health, development, or behavior, it's essential to share your observations and concerns with the parents and refer them to their local health care provider for an evaluation. Information you contribute is just as important as that collected by health professionals. Regularly review your observations of the children at play, resting, eating, and toileting—plus the anecdotal information you have gathered from families and staff about each child's health. You can often uncover potential health problems if you make check-ups an ongoing process.

---

[4] Maria Anderson and Paula F. Goldberg. *Cultural Competence in Screening and Assessment: Implications for Services to Young Children with Special Needs Ages Birth through Five.* Minneapolis: National Early Childhood Technical Assistance System, December 1991, p.4.

Checking for Good Health Practices In Your Program

An important part of prevention is maintenance. Every day you take steps to keep children well when you keep these health concerns in mind.

- ❖ The environment needs to support children's total well-being.

- ❖ Toys and equipment should be as germ-free as possible.

- ❖ Diapering and toileting practices need to be hygienic.

- ❖ Personal hygiene practices should serve as models for the development of self-help skills.

- ❖ Sleeping and rest periods should take place in healthy environments. Infants should be placed on their backs to sleep to reduce the risk of Sudden Infant Death Syndrome (SIDS).[5]

- ❖ Feeding and eating should provide children with appropriate nutrition and should support the development of self-help skills.

- ❖ Illnesses that do occur need to be managed so as to support the sick child and prevent the spread of disease to others.

Health care professionals also recommend that anyone who is exposed to blood—whether it is in an infant's stool, a toddler's nosebleed, a skinned knee, or under any conditions at all—adopt the universal precautions developed by the Centers for Disease Control and the Occupational, Safety, and Health Administration (OSHA). These include wearing gloves, disinfecting blood-contaminated areas and cleaning supplies, disposing of blood-contaminated materials and diapers properly, and washing hands after exposure.[6] We can't always tell that a child is sick by appearances alone. Some diseases can be carried a long time before symptoms appear.

By being conscientious about procedures that promote wellness, you can do a lot to keep children healthy. In Appendix C you will find a checklist that can help you make sure your program promotes good health.

Responding to Child Abuse and Neglect

Child abuse and neglect can occur in any family, regardless of income or background. Because your legal responsibilities and the possible repercussions of your actions are so significant, you need to know exactly what child abuse and neglect are. The Child Abuse, Domestic Violence, Adoption, and Family Service Act of 1992 (Public Law 102-295) defines child abuse and neglect as:

---

[5] Countries where infants are placed on their backs to sleep have found a 50 percent reduction in the rate of SIDS. The American Academy of Pediatrics campaign to prevent SIDS deaths is called "Back to Sleep."

[6] American Public Health Association and the American Academy of Pediatrics. *National Health and Safety Standards: Guidelines for Out-Of-Home Child Care Programs.* Arlington, VA: National Center for Education in Maternal and Child Health, 1992, pp. 75-76, HP38.

"...Physical or mental injury, sexual abuse or exploitation, negligent treatment, or maltreatment of a child under the age of 18 (except in the case of sexual abuse) or by the age specified by the child protection law of the State by a person who is responsible for the child's welfare, under circumstances which indicated that the child's health or welfare is harmed or threatened...."

What does all this mean? Most experts agree that there are four types of abuse:

❖ **physical abuse,** including burning, kicking, biting, pinching, or hitting a child;

❖ **sexual abuse,** including using a child for another's sexual gratification through such activities as fondling, rape, sodomy, and using a child for pornographic pictures or film;

❖ **emotional abuse or maltreatment,** including blaming, belittling, ridiculing, and constantly ignoring a child's needs; and

❖ **neglect,** including failing to provide a child with food, clothing, medical attention, or supervision.

Following is a list of physical and behavioral indicators of child abuse. Remember, though, that there is no single sign or cue that can tell you with certainty that a child is abused. Repeated or multiple signs, however, should be regarded as "red flags."

You should check children daily for any of the following **physical signs:**

❖ bruises and welts (especially on the face, back, back of legs, or buttocks; unusual patterns that might indicate use of a buckle or other object; clusters that might indicate repeated contact; wounds in various stages of healing);

❖ burns (glove or donut-shaped marks that might result from immersion; cigarette or rope marks; dry burns that might indicate application of a hot surface);

❖ cuts, scrapes (especially on the face or genitalia);

❖ broken bones (especially in various stages of healing);

❖ head injuries (black or bruised eyes or jaw; bleeding beneath the scalp);

❖ bleeding or discharge (in genitalia or anal area; in urine, throat, or mouth);

❖ pain (difficulty walking, sitting, or urinating);

❖ constant hunger or abnormal weight loss/drowsiness; and

❖ vomiting (without signs of flu or other illness).

Check also for these **behavioral signs:**

❖ unhappiness (seldom smiles; has deep fear of adults; reacts with emotion to unpleasantness; flinches in the presence of others; has excessive tantrums);

❖ aggression (is disruptive; exhibits angry behavior; has poor peer relationships);

❖ withdrawal (is unwilling to participate in activities; hugs self; refuses to have clothes or diapers changed; shows loss of appetite);

❖ acts inappropriately for age, either as one who is considerably older or younger (shows keen interest in sexual matters; excessively seeks or shuns affection from adults; has delayed growth/development);

❖ is frequently absent or late (parents habitually arrive early/late to drop off and/or pick up);

❖ lacks adequate/appropriate clothing/hygiene;

❖ hurts self or others; and

❖ touches others in a sexual way or masturbates excessively.

Observing any of these signs should lead you to wonder whether a child may be a victim of abuse or neglect. If you know the family well, you can often determine if the observed signs come from probable abuse or from something else. Some problems may be temporary and readily handled by families; others may be chronic and require your intervention. Consider, too, that the risks of child abuse increase when families are under stress from marital, economic, or social pressures.

If you have any reason to suspect that a child is being abused or neglected, you are legally required to report your suspicions to the appropriate authority (e.g., Department of Social Services, the Department of Human Resources, the Division of Family and Children's Services, or Child Protective Services of your local city, county, or state government). Every one of the 50 states has laws governing the reporting of suspected child abuse. Your own program should have a written policy in place.

You'll notice that in this discussion we keep mentioning the word suspect. Even though you'd be far more comfortable in making your report if you had proof, the law is very clear that you must report your suspicions—even if your suspicions should later prove to be wrong.

Undoubtedly, this is an uneasy position for you. You might think, "What if I'm wrong? What if there is a logical explanation for the symptoms I've observed? I might be ruining a family's reputation. In all likelihood, I'll never regain that family's trust. And what about the child? Might I not, through a false accusation, be making matters worse?"

No one can know whether all or none of these "worst case" scenarios will come true. The fact is, though, that you can't afford to risk that your suspicions might be correct. It is your professional responsibility to protect all children from harm.

Responding to Sick Children

Although prevention goes a long way in keeping children well, it's impossible to prevent childhood illnesses from occurring. When children are sick, they need your comfort, concern, and—above all—your knowledge of good health practices. This section examines ways to respond to children who are temporarily ill; children who have long-term illnesses; and children experiencing health emergencies.

Caring for Children Who Are Temporarily Ill

Despite every effort on your part, young children typically get sick five to twelve times a year. One recent study found that on any given day, 17% of the children in care arrive feeling ill. Fortunately, most instances are not serious.

Much of your approach to dealing with sick children is a management issue. You need to have a policy in place that outlines step-by-step procedures to follow when a child becomes ill. Your first move is to decide which illnesses require you to send children home and which illnesses you can deal with in your daily routine. Some programs have neither the staff nor the space to care for a child who is too ill to participate fully. Generally, however, most programs try to allow mildly sick children to stay. Keeping them with you is often the most compassionate choice for the child and the family.

The American Academy of Pediatrics takes the position that there are very few illnesses for which children should be sent home. Their stand is based on the fact that many common childhood diseases, such as earaches, are not contagious. Still other diseases—such as the so-called common cold—are spread before symptoms first appear. By the time you know a child has a cold, the other children will already have been exposed to it. Sending the sick child home does nothing to prevent the further spread of the illness.

Your best strategy for stopping the spread of a cold or other disease is to be especially sure to carry out the sanitation and hygiene practices described earlier in this chapter. As long as you wash your hands every time you attend to a sick child and make sure tissues and wipes are disposed of carefully—as long as you are sure that dirty clothing and linens are appropriately handled and washed, and that the sick child's hands, crib or bed, and playthings are kept clean—you can help prevent the spread of germs.

When then, is a child too sick or too contagious to remain at your program? Your state licensing program has specific "sick child" policies that identify diseases that require you to send children home. The list also identifies those diseases that must be reported to your state department of public health. In general, these include highly contagious diseases such as bacterial meningitis, Hepatitis A, measles, salmonella, and the like. Check your local health department requirements.

Most health authorities—including the Centers for Disease Control and the American Academy of Pediatrics—recommend that children be excluded from care if any of these symptoms are present:

❖ fever (oral temperature of 101°F or higher, rectal temperature of 102°F or higher, armpit [axillary] temperature of 100°F or higher), accompanied by behavioral changes and other signs of illness;

❖ pinkeye (purulent conjunctivitis) with white or yellow eye discharge (until 24 hours after treatment has been initiated);

❖ chicken pox (until 6 days after onset of rash or sores have dried);

❖ pertussin (until 5 days after antibiotic treatment has begun);

❖ mumps (until 9 days after onset of gland swelling);

❖ Hepatitis A (until one week after onset of illness);

❖ measles (until 6 days after onset of rash);

- rubella (until 6 days after onset of rash);
- head lice (until the first treatment is initiated) or scabies (until after all treatment is completed);
- tuberculosis (until health official provides permission);
- impetigo (until 24 hours after treatment has been initiated);
- strep throat (until 24 hours after treatment has been initiated and fever is gone);
- uncontrolled diarrhea;
- uncontrolled coughing;
- difficult or rapid breathing;
- vomiting two or more times within the past 24 hours;
- mouth sores with drooling; and
- rash with fever or behavior change.

Sick children who remain in care need adequate rest, an appropriate diet (usually including increased liquids to prevent dehydration), medication as ordered (with written instructions from the child's physician on dispensing the medicine, as well as written permission from the parent to do so), and both close supervision and emotional support. Your chief role is to make the sick child as comfortable as possible without neglecting the other children in your program.

Caring for Children with Long-Term Illnesses

Long-term conditions can range from mild allergies to terminal illnesses. Chronic health problems may include cancer, asthma, diabetes, anemia, sickle cell disease, epilepsy, heart-related problems, and kidney or liver-related problems.

If you have a child with a long-term health problem in your care, talk to the child's parents and doctor to find out as much as you can about the child's condition. Read up on the disease. Send for information from a professional organization, such as the American Diabetes Association. Do a literature search on the Internet (use MEDLINE or another medical database). Ask your local librarian for help.

As with all children, sick children long to be a part of the group. And for the most part, children with chronic health conditions can participate fully. It's important that you and everyone in your program make the sick child feel as "normal" as possible. Try to avoid making a child feel as if he or she is constantly being "sanitized."

No matter what the impact of the child's illness, you'll want to develop and have on hand a written health plan for the child. Working with the child's family and health care provider, detail all accommodations that you need to make to your program and list out the medications and procedures you need to follow every day and in a health emergency.

Responding to Emergencies

What do you do when an emergency arises? As with safety emergencies, your best strategy is to be prepared. Health experts recommend having emergency plans in place and accessible. If you care for infants and toddlers with chronic health problems, you must be ready to swing into action at the first sign of distress.

For every child with a chronic health problem, you'll need to do the following.

- ❖ **Know what to expect.** Talk to the child's family and doctor about the types of crises that might occur.

- ❖ **Become knowledgeable about what causes these crises**, how often they are likely to occur, and how long each one is likely to last.

- ❖ **Learn the signs of an approaching crisis** and also how the child is likely to behave just prior to the crisis.

- ❖ **Get trained** by a family member, the child's doctor, or the American Red Cross on the procedures you should follow in a crisis.

- ❖ **Have a written plan for dealing with the crisis**, listing simple step-by-step directions that you would be able to follow, even under stress.

- ❖ **Train other staff and volunteers** in emergency procedures, including using gloves for contact with blood. Post instructions for when to call for emergency assistance and the phone numbers.

- ❖ **Identify—in the child's health plan—activities that should be avoided** and/or dietary restrictions that might bring on an emergency. Post reminders prominently so that everyone knows, for example, that Leo should not eat citrus fruits because he is severely allergic.

In addition to having plans related to children's chronic conditions, you'll want to make sure that you have symptom-based plans that tell you what to do if any child in your program experiences an emergency. Contaminated food, for example, can make your entire group ill. You'll therefore want to know how to respond, should one or more children experience stomach cramps and diarrhea or vomiting. Likewise, you need to know what should be done for a child who faints, has convulsions, or chokes. You'll probably find it most efficient to combine this effort with the development of your plans for safety-related emergencies, since much of the information will be the same. You can consult Chapter 8 for further guidance on writing emergency plans. (As always, don't forget to share your plans with the children's families. Include their ideas and make sure they are comfortable with these plans.)

Helping Children Develop Good Nutrition and Other Health Habits

From the time an infant begins nursing or taking a bottle as she is lovingly held in her parent's arms, the child learns about nutrition. If these same feelings of warmth and comfort carry over to mealtimes at your program, children learn to associate nutrition with caring and pleasure. This association is the first step on the road to lifelong good nutrition.

The tone you set and the foods you offer children set the stage for permanent nutrition habits. As examples, think about the ways in which these staff are helping children develop positive habits through eating experiences.

Linda picks up four-month-old Julio and sits with him in the rocker. She nestles Julio in the crook of her left arm and holds the bottle for him with her right hand. As she feeds the baby, she looks him intently in the eyes and talks to him in a low, soothing tone, commenting in Spanish on how hungry he is. She rocks the chair and begins singing a Guatemalan folk song Julio's mother told her she sings to him.

Eight-month-old Jasmine has been eating mashed cooked fruits for three months now. Janet introduced Jasmine to orange slices several days ago. After an initial nasty expression, Jasmine has been screeching for orange slices at every meal, which Janet gladly gives her. Even though the child has had no physical reactions to the orange, Janet is going to wait a few more days before starting Jasmine on another raw fruit.

Willard (11 months) enjoys feeding himself cubes of cheese and eating applesauce with a spoon. Grace lets him spend unhurried time feeding himself and babbling to his food.

Matthew (26 months) is helping Mercedes place five plates on the table for lunch. They will eat lunch family style, joining Mercedes's great nieces who are visiting from Brazil. Mercedes offers the serving bowls to each child one at a time. The children use the small spatula and ladles to help themselves to chicken kabobs, mashed cassava, and carrots. Matthew tries to pour milk from a small pitcher into his glass, with Mercedes's assistance. During lunch, they talk excitedly with one another. When Matthew is through eating, he clears his plate over the trash basket and carries it into the kitchen.

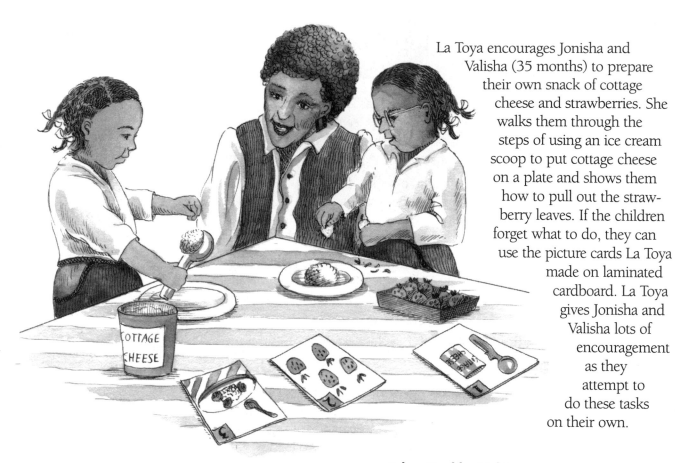

La Toya encourages Jonisha and Valisha (35 months) to prepare their own snack of cottage cheese and strawberries. She walks them through the steps of using an ice cream scoop to put cottage cheese on a plate and shows them how to pull out the strawberry leaves. If the children forget what to do, they can use the picture cards La Toya made on laminated cardboard. La Toya gives Jonisha and Valisha lots of encouragement as they attempt to do these tasks on their own.

Other Healthy Habits

In addition to helping children develop good nutrition habits, you can encourage children to learn and use lifelong self-help skills to promote their own good health. Chief among these skills are:

- ❖ **washing hands** before handling food and after sneezing, cleaning up, handling pets,[7] and toileting (wiping hands with damp paper towel moistened with a liquid soap, rinsing hands under running water while rubbing hands back and forth, drying hands with paper towel, turning off faucet with paper towel, and discarding towel in trash);

- ❖ **brushing teeth** after eating;

- ❖ **sneezing and coughing into one's elbow** and away from people;

- ❖ **blowing one's nose into a tissue,** discarding the tissue, then washing hands;

- ❖ **disposing of trash correctly,** dropping used paper cups, paper towels, and tissues in a lined plastic receptacle with a pedal-operated lid or into a metal receptacle lined with plastic; and

- ❖ **putting on outerwear** for going outside in cool, cold, or rainy weather.

---

[7] Only pets that do not carry diseases and are not dangerous should be included in your program. Avoid turtles, iguanas, lizards, parrots, and aggressive dogs such as pit bulls.

Young infants like Julio experience good health habits when someone takes care of their health needs. This builds a foundation for developing lifelong self-help skills.

Mobile infants take pride in doing the same things that important adults in their lives do. When Abby, for instance, sees Brooks and her parents washing their own hands, brushing their teeth, or disposing of a used paper cup in the trash, she wants to copy their actions.

Toddlers can acquire self-help skills as part of their everyday routines. Valisha, for example, can help mash the potatoes for her lunch, pour juice from small pitchers for an afternoon snack, take off and hang up her coat when she comes inside from outdoor play, and throw away used paper towels and tissues.

Here are some strategies you can use to encourage the children in your care to develop self-help skills.

- **Model good practices.** Even infants can begin to learn health habits.

- **Involve children in healthy routines.** Ask children to wipe up spills or throw away used paper cups, napkins, and tissues. Eventually, children will take on responsibility for these actions.

- **Ask families to join you.** Involve parents in what you are doing, and ask them to be role models for their children. Children will soon learn that both you and their families value health habits.

- **Read books about health habits with children.** Many delightful picture books focus on healthy routines. Books such as *Teddy Bears Cure a Cold* (Suzanna Gretz), *The Philharmonic Gets Dressed* (Karla Kushin), or *Going to the Potty* (Fred Rogers) help children understand that everyone practices health habits.

- **Give children dramatic play opportunities.** As they dress a baby doll, feed it a bottle, or prepare a pretend meal, children practice self-help skills. Pretend experiences lay the groundwork for real life successes.

- **Encourage and praise children's efforts.** Sincere feedback lets children know that you appreciate their attempts at self-help skills. It contributes to both their confidence and competence.

Using strategies such as these, children are more likely to develop positive health habits and practices. Ultimately, children will become responsible for their own well being—which is a goal that you, families, and the children themselves most likely share.

Using Partnerships to Enhance Children's Health

You can see that keeping infants and toddlers healthy is a big, big job. In fact, to do this job well, you can't possibly do it alone. The responsibilities are too many and too great for any one person or any one program.

The solution rests in reaching out to other individuals and organizations in your community. There are many places to go for help. Here are some thoughts.

❖ Create links among child care programs, families, and resource and referral agencies to ensure communication about health issues.

❖ Work with child care health consultants who offer training on health issues, ranging from the best placement of changing tables to sick child care policies.

❖ Conduct training for families on ways to use community resources.

❖ Contact your local and state health department and community resources (such as Child Find) about conducting screenings and identifying and helping children with health impairments.

❖ Obtain Spanish and English videos, stickers, and posters on Sudden Infant Death Syndrome (SIDS) by calling 800-505-CRIB for materials on "Back to Sleep" positions for infants.

❖ Contact local and state chapters of the American Academy of Pediatrics, the American Dental Association, the Association of Dental Hygienists, and the American Academy of Pediatric Dentists for informational material.

❖ Contact professional organizations (the American Academy of Pediatrics; American Public Health Association; the American Red Cross; the Association for the Care of Children's Health; the National Association for the Education of Young Children; the Children's Defense Fund) and government agencies (Maternal and Child Health; Medicaid/EPSDT; Food and Nutrition Service) for information on parent education and children's health issues.

❖ Contact local community health centers, mental health providers, hospitals, maternal and child health programs, and HMOs about serving as resources for families and the program.

❖ Link up with national health campaigns such as The Healthy Mothers, Healthy Babies Coalition, *Sesame Street's* lead poisoning campaign, and the National SAFE KIDS Campaign.

❖ Use area health education centers, nursing schools, colleges, police and fire departments, health fairs, and public libraries as resources to educate families, colleagues, and yourself on health issues.

You serve children best when you work as a team with their families and community agencies.

❖   ❖   ❖

Sharing Thoughts About
Children's Health

Dear Families:

As a parent, you have every right to assume that your child will be well and happy while in our care. And we want you to know that your child's health is very important to us, too. We work very hard to stop the spread of germs by following good health practices.

We believe that children's health is more than just their physical well-being. It also includes emotional and social wellness. A child who eats nutritious meals, gets plenty of rest, can explore in an environment that is relatively free of germs, and feels valued and secure, is one who can focus on the important job of learning.

How We Can Work Together

We do many things to promote your child's good health. And in everything we do, we welcome and need your support. Here are some examples.

❖ *We work with you to screen your child for possible health problems*, including those related to vision, hearing, and developmental delays. We would like to have your participation during screening so your child will feel comfortable.

❖ *We work with you to make sure your child gets all of his or her shots and other needed medical attention.* At these times, and at other times as well, we need to have the most current information about your child's health situation.

❖ *We practice and teach children personal hygiene,* including hand washing, toileting, tooth brushing, and other self-help skills, just as you do at home.

❖ *We feed your child nutritious meals and snacks.* If your child develops a food allergy, please let us know so we can post this information for everyone to see.

❖ *We make sure that children who are ill are supported,* and that others are not exposed to infection. We will, of course, let you know if a child in the program has a contagious disease (such as chicken pox).

❖ *If your child is supposed to take medication, we do need written permission.* If a health emergency arises, we also need to have a release form on file.

We regard you as our full partner in all of the health-related activities we do. We need to work together and be constantly watchful. Your child's health depends on it!

Sincerely,

©1999, Teaching Strategies, Inc., Washington, DC. Permission granted to reprint, for non-commercial uses only, by programs implementing *The Creative Curriculum for Infants & Toddlers.*

Algunas ideas acerca de la salud de los niños

Estimadas familias:

Como padres de familia, ustedes tienen el derecho a asumir que su hijo(a) sea feliz y esté bien mientras se encuentre en nuestro cuidado. Nosotros deseamos que sepan que la salud de su hijo(a) también nos es muy importante. Mediante unas buenas prácticas de salud, nosotros trabajamos fuertemente para evitar la propagación de gérmenes.

Nosotros creemos que la salud de los niños consiste en mucho más que el bienestar físico, pues el bienestar emocional y social también hacen parte de la salud. Un niño que consume alimentos nutritivos, descansa suficiente tiempo, puede explorar en un ambiente relativamente libre de gérmenes y se siente valorado y seguro, puede concentrarse en el importante trabajo de aprender.

Cómo podemos trabajar juntos

Nosotros hacemos mucho para promover la buena salud de sus hijos. Y, en todo lo que hacemos, les damos la bienvenida y les solicitamos su apoyo. Los siguientes son unos cuantos ejemplos:

❖ *Trabajamos con ustedes para detectar posibles problemas de salud de sus niños,* incluyendo aquellos relacionados con la visión, el oído y los retrasos en el desarrollo. Nos gustaría que durante dicha detección ustedes estuvieran presentes para que los niños se sientan cómodos.

❖ *Trabajamos con ustedes para garantizar que sus hijos reciban todas las vacunas y demás atención médica necesaria.* Hoy en día y, de hecho, en cualquier otro momento, necesitamos contar con la información más actualizada sobre el estado de salud de sus hijos.

❖ *Nosotros practicamos y les enseñamos a los niños higiene personal,* incluyendo lavarse las manos, ir al baño, lavarse los dientes y otras destrezas autónomas, tal como ustedes lo hacen en su hogar.

❖ *Nosotros les ofrecemos a sus hijos nutritivos alimentos y meriendas.* Si su hijo(a) es alérgico(a) a algún alimento, permítanos saberlo para anunciarlo y que todos lo sepan.

❖ *Nosotros confirmamos que a los niños enfermos se les apoya y que los demás no estén expuestos a infecciones.* Nosotros, por supuesto les haremos saber si algún niño del programa tiene alguna enfermedad contagiosa (como el sarampión).

❖ *Si su pequeño(a) debe tomar medicina, necesitamos la autorización por escrito.* Y, en caso de emergencia, también necesitamos contar con una autorización en nuestros archivos.

Nosotros les consideramos nuestros socios en todas las actividades de salud que realizamos. Necesitamos trabajar juntos y mantenernos alerta. ¡La salud de sus hijos depende de ello!

Les saluda atentamente,

©1999, Teaching Strategies, Inc., Washington, DC. Se permite la reproducción, únicamente con fines no comerciales, a los programas que ponen en práctica *The Creative Curriculum for Infants & Toddlers.*

Guiding Children's Behavior

C hildren need adults to guide them—to help them learn what is acceptable behavior and what is not. Getting infants and toddlers to stop doing something or to do something else is not difficult. Because we adults are so much bigger and more powerful than they are, we can move children where we want them to be and make them behave. But is this all we want? Wouldn't we prefer that children develop self-control and learn to balance their own needs with the needs of others?

In *The Creative Curriculum,* we place great importance on helping young children develop inner controls and positive social skills. We believe that when young children begin learning how to control their own behavior, it is more likely they will grow into people who can make good decisions. We also recognize that children who know how to relate to others in positive ways and can make friends tend to be happier and more successful in life.

In this chapter, you will learn about:

  ❖ taking a positive approach to guiding behavior;
  ❖ responding to challenging behaviors, such as temper tantrums and biting; and
  ❖ helping children relate positively to each other.

Taking a Positive Approach

When you have realistic expectations of children and gently guide their behavior in ways that show respect and help children feel good about themselves, you are taking a positive approach. Your positive approach can help young children learn for themselves, over time, what behavior is acceptable and what is not.

Positive guidance can take many forms. Sometimes you take steps to prevent dangerous or unacceptable behavior. You *prevent dangerous behavior* when, for example, you cover an electrical outlet so children cannot hurt themselves. You *prevent unacceptable behavior* when you plan your daily schedule so children have plenty of time outdoors to practice their gross motor skills and burn up energy. Other times you may intervene to *redirect children's behavior*. For example, you give an infant a rubber toy to chew on instead of the piece of paper that had been lying on the floor, or remind a toddler to climb on the climber instead of the table. At still other times, you intervene directly to *stop a dangerous behavior*, such as kicking or biting.

The first steps in providing positive guidance and promoting self-discipline are understanding child development and building trusting relationships. When you know what children (in general) are like at different ages, you will have realistic expectations and can meet their needs in caring ways. For example, when La Toya organizes lunch so that everything is ready when the children sit down, she decreases the chances that children will end up crying, climbing on the table, or pushing one another because they are hungry and frustrated. As a result, instead of focusing on maintaining order, she and the children can enjoy the smell of an orange and talk about the morning's events as they eat lunch together. Because children feel close to her, they will imitate her actions and look for her approval. La Toya's smile of encouragement when Valisha shares a piece of her orange will inspire Valisha to do it again another day.

How you guide a child's behavior depends in large part on the child's age and temperament. Because children grow and change so rapidly during their first three years, the strategies you use to guide their behavior must change, too.

Guiding the Behavior of Young Infants

Guiding the behavior of young infants begins when you and a child's parents gently set patterns and respond in respectful, caring ways. You help an infant learn how it feels to manage her own feelings and behavior when you, for example, pick her up to comfort her or begin to encourage her to sleep by following the same ritual. Guiding the behavior of young infants also means keeping them safe. (For additional information, see Chapter 8, Ensuring Children's Safety.) Here are some suggestions:

❖ **Establish and follow rituals, providing as much continuity with a child's home as possible.** Singing the same songs or rocking a tired baby before laying her down helps her begin learning how to organize her own behavior.

❖ **Use your face, voice, touch, and motion to help a young infant manage or regulate stimulation and feelings.** Holding a young infant, looking in her eyes and talking quietly to her may help her calm herself and be able to focus briefly on something that catches her interest. Observe and take steps throughout the day to ensure that children aren't overwhelmed by the noise and confusion of group life.

❖ **Stay nearby when babies are laying or sitting close to each other.** Be sure everything within reach is all right for children to play with and mouth.

Guiding the Behavior of Mobile Infants

Mobile infants are on the go and want to explore everything. Your challenge is to set limits they can understand in ways that show respect and help children gain a sense of competence. Here are some suggestions.

❖ **Use simple, clear language to communicate which behaviors are acceptable.** Let your expression and tone of voice emphasize your message as Grace did when she explained to Willard, "You may use the crayons on the paper."

❖ **Use "No" sparingly.** Save this for dangerous situations so it will be effective.

❖ **Give children many opportunities to move and be active throughout the day.** Children who are engaged are less likely to get into dangerous situations and conflicts. They are more likely to experience mastery.

❖ **Use familiar signals to let children know when it's time to move from one activity to another.** For example, give a two-minute warning when it's time to clean up. Dim the lights and play soft music when it's time for nap. When children have a sense of what to expect, they tend to feel secure and calm during transitions. With less confusion, problem behaviors tend to decrease.

❖ **Plan the day so there are no long waits between routines and activities.** If children have to wait for a few minutes, sing a song, do a fingerplay, or tell a story to help the time pass in an interesting, relaxed way.

❖ **Look at a situation through children's eyes before intervening.** Be aware, for example, that what looks like one child grabbing a toy from another may be a "taking away-giving back" game.

❖ **Give children the chance to work things out themselves—if no one will be hurt**. A child may briefly react and then decide she doesn't care when someone picks up a toy she had been playing with. In situations like this, your involvement creates unnecessary tension.

Guiding the Behavior of Toddlers

Toddlers' behavior can, at times, stretch your patience. It is also exciting to watch toddlers who feel confident take initiative to learn about themselves and their world by testing limits. Here are some suggestions that can help you guide toddlers' behavior in positive ways so they feel competent as they learn the rules and how to follow them.

❖ **Encourage toddlers' growing sense of independence.** Invite them to participate in daily routines. Give them many chances to make choices. Set up the environment so children can hang up their own coats and reach the sink to wash their own hands.

❖ **Set a few, simple clear rules**—knowing that children may need your help to follow them. Rules such as, "Sit at the table when you cut with scissors" give children a sense of order and security as well as the opportunity to develop self-discipline. Over time, and after many reminders, children will learn to take their scissors to the table.

❖ **Understand that toddlers are not yet ready to share.** When they don't share, they aren't being greedy or mean. They need time to develop a sense of ownership and to learn to share. Model and encourage sharing but do not insist on it. Have duplicates of favorite toys available to help avoid conflicts.

❖ **State rules positively rather than negatively.** Give children an alternative way to behave. For example, you might say, "Please walk" instead of "Don't run."

❖ **Share your feelings about certain behaviors.** "I know that you are angry and that's O.K. But I don't want people to hurt each other. I'm going to help you so you don't hit."

❖ **Give children alternative ways to express their anger.** "If you feel angry, tell us. Say, 'I'm mad!' so we will know how to help you."

❖ **Ask toddlers silly questions so they have lots of opportunities to say, "No."** Matthew loves Mercedes to ask questions such as, "Do we eat a shoe for dinner?" or "Is it time to go to sleep after breakfast?"

❖ **Pay close attention to a child who is likely to hit or bite.** Look for opportunities to help a child stop a behavior before another child gets hurt.

❖ **Acknowledge when children show self-discipline.** Barbara did this when she saw Leo—who was about to throw a block—catch her eye, and then put the block down on the floor. "That was good stopping, Leo."

❖ **Avoid talking with other adults about a toddler's challenging behavior in front of the child.** Toddlers are very aware when they are the topic of conversation. Being talked about can be uncomfortable.

When you take a positive approach to guiding children's behavior, you help children learn self-control and promote their self-esteem. But how do you do this when their behaviors challenge your patience or upset you? We address that question next.

Responding to Challenging Behaviors

When faced with an outbreak of crying, hitting, kicking, temper tantrums, or biting, all caregivers/teachers of infants and toddlers have, at one time or another, found themselves thinking, "What do I do now?" Here are some ideas to consider.

Review your goals for children. Ask yourself, "What do I want to teach children about themselves and their feelings?" La Toya, for example, wants children to receive the message that their feelings are legitimate and respected. She also wants to help them understand what is acceptable behavior as well as what is not.

Be realistic. Base your expectations of behavior on what you know about child development. Infants and toddlers have immediate and intense feelings of joy and excitement, as well as feelings of anger and frustration. They do not yet have the ability to stop and think about how to express their feelings in acceptable ways. Therefore, you can expect that sometimes children will lose control and display behavior that is difficult to handle.

Be aware of your own feelings. Infants and toddlers express their emotions openly and intensely. They have a way of reaching back and stirring up deep feelings in us such as happiness, anger, and frustration that echo back to our own childhoods. Helping a young child learn to manage her feelings means being aware of who is feeling what.

Maintain a calm atmosphere. Strong emotions can be frightening for children and adults. Increased tension often increases the likelihood of negative behavior. To calm a child, first calm yourself. Take a deep breath. Talk with a colleague.

Consider what the child is feeling. To help you figure out how to respond in a positive way, ask yourself, "What is this child saying?" When children cry, withdraw, hit, bite, or lie on the floor kicking and screaming, they may be telling you, "I am lonely," "I am scared," "I am overstimulated by too many exciting things to do," "I am angry," or, "I need you to set some limits for me."

When you intervene, do so in ways that acknowledge children's feelings and give them acceptable ways to behave when an incident does occur. Here is an example of what La Toya said and did after Valisha kicked Eddie (who had taken all the farm animals off the shelf and was playing with them).

- ❖ She acknowledged that Eddie was kicked. "That really hurts, Eddie, doesn't it?"
- ❖ She described what happened. "Valisha, you kicked Eddie and that hurts him."
- ❖ She acknowledged Valisha's feelings. "I think you're angry, Valisha, because Eddie has all the farm animals and you want some too."
- ❖ She stated what is not acceptable. "I can't let you kick because kicking people hurts."
- ❖ She stated what is acceptable. "You can kick the ball if you want to kick something. Or you can tell us in words how angry you are."
- ❖ Finally, she helped Valisha come up with a solution. "How can you let Eddie know that you want some of the animals? That's a good idea. You can ask him for some."

Talk with others. Colleagues and a child's parents can help you put together a picture of what is happening in a child's life. Events at home or in the neighborhood may be upsetting a child. Perhaps something has happened in child care—such as the absence of a primary provider—that may leave a child feeling sad or angry.

When a child's behavior is especially upsetting, talk about it with parents and colleagues. Review the steps you have taken. Indeed, it sometimes happens that after adults talk together about a child's behavior, the behavior disappears. It is as if the act of talking the subject through helps the adults relax and be more available to a child in a way they couldn't when tension was running high.

Since temper tantrums and biting are challenging behaviors among infants and toddlers, we discuss each of these separately.

Temper Tantrums

Temper tantrums are no fun for anyone. They can leave children feeling exhausted and frightened at their loss of control. They can also leave adults feeling angry, incompetent, and even embarrassed, if they occur in public.

If children could tell us what a tantrum feels like, they would probably describe it as a storm of frustration and rage that sweeps in and overwhelms them. It's important to remember that life can be very frustrating for toddlers. Developmental theory tells us that they are learning about limits. They often struggle to accept the limits you set for them as well as the limits of their own abilities. In addition, they frequently find themselves caught between wanting to be a "big kid" and to be a baby. One minute they want you to hold them in your arms. The next, they become upset because they can't tie their own shoes, carry a heavy bag of groceries home from the store, or tell you something because they don't have all the words they need.

Once a tantrum begins, there is often little you can do except keep a child from hurting himself or someone else, and assure the child that you are there. After he has calmed down, acknowledge his feelings in ways that show you accept him and his feelings. Do not shame him. "Not being able to finish that puzzle really frustrated you! It can be scary to be so angry." Suggest other ways to deal with the frustration: "Next time, maybe you should try the animal puzzle instead. Or you can ask me to help you."

It's best to focus your energies on prevention. Planning ahead to minimize temper tantrums will help avoid what can be a very stressful experience for children—and for you.

Minimize frustrations. Create an environment that is as frustration-free as possible. Set up an interesting, safe space that children can explore freely without constantly having you say, "No." Make sure the toys, games, and puzzles you offer match the abilities of the children in your care. Always have on hand familiar toys and puzzles that children have successfully played with in the past.

Give toddlers plenty of opportunities to feel competent. A child who feels competent is less likely to have tantrums. Invite toddlers to help you with everyday chores, such as setting the table or folding the laundry. Offer them many opportunities to make choices about what to wear, eat, and play with. Label shelves with pictures so children can find what they want and help put toys away. Read children's cues to help you understand what they want to communicate and respond accordingly.

Give toddlers a chance to be babies, too. Keep in mind that toddlers need hugs and cuddles. Be there to offer them when they are needed.

Anticipate children's physical needs. You can often turn the tide and ward off a tantrum by doing things such as serving lunch before children get too hungry, helping children take naps before they start falling apart, and giving them a chance to play outdoors when they are ready for active play.

Biting

Biting is very common in group settings of young children. Yet whenever it happens, it is always disturbing to parents and caregivers alike. As with tantrums, it's best to focus your energies on prevention. Understanding the reasons for biting will help you come up with effective strategies to prevent it.[1]

The chart that follows identifies some typical situations when children tend to bite and what you might do to prevent this behavior from happening.

Why Children May Bite	Strategies to Help Prevent Biting
They have a strong need for independence and control. The response to biting satisfies these needs and reinforces the behavior.	Give choices throughout the day and reinforce positive social behavior. If children get attention when they are not biting, they will not have to use this negative behavior to feel a sense of personal power.
Teething causes their mouths to hurt.	Offer children teething toys or frozen bagels to mouth.
They are experimenting. An infant or young child may take an experimental bite out of a mother's breast or caregiver's shoulder. They may simply want to touch, smell, and taste other people to learn more about them.	Provide a wide variety of sensorimotor experiences (such as fingerpainting, playing with dough, preparing and eating food, or engaging in water and sand play) to satisfy this need.
They are exploring cause and effect: "What will happen when I bite?"	Provide several different activities and toys that respond to children's actions and help them learn about cause and effect.
They are trying to approach or interact with another child.	Give children many opportunities to interact with one another. Guide their behavior as necessary, paying special attention to positive interactions.
They feel frustrated or angry. Some children lack skills to cope with situations and feelings such as wanting another child's toy or an adult's attention. When frustrated or angry, they bite.	Watch for signs of rising frustration and potential conflict. You can often intercept a potentially harmful incident by responding to children's needs promptly.
They are asking for attention.	Give children lots of attention throughout the day.
They are imitating behavior.	Model loving, supporting behavior. Offer children positive alternatives for negative behavior. Never bite a child to show how it feels to be bitten.
They feel threatened. When some children feel they are in danger, they may bite in self-defense. Other children may be overwhelmed by their surroundings and the events in their lives and bite as a means of gaining control.	Provide support and assurance so that the child recognizes that he and his possessions are safe.

---

[1] Based on Donna Witmer, "Children Who Bite," *Scholastic Pre-K Today,* March 1992; and Fact Sheet, *Biters: Why They Do It and What to Do About It.* National Association for the Education of Young Children, June 1996.

Unfortunately, no matter how attentive you are, it is likely that sooner or later a child in your program will bite another. Here's what you can do at that moment.

Respond to the situation promptly. As soon as an incident takes place, you must take immediate action.

- ❖ **Comfort the child who was bitten.**
- ❖ **Wash the wound.** Apply an ice pack to help keep bruising down. If the skin is broken, follow the universal precautions for handling blood, which include wearing nonporous disposable gloves, and recommending that parents notify their pediatrician and follow his or her advice.
- ❖ **State clearly that biting is not all right.** Speak firmly and seriously.
- ❖ **Invite the child who bit to help you care for the bitten child.** This gives the child the opportunity to be a helper and leave the role of aggressor. Use these moments to offer the biter support and to teach caring behavior. Remember that, from the biter's point of view, it's scary to be so out of control that you end up hurting someone.
- ❖ **Help the child who bit understand that there are other ways to express anger,** such as using words or growling like a tiger.

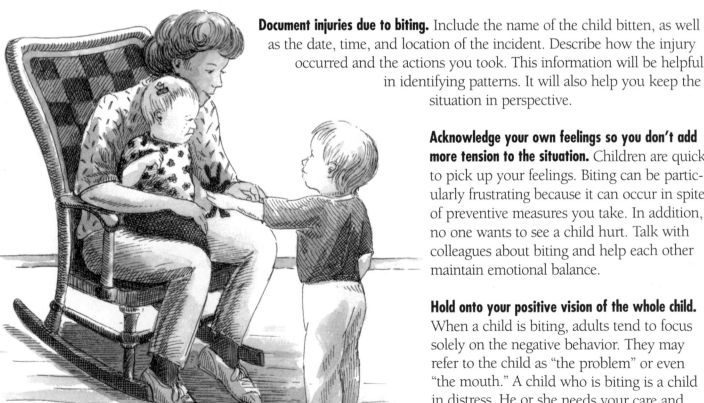

Document injuries due to biting. Include the name of the child bitten, as well as the date, time, and location of the incident. Describe how the injury occurred and the actions you took. This information will be helpful in identifying patterns. It will also help you keep the situation in perspective.

Acknowledge your own feelings so you don't add more tension to the situation. Children are quick to pick up your feelings. Biting can be particularly frustrating because it can occur in spite of preventive measures you take. In addition, no one wants to see a child hurt. Talk with colleagues about biting and help each other maintain emotional balance.

Hold onto your positive vision of the whole child. When a child is biting, adults tend to focus solely on the negative behavior. They may refer to the child as "the problem" or even "the mouth." A child who is biting is a child in distress. He or she needs your care and support to get through a tough time, during and following an incident.

Make and carry out an ongoing prevention and intervention plan. Here are some positive steps you can take.

❖ **Observe to try to identify patterns of instances when biting occurs.** For example, is a child more likely to bite before lunch? Or when things get very loud and confusing?

❖ **Ask parents about what might be going on at home.** Find out if there have been any changes recently. Talk together about how you might help a child stop biting.

❖ **Decide on a plan.** For example, if you notice that a child tends to bite when things get hectic, plan to spend extra one-on-one time with her and make sure to include her on many small group walks.

❖ **If you work in a center, have someone focus on the child who is biting, ideally someone who knows and enjoys this child.** This person should be available to the child all day, to provide support, encourage positive behavior, and of course, to be ready to step in quickly and help the child stop biting. If you work on your own, you may need to adapt your plans for the day so you can give the biter the attention needed. You may, for example, decide not to offer fingerpainting—which requires your supervision—and instead provide colored markers that children can use more independently. Alternatively, you may decide to bring in an extra adult to help out for awhile.

❖ **Observe.** Keep track of how things are going. Adapt your plan as necessary.

Help parents understand the situation. Because biting can upset all parents in a program, it's often helpful to address this issue before it occurs. Discuss with parents the many reasons why children may bite and describe various preventive steps you can take. Share strategies to prevent and deal with biting that parents can use at home. Invite parents to share their strategies with you. Always remember that biting the child back "to see what it feels like" is never an option. If biting does occur, talk with parents directly and openly. Acknowledge their feelings. Consider inviting a community health specialist to meet with parents to address health concerns.

Seek help if biting continues or grows more vicious. Though most episodes of biting fade in a few weeks, there are times when biting signals that a child needs special assistance. If you become concerned, call in a community resource person, such as a developmental specialist, to help you explore interventions a child may need if the approaches we outlined do not help.

While guiding children's behavior may sometimes appear to be taking up too much of your time, it is an important part of your work with infants and toddlers. As you help children learn to control their behavior, you also build a solid foundation for their positive interactions with others.

Helping Children Relate Positively to Each Other

Children begin to learn about relationships from the time they are born. They learn about caring for others, using as models the way others care for them. When you treat children in loving and consistent ways and show how much you value and respect them, you promote positive attitudes toward others—what is also called **prosocial behavior**.

Day after day, you have many opportunities to teach children about getting along with each other. Here are examples of some of the things you can do.

Remember that children look to you as a model. The infants and toddlers you care for are very aware of what you do. How you interact with each child, with colleagues, and with parents teaches children more powerfully than any words you might say about how to get along with other people.

Mirror the behavior of infants and toddlers. When you smile at an infant who's smiling at you, or reflect back the funny expression on a toddler's face, you confirm a child's self-image and what he or she experiences. Because infants and toddlers are so aware of their special adults—including you—mirroring is a powerful way to support children as they create a sense of self and to show them the pleasure of relating to other people.

Respect each child's style of interacting. Some children jump immediately and enthusiastically into activities. Others need time to watch and may eventually need some gentle encouragement. You can respond in the most helpful way when you are aware of each child's style, and understand that it may be culturally based.

Arrange your environment so that children have opportunities to spend time alone or in small groups during the day. Living all day in a large group can be stressful for children and for you. Time away from the large group offers a chance for social interactions that may not take place when everyone is together. Examples of physical spaces that give children a break from group life and promote one-on-one interactions are a large cardboard box or a comfortable chair with room for two. Examples of activities during which you and one or two children can enjoy being together are taking short walks in the neighborhood or preparing a snack.

Acknowledge children's positive interactions. Comment when you see a child interact in cooperative and helpful ways. For example, when two six-month-olds are sitting on a blanket together, you might say, "You are getting to know each other. You touched her face very gently." When Jonisha draws a picture for Valisha, La Toya might comment, "That was very thoughtful. What good sisters you are."

Give children opportunities to help you. Children feel proud of themselves and begin to understand how to be contributing members of a community when you invite them to help you. When Mercedes asks Matthew to carry a letter to the mailbox or help set out his mat at naptime, he feels good about helping.

Encourage children to help one another. Throughout the day, offer children opportunities to assist each other. Invite one child to help look for another's missing sock. Acknowledge when a child uses words or gentle pats on the back to comfort another child.

Read books with themes of helpfulness and friendship. There are wonderful books, such as *Grampa Can Fix It* and the *Max* books, you can read to toddlers. Children also love homemade books about familiar events and people they know—for example, *Valisha Helps Jonisha Find Her Shoe.*

Include equipment and materials that promote interaction and cooperation in both your indoor and outdoor environments. To set the stage for children to interact with one another, you might provide a wooden rocking boat that two or more children can sit in and rock, set out large sheets of butcher paper for children to color or paint on together, or provide opportunities for water and sand play.

Allow children time to work out their differences—but be ready to step in if you are needed. When you wait a few minutes before stepping in, you give two toddlers a chance to discover there is room for both of them to sit on the sofa together. Keep your eye on them so you can be there if you see one or the other about to be pushed off.

Guiding behavior is something you do throughout the day when working with infants and toddlers. We discuss how you guide behavior as part of daily routines and activities in the remaining chapters of this book.

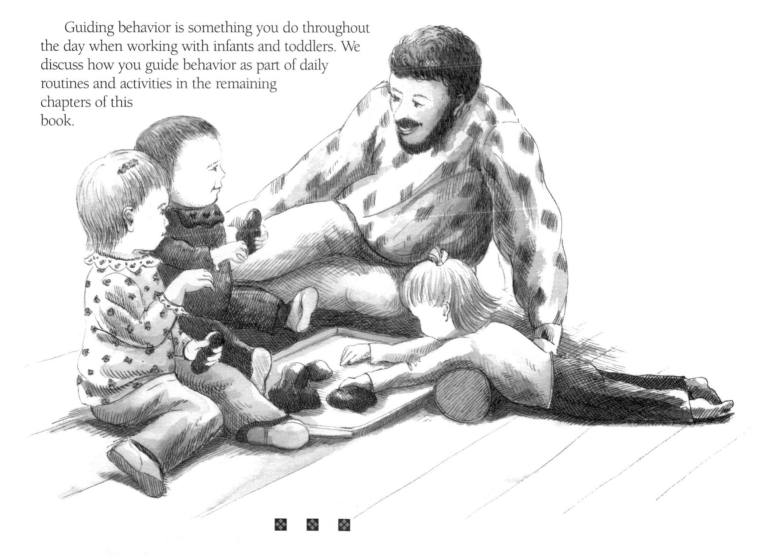

— ◼ —
Sharing Thoughts About
Guiding Children's Behavior

Dear Families:

Young children need adults—to help them learn what is acceptable behavior and how to relate positively to others. We focus on social skills and self-discipline because we know that children who practice these behaviors are more successful in life. Researchers also tell us that children who learn to take personal responsibility for their actions are better able to make good choices in life.

We take a positive approach to guiding behavior. We try to prevent problems, for example, by giving children time outdoors each day to burn up energy. At other times, we try to redirect children's behavior, for example, by giving an infant a rubber toy to chew on instead of the piece of paper from the floor. And, when necessary, we intervene directly to stop hitting or biting.

How We Can Work Together

Guiding children's behavior is a very important responsibility we share. Here are some approaches we can both use.

❖ *Model how we want your child to relate to others.* When we treat your child with love and respect, we set the stage for future relationships. Watching us work together in respectful ways also teaches your child how people should behave towards one another.

❖ *Give your child every opportunity to develop a sense of responsibility.* Young children love to help with everyday chores such as putting napkins on the table. They also like to have choices such as: "Do you want milk or juice with your crackers?" or "Shall we read the book about the bear or the one about the train?"

❖ *Help your child express feelings in acceptable ways.* We can talk about what your child might be feeling to introduce the practice of expressing feelings in words. We can also offer activities like pounding playdough and playing with puppets. When we have to step in, we should always give a positive alternative—"I can't let you hit because someone will get hurt. If you are angry, growl like a lion or kick the ball."

Let's talk about any challenging behaviors, such as biting and temper tantrums. Together, we can figure out how best to deal with them. We can look for patterns in these behaviors to help us better understand what your child might be experiencing. This will help both of us respond in ways that strengthen your child's self-control and self-esteem.

By working together, we can help your child develop the social skills and self-control that are so essential for success in life.

Sincerely,

©1999, Teaching Strategies, Inc., Washington, DC. Permission granted to reprint, for non-commercial uses only, by programs implementing *The Creative Curriculum for Infants & Toddlers*.

Algunas ideas sobre cómo guiar
el comportamiento de los niños

Estimadas familias:

Los niños pequeños necesitan que los adultos guíen su comportamiento para aprender lo que es y no es aceptable, y para ayudarlos a relacionarse positivamente con los demás. Nosotros nos concentramos en las destrezas sociales y en el autocontrol, porque sabemos que aquellos niños que aprenden a relacionarse con otros en formas positivas y a hacer amigos, tienen más exito en la vida. Además, los niños que aprenden a asumir la responsabilidad de su comportamiento, están mucho más capacitados para hacer buenas elecciones en su vida.

En cuanto a la orientación del comportamiento infantil, nosotros asumimos un enfoque positivo, tratatando de prevenir los problemas. Otras veces, tratamos de reorientar el comportamiento infantil, y cuando es necesario, intervenimos directamente, para detener los golpes o los mordiscos.

Cómo podemos trabajar juntos

Guiar el comportamiento infantil es una importante responsabilidad que todos compartimos. Los siguientes son unos cuantos enfoques que, conjuntamente, podemos emplear.

❖ *Modelen la manera en que desean que sus hijos se relacionen con los demás.* Los niños aprenden sobre las relaciones sociales, a partir de de los adultos importantes en su vida. Al tratarlos con amor y respeto, creamos la base para las relaciones futuras. Además, cuando ellos observan esto, aprenden cómo deben comportarse unas personas con otras.

❖ *Bríndenle a sus hijos todas las oportunidades posibles de adquirir el sentido de responsabilidad.* A los pequeños les fascina colaborar con las tareas diarias y les encanta poder escoger entre opciones. Por ejemplo: "¿Deseas jugo o leche con las galletas?" o "¿Quieres leer el libro del osito o el del tren?".

❖ *Ayúdenle a sus hijos a expresar sus sentimientos en formas aceptables.* Podríamos hablar acerca de lo que pudieran estar sintiendo sus pequeños, con el fin de introducir la práctica de expresar los sentimientos oralmente. Cuando debamos intervenir, debemos hacerlo siempre ofreciéndoles una alternativa positiva: "No puedo permitirte que golpees, porque puedes herir a alguien. Si estás furioso(a), ruge como un león o patea la pelota".

❖ *Hablemos sobre los comportamientos desafiantes como morder o gritar con furia.* Juntos podremos establecer la mejor manera de manejarlos. Cuando dichos comportamientos ocurran, podemos intentar descubrir patrones, con el fin de comprender mejor lo que los niños sienten. De esta manera, conjuntamente, podremos responder en formas que fortalezcan el autocontrol y la autoestima de su hijo(a).

Trabajando juntos, podremos ayudarle a sus hijos a adquirir las destrezas sociales y el autocontrol esenciales para que tengan éxito en la vida.

Les saluda atentamente,

©1999, Teaching Strategies, Inc., Washington, DC. Se permite la reproducción, únicamente con fines no comerciales, a los programas que ponen en práctica *The Creative Curriculum for Infants & Toddlers*.

Part III Routines

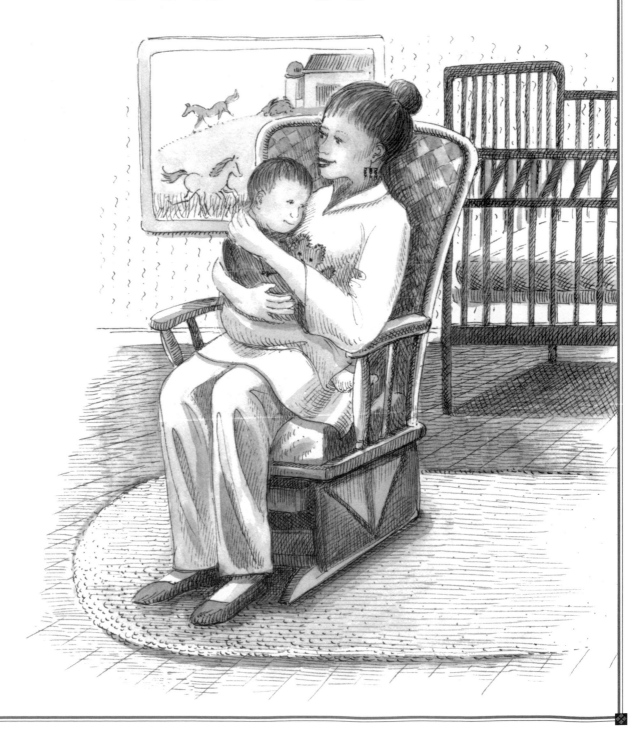

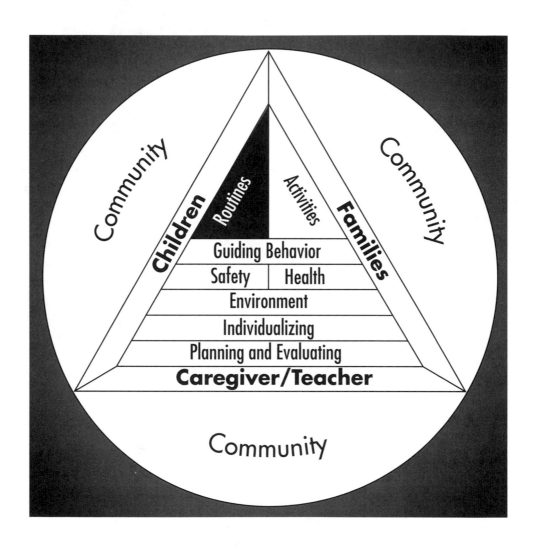

Routines

Hellos and Good-byes
Diapering and Toileting
Eating and Mealtimes
Sleeping and Naptime
Getting Dressed

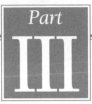
Putting Quality Into Action: Routines Day By Day

The best thing about routines, as seen through the eyes of infants and toddlers, is that they happen day after day, often several times a day. They are predictable, enabling children to learn what to expect. At the same time, they vary enough to hold children's attention and interest.

For adults, daily routines are opportunities to build relationships with children. The one-on-one time you spend easing hellos and good-byes, feeding, diapering, dressing, and soothing a child to sleep help infants and toddlers learn to trust and feel secure with you. As children gain new skills and can participate more actively in daily routines, they develop a sense of their own competence. Routines are also times to nurture children's curiosity and guide them as they make increasing sense of their world.

Because children are unique individuals, they may experience the same routine in different ways. Leo, for example, may have a full-fledged temper tantrum to protest his mother's leaving, while Gena, who also doesn't want her mother to go, may quietly watch her walk out the door. Matthew may eye the potty seat in the bathroom curiously, while Jonisha proudly uses the toilet on her own, remembering to flush and to wash her hands. Julio may fall asleep as snack is being prepared, while Valisha intently practices using a plastic knife to cut slices of banana and pear. The decisions you make about how to respond to children should be based on what you know about each child's developmental level, interests, and temperament.

As children participate in daily routines, they learn to think, collect new information about themselves and their world, and develop skills. For young children, all learning is integrated: physical skills affect social skills and vice versa. Therefore, when Jasmine is asked if she wants "a cracker" or "yogurt," she not only learns the names of things, she also learns about making choices. Similarly, when Matthew learns to put on a jacket by himself, he develops fine motor skills, explores concepts such as *in* and *out,* learns about cooperation (when an older friend shows him the flip-flop method), and confirms his sense of independence. Everyday routines help children grow and learn in all areas.

In Part III, we look at five routines:

- ❖ hellos and good-byes;
- ❖ diapering and toileting;
- ❖ eating and mealtimes;
- ❖ sleeping and naptime; and
- ❖ getting dressed.

For each routine, we discuss its importance to children and families and offer suggestions under the following headings.

Questions to Consider

As you work everyday with children, you make decisions. Thoughtful decision making will help you make the most of each moment. Routines are not just something to get through; they are an integral part of the curriculum. In this section, we identify some of the questions that typically arise and offer suggestions for addressing them. These questions may relate to how to set up your environment, what supplies and materials you need and how to arrange them, what procedures will enable you to work efficiently, how to ensure children's health and safety, and how to involve children's families.

A Child's Eye View

Every routine offers opportunities to build relationships with children and support their growth and learning. To highlight the range of possibilities, we consider how the routine might vary for young infants, mobile infants, and toddlers. We present this information in a series of charts that identify some typical behaviors you might observe. Then, we consider the following.

What the child might be experiencing. To respond appropriately, you must try to determine what is behind a child's behavior. You combine your knowledge of how infants and toddlers grow and learn with your observations of children in your program to help you determine what the child may be feeling or thinking.

How you can respond. There are many ways to respond to children's actions. When you decide to step back and observe as a child plays peek-a-boo, you give her the opportunity to explore hellos and good-byes at her own pace. During lunch time, when you ask a question such as, "What do you think we'll see when we peel this orange?" you stretch a child thinking. In this section we offer suggested responses based on what a child may be experiencing.

Sample letters to families. These letters explain why you focus on the routine in your program and invite families to be your partners in making routines rich experiences for children. Letters are in English and Spanish.

❖ ❖ ❖

Hellos and Good-byes

— ◆ —

Leo sits on the floor in front of his family pictures that Barbara has covered with clear Contact™ paper and hung at child-level on the wall. He runs his fingers over the pictures of Virginia, Elmer, Leo, and their dog Isabelle, all standing in front of their house. "What are you doing?" asks Barbara, as she comes over to join him. "Mommy and Daddy," he says, looking up at her with a smile.

— ◆ —

Infants and toddlers usually arrive at programs with their families. Each day in your program begins with families and children saying hello to you and good-bye to one another. Each day ends as families and children reunite and say good-bye to you.

Learning to separate from and reunite with people we love is a lifelong process. It is not a goal to be achieved in the first week or month or even year of child care.

Separations and reunions can bring out deep feelings in everyone involved. Some of these feelings can be uncomfortable, and it is natural to want to avoid them. It is not surprising that you and children's parents may often conspire to get through the beginning and end of the day as quickly as possible.

In part because hellos and good-byes arouse such strong feelings, they can provide valuable learning for infants and toddlers. Infants can learn about trusting others when the important adults in their lives say good-bye and return as promised. Toddlers can learn about what it means to be a separate person who has deep attachments to others. Caring adults can support this kind of learning.

Questions to Consider

How do you set the stage for hellos and good-byes in your program? Here are some questions and suggestions to guide your thinking as you make decisions.

"How can I support children and their families when it comes time to say hello and good-bye?"

Look at your program through the eyes of children and their families. What do you already do to ease their anxiety about separating and reuniting? What else might you do? Consider the following ideas.

Spend some time with each child and his or her family before the child is left in your care for the first time. Invite parents and other family members to visit your program with their child. Offer to conduct a home visit ahead of time so that they and their child can get to know you. As parents get to know you, they will feel more comfortable when it's time to say good-bye each day. Then too, children will feel more at ease when they see you spending time with their families.

Arrange a transitional period with families. Children need a little time to get to know you and to feel comfortable in this new setting. They can do this best when they are with the people they trust the most. Let families know how important this transitional period is and help

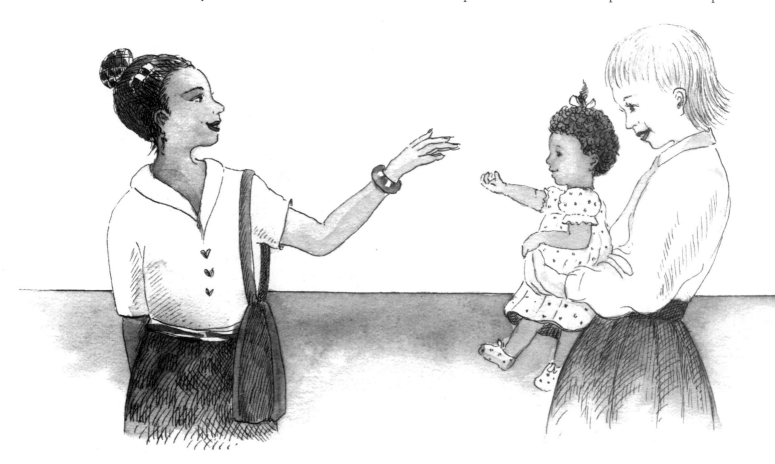

them plan ahead so they can take the time needed to ease their child into your program. During the first week or two, encourage families to stay with their child in your program, play together, say good-bye, and then return, gradually increasing the amount of time they are away.

Hang a welcome sign up at the beginning of the year with the names (and photos) of children and members of their families. It's a good idea to keep the sign up for a month or two. In addition to communicating the message of welcome, photos will help families get to know one another's names and the names of each other's children. You can also make a list of names for families to take home. This will prove especially helpful when children enter your program during the year.

Greet families each morning. Say "good-bye" each afternoon. If you are busy with another child or family, signal that you will be there as soon as you are finished. Give each family a warm hello and share what you will do that day. Be sure to say "good-bye" as each family departs.

Pay attention to and participate in rituals children and their families develop. Be available to hold an infant after a parent gives him or her a good-bye kiss. Walk a toddler to the door to wave good-bye. If families haven't developed a ritual, consider helping them do so. Rituals help children—and adults—feel more secure because they know what to expect.

Hang children's pictures in their cubbies, and label drawers so parents can find their children's belongings and whatever else they may need. Parents will probably feel more comfortable at your program if they can find a cup to get their child a drink of juice, or if they can find their child's belongings in a labeled cubby. When family members are comfortable, they'll be better able to help their children feel more comfortable, too.

Set out an interesting object or activity every morning. A flowering plant, photos you took during a neighborhood walk, or a new toy displayed where everyone can see it, can give parents and children something to explore together as children settle in for the day. Because these transition times often leave adults and children unsure of what to do next, having something to focus on is especially comforting.

Keep in touch with parents about how things are going for them and their children. Keeping the doors of communication open can help parents feel more at ease about sharing any questions or concerns they may have about hellos and good-byes.

"How can I help children feel connected to their families throughout the day?"

Learning how to express and deal with feelings about hellos and good-byes doesn't just happen in the morning and afternoon. When you offer opportunities for children to feel attached to their parents throughout the day, children can gain a sense of security and better understand that they are individuals—attached to, yet separate from their parents. Here are some ways you can help children feel in touch with their parents when they are apart.

Encourage families to bring a child's special blanket or stuffed animal from home. These items, sometimes called transitional objects or "loveys," help young children feel more secure when they are away from those they love. Respect a child's needs and wishes to hold onto her special object. Ivan did this when another child wanted Gena's toy lamb, Franklin: "I explained that Gena wanted to hold Franklin close and helped Tim find a toy to play with." Label these items to prevent them from getting lost. Identify a place to keep them when children aren't using them. Remind parents to take these objects home at night to avoid making a trip back or facing a miserably unhappy child.

Include pictures of children and their families in your environment. Ask parents to bring in photos, or photograph families yourself in your setting or during a home visit. Laminate the photos or cover them with clear Contact™ paper and display them on the wall at children's eye level. You can also fill a basket with family pictures so children can literally "carry" their families around with them. Make a photo album or book of family pictures. Better yet, try all of these ideas and your own, too.

Place toy phones or old real ones near family pictures. Invite children to make pretend calls to their parents. Make a call yourself, if you think it will be helpful.

Talk about children's parents throughout the day. Comments such as, "How did you and mommy get here today?" and, "Your daddy told me you helped wash the car over the weekend," can help children feel close to their parents.

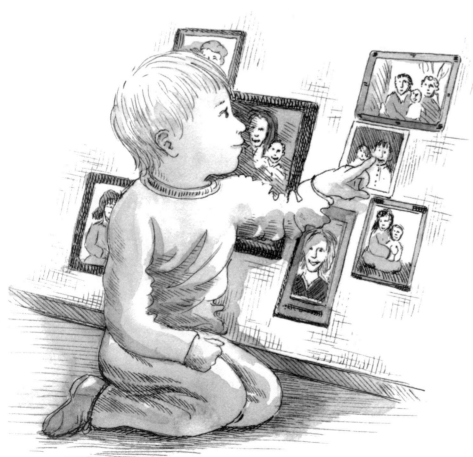

Make daily routines an important part of each day. Invite children to participate in the kinds of activities they do at home with their parents, such as putting on their coats and carrying a letter to the mailbox. You can also invite parents to join their children for lunch or snack as often as possible.

Have parents record a favorite bedtime story or song that children can listen to, especially before a nap. Children will find these sounds of home soothing.

Photograph family members in your setting. Display pictures of family members playing and reading with their children. These photos can help make parents a constant part of your program. They also are a concrete way to help children feel connected to their parents during the day.

"How can I help children gain some sense of control over hellos and good-byes?"

Here are some suggestions of ways you can help children begin to feel more comfortable and competent as they experience hellos and good-byes.

Create an environment in which children can feel competent throughout the day. Children gain a sense of mastery when they can hang up their own coats, reach the sink to wash their hands, help spread cottage cheese on crackers, or find a paper towel to wipe up the juice they spilled. These feelings help them to feel capable of handling separations.

Offer activities that allow children to express their feelings about hellos and good-byes. You want to give children the message that it is okay to feel whatever they feel. Activities such as playing musical instruments, dancing, painting, and playing at the water table or with puppets provide acceptable ways for children to explore and express their emotions.

Encourage play that helps children gain a sense of mastery over separating and reuniting. Encourage peek-a-boo games. Offer many opportunities for children to appear and disappear by playing in tunnels, cardboard boxes with doors that open and close, or tents made by draping a blanket over a table. Provide props such as hats, briefcases, cloth bags, and empty food boxes to encourage toddlers to pretend they are leaving for work or going shopping and coming home again.

Read books with children about comings and goings. Books such as *Are You My Mother?* by P.D. Eastman (*Eres tú mi mama?*) and *Goodnight Moon* by Margaret Wise Brown can help children understand separation as they hear about others saying hello and good-bye. (In the first book, a little bird falls from the nest and asks everyone, "Are you my mother?" until he finally finds her. In the second book, a bunny says goodnight to all the objects in the bedroom.) Consider writing your own books. *Jonisha and Valisha Say Good-bye* is the twins' favorite of all the books at La Toya's house.

Hold the vision of children as competent. Children can sense when you have confidence in their ability to handle hellos and good-byes. Your feelings about them help to shape their sense of themselves.

A Child's Eye View of Hellos and Good-byes

In the charts that follow, we consider typical behaviors you may observe, what children may be experiencing, and how you might respond to build relationships and promote learning.

Young Infants		
What You Observe	**What the Child May Be Experiencing**	**How You Can Respond**
Seeming not to notice when her parents leave	This doesn't necessarily mean she won't notice they're gone at a later time. At this time, though, she may be distracted. For example, she may feel hungry or be listening to the sound of other children playing. Or she may not yet have a sense of her parents as separate people.	Encourage her parents to say good-bye. Over time, she will learn what the term means. This understanding should help make her feel more secure because she knows her parents won't disappear without warning.
Crying strongly when his parents leave	He may understand that his parents are separate people and he wants to be with them.	Show you understand his feelings: "You probably feel sad when Mommy leaves." By listening to him, you show respect. You also help him learn that, no matter what he feels, he can tell you.
Breaking into tears when she spots her parents at the end of the day	She may be showing how deeply she trusts her parents. When they arrive, she feels safe to share any and all her feelings and to ask her parents to comfort her. She may also be hungry or tired. On the other hand, she may be relieved that they've returned.	Help parents understand this hard-to-take declaration of love and trust. Help them realize that crying doesn't mean their child doesn't want to see them. By helping parents feel more at ease, you encourage them to respond to their child in ways that tell her she is safe and loved.

Mobile Infants		
What You Observe	**What the Child May Be Experiencing**	**How You Can Respond**
Withdrawing and sucking her thumb after her grandfather leaves	She may feel very upset about her grandfather leaving. On the other hand, her behavior may be unrelated to separation. She may not feel well or she may be tired, and this is a way to let you know she needs a low-key morning or an early nap.	If you think that her behavior is related to separation, encourage her grandfather to develop a good-bye ritual. Knowing what to expect will help her feel more in control of partings.
So busy practicing climbing up and down the slide that he does not say good-bye	He may be feeling the joy of exploring a new skill.	Encourage his parents to say good-bye (because he may become more aware of their departure after they have left). Hearing a good-bye—even if he is busy on the slide—teaches him he can trust his parents to let him know they are going.
Ignoring her parents when they arrive at the end of the day	She may be happily and deeply involved in what she is doing. She may also be expressing feelings about being left or about something that happened earlier in the day. She may also be trying to gain a sense of control over the situation.	Assure parents that their being ignored doesn't mean she is happier in child care than with them at home. Encourage parents to spend a few minutes talking about what she is doing and about her day. This will help her reconnect in a way that gives her a sense of control and begins the transition to home.

Toddlers		
What You Observe	**What the Child May Be Experiencing**	**How You Can Respond**
Clinging, kicking, and screaming as his parents begin to say good-bye	He may feel very sad about their leaving. He knows he needs his parents and may feel afraid when he is separated from them.	Encourage his parents to develop a good-bye ritual to help him feel more in control. Then help him find something comforting to do after his parents leave. Promote his sense of competence throughout the day, for example, by offering him realistic, manageable choices and inviting him to help with "real work," such as watering the plants.
Crying and protesting when her aunt leaves, although she has taken comings and goings in stride for sometime now	She may be experiencing a normal, bumpy stage in dealing with separation. Perhaps she has just realized that this intriguing place with its toys and nice people will be an everyday thing. Now that its newness is gone, she misses those she loves. Also, she may have something else going on in her life that is upsetting her.	If you feel confident that she'll soon take hellos and good-byes in stride, she'll pick that up. Focus on being supportive and helping her feel good about herself. Remind yourself—and her aunt—that learning to deal with separation involves ups and downs. Talk with her aunt about whether something is happening at home or in child care that may be upsetting, and if so, make a plan to address it.
Saying good-bye to his parents cheerfully and going off to play with a friend; greeting his "Gamma" with a hug at the end of the day; waving good-bye to you and happily walking out the door	He can usually keep a picture of people in his mind, even when separated from them. This gives him a good sense of security and comfort.	Encourage his sense of competence by continuing to provide reminders of his family throughout the day. Appreciate with his parents how—by working together—you have helped him feel good about his growing independence. Recognize, however, that on some days, he may still have difficulty saying good-bye.

Sharing Thoughts About
Hellos and Good-byes

Dear Families:

Every day you and your child say good-bye to one another in the morning and hello again in the afternoon. These hellos and good-byes are children's first steps on a lifelong journey of learning how to separate from and reunite with important people in their lives.

Learning to say hello and good-bye to people we love is a process, not a goal to be achieved in the first week or month or even year of child care. Indeed, after many years of experience, we adults sometimes find it difficult to separate and reunite.

We focus on hellos and good-byes in our program because they are such a major part of your child's life—today and always. Being able to separate is necessary if children are going to develop as independent, competent people. Being able to reunite is necessary to building and maintaining caring, long-term relationships.

How We Can Work Together

❖ *Try to spend some time each morning and afternoon here with your child.* Your presence will help make the transition between home and child care easier for your child.

❖ *Remember always to say good-bye.* By saying good-bye, you strengthen your child's trust in you. Your child can count on the fact you will not disappear without warning. When you let us know you are about to leave in the morning, we can help you and your child say good-bye.

❖ *We can work together to create a hello and good-bye ritual.* This may be as simple as walking to the door with your child or giving your child a giant hug before you leave. Having a ritual offers you both the comfort of knowing what to do.

❖ *Be aware that sometimes good-byes and hellos will be "bumpier" than others.* As we all know, good-byes and hellos can stir up many deep feelings. These feelings, combined with your child's stage of development and other factors such as being hungry or tired, can make saying good-bye and hello difficult at times.

❖ *Bring in family photos and other reminders of home that you want to share.* Seeing these special objects will help your child feel connected to you throughout the day.

By working together, we can help your child feel comfortable, secure, and competent in child care.

Sincerely,

©1999, Teaching Strategies, Inc., Washington, DC. Permission granted to reprint, for non-commercial uses only, by programs implementing *The Creative Curriculum for Infants & Toddlers.*

Algunas ideas sobre
los saludos y las despedidas

Estimadas familias:

Diariamente, ustedes y sus hijos se despiden en la mañana y se saludan nuevamente en la tarde. Estos saludos y despedidas constituyen los primeros pasos de un viaje que dura toda la vida, de aprender a separarse y a reunirse con las personas importantes en nuestra vida.

Aprender a saludar y a despedirse de quienes amamos es un proceso, no un fin que deba lograrse durante la primera semana o el primer mes, ni siquiera durante el primer año del cuidado infantil. De hecho, después de varios años de experiencia, incluso los adultos encontramos dificultades para separarnos y reunirnos nuevamente.

En nuestro programa nos concentramos en los saludos y las despedidas por constituir —hoy y siempre— un aspecto primordial de la vida de su hijo(a). Poder separarse es necesario, si se desea que los niños sean independientes y competentes. Y, poder reunirse es necesario para construir y mantener relaciones afectivas a largo plazo.

Cómo podemos trabajar juntos

❖ *Traten de pasar un tiempo con su hijo(a) aquí, cada mañana y tarde.* Su presencia contribuirá a facilitarle a su niño(a) la transición entre el hogar y la guardería.

❖ *Recuerden despedirse siempre.* Al despedirse, ustedes fortalecen la confianza de sus hijos en ustedes, pues ellos podrán contar con que ustedes no desaparecerán sin avisarles. Si nos permiten saber que se encuentran próximos a irse en la mañana, podremos ayudarles a ustedes y a sus hijos a despedirse.

❖ *Podemos trabajar juntos para crear un ritual de saludos y despedidas.* Esto puede ser tan sencillo como caminar con su hijo(a) hasta la puerta, o darle un fuerte abrazo antes de marcharse. Un ritual les ofrece a ambos la comodidad de saber qué hacer.

❖ *Mantenga presente que algunos saludos y despedidas son más "difíciles" que otros.* Como es sabido, las despedidas y los saludos pueden revolver diversos sentimientos profundos. Estos sentimientos, combinados con el nivel de desarrollo del niño y con otra serie de factores, como el estar cansado o hambriento, pueden hacer más difícil en ciertas ocasiones despedirse y saludarse.

❖ *Traigan fotografías familiares u otro(s) objeto(s) que recuerden su hogar.* El ver estos objetos
especiales le ayudarán a su hijo(a) a mantenerse conectado con ustedes durante el día.

Si trabajamos juntos, podremos ayudarle a su hijo(a) a sentirse a gusto, seguro(a) y competente en la guardería infantil.

Les saluda atentamente,

©1999, Teaching Strategies, Inc., Washington, DC. Se permite la reproducción, únicamente con fines no comerciales, a los programas que ponen en práctica *The Creative Curriculum for Infants & Toddlers*.

Diapering and Toileting

— ◈ —

"I'm going to change that wet diaper," says Grace before she gently picks Willard up and places him on the changing table. "Those are bright blue pants you are wearing today. Did your Daddy put them on you this morning?" "Daddy," says Willard. "We're going to put those bright blue pants right back on as soon as we're finished, okay?" As Grace pulls off Willard's pants, he touches his tummy. "Your tummy," she says. "Are you giving your tummy a little pat?"

— ◈ —

I f a child is changed six times a day until he's thirty months old, he will have had his diaper changed more than 5,400 times. Anything a child experiences 5,400 times is an important part of his life—and of those who change him.

Diapering offers you a chance to focus all your attention on a single child. It is a time you can talk together, sing a song, or play a game of "Where are your toes?" When you can approach diapering as an activity to be experienced together rather than an unpleasant task to hurry through, you teach children an important lesson: that their body functions are a normal, healthy part of everyday life. You can also use diapering as an opportunity to help children learn about many other things, such as the names of parts of their bodies and clothes, and concepts such as up and down, wet and dry, and cool and warm.

Sooner or later, typically between two-and-a-half and three, children reach the point when they are ready physically, cognitively, and psychologically to begin using the toilet. If you—and a child's parents—follow children's leads, are supportive, work together, and avoid getting into power struggles with toddlers, you can help make mastering the skill of using the toilet a pleasant and educational experience. Children will learn to feel good about their bodies and accept their body products as natural parts of themselves. They will develop new fine motor skills as they learn to buckle and button. They will also learn about the pleasure and sense of achievement that comes with wearing "big kid" underpants and gaining self-control.

Questions to Consider

Here are some questions to consider as you decide how best to make diapering and toileting in your program as efficient and pleasant as possible.

"How can I manage the group so that diapering is a time to focus on one child?"

Though of course there will be times when you will want or need to change a child quickly, in many instances, you can make diapering a special time by planning ahead. Here are some strategies to consider.

Coordinate with your co-workers so you can spend unhurried time with a child when changing his or her diaper. Assuming that each child has a primary caregiver, that person has the basic responsibility for changing one or more certain children. You'll need to cue one another when one of you is going to change a child so the other can keep an eye on all the remaining children, and also to let each other know when it's necessary to finish up quickly and return to the group.

Follow a set procedure for changing diapers to assure children's safety and health. As you follow these steps, remember to talk with the child and take advantage of this one-on-one time you have to be together.[1]

- Put a nonabsorbent, disposable cover on the diapering surface. Check to be sure the supplies you need are ready and within reach, so that you can always keep one hand on the child. If you plan to use diaper cream, put a dab on disposable paper. Put all containers away.
- If you use disposable nonporous gloves, put them on now.
- Pick up the child. If the diaper is soiled, hold the child away from you.
- Lay the child on the diapering surface. Never leave the child unattended.
- Remove the soiled diaper and clothes. Put them aside.
- Clean the child's bottom with a moist disposable wipe. Wipe from front to back, using the towelette only once. Repeat with fresh wipes, if necessary, until the child is completely clean. Pay particular attention to skin folds.
- Leave the wipes in the soiled disposable diaper.
- Do not use any kind of powder; inhaling it can be dangerous. Use cream or other skin care products only if parents request it.
- Fold the disposable diaper with the soiled wipes inward, reseal it with its own tape, and discard it into a lined, covered step can, using the foot pedal. Put cloth diapers in a sealed plastic bag or container to be taken home.
- If you used disposable gloves, discard them now into the step can.
- Wipe your hands with a moist, disposable wipe. Dispose of it in the step can.

---

[1] Caryl A. Haddock, Serena Dee, Abby S. Kendrick, and Yvette Yarchmink, Eds. *Health and Safety in Child Care: A Guide for Child Care Providers in Massachusetts,* 2nd Edition. Commonwealth of Massachusetts: Massachusetts Department of Health, 1995, p. 57. Reprinted with permission.

- ❖ Diaper and dress the child in clean dry clothing. Children should always wear outer clothing over a diaper to further contain urine or feces. Now you can hold the child close to you.
- ❖ Wash the child's hands with soap and water (or a disposable wipe). Help the child return to the group.
- ❖ Dispose of soiled items. Label and securely tie the bag for cloth diapers and put it out of children's reach for parents to take home. (Do not rinse diapers in a toilet; bulky stool in the cloth diaper, may, however, be emptied into the toilet.)
- ❖ Put soiled clothes in a labeled and securely tied plastic bag to be taken home. (Children should not handle soiled clothing.)
- ❖ Remove the disposable cover from the diapering surface and discard it into the lined, covered step can.
- ❖ Wash and rinse the diapering area with soap and water if there is visible soiling. Otherwise, sanitize with bleach solution made fresh daily.
- ❖ Wash your own hands thoroughly with soap and running water.
- ❖ Record the diaper change. Report any concerns to parents (unusual color, odor, frequency, consistency, or rash).

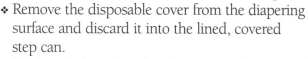

Remain aware of the rest of the group as you change a diaper.
Watch through the corner of your eye, listen, and use your sixth sense to recognize when you are needed. This is vital if you are the sole adult in a program.

Be sure your environment is safe.
Use the checklist for safety in the changing area (see Chapter 8, Ensuring Children's Safety). Check each day to be sure that all children will be safe as they play while you change a diaper.

Schedule regular times to check children's diapers each day—of course, changing children in between as needed. *The National Health and Safety Performance Standards Guidelines for Out-of-Home Child Care Programs* recommends that diapers be checked at least hourly for wetness and feces.[2] Following this type of schedule will help you guide other children into activities that do not require your active participation, leaving you free to pay attention to the child you are changing.

---

[2] American Public Health Association and the American Academy of Pediatrics. *National Health and Safety Standards Guidelines for Out-of-Home Child Care Programs.* Arlington, VA: National Center for Education in Maternal and Child Health, 1992, p. 70.

"How can my space help children feel competent as they master the new skill of using the toilet?"

Think of the many ways you can arrange your bathroom space to encourage children to use the toilet and wash their hands. Here are are some ideas to consider.

Adapt your bathroom as necessary to help children feel more independent. If you have child-sized toilets and sinks, that's great. If not, offer children the option of using a potty chair that sits on the floor or a potty seat on the toilet. (*The National Health and Safety Performance Standards* recommend you provide child-sized toilets or safe and cleanable step aids and modified toilet seats secured to adult-sized toilets. It discourages using potty chairs because they are difficult to maintain. If you use them, be sure you can clean and sanitize them easily.) There are many different types of potty seats designed to meet the needs of children with various disabilities. Families and therapists can advise you on selecting appropriate equipment. If you have a child in a wheelchair or using a walker, be sure to allow enough space in the bathroom. You'll also need handrails to make the transfer from a wheelchair to the toilet an easy one.

Provide steps so children can reach the sink, turn on the water, and wash their hands when they are through. Place paper towels close to the sink so children can dry their hands. Finally, display pictures of children doing a variety of activities, including using the toilet. (See Chapter 9, Promoting Children's Health, for more information about handwashing.)

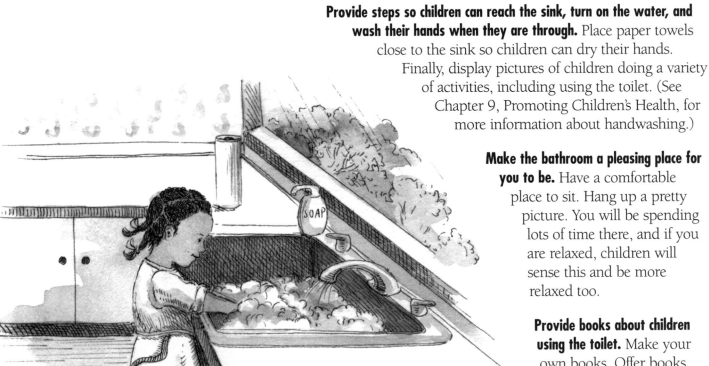

Make the bathroom a pleasing place for you to be. Have a comfortable place to sit. Hang up a pretty picture. You will be spending lots of time there, and if you are relaxed, children will sense this and be more relaxed too.

Provide books about children using the toilet. Make your own books. Offer books such as *Going To The Potty* (Mr. Rogers). Children will enjoy and learn from reading about another child's feelings, successes, and accidents.

"How can I work with parents to support children as they learn to use the toilet?"

Be aware that parents—and you—are likely to have strong feelings about, and perhaps different strategies for toilet learning. One's approach to toilet learning is largely shaped by childhood experiences and culture. For example, many believe that teaching a child to use the toilet means the adult taking responsibility for getting the child to the bathroom at the right time. People with this idea begin toilet training a child around the child's first birthday. Others believe that learning to use the toilet should begin when a child is ready to assume responsibility for his or her own use of the toilet, typically around 30 months of age. Sometimes other issues are at stake. Ivan, for example, worked with a mother who toilet trained her son at 20 months—it was an area of his life where he could excel.

Ask parents how they are helping their child learn to use the toilet at home. Listen carefully, and try to understand families' perspectives when they do things differently than you do. Ask questions to help you understand what is going on.

Share your approach to toilet learning with families before they enroll. Ask parents who are considering putting their child in your program what their approach to toilet learning is, or what they think it will be. Depending on the extent of your differences, parents may decide to look elsewhere for care or you may suggest they do so. More likely, though, your discussion will serve you both by alerting you to differences you will have to negotiate when the time comes.

Discuss the signs that indicate a child is ready. You can hold a parent meeting or offer a workshop on this topic for parents whose children are starting to use the toilet. These signs include:

- staying dry for long periods of time;
- wanting to sit on the toilet with their clothes on;
- telling you they have urinated or had a bowel movement or are going to (though usually too late to get them to the bathroom in time);
- being able to remove their clothing by themselves or with a little assistance;
- being able to push when having a bowel movement; and
- saying they want to use the toilet and talking about their "pee" and "poop" or whatever words they have been taught at home.

Share with parents the steps you take to help a child learn to use the toilet. These steps generally include the items that follow.

- Watch for signs children are ready.
- Encourage children persistently and calmly, but without shame and undue pressure, to use the toilet.
- Remind children to go to the toilet frequently. That way they won't get so involved in what they are doing that they forget and have an accident. Take advantage of group potty time so children can see and learn from one another.

❖ Applaud children's successes without overdoing it.
❖ Allow children to see what they have produced and invite them to help flush it away if they choose to.
❖ Treat accidents matter-of-factly.

Help families be realistic in their expectations of how toilet learning will go. Point out that accidents are par for the course and should be treated in a matter-of-fact way. Explain that even children who can use the toilet successfully may need to wear diapers at night for a time, or may temporarily regress in response to stresses in their lives. Explain that boys and girls differ in how readily they learn to use the toilet. Girls usually become successful "toilet users" at a younger age because they can more easily control voiding urine. Finally, remind parents that all children are different and that it is important not to expect one sibling's experience with toilet learning to be the same as another's.

Set a relaxed tone. Assure parents that over time, their children will learn to use the toilet. We all did.

Make resources available for parents who may be feeling a little confused or overwhelmed. Some parents will be easy-going about toilet learning, while others will want to learn everything about it that they can. Display books or articles you think would be helpful. Encourage parents to share their experiences with one another.

Negotiate differences in your approaches, if necessary. Keep in mind that, from a child's perspective, a sense of continuity is very helpful. Things don't have to be done exactly the same at home and in child care, but children need to know what to expect. For example, La Toya feels it is not realistic in a group setting for her to assume responsibility for getting a child to the toilet on time, even though parents may choose to do so at home. Usually she and parents decide together that a child will continue wearing diapers for a few more months at the program, even though the child goes diaperless during weekend days at home. La Toya's experience has been, "When I take time to work through differences with parents, children sense this and everything turns out just fine."

Discuss toilet learning with parents regularly. Exchange observations about what is happening at home and in child care. Share strategies that are particularly helpful to a child. Give parents encouragement as necessary. Above all, keep your sense of humor.

Post a chart or daily notes to back up your daily conversations. Include information about when a child last went to the toilet and whether he or she has had a bowel movement. Note any "accidents" that have occurred. Notes help create an awareness of patterns that may exist. They also serve as reminders to take home wet or soiled clothes and replace them with fresh items.

A Child's Eye View of Diapering and Toileting

In the charts that follow, we consider typical behaviors you may observe, what children may be experiencing, and how you might respond to build relationships and promote learning.

Young Infants		
What You Observe	**What the Child May Be Experiencing**	**How You Can Respond**
Fussing or crying Squirming in your arms	He may be uncomfortable because his diaper is wet or soiled.	Check his diaper. If that is the problem, change it promptly to show him you are listening and care about his comfort. Promote a sense of self-respect and competence by inviting him to participate in the process. Explain: "I am going to pick you up now." Wait for him to look at you before doing so.
Looking at you as you change her diaper	She probably enjoys being with you. She may be curious about what you are doing. She may want to "talk" with you.	Look at her and smile. Talk with her about what you are doing. Explain: "I'm going to lay you down here. First, let's take off your purple socks." Reinforce the pleasure of interesting sounds and communicating with another person when you say to her: "Your snaps go pop, pop, pop."
Trying to roll over as you change his diaper	The paper covering the changing table may be scratchy. He may want to see something across the room. He may be protesting having to lie still.	Make the changing table's surface as comfortable as possible. Acknowledge his feelings: "I know it is hard for you to lie still." Offer him a job to hold his attention: "Will you please hold your clean diaper?"

Mobile Infants		
What You Observe	**What the Child May Be Experiencing**	**How You Can Respond**
Resisting lying down on her back	As she begins to walk, she may be feeling so driven to be upright and explore that it is actually uncomfortable to be placed flat on her back.	Show that you understand how she feels by changing her in a standing position, if possible. Acknowledge her desire to be standing upright and exploring: "I know you want to keep moving, so we'll change you just as quickly as we can."
Reaching into his diaper to explore his bowel movement as you get ready to change him	He may be curious about what he has produced and is learning about it through his senses—the way he learns about everything else.	Explain that his "poop" is not for playing with, but for flushing away. Help him wash off his hands without making a big deal of it. Provide a variety of sensory experiences throughout the day, including some with smells.
Trying to fasten the buckles on her overalls after you change her	She may feel competent about her developing skills and want to participate in the changing process.	Acknowledge her efforts: "You just about have that buckle fastened." Offer help in a way that encourages her participation: "I'll hold this button part and you put the loop around it." If she is having trouble with the buckles, suggest that her parents dress her in clothes with easier closures, such as Velcro™, so she can experience success. Offer her other opportunities to develop fine motor skills, such as turning the water off and on when she washes her hands and helping to open a new box of diapers.

Toddlers		
What You Observe	**What the Child May Be Experiencing**	**How You Can Respond**
Touching his genitals as he prepares to sit on the potty	He may be curious about his body and its various sensations. He may be exploring a new topic of interest—the difference between girls and boys—or just aiming!	Continue to help him accept and feel good about his body. Use the same words his family uses at home. Discuss with parents the words they use at home, and use the same words at your program.
Using the toilet successfully	She may be feeling pride and pleasure in being a "big girl."	Encourage a repeat performance by expressing your pleasure without overdoing it and adding unnecessary pressure. You might just say: "Good job!"
Wetting or soiling himself after using the toilet successfully	He may feel embarrassed or ashamed.	Take a matter-of-fact approach: "Accidents happen. Let's clean you up." If they continue or occur with increasing frequency, talk with his parents about whether something at home or in child care is adding stress to his life. If possible, address the stress-producing situation.

Sharing Thoughts About
Diapering and Toileting

Dear Families:

If your child is changed six times a day for two-and-a-half years, he or she will have had a diaper change more than 5,400 times. Anything experienced 5,400 times is an important part of your child's life—and of yours. Over time, your child will be doing the growing and learning he or she needs to begin using the toilet—a milestone we will celebrate together!

We focus on diapering and toileting in our program because they are such rich opportunities for spending one-on-one time with your child in our group setting. Through these daily routines we can help your child learn to feel good about his or her body. We can also help your child feel proud and competent about using the toilet and about becoming more independent.

How We Can Work Together

❖ *Please provide us with fresh diapers and dry clothes for your child.* This will free us to focus on your child's needs during diapering and toileting, rather than on searching for supplies.

❖ *Let's talk together about approaches to helping children learn to use the toilet.* How we each do this is, in large part, determined by our own childhood experiences and our culture. Talking together will let us build on the similarities in our approaches and work out any differences we may have.

❖ *Keep in touch with how things are going.* This will allow each of us to have a clear picture of how your child is doing. We can then make decisions about ways to give your child the support he or she needs.

❖ *Remember that accidents are to be expected.* Learning to use the toilet takes time. Even children who can use the toilet successfully may have accidents in response to stresses at home or in child care, such as the birth of a new sibling or the prolonged absence of the child's favorite caregiver. Having realistic expectations allows us to respond to accidents matter-of-factly and address issues causing stress, as necessary.

By keeping a sense of perspective and a sense of humor, we can give your child the time and support needed to learn to use the toilet.

Sincerely,

©1999, Teaching Strategies, Inc., Washington, DC. Permission granted to reprint, for non-commercial uses only, by programs implementing *The Creative Curriculum for Infants & Toddlers.*

Algunas ideas sobre el cambio del pañal y sobre ir al baño

Estimadas familias:

Si a su hijo(a) se le cambia el pañal seis veces al día durante dos años y medio, quiere decir que a él/ella se le cambiará el pañal más de 5.400 veces. Cualquier clase de experiencia que tenga lugar 5.400 veces, constituye una parte importante de la vida tanto de su niño(a) como de la suya. En el debido tiempo, los niños crecen y aprenden lo que necesitan para comenzar a ir al baño. ¡Lo que celebraremos juntos!

En nuestro programa nos centramos en el cambio del pañal y el uso del baño por ser ricas oportunidades que tenemos en nuestro ambiente de grupo, de compartir tiempo en forma individual con su hijo(a). Mediante estas rutinas diarias podremos ayudarle a su niño(a), a aprender a sentirse a gusto con respecto a su propio cuerpo. También contribuiremos a que se sienta orgulloso(a) y competente para hacer uso del baño y con respecto a su mayor autonomía.

Cómo podemos trabajar juntos

❖ *Por favor traigan pañales y una muda de ropa limpia para su niño(a).* Así, podremos centrarnos en las necesidades del niño, cuando necesite que se le cambie el pañal o ir al baño, en lugar de tener que buscar recursos.

❖ *Hablemos acerca de los enfoques para ayudar a los niños a utilizar el baño.* El enfoque de cada uno está, en gran parte, determinado por nuestras experiencias infantiles y nuestra cultura. Hablar de ello, nos permitirá trabajar con base en las similitudes de nuestros enfoques y resolver las posibles diferencias que tengamos.

❖ *Manténganse al tanto de cómo marchan las cosas.* Esto nos permitirá a todos, tener una idea clara de cómo le va a su niño(a). Luego, podremos tomar decisiones con respecto a las maneras en que podemos brindarle el apoyo que necesita.

❖ *Recuerden que pueden ocurrir accidentes.* Aprender a ir al baño toma tiempo. Incluso los niños que lo utilizan con éxito, pueden tener accidentes como reacción a las tensiones en el hogar o en la guardería, como en el caso del nacimiento de un hermano, o la ausencia prolongada de la persona preferida encargada del cuidado del niño. Tener expectativas realistas nos permitirá responder a los accidentes y ocuparnos de lo que pudiera causar tensión, en la medida en que sea necesario.

Al mantener tanto un sentido de perspectiva como sentido del humor, podremos ofrecerle a su niño(a) el tiempo y el apoyo necesario para aprender a ir al baño.

Les saluda atentamente,

©1999, Teaching Strategies, Inc., Washington, DC. Se permite la reproducción, únicamente con fines no comerciales, a los programas que ponen en práctica *The Creative Curriculum for Infants & Toddlers*.

Eating and Mealtimes

— ■ —

"Here Matthew. Will you please carry these spoons over to the table?" asks Mercedes. "We need them to eat our lunch." Matthew takes two spoons from Mercedes and reaches up to put them on the edge of the kitchen table. He climbs up on a chair. "My like beans," says Matthew, as Mercedes spoons some rice and beans on his plate. "Me too," says Mercedes as she sits down next to him.

— ■ —

Eating involves much more than providing fuel for our bodies. Mealtimes and related activities—such as setting the table, washing hands before sitting down to eat, carrying on a conversation with others, and brushing teeth—give children opportunities to develop self-help, communication, and social skills. Mealtimes are also times to practice fine motor skills and develop good nutrition and health habits.

When Linda holds Julio in her arms to give him his bottle, she is telling him, "You can trust me to take good care of you." When Janet puts a spoon and a plastic dish of mashed sweet potato on Jasmine's high chair tray, she is saying, "Go ahead. Here's a chance to practice feeding yourself." When La Toya talks with children about how the green beans are the same color as the playdough they made, reminds them that their chairs are for sitting on, and helps them to brush their teeth, she is teaching concepts, social skills, and supporting their development of healthy habits.

Eating and mealtimes also offer opportunities to build on your partnership with families. At home, the foods families eat reflect personal tastes as well as the family's culture or heritage. Parents need to know that in your program, the meals their children eat also stay within the family culture (and meet the children's nutritional needs, too). In addition, for children younger than three, there are special eating issues that you and parents must discuss together. These issues may include nursing, weaning, introducing solid foods, allergies, and what to bring to child care for a child's lunch.

Questions to Consider

You'll have to make many decisions about mealtimes and eating. Here are some questions and suggestions that can help you.

"How can I work with families to be sure there is continuity between mealtimes in the program and what children are used to at home?"

Communicating with families is necessary to create familiar and pleasant mealtimes. Here are some suggestions for you to consider.

Recognize that certain topics can call up very deep feelings. Depending on children's ages, discuss topics such as nursing, weaning, and introducing new foods at the very beginning of your relationship with families. Respect parents' wishes and follow them whenever possible. For example, do not give extra bottles to an infant whose mother wants to continue nursing. If differences arise, discuss them with families. Welcome mothers to come to the program at any time to nurse their infants. Provide a comfortable place where they can be together without interruption.

Talk with each child's parents about what their child eats at home and in child care. When appropriate, discuss parents' plans for introducing solid foods. Ask parents about foods their toddlers eat at home. Share your program's menus. If parents provide their child's lunches, offer suggestions of safe and nutritious foods to bring. Respect and follow parents' special food requests as closely as possible, whether for health, cultural, or personal preference reasons.

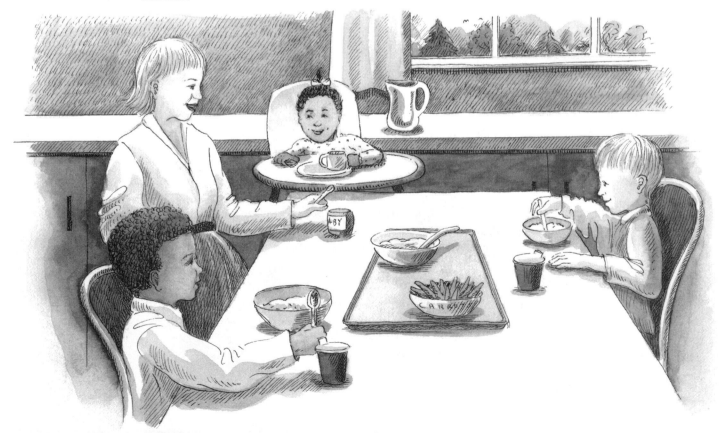

Keep and post records of what and how much children eat during the day. Giving parents a brief note with this information will help them plan their children's meals and snacks for the rest of the afternoon and evening.

Work hand-in-hand with families when it comes to introducing foods to infants. With the knowledge and approval of parents, introduce new foods gradually. Children need time (usually five days) to be sure that they aren't showing signs of allergic reactions.

Experts recommend introducing semi-solid foods (such as rice cereal) first, when infants are at least four months old and their digestive tracts are able to break down solid foods. Then, at about six to eight months, you can offer fruits and vegetables. At about eight to nine months, most infants are ready to taste foods with lumps. You can give table foods at about nine months, and offer eight- to ten-month-olds finger foods.

"What health and safety concerns do I need to consider?"

Be sure families know you take health and safety concerns seriously. Here are some points to consider and to share with families, whether you provide food for children in your program or parents prepare and bring food for their child.

Avoid serving foods that may cause choking. Children under three should not eat certain foods because they present choking hazards. Hot dogs and peanuts are the most frequent causes of choking in children younger than three. Other foods that can cause a young child to choke include: raw carrots, raisins (and similar dried fruit such as cherries or cranberries), popcorn, whole grapes, blueberries, whole olives, corn, uncooked peas, nuts, peanut butter, crumbly cookies or crackers, jelly beans, and hard candy.

Follow practices that promote good nutrition. Other food health precautions include the following.

❖ Don't give honey to infants under 12 months of age because it may carry bacteria that can cause food poisoning.

❖ Give infants under 12 months only formula or breastmilk—no cow's milk. Between one and two years of age, children can have whole milk. After two, low-fat milk is okay.

❖ Avoid giving infants under 12 months white table sugar, artificial sweeteners, corn syrup, egg whites, fried foods, shellfish, raw onions, and processed meats.

❖ Delay offering infants tomatoes and pineapple during the first year of life. The high acidity in these foods can harm delicate mouth tissues.

Be aware of any allergies that children may have. If you observe or learn from parents that a child is allergic to a particular food (chocolate, strawberries, peanut butter, and tofu are among the most common food allergies), make sure this information is circulated and posted where everyone—including volunteers—can see it.

"How can I organize mealtimes so that I can sit down and talk with the children instead of running around?"

An important part of children's mealtime experiences is being with you. You can model good manners and the pleasures of social interaction over food. For young infants, who need to be fed on demand and to be held when you give them a bottle, mealtime is one-on-one time with you. For a group of mobile infants, toddlers, or a mixed-age group, family-style dining is a good way to organize mealtimes. In this arrangement, everyone sits together around the table—on chairs, in high chairs, or on your lap, depending on children's ages—so they can see and interact with each other. In programs where food is provided, it can be served in plastic dishes. You help children, as necessary, allowing those who can to help themselves. Alternatively, when children bring their lunches from home, you all can sit together and eat. Here are some suggestions to help make family-style dining a positive experience for children—and for you.

Plan ahead. Think about how to arrange your tables to make mealtimes manageable, based on the number of tables you need, your staffing, and the age of the children. If you are in a setting with other adults and are caring for mobile infants and toddlers, you may want to serve meals at child-sized tables that seat three or four children and one adult. If you are the only adult in the setting, consider seating yourself and the children together at one large table so you can participate and oversee things. Be sure to have everything you need on hand—food, plates, spoons, and so forth. This way you won't have to leave the table to look for missing items.

Create a calm and pleasant atmosphere. Transitions that help set a quiet tone include reading a book or doing another quiet activity. Attractive placemats tell children that mealtimes are special.

Keep waiting time as brief as possible. Invite one or two children to help you set the table while others are playing. Have the food ready when the children get to the table. If hungry children have to wait, confusion and conflicts are bound to occur.

Model good manners. Say "please" and "thank-you," and encourage children to do the same to you and to one another. Ask children to wait to begin eating until everyone is served. Be flexible about this, however, since the younger the child, the harder it will be to wait.

Invite parents to join their children for snacks and meals whenever they can. With extra hands available to help, each child can get more attention. Having family members present can also ease separation and help children make the connection between eating at home and at child care.

Make cleaning up as easy as possible. Spills and messes are bound to occur. What can you do to focus on the children rather than on keeping everything neat and tidy? You can locate your eating space in an area with an easy-to-clean floor, have the children wear bibs, place extra napkins and paper towels nearby, and invite children to help clean up spills. These are simple solutions to help you remember what's really important.

Encourage relaxed, friendly conversation. Talk together during mealtimes about familiar topics of interest to the children, such as the taste and smells of the food you are eating, activities you did earlier in the day, or plans for the afternoon. Encourage children to let you know what they want and need during mealtimes.

Create an after-meal ritual with mobile infants and toddlers. For example, encourage children to stay at the table and talk with each other until everyone has finished. If the children can't wait, let them leave the table to brush their teeth or work on a puzzle until all have finished the meal.

Consider the best time for you to eat. Although you want to be a good model for children, you may find that trying to eat at the same time you're supervising a group at the table is too much. You may prefer having your lunch during a more quiet time, which is certainly understandable. Janet has figured out a compromise that works for her. She eats some of her lunch with the children and saves the rest for later while the children are napping.

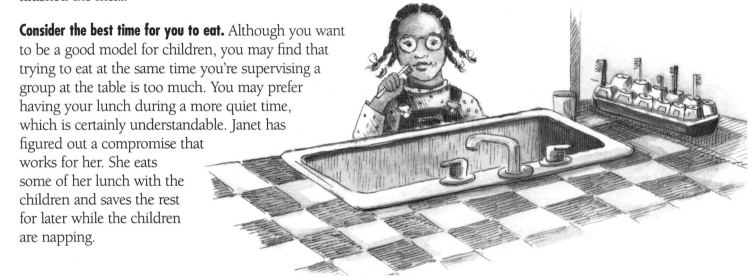

"How can I promote children's growing independence during snack and mealtimes?"

When children leave the table, they should have had enough to eat. They should also feel good about themselves and about their growing abilities. Here are some ways you can promote these positive feelings.

Use plates and eating utensils that are unbreakable, safe, and easy to handle. Small plastic pitchers for pouring juice or milk and plastic serving bowls encourage children to serve themselves. Special seats, utensils, deep-sided bowls, and mugs with two handles are adaptations that can help children with special needs to be independent, too.

Avoid struggling over food. Encourage children to try new foods, but don't force them to eat something they really do not want. Talk about new foods, serve them in attractive ways, and taste everything yourself. Don't worry if toddlers eat just one or two foods at a time. Research has shown that they will get the nutrients they need over the course of a week or even a month——if not in a single meal.

Encourage children to participate in whatever ways are appropriate for their level of development. Place an infant seated on your lap so he can hear and see the other children. Offer a mobile infant a chance to use her fingers to feed herself. Invite toddlers to help you set the table and do other mealtime-related tasks.

Offer activities that promote new mealtime skills throughout the day. For example, include plates and eating utensils in the dramatic play area. Toddlers can role-play mealtime events. You can also provide small pitchers and cups for water play. Children can use these to practice pouring liquids.

Recognize children's skills and new accomplishments. Don't forget to make a positive comment when you see a child just learning to hold a bottle, drink from a cup, or spread cottage cheese on a cracker. Your praise can encourage children to improve their skills and learn new ones.

A Child's Eye View of Eating and Mealtimes

In the charts that follow, we consider typical behaviors you may observe, what children may be experiencing, and how you might respond to build relationships and promote their learning.

Young Infants		
What You Observe	**What the Child May Be Experiencing**	**How You Can Respond**
Fussing	He may be hungry.	Set the infant on your lap as you give him a bottle. From that position, he can experience the sights, sounds, and smells of mealtime.
Cooing or babbling while eating a banana	She is expressing pleasure and interest in what is happening.	Talk with her about what's going on: "We're having some banana for snack today."
Reaching in his bowl to grab a handful of pureed sweet potatoes; tasting and smearing the food all over his high chair tray	He is exploring the taste and texture of this food.	Even if it makes a mess of face, hair, and high chair, you'll want to encourage touching and tasting as a way to learn. You may suggest he use a spoon, but don't be surprised if he continues to eat with his hands.

Mobile Infants

What You Observe	What the Child May Be Experiencing	How You Can Respond
Throwing the banana you hand him on the floor or turning his body away	He may be saying that he has had enough to eat or doesn't like bananas.	Ask if he has finished eating. Offer him another banana slice. If he still is not interested, wipe his hands and face and guide him to another activity.
Grabbing a cracker from another child	She may not know how to ask for something she wants or how to share.	Explain that the cracker belongs to another child. "That's Eileen's cracker. Here's one for you."
Getting up from the table	He has finished eating.	Help him think about what to do next. "I guess you're finished eating. Let's clean up and wipe your hands and face. Then you can play."

Toddlers

Watching as you set the table	She is curious about what you are doing.	Give her a way to participate. "Let's wash your hands. Then you can help me put the napkins and plates on the table."
Pouring juice carefully and eating cooked vegetables with a spoon	He is proud of serving and feeding himself.	Build his confidence by commenting on his growing skills: "Good job! You ate all your vegetables with your spoon!"
Finishing her milk and the last bit of food on her plate	She has finished eating and may still be hungry.	Ask if she wants more food, and if so, provide it. If not, remind her of what to do: "Put your plate in the dirty plate bin. Then you can wash your hands and face and brush your teeth." Encourage her to do a quiet activity until everyone has finished eating.

Sharing Thoughts About Eating and Mealtimes

Dear Families:

Picture your child eating a meal or snack in child care. What is he or she experiencing? For one thing, your child is getting the kinds of foods he or she needs to be healthy and strong. But there is so much more. Eating snacks and meals—and for older children, doing related activities such as setting the table, cleaning up, and brushing their teeth after eating—give your child a chance to feel cared for, and to develop self-help, communication, and social skills. Mealtime is also a chance for children to begin practicing good nutrition and health habits.

Children's experiences and the attitudes they form today will help shape their eating habits in the future. By modeling healthy practices and making eating a pleasurable and social time, together we can lay the groundwork for nutritional and enjoyable eating for the rest of their lives.

How We Can Work Together

❖ *You are welcome to join us for a snack or meal whenever you can.* Your child will love having you with us. So will we! In addition, you'll have a chance to see how we do things so you can ask questions and make suggestions. Of course, if you are nursing your child, please come anytime. We will find a comfortable place where you can feed your baby without interruption.

❖ *Please share with us what your child experiences during mealtimes at home.* What does your child eat and drink? What kinds of things do you talk about? How does your child participate? This kind of information will help us give your child a sense of continuity by talking about family meals and serving some of the same foods.

❖ *Give us any information we need to keep your child healthy.* Let us know, for example, whether your child has any allergies or perhaps a tendency to choke. Keep us informed of any changes. Check to be sure we post this information so that any adult working in our program who may feed the children will know it, too.

❖ *Please ask us for menus and ideas for mealtimes.* Sometimes it's hard to come up with ideas for lunches. We'll be glad to give you some tips. We welcome your ideas as well.

Together, we can make mealtimes an enjoyable and valuable learning experience for your child.

Sincerely,

 ©1999, Teaching Strategies, Inc., Washington, DC. Permission granted to reprint, for non-commercial uses only, by programs implementing *The Creative Curriculum for Infants & Toddlers.*

Algunas ideas acerca de
la comida y las horas de comer

Estimadas familias:

Imagine a su hijo en la guardería comiendo o merendando. ¿Qué es lo que experimenta? Para empezar, está recibiendo alimentos necesarios para mentenerse fuerte y saludable. Pero, se trata de mucho más. Comer y merendar —y para los niños mayorcitos, llevar a cabo otras actividades relacionadas como poner la mesa, recoger y limpiar, y lavarse los dientes después de comer— les brinda a los niños tanto la oportunidad de sentir que se les atiende, como de adquirir autonomía, desarrollar la comunicación y destrezas sociales. Las horas de comer, también les brindan a los niños la oportunidad de comenzar a practicar buenos hábitos de nutrición y salud.

Las experiencias de los niños y las actitudes que adopten hoy en día, les ayudarán a conformar sus hábitos alimenticios futuros. Al modelar prácticas saludables y convertir la hora de comer en un tiempo placentero y de socialización, juntos podremos darle los cimientos a una alimentación nutritiva y grata para el resto de sus vidas.

Cómo podemos trabajar juntos

❖ *Ustedes son bienvenidos a compartir con nosotros una merienda o comida cuando puedan hacerlo.* A sus hijos les encantará que ustedes estén con nosotros. ¡Y también a nosotros! Además, ustedes tendrán la oportunidad de ver lo que hacemos y cómo, y podrán hacernos preguntas y sugerencias. En nuestro salón, encontraremos un lugar en el que se pueda alimentar a su bebé sin interrupciones.

❖ *Por favor, compartan con nosotros las experiencias de los niños en el hogar a la hora de comer.* ¿Qué come y bebe su hijo(a)? ¿De qué hablan? ¿Cómo participa su hijo(a)? Esta clase de información nos permitirá ofrecerle a los niños un sentido de continuidad al hablar de las horas de comer familiares y servir algunas de las mismas comidas.

❖ *Provéannos la información necesaria para mantener saludable a su hijo(a).* Déjennos saber si, por ejemplo, su niño(a) tiene alguna alergia o, quizá, tendencia a ahogarse, y manténgannos informados sobre cualquier cambio. Verifiquen, para estar seguros, que exhibimos esta información, de manera que cualquier adulto que trabaje en nuestro programa y que pudiera alimentar a su hijo(a), también esté al tanto.

❖ *Soliciten menús e ideas para las horas de comer.* A veces, es difícil imaginar qué almuerzos nutritivos disfrutará su hijo(a). Nos encantaría hacerle unas cuantas sugerencias, así como recibir sus ideas.

Juntos, podremos convertir las horas de comer en experiencias de aprendizaje gratas y valiosas para todos nosotros.

Les saluda atentamente,

©1999, Teaching Strategies, Inc., Washington, DC. Se permite la reproducción, únicamente con fines no comerciales, a los programas que ponen en práctica *The Creative Curriculum for Infants & Toddlers*.

Sleeping and Naptime

— ■ —

Barbara notices Leo lying on the blue pillows in the reading corner rubbing his eyes. "Leo, you look a little sleepy. Your daddy told me you didn't sleep very well last night." Leo looks up at her. "I think maybe you could use an early nap today." Barbara checks in with Carol who is making playdough with three children. Carol says they are almost finished and that she will watch things while Barbara takes Leo into the nap room. Barbara goes over and picks Leo up. "Let's go sit together in the rocking chair."

— ■ —

Sleeping and naptime ensure that children get the rest they need during their active day in child care. Even for those who do not sleep, naptime can serve as a break from group life. It gives children some relaxed time on their own to rest or look at a book. Naptime also provides a quiet time when you can relax, meet with colleagues, and refocus your attention and energy so you can be more available to children.

In addition to meeting children's physical needs, sleeping and naptime also give children of all ages an opportunity to experience trust in their world and in themselves. When Barbara rocks Leo to sleep, and Abby wakes up in the familiar setting of her own crib at Brooks's house with her blanket from home, they experience their world as safe and predictable. When you give individual children the support and time they need to fall asleep and wake up, they learn to trust themselves as they negotiate the path from being awake to asleep and back again.

Finally, discussing sleeping and naptime with families gives you the opportunity to strengthen your relationship. You can share information about a child's patterns of falling asleep and waking up, exchange strategies about helping a child fall asleep, or work through differences you may have on issues such as whether a child should be awakened if he or she sleeps past a certain time.

Questions to Consider

How will you set the stage for sleeping and naptime in your program? Here are some questions and suggestions to guide your decisions.

"How can I create an environment that encourages sleeping?"

An environment that is too stimulating can make it difficult for children to fall asleep. Here are some suggestions of ways to lessen stimulation and promote sleep.

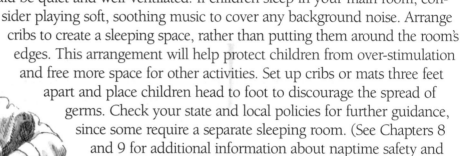

Make space where children can sleep quietly and safely. If children sleep in a separate room, it should be quiet and well-ventilated. If children sleep in your main room, consider playing soft, soothing music to cover any background noise. Arrange cribs to create a sleeping space, rather than putting them around the room's edges. This arrangement will help protect children from over-stimulation and free more space for other activities. Set up cribs or mats three feet apart and place children head to foot to discourage the spread of germs. Check your state and local policies for further guidance, since some require a separate sleeping room. (See Chapters 8 and 9 for additional information about naptime safety and health concerns.)

Be sure each child sleeps in the same place each day. Infants will feel more secure when they are placed in the same crib day after day. Two year olds will be comforted by the routine of being on the same mat or cot in the same location.

Provide children with clean sheets and blankets. You may provide and launder these regularly or parents may do so, depending on your situation.

Encourage families to bring in comfort objects from home, such as a child's blanket or stuffed animal. Holding onto these reminders of home is soothing and can help children feel secure enough to fall asleep.

"When and for how long should children sleep each day?"

From birth, children differ in how much sleep they need, how soundly they sleep, and the regularity of their sleep patterns. They also differ in the length of time it takes them to wake up and in their moods upon awakening.

Typically, the younger a child is, the more sleep he or she needs. Infants such as Julio need more sleep than toddlers like Matthew. Children also need to be able to sleep according to their personal schedules. Sometime during their second year, children change from sleeping in the morning and afternoon to sleeping only during the afternoon. During this transition, two naps a day can be too many, while one isn't enough. This can be a challenging time when children can easily become overtired and adults frustrated. It is helpful if you can remain flexible and plan your day to give children the option of one or two sleep periods. Over time, most two year olds such as Gena and Valisha will typically sleep one time each day during regularly scheduled after-lunch naps.

"Why do some children find it so difficult to fall asleep?"

Do you know a child who fights sleep? The reasons for this are many and depend in large part on a child's temperament and stage of development. Here are some common reasons for resisting sleep.

Sleeping means being still. Infants on the verge of walking and those who are new walkers want very much to be upright and to move. Being picked up and placed in a crib to sleep is exactly what they do not want. You may find children at this stage standing in their cribs protesting sleep and sometimes moving their legs as if they are walking, even as they fall asleep.

Sleeping means "losing touch" with the world. The world is filled with many fascinating things to do. Some children find it hard at times to "disengage" and fall asleep.

Falling asleep can be experienced as a kind of separation. When children close their eyes and fall asleep they may feel as if they are saying "good-bye" to the people and things in their world. Children like Leo, who are struggling with separation, often fight sleep.

Toddlers may be asserting their independence and trying to act more grown up. Refusing to nap when you ask them to is one way toddlers can take charge and demonstrate their growing independence. They may also be very aware of older siblings who no longer nap and may even say, "Napping is for babies."

Overstimulation, stress, and being overtired can make it hard to relax and fall asleep. Have you ever found it hard to unwind after a particularly busy or stressful day? Or when you are overtired? Children, too, can become so wound up that they find it difficult to slow down and sleep.

Stalling gives a child more one-on-one time with his or her special adult. Some children want or need extra attention. They learn that not cooperating at naptime is a way of engaging an adult.

Children may sense the tension of the adult who wants them to sleep. Have you ever noticed that the more you want children to nap, the less likely some of them will do so? As Barbara has discovered, "It's like they have radar. They can sense my worry that they won't fall asleep and this makes it hard for them to relax."

A child may not be tired. Some children need less sleep than others. Knowing this, you can offer alternative options to sleeping, such as playing quietly.

"What can I do to help assure children get the sleep they need?"

Here are some suggestions of strategies you can use to help children get the rest they need.

Take children outdoors each day. Daily exercise and time in the fresh air and sunshine help children relax enough to go to sleep.

Watch for cues throughout the day that tell you a child is tired. The better you know a child, the easier it will be to tell when that child needs a nap. Children's cues may include crying their "I'm tired" cry, rubbing their eyes, or being more fussy, cranky, or easily frustrated than usual.

Establish a regular routine. Create a relaxed mood by planning a quiet activity—such as reading a story or playing soft music—before naptime. This will help toddlers quiet down and know that it will soon be time for a nap.

Develop naptime rituals that you do each day with individual children to help them fall asleep. Talk with families about what they do at home so you can offer similar routines. These may include singing a lullaby, playing a tape of a parent singing or reading, rocking with a child for a few minutes, or rubbing a child's back. For some children, the routines may be simply putting them in their cribs and saying, "Night night," or "Sleep well."

Be aware of children's individual styles as you plan naptime. Helping a group of children sleep is a bit like doing a juggling act. Knowing how individual children fall asleep and wake up can help you decide how best to manage this routine. Barbara and her co-workers at the Head Start Center find it works best to help the soundest sleepers get settled first and then focus on the children who need more attention and time.

"What do I do when a child cries at naptime?"

There really is no magic formula about how long to let a child cry before picking him or her up. How you respond to a child who cries depends in large part on what you know about that individual child. Here are some points to consider when faced with a crying child at naptime.

Look for patterns (with families' help) to understand why a child may cry at naptime. Is a child crying to release tension before he can fall asleep? Is he overtired? Is he fearful? Comparing notes on a child's behavior at bedtime and naptime can help you and families better understand the reasons for crying. Some children just need to cry a short time before they fall asleep.

Listen to the intensity of the cry. Is the child letting off steam or merely protesting for a few minutes? Is the crying winding down? Does the child seem to be in serious distress? Does the child stop crying and settle down if you sit with him for a few minutes? Are things going along relatively smoothly, or has there been any upset at home? Also, consider the effect of crying on other children. Will it upset any children or start other children crying? Your answers will help you decide how long to let a child cry.

Avoid making naptime a battleground. When children associate naptime with tension and anger, it is only natural that they should cry.

"What do I do when children don't sleep?"

As children get older, they begin to nap on more of a schedule, giving you a little time to yourself. You can expect, however, that there will be days when one or more children aren't going to fall asleep as planned. It's natural to feel frustrated when this happens, and your tension will make it difficult for children to relax. Here are some suggestions for addressing the problem.

Reflect on what a child might be experiencing to help you decide how to respond. Try to understand why a child is having trouble sleeping to help you decide how to help the child. For example, Grace is aware that Willard is just about to begin walking on his own. She knows it is hard for him to stop to sleep. She has been making an extra effort to do quiet, relaxing activities when she sees he is getting tired. Yesterday, when he didn't sleep at all and became very cranky, she talked to a colleague at the Kendrick Center who reminded her that he was going through a stage that wouldn't last forever. In another example, when Matthew recently had trouble sleeping, Mercedes realized that, because it had been cold and rainy for several days, he had been cooped up inside. The next day, with a cold rain falling, she got out the cloth tunnel and made up a jumping game which Matthew loved. After the exercise, sleep came easily.

Plan your day so you can do what's necessary and get a break, even if some of the children don't sleep. On days when you need to do something such as attend a staff meeting or meet with a parent, try to arrange for a substitute to watch the children at naptime. This can help you feel less pressure over naps and allow you to meet your other responsibilities. In center-based programs and family child care programs where there is more than one adult, rotating the times each adult goes for lunch permits everyone to get a break, even if some children stay awake. As some toddlers begin outgrowing naps, many programs make a rule that children should lie on their mats at least 10 to 15 minutes. Toddlers often will fall asleep once they are quiet. Children who do not sleep are encouraged to read or play quietly so they don't wake the other children.

Take a look at the big picture, if no one sleeps. If, day after day, none of the children are sleeping, there is usually something program wide that needs adjusting. Here are some questions to ask yourself: Are you giving children enough time for outdoor play and exercise each day? Have you planned your daily schedule so that naptime is too early? Do you give children ample wind-down time after lunch and a busy morning? If answering these questions still doesn't help the problem, try asking a colleague to observe. Often another pair of eyes can help you see things you may not be able to see on your own.

"How can I work with families around sleep issues?"

Here are some suggestions of ways to work together to make sleeping a positive experience for children.

Exchange information each day about children's sleep patterns. You and children's parents each need to know how long a child slept, when he or she last slept, and any changes in sleep patterns, so you can plan accordingly. Knowing Matthew had a restless night means Mercedes can be on the lookout for signs of tiredness and offer a quiet activity or an earlier-than-usual nap. Knowing Abby had a two-hour nap means her father might stop to do some food shopping on the way home, since Abby is well rested.

Ask families about how their child sleeps at home. In some families, children sleep on a schedule and always in their cribs. In other families, children may sleep whenever they fall asleep and wherever they are. Some children may sleep on a mat on the floor or in a hammock. Knowing children's habits can help you plan so that you can offer as much continuity and comfort as possible.

Work together to resolve differences. Some parents may ask you to limit the amount of time their child sleeps at the program so he or she will go to sleep easily at home. You may feel it is not right to awaken a sleeping child. Other parents may want their child to sleep a long time during the day so they can have time with him or her at night. You may feel that children need to go to bed early so they are rested when they arrive at your program. To avoid a power struggle, talk about your differences and come up with a plan that is workable for both of you—always considering the child's best interests.

Be available to support parents whose children have sleep problems. Assure parents that sleep problems are common—especially during the second year of life—and that they pass. Explain that parents need not worry that their child will suffer from lack of sleep; children do get the sleep they need. Encourage parents to talk with one another so they can share experiences and strategies and know they are not alone.

A Child's Eye View of Sleeping and Naptime

In the charts below, we consider typical behaviors you may observe, what children may be experiencing, and how you might respond to build relationships and promote learning.

Young Infants		
What You Observe	**What the Child May Be Experiencing**	**How You Can Respond**
Rubbing his eyes	He may be sleepy.	Describe what you think he is feeling: "You look sleepy." Though he will not yet understand your words, when you respond to his needs he will learn that he can trust you. Then consider what this child needs to fall asleep. For example, does he want to sit in your lap in the rocking chair and rock? Or does he need to lie in his crib and cry for a few minutes to release tension before he sleeps?
Falling asleep in the stroller during a neighborhood walk	She is tired and needs to sleep.	Let her sleep. Even though she may not be learning as she sleeps, she will be more alert and better able to take advantage of other learning opportunities when she awakes and is rested.
Waking up crying	He may be hungry or uncomfortable because he is wet. Or he may need some comforting as he makes the transition between being asleep and awake.	Talk gently and pick him up. Check his diaper and offer him a bottle if you think he is hungry. Assure him that everything is all right: "You will be OK. Shall we read a book together while you wake up?"

Mobile Infants

What You Observe	What the Child May Be Experiencing	How You Can Respond
Protesting strongly when you put him in his crib—even though you know he should be tired	He may be so driven to be up and moving and doing that he is feeling uncomfortably restrained.	Describe what you think he is feeling: "It's hard to stop playing." Sing a soothing song or rub his back gently. Offer him his "lovey" from home if he has one. Explain: "Now it's time to rest. Later you can play some more." Let him cry for a brief time if he needs to do so to wind down. If his protests persist and he shows no sign of settling down, you may want to get him up and let him play. Offer him a nap later in the day. He will sleep when he needs to sleep.
Stirring and beginning to call for you after sleeping for only a short time	She may be rested and ready to get up. Or she may still need more sleep.	If you think she is ready to wake up, get her up and spend some quiet time with her until the others wake up. If you think her sleep has been interrupted and that she is still tired, help her fall back to sleep by gently laying her back down and patting her back.
Appearing to be very sleepy soon after arriving at child care	He may have a long commute to child care or he may not have slept well the night before. He may be in between needing one nap and two.	Adapt your plans to allow for his sleeping. For example, change your morning plans as necessary so you can offer him a nap. Be sure there is stroller space for him if he gets tired during a walk. If he can sleep when he is tired, he can enjoy and take advantage of various experiences when he is more rested.

Toddlers		
What You Observe	**What the Child May Be Experiencing**	**How You Can Respond**
Squirming on her mat and having trouble getting settled	She may need to go to the bathroom. Alternatively, she may be overstimulated by sounds and sights in the room.	Ask if she needs to go to the bathroom and let her go if necessary. Dim the lights and play quiet soothing music. Sit with her and talk quietly as you rub her back or cover her with a blanket. Be sure she has her "lovey" from home.
Moving off his cot and making a lot of noise that disturbs the other children	He may not feel tired or may need help settling down. He may be asserting his growing independence by testing to see how you will respond.	Step in immediately. Explain: "The other children are sleeping. Now it is time to be quiet and lie down on your cot so you don't wake them up." Help him relax and settle down.
Staying awake at naptime	She may have outgrown the need for a nap.	Encourage her to lie down on her cot for 10 to 15 minutes to see if she will fall asleep. If she remains awake, explain: "You can play quietly or read on your mat until the other children wake up."

Sharing Thoughts About Sleeping and Naptime

Dear Families:

Having enough sleep makes it more likely that children will enjoy and benefit from learning opportunities throughout the day. Other than satisfying the need for sleep, sleeping and naptime enable children to develop trust and competence as they move from being awake to falling asleep and waking up again. As we—with your help—learn your child's individual style of preparing for sleep and waking up, we can offer the support he or she needs. For example, while some children like to be rocked or have their backs rubbed, others prefer to be left alone as they drift into sleep.

How We Can Work Together

❖ *We can communicate each day.* By keeping each other informed about the length of time your child sleeps and any changes in his or her sleeping patterns, we each can plan better. For example, if we know your child didn't sleep well the night before, we can offer an early nap, if necessary. If you know your child took a long nap and is well rested, you may decide it is all right to stop and buy groceries on the way home. Do you think your child is getting enough rest during the day? Let us know.

❖ *Please share with us ways that you help your child fall asleep.* If we know, for example, that you sing a certain song or rock your child for a few minutes before placing him or her in the crib, we can do the same thing. This will help your child experience some of the safe and secure feelings he or she has with you and make it easier to fall asleep.

❖ *Please bring your child's "lovey" from home.* Having a special blanket, stuffed animal, or other object from home can make falling asleep easier for a child. If your child has such an object, please label it with your child's name and bring it in. We'll take care it doesn't get lost and help you remember to take it home at night.

Together, we can help make sleeping and naptime a pleasant and restful experience for your child.

Sincerely,

©1999, Teaching Strategies, Inc., Washington, DC. Permission granted to reprint, for non-commercial uses only, by programs implementing *The Creative Curriculum for Infants & Toddlers.*

Algunas ideas sobre
el sueño y la siesta

Estimadas familias:

Dormir suficiente tiempo hace más probable que los niños disfruten y se beneficien de las oportunidades de aprendizaje diarias, pues además de satisfacer la necesidad de descansar, el sueño y la siesta les permiten a los niños sentirse confiados y competentes, a medida que aprenden a estar despiertos, a dormirse y a despertarse nuevamente. Con su ayuda, aprenderemos sobre el estilo individual en que su niño(a) se prepara para dormir y despertarse, y podremos brindarle el apoyo que necesita. Por ejemplo, mientras que a algunos niños les gusta que los mezan o que les acaricien la espalda, otros prefieren quedarse solos mientras se duermen.

Cómo podemos trabajar juntos

* *Podemos comunicarnos diariamente.* Al mantenernos informados sobre la cantidad de tiempo que duerme su hijo(a) y sobre cualquier cambio en sus patrones de sueño, tanto usted como nosotros podremos planificar mejor. Por ejemplo, si su niño(a) no durmió bien la noche anterior, podríamos ofrecerle una siesta más temprano. Si, en cambio, durmió una larga siesta, usted podría decidir ir al supermercado en su camino a casa, ya que su hijo(a) habrá descansado suficiente tiempo.

* *Por favor compartan con nosotros la manera en que usted le ayuda a su hijo(a) a dormir.* Si, por ejemplo, usted le canta cierta canción, o le mece por unos cuantos minutos antes de colocarlo en su cuna, podremos hacer lo mismo. Así, su niño (a) podrá experimentar la seguridad y tranquilidad que siente con ustedes y le será más fácil dormirse.

* *Le damos la bienvenida a su objeto "preferido".* Si su niño(a) está apegado a algún objeto en especial, márquenlo con el nombre del niño y tráiganlo. Se lo cuidaremos para que no se pierda y se le recordaremos a la hora de irse a su hogar.

Juntos, podremos convertir el sueño y la siesta en una grata experiencia para su hijo(a).

Les saluda atentamente,

©1999, Teaching Strategies, Inc., Washington, DC. Se permite la reproducción, únicamente con fines no comerciales, a los programas que ponen en práctica *The Creative Curriculum for Infants & Toddlers*.

Getting Dressed

— ◆ —

As Brooks lifts Abby's wet shirt over her head, Abby breaks away and runs to the other side of the room. Brooks walks over and says calmly, "We need to put a dry shirt on you. It's cold in here." She leans over Abby and begins to put on her shirt. "This will only take a few seconds," she says as Abby tries to pull away. "Help me count one... two... three. There, we are done."

— ◆ —

Dressing offers pleasant—and sometimes challenging—moments to enjoy being with infants and toddlers. You can use these moments to promote cooperation, introduce names of body parts and colors, give children the chance to develop and practice self-help skills, and help them learn to make decisions.

Young infants often may lie on their changing tables as you do the work of pulling legs through pants and freeing an arm from a sleeve. However, they are making some important discoveries: about parts of their bodies; where their bodies begin and end; and even about trusting others. Over time, they will become more active partners in dressing.

Mobile infants like Willard and Abby, who love to move and do, may often protest having to stop and be dressed. How can you deal with their protests? Try to involve them in the process. If their protests continue, be firm, respectful, and finish dressing them as quickly as possible. Also, keep your sense of humor, even if you turn around to find a child pulling off the overalls you just struggled to pull on. (Undressing is easier than dressing for children. With practice, they will develop the fine motor skills they'll use one day to put their clothes on.)

Toddlers may also protest the restrictions of dressing. Yet, as they practice new skills—such as pulling on their socks and opening and closing Velcro™ fasteners—and learn names for parts of their bodies and colors of their clothes, they feel proud and competent. In addition, when you ask them to choose between changing their paint-spattered shirt now or after snack, they begin to see themselves as capable decision-makers.

Questions to Consider

Here are some questions and suggestions to guide your daily decision-making.

"How can I use dressing to promote children's sense of competence and independence?"

Your challenge is to promote children's confidence in their own abilities, while sometimes needing to dictate exactly how they will move their bodies as you dress them. Here are some strategies to help you meet this challenge.

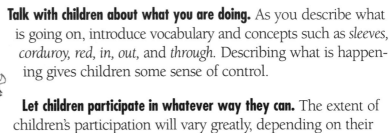

Talk with children about what you are doing. As you describe what is going on, introduce vocabulary and concepts such as *sleeves, corduroy, red, in, out,* and *through.* Describing what is happening gives children some sense of control.

Let children participate in whatever way they can. The extent of children's participation will vary greatly, depending on their level of development. While Jasmine might lift her arm as Janet puts on her sweater, Valisha and Jonisha may be able to put on their shoes and secure the Velcro™ fasteners.

Step in to prevent frustration when children attempt a task that may be too difficult. Although children really try very hard to master new skills, sometimes they choose a skill that is way beyond them. For example, Jonisha insists on buttoning her sweater by herself, like her older brother Daniel does. When she can't do this, she becomes frustrated. At this point, she needs La Toya to step in, free her from the unrealistic pressure she has put on herself, button the sweater, and explain that when Jonisha gets older—like Daniel—she will be able to button her sweater herself.

Give children clear-cut choices whenever possible. Offering children choices they can manage serves two purposes. It provides a much-needed sense of control, and more importantly, it provides decision-making practice. Examples of choices you might offer include: "Do you want to get dressed here in the nap room or in the living room?" and "Do you want to wear your green socks with butterflies or the purple ones?"

Be aware that children's temperaments may shape the way they experience dressing. For example, intense children like Matthew sometimes respond very strongly to any change—even putting on a new pair of pants. When you work with this type of child, be sure to have an extra set of familiar clothes available. Other children may fuss because they are sensitive to touch and may find certain textures uncomfortable. You'll want to have soft, well-worn cotton clothing on hand for these children.

"How can I promote children's dressing skills throughout the day?"

Dressing oneself requires mastering many different motor skills. For example, to put on a sock or to slip their arms into the sleeves of a sweater, children need to be aware of their bodies and to be able to control their body movements. Eventually, children need to be able to manipulate snaps, buttons, zippers, and buckles with their fingers. All the motor experiences you offer children— such as threading beads (eye-hand coordination) or dancing (awareness of different body movements) —will help them master dressing. In addition, there are some activities related to dressing that you can offer.

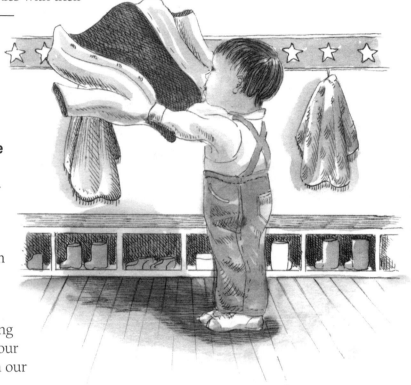

Select dress-up clothes and props with large, easy-to-manage fasteners. Children can practice snapping, buckling, zipping, and buttoning as they stretch their imaginations during pretend play.

Make practice boards. Mount a zipper, snaps, and Velcro™ fasteners on a board. Attach an old shoe with fasteners to a board.

Sing songs and do fingerplays about dressing. Children usually enjoy going through the motions while singing with you: "This is the way we snap our snaps, snap our snaps, snap our snaps" (or "zip our zippers," "button our buttons," and so forth).

"How do I handle a mobile infant or toddler who is protesting getting dressed?"

You can count on the fact that some mobile infants and toddlers will protest getting dressed. Here are some suggestions of what to do.

Encourage children to help you. Give children a task as you dress them. For example, ask them to hold their shoes, or to reach up to the ceiling as you pull on their sweater. Children who are a year old can usually take off their own hats and pull off their socks and shoes. By 18 months, they usually can unzip their jackets.

Acknowledge children's feelings. For example, explain that you know a child wants to play, but that you need to change his wet shirt first so he doesn't get cold.

Be quick. In some situations, the faster dressing is over with, the better it will be for all concerned!

Talk with parents about strategies they use to make dressing easier. Don't forget that parents share the challenge of dressing active, protesting children. Ask for any ideas they use to make dressing easier and more pleasant for all.

Above all, avoid turning protests about dressing into a power struggle. Try to understand why children sometimes struggle against the restrictions that are part of getting dressed and undressed. Once you recognize that they are not trying to make your life difficult, you'll be better able to focus on the dressing process itself, rather than your frustration.

A Child's Eye View of Getting Dressed

In the charts below, we consider typical behaviors you may observe, what children may be experiencing, and how you might respond to build relationships and promote learning.

Young Infants		
What You Observe	**What the Child May Be Experiencing**	**How You Can Respond**
Looking up at you as you put on her pants	She may be interested in you. She may want to communicate with you.	Take time to explain what you are doing: "I'm snapping closed your bright red pants."
Fussing as you remove his shirt over his head	He may not like having his head covered, even temporarily.	Remove the shirt quickly. Soothe him by taking a few minutes to talk together, or play "Where is your tummy?" When you put a shirt back on, choose one with buttons or snaps down the front.
Moving her arms and kicking her legs in the air after you remove her clothes	She may be enjoying the sensations of air flowing over her exposed skin and the freedom to move without the restrictions of clothes.	Talk with her: "It feels good moving your arms and legs through the air, doesn't it?" Give her a few minutes to enjoy the freedom of movement. Hold her securely on the changing table to prevent her from rolling off.

Mobile Infants		
What You Observe	**What the Child May Be Experiencing**	**How You Can Respond**
Squirming as you try to dress him	He may be feeling restrained.	Finish as quickly as possible. Explain: "I know you want to play. Let's get this shirt on quickly so you can get going." Try to involve him by offering him a job, such as holding his shirt or singing a song with you to help make dressing go faster.
Giggling as you play "This Little Piggy Went to Market" with her toes	She may be enjoying having some one-on-one time with you.	Continue playing. Focus on enjoying a few minutes with her and knowing that you are doing an important part of your job.
Pulling off the overalls and socks you just struggled to put on	He may be declaring his independence. He may be practicing dressing skills.	Appreciate the humor in the scene. Give him time to enjoy his accomplishment before you dress him again. Provide opportunities to practice with snaps and other closures throughout the day.

Toddlers		
What You Observe	**What the Child May Be Experiencing**	**How You Can Respond**
Insisting "Me do!" as you begin to dress her	She may be firming up her emerging sense of self by making her wishes known.	Talk with her parents about choosing clothes that encourage her independence, for example, shoes with Velcro™ fasteners and pants with elastic waists. Give her chances to undress and dress herself. Step in to offer guidance or to take over if she begins to get frustrated.
Turning dressing into a game of chase	He may be having fun playing with you. He may be asserting his independence by taking control over the activity.	Try to turn dressing into a game. Ask: "Let's see how fast we can get these pants on you." Respect his independence by allowing him to choose what he wants to wear (from two acceptable choices) and suggesting he do certain tasks himself. If necessary, insist firmly that it is time to get dressed and dress him as quickly as possible.
Pulling her shirt over her head and breaking out into a big laugh, while being changed into clean clothes.	She may be feeling proud and competent.	Acknowledge her accomplishment: "You put your shirt on. Good going!" Share your pleasure in her accomplishment with her parents.

Sharing Thoughts on Dressing

Dear Families:

Infants and toddlers are dressed and undressed throughout the day—every day—at home and in child care. And yet dressing is one routine that adults—and children—often want to get through as quickly as possible. Let's face it: dressing a squirming infant or a protesting toddler is no simple task. You can imagine that being an infant who must lie still or a toddler who must stop what he or she is doing to get dressed is no fun, either.

We focus on dressing in our program because we believe that by giving this routine some special attention, it can become a valuable learning experience. Equally important, dressing offers many opportunities just to spend time together with children.

How We Can Work Together

❖ *Please leave an extra set of your child's clothes with us.* Having spare clothes on hand makes it easier for us to dress your child and assure that he or she is always dry, warm, and relatively clean. When clothes are labeled, we can spend our time with your child instead of trying to figure out which clothes belong to whom. Wearing familiar clothes will help your child experience the safe and secure feelings of home here in child care.

❖ *Dress your child for active, sometimes messy play.* Clothes that need to be kept clean can interfere with children's enjoyment of activities such as climbing, food preparation, or painting. If you want to bring your child to child care in "good" clothes, we'll be happy to help your child change into clothes that will allow him or her to "move and do" throughout the day. Of course, we'll do our best to take care of your child's good clothes.

❖ *Choose clothes for your child that are easy to manage.* Pants with elastic waists, shoes with Velcro™ fasteners, and overalls with straps that stretch make it easier for your child to dress him or herself. This skill can make your child feel competent.

❖ *Communicate with us. How do you handle dressing at home?* Do you offer your child lots of help? Or do you encourage your child to learn to dress independently? By sharing our approaches, we can learn from one another and strengthen our partnership to benefit your child.

Together, we can make dressing a positive learning experience for your child.

Sincerely,

©1999, Teaching Strategies, Inc., Washington, DC. Permission granted to reprint, for non-commercial uses only, by programs implementing *The Creative Curriculum for Infants & Toddlers.*

Algunas ideas acerca de vestirse

Estimadas familias:

A los niños pequeños se les viste y se les desviste varias veces al día —todos los días— en el hogar y en la guardería. Sin embargo, vestirse constituye una rutina que los adultos —y los niños— desean llevar a cabo lo más rápidamente posible. Veamos. Sin duda, vestir a un niño que se retuerce o a uno que protesta, no es tarea fácil. Y no es difícil imaginarse que, para un niño pequeño quedarse quieto, o dejar de hacer lo que esté haciendo por vestirse, tampoco sea agradable.

En nuestro programa nos centramos en vestirse, porque creemos que prestarle atención especial a esta rutina, puede convertirla en una valiosa experiencia de aprendizaje. De similar importancia es que, vestirse les ofrece a ustedes y a sus hijos múltiples oportunidades de estar juntos.

Cómo podemos trabajar juntos

❖ *Por favor, traigan una muda extra de ropa para su hijo(a).* Contar con ropa adicional a la mano, nos facilitará cambiar a su niño(a) y garantizar que siempre esté seco, no sienta frío y esté relativamente limpio. Si la ropa está marcada, podremos pasar más tiempo con su hijo(a), en lugar de estar tratando de averiguar qué ropa le pertenece. Usar ropa conocida le ayudará a su niño a experimentar en la guardería, la sensación de seguridad y de tranquilidad del hogar.

❖ *Vistan a sus hijos para el juego activo, en el que a veces se ensucian.* Usar ropa que no se pueda ensuciar puede interferir con el placer de actividades como escalar, preparar alimentos o pintar. Si desean traer al niño con ropa "buena", con gusto le ayudaremos a cambiarse y a ponerse ropa con la que se pueda "mover y actuar" todo el día. Por supuesto, también le cuidaremos su ropa buena.

❖ *Elijan ropa fácil de manejar.* Los pantalones de cintura de elástico, los zapatos de apuntar con "velcro" y los "overoles" con tirantes que se estiran, le facilitarán al niño vestirse solo(a). Esta destreza contribuye a que se sienta capaz.

❖ *Comuníquense con nosotros.* ¿Cómo manejan en su hogar el vestirse? ¿Le ofrecen al niño demasiada ayuda? O, ¿le animan a vestirse autónomamente? Al compartir nuestros enfoques podremos aprender mutuamente y fortalecer nuestra labor conjunta para beneficiar a su hijo(a).

Juntos, podremos convertir el vestirse en una grata experiencia de aprendizaje para su hijo(a).

Les saluda atentamente,

©1999, Teaching Strategies, Inc., Washington, DC. Se permite la reproducción, únicamente con fines no comerciales, a los programas que ponen en práctica *The Creative Curriculum for Infants & Toddlers*.

Part IV Activities

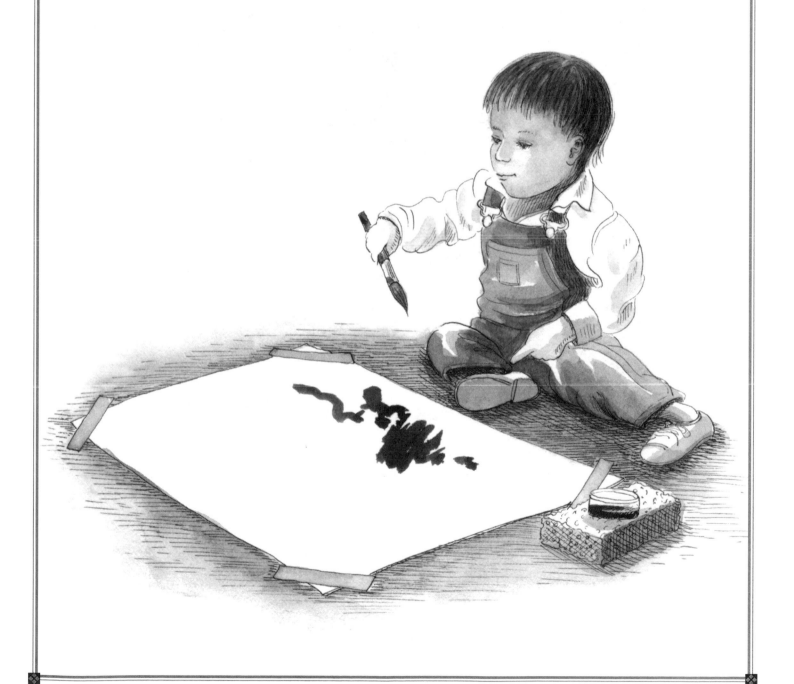

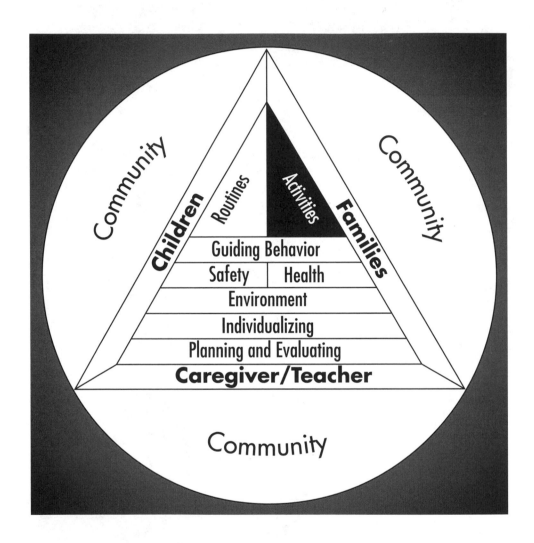

Activities

Playing with Toys
Dabbling in Art
Imitating and Pretending
Enjoying Stories and Books
Tasting and Preparing Food
Exploring Sand and Water
Having Fun with Music and Movement
Going Outdoors

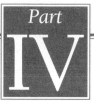
Putting Quality Into Action: Activities Day By Day

When you hear the word "activities" what are your first thoughts? Do you think about planning an activity for a specific time of day, gathering materials, introducing the activity to a group, and conducting the experience? When we think of activities for infants and toddlers, we see a very different kind of experience. Activities are part of everything you do with infants and toddlers throughout the day, and like everything you do, activities are opportunities to build trust and strengthen your relationship with each child.

For infants and toddlers, routines and activities are interrelated. When you feed an infant, allowing him to mush the carrots on his tray, you are providing a "tasting and preparing food" activity. When you put on a tape, hold an infant in your arms, and march around the room with two toddlers, you are "having fun with music and movement." There will, of course, be times when you plan activities, especially as children get older and develop new skills. But with infants and toddlers, you are "planning for possibilities" for your never know how they will respond or what will really capture their attention.

What makes caring for infants and toddlers a deeply satisfying profession is your ability to appreciate and find joy in the everyday discoveries that delight a child—the sound a rattle makes; the colorful patterns on your dress; the ball that unexpectedly rolls across a child's path; the ants marching across the pavement. We include activities in *The Creative Curriculum* as a way to help you plan experiences that you can share with infants and toddlers. We discuss the variety of materials you can put out to encourage infants and toddlers to observe, explore, and learn about the world around them.

The next eight chapters present the following activities:

- ❖ Playing with Toys
- ❖ Dabbling in Art
- ❖ Imitating and Pretending
- ❖ Enjoying Stories and Books
- ❖ Tasting and Preparing Food

❖ Exploring Sand and Water
❖ Having Fun with Music and Movement
❖ Going Outdoors

As you read about these activities, consider the children in your group—their age, and how each child might respond. With very young infants, you are building a relationship of trust. To develop a sense of safety and security, you spend time talking, touching, holding, and responding promptly to each child's needs. Activities for young infants are opportunities to share the sights, sounds, the textures, tastes, and smells that make up this wondrous new world.

Mobile infants are learning that they can explore and reach the objects and people that fascinate them. Activities for this age group require a safe environment and a selection of materials that will attract children's attention and inspire their curiosity. This type of planning allows you to watch and notice what seems to interest each child before you decide how to respond.

Activities for toddlers should build on their many interests and their new skills. Because toddlers are developing a concept of who they are and what they can do, it is important to plan activities that challenge toddlers to use their new skills and enable them to feel successful.

In each chapter we discuss two types of decisions caregivers/teachers make when planning for activities.

Setting the Stage

Some advanced planning is needed for most activities so that you have the materials you need and the children will be safe. Preparing ahead also gives you more time to spend with each child.

Encouraging Children's Play and Learning

In this section we discuss how young infants, mobile infants, and toddlers are likely to respond to different activities. We suggest ways to enjoy the experience with a child by taking time to watch, following a child's lead, and knowing when and how to extend the experience.

Each activity chapter concludes with a sample letter entitled "Sharing Thoughts" (in English and Spanish). The letters are to help you share with families what goes on in your program and to inspire them to share similar experiences at home with their child.

❖   ❖   ❖

Playing with Toys

— ◈ —

As Julio lies on the changing table, Linda taps her finger against the mirror fastened to the table's side. Hearing the sound, Julio moves his head toward the mirror. Slowly, Linda swings her finger to and from the mirror's edge, while Julio tracks her moving finger intently with his eyes.

— ◈ —

Try to think of a world without toys. Can you? Probably not. That's because toys take many forms. Some toys, like hardwood blocks, are store-bought. Others, such as empty milk cartons covered with Contact™ paper, are home-made versions of their more expensive counterparts. For infants and toddlers, an empty box can be just as exciting as anything you can buy.

Some of the very best toys for young children are already in your home or program, serving other purposes. An unbreakable wall mirror, plastic measuring cups that nest together, and a wooden spoon that can be banged against a metal pot (like a drum) are all wonderful toys. In fact, any object that young children can explore, put together, take apart, push or pull, stack, and create with becomes a toy in a child's hands.

The best thing about toys is that they are appealing to young children who learn by playing with them. Abby, for example, learns about size, shape, and sequence as she stacks rings on a peg. As Leo pulls the string on a wheeled toy, he learns about problem solving, cause and effect, balance, and eye-hand coordination. By rolling a ball back and forth with a friend, Matthew develops social skills. Toys are natural teachers.

Setting the Stage for Toys

Although you won't have to "prepare" children for playing with toys, you will have to make many decisions about toy selection, display, and arrangements. The key is to match toys to children's capabilities, interests, and needs.[1]

"What toys are appropriate for young infants?"

Toys that engage infants in a range of age-appropriate sensory and motor experiences can help them begin to explore and understand their world. You encourage active exploring by giving young infants toys that are interesting to look at, safe to mouth, easy to grasp, and fun to bang, shake, and drop.

Mobiles. Infants like patterns, circles, and areas of high contrast, especially black against white. Think about hanging a mobile over a newborn's crib or changing table. Experts recommend that you hang the mobile at the point where an infant's eyes focus best. For infants under three months, a mobile should be about 14 inches from the child's eyes. As infants grow and their eyesight improves, you can gradually raise the mobile. Mobiles promote the development of vision and hearing by drawing an infant's attention to a particularly interesting sight or sound. At about four months, infants will begin to reach for the mobile and this promotes eye-hand coordination.

Mirrors. From the age of about two months, children are captivated by mirrors. Watching their image appear and disappear in a mirror helps them learn to focus and promotes a beginning sense of self. You can position stable, unbreakable mirrors on the sides of cribs, changing tables, and on the bottom of walls in play spaces where infants can continually admire themselves.

Cuddly toys. Stuffed animals, hand puppets, and soft, washable, one-piece rag dolls delight young infants and help them begin to learn concepts like hard and soft, bright and dark, big and little. Bright colors, boldly contrasting patterns, painted-on faces, and sounds are more important at this early age than realistic features or correct anatomy.

Grasping toys. From about three months on, children love to grab, shake, mouth, drop, and explore objects like rattles and soft teething rings they can hold in their fists.

Through many experiences with a range of safe, developmentally appropriate toys, infants learn that the world is an interesting place filled with things to be explored.

---

[1] For detailed information on selecting developmentally appropriate toys, see Martha B. Bronson, *The Right Stuff for Children Birth to 8: Selecting Play Materials to Supplement Development.* Washington, DC: National Association for the Education of Young Children, 1995.

"What toys are appropriate for mobile infants?"

Mobile infants still enjoy toys that they can explore with all of their senses. Willard, for example, finds that an oversized stuffed dinosaur is easier to hug than a small rubber one. As Abby yanks on large pop-it beads or inserts a circle into a foamboard, she learns how to squeeze, twist, push, and pull. Puzzles, block towers, and large pegs in a peg board are great fun to take apart, though the mobile infant may not yet be able to put them together. Other toys for mobile infants include the following.

Balls. According to Dr. Burton White of Harvard University, the single best toy for a child between the ages of seven months and two years is a plastic, inflatable beach ball.[2] Mobile infants love to carry, throw, and retrieve balls. Clutch balls with indented surfaces can be easier to handle than smooth balls. Other good choices include balls with chimes and visible objects rolling inside, or weighted balls and oddly shaped ones, such as footballs, which roll in unpredictable ways, and yarn balls, hung from the ceiling for babies to bat.

Puzzles. Puzzles are actually grasping toys. By exploring the puzzle pieces and discovering how the shapes fit together, infants develop eye and hand coordination. For mobile infants, select puzzles that have only two or three pieces and can be held by knobs. (You can glue empty spools on puzzle pieces to serve as knobs if they do not come that way.) The puzzles themselves should be colorful and show objects, people, and animals familiar to the child.

Activity toys. Many toys for mobile infants provide practice in wrist control and the use of small muscles in the fingers and thumb. To illustrate, activity centers that can be attached to furniture provide opportunities for children to open doors, turn dials, pull on knobs, and push buttons.

Other popular activity toys include stacking rings, nesting cups, foam boards, shape sorters, busy boxes that can be poked and pulled at, surprise boxes that pop-up, measuring spoons, and plastic pitchers children can fill with objects. Playing with these objects helps mobile infants to broaden their understanding of the world. Stacking rings and nesting cups, for example, teach children about size and that different sized objects can be put in a specific order.

Push and pull toys. When infants learn to crawl, they also learn to move their toys as well as themselves. For example, sturdy carriages and shopping carts are especially appropriate for children beginning to walk because they offer much-needed balance. More experienced walkers enjoy push and pull toys, such as plastic lawnmowers or carpet sweepers. Toys that play music or make sounds as they move can enhance the play experience by encouraging the child to move in order to make the sound (teaching cause and effect).

Transportation toys. These are, in many ways, a combination of grasping and pushing toys. They include one-piece molded replicas of cars (6 to 8 inches long), buses, trains, trucks, and airplanes attached to large wheels or rollers. Indoors, mobile infants like to lift and

---

[2]Burton L. White. *The First Three Years of Life,* Revised Edition. New York: Prentice-Hall, 1986, p. 146.

push these vehicles across the floor. Outdoors, they love to straddle "ride-on" toys and move about using their feet as the car's motor.

Experience with transportation toys promotes an understanding of movement through space: larger toys move differently compared to smaller toys. Use of transportation toys also fosters planning: to go from here to there, I need to push the toy or move my feet.

Blocks. At first, mobile infants prefer to carry, pile, knock down, and even throw blocks. For these reasons, foam, cloth, and washable blocks are best. Later on, you can introduce firmer blocks, made of lightweight wood for stacking. Stacking blocks should be cube shaped, brightly colored or patterned, and easily grasped (2 to 4 inches). A selection of 20 to 25 blocks for a mobile infant is sufficient. By stacking blocks made of different kinds of materials, children learn concepts such as hard and soft, and what different sounds blocks make when they fall.

Outdoor play equipment. Nearly all of the toys mentioned so far can be brought outside to provide new experiences. Non-walkers enjoy swings as well as crawling platforms made of foam and vinyl. In addition, mobile infants like play equipment that allows them to get up and down and that can be used as a slide. Sturdy equipment that several children can use at once and that can be used both indoors and outdoors is a good investment.

Mobile infants with more developed physical skills enjoy low, carpeted climbers, lofts with side rails, tunnels, and obstacle courses. Outdoor play equipment of this sort challenges children to climb, slide, twist, and roll.

"What toys are appropriate for toddlers?"

Toddlers continue to use all of the toys mobile infants use. However, toddlers use the toys in more sophisticated ways. For example, toddlers can stack more blocks in addition to pretending that the blocks are something else like cars zooming along the road. In order to continue supporting children's ongoing development, select toys that stimulate toddlers' understanding of themselves in relationship to the world around them.

Mirrors and dolls inspire toddlers to engage in pretend play. Free-standing mirrors allow toddlers to admire themselves as they put on a hat or jacket. Boys and girls alike enjoy washing, feeding, dressing, and undressing dolls. Toddlers seem to prefer dolls about 12 to 15 inches long that they can carry in one hand, cradle in their elbow, or tuck under their arm. Dolls should reflect the ethnic backgrounds of the children in your program.

Push and pull toys often enhance toddlers' pretend play. They enjoy pushing a carriage full of dolls, mopping and sweeping with child-size tools, and pulling a wagon.

Soft, fuzzy stuffed animals are popular with toddlers, as are rubber, wood, vinyl, and plastic figures. Leo and Matthew like to carry around and dramatize stories using farm animals, exotic species, and even imaginary monsters.

Puzzles and matching games provide opportunities for toddlers to develop and apply thinking skills. Most toddlers can handle 4- or 5-piece puzzles (with and without knobs, made out of rubber and wood). Older toddlers who enjoy puzzles may want the challenge of more complicated puzzles, with as many as 12 pieces. As older toddlers become more skilled in sorting and matching, they love playing games in which they put giant dominoes (2 to 4 inches in size) together or match picture pieces to lotto boards.

Activity toys encourage toddlers to work on many emerging skills. For example, more advanced shape boxes, nesting cups, and stacking rings (with 5 to 10 pieces) enable toddlers to learn about shapes, colors, cause and effect, and sequence. As they play with these toys, toddlers also improve their eye and hand coordination. Pegboards and magnetic boards provide toddlers with opportunities to use their improved fine motor skills for exploring concepts such as shape, size, and color.

Toddlers also enjoy the surprise of reaching into mystery bags and boxes to discover objects that must be identified by their shape, texture, or smell. Gena, who has a difficult time reaching into "feelie" bags, likes to close her eyes and have Ivan surprise her with an object he rubs against her skin or one that she can sniff and then identify.

Toddlers naturally gravitate to toys that promote their independence. Self-help boards, cards, or frames for practicing fastening and unfastening Velcro™ strips, snaps, buckles, hooks, and zippers are always favorites. Learning to lace and string large wooden or plastic beads also provides children with experiences doing things on their own.

Transportation toys continue to hold toddlers' interest, although children this age usually prefer smaller (2 to 4 inches) or larger (12 to 15 inches) models than do mobile infants. Toddlers especially like ride-on trucks that they can climb into and imitate their parents. With their increased fine motor skills, toddlers enjoy handling moveable accessories: steering wheels that turn; bulldozing shovels that pick up and dump; cherry pickers that reach high; and knobs, levers, buttons, and wheels of all sorts.

Blocks are popular with toddlers who begin to use them for construction, rather than just stacking. To build stable constructions with blocks, toddlers need heavier, sturdier blocks for stacking than those used by mobile infants. Hardwood unit blocks are the universal favorites because of their weight, durability, and the many ways they can be used. While toddlers don't need the specialized shapes (such as arches or triangles) that preschoolers enjoy, they should have at least 40 to 60 blocks per builder in a group. With a good supply of blocks handy, children can experiment fully with constructions.

Older toddlers like to build with hollow blocks, and those made of heavy cardboard or sturdy foam. Toddlers of all ages also enjoy putting together interlocking blocks. Younger toddlers seem to prefer bristle blocks which fasten together much like Velcro™. More skilled older toddlers enjoy using Duplos™, which are larger versions of the popular Legos™. A selection of 20 to 30 blocks per child will give toddlers a rich building experience.

Outdoor toys and equipment for toddlers promote gross motor skill development. Tunnels, swings, riding toys, and climbers continue to provide physical challenges and excitement. Large cardboard boxes that toddlers can use as caves or hideaways, make wonderful climbing spaces. Balls of varying shapes, colors, textures, and sizes are great for kicking, batting, throwing, and (occasionally) catching. As toddlers get to be close to age three, they can learn to manage pedals and try a beginner's tricycle.

"Are home-made toys just as appropriate as those I can purchase?"

As mentioned earlier, some of the most popular items are not in fact toys, but "beautiful junk." For example, you can use empty hosiery packaging (such as L'Eggs™ egg shaped containers) as shakers, or empty freezer containers as nesting cubes. Here are a few "recipes" for homemade toys that you might want to add to your program for toddlers.

A bag collection. With the help of families, collect paper shopping bags from grocery stores, drug stores, and the like. Hang the bags on low hooks that children can reach. The toddlers can then take a bag to carry a toy around or to use in their pretend play.

Shape sorters. Cut out holes in the plastic lid of a wet baby wipes box or a coffee tin, taping sharp edges. Let toddlers fit empty spools, clothespins, cards, and other "stuff" through the holes.

Drop and dump toys. Put objects such as large hair curlers, bean bags, gelatin boxes, or squeeze toys into a plastic pitcher, small waste basket, or rubber pail. You can even tie a rope to a ceiling hook and suspend the pail in the air at a height that reaches the toddler's waist. Place a rubber wash basin under the pail and let toddlers dump the objects into the basin and then refill the pail.

Lotto games. Make matching games that feature people and objects from the child's world. Use photos, catalog pictures, post cards, and the like. To get duplicates of items (for the lotto card and the marker), make color photocopies. Paste the pictures on cardboard "lotto cards," then laminate them. Let toddlers begin with two or three squares to be matched; add items as the children's skills grow.

Cardboard blocks. Fill empty milk cartons with newspaper squares or crumpled paper grocery bags and cover with Contact™ paper. "Brick" paper makes these blocks look like the store-bought ones.

Old equipment. Broken telephones, old computer keyboards, and other adult-like items are especially appealing to toddlers, who love to imitate the grown-ups in their lives.

"What adaptations are needed for a child with a disability?"

Depending on the type of disability, some children find it difficult to play with toys. Consequently, they may spend large parts of their days observing the play of other children instead of actively joining in. Simple adaptations to toys can open a new world of play and exploration for children with varying types and degrees of disabilities. You may find, to your surprise, that toys chosen for the child with a disability also become favorites for other children in your program.

Some easy-to-implement, low-tech modifications to materials and your environment can make all the difference. Here are some suggestions.[3]

Handles or built-up knobs. Glue wooden knobs or corks to puzzles and other toys to assist children with limited fine motor skills. Add foam curlers to build up the handles of spoons, brushes, crayons, and markers.

Activity frames. Activity frames are similar to the "Baby Gyms" that are used for infants. Hang toys from the frame so that the children have easy access to them. These devices allow children with severe motor impairments to use toys that would otherwise be out of reach or would be dropped. The frames can be placed on the floor, attached to a table, or attached to a wheelchair or stander.

Grasping aids. Velcro™ is a wonderful invention for children who have trouble grasping objects. You can construct a number of different grasping devices with this material.

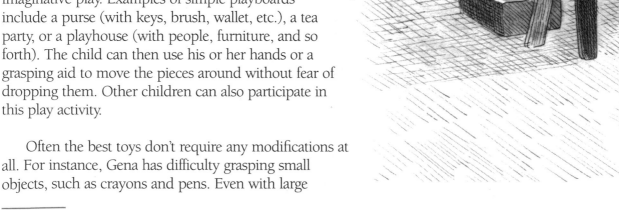

- ❖ A **stick holder** is a small stick with a piece of soft Velcro™ wrapped around one end. Attach a piece of rough Velcro™ to toys, such as toy people or cards. The child will then be able to use the stick to manipulate and pick up the toys.

- ❖ A **palm holder** is a piece of terrycloth with Velcro™ attached to it. The holder is placed around the child's palm (for children who have little or no grasping skills).

- ❖ A **Velcro™ mitt** is a mitten with Velcro™ attached to it.

Playboards. You can attach toys to a firm surface (such as foam core, a pegboard, or indoor-outdoor carpet) with Velcro™, string, or elastic. This creates a variety of playboards that allow children to participate in imaginative play. Examples of simple playboards include a purse (with keys, brush, wallet, etc.), a tea party, or a playhouse (with people, furniture, and so forth). The child can then use his or her hands or a grasping aid to move the pieces around without fear of dropping them. Other children can also participate in this play activity.

Often the best toys don't require any modifications at all. For instance, Gena has difficulty grasping small objects, such as crayons and pens. Even with large

[3] Assistive Technology Training Project Staff. *Infusing Assistive Technology into Early Childhood Classrooms*, Draft Version. Phoenix, AZ: Assistive Technology Training Project, Fall 1996.

crayons, she is too weak to draw on paper effectively. One day Ivan found some special "animal markers" at a discount store. (These markers are egg-shaped with different animals on each cap.) They were the perfect size for Gena to grasp and use. She can also grasp the cap and work on getting it on and off the marker. A funny thing happened when Ivan brought them out for Gena—all the children gathered round and wanted to play with "Gena's markers." All of a sudden, Gena was the focal point of a play activity in which she could fully participate. Ivan also used these markers to talk about colors and different animals and the sounds they make.

Other strategies to help children with special needs are to attach play materials to steady surfaces, to enlarge materials (such as large puzzle pieces) for visually impaired children, and to simplify the game or toy (for children with processing problems).

Remember that the child's family and therapists are great resources. If possible, invite the child's physical or occupational therapist to visit your program and suggest ways to adapt your space and toys to meet the child's unique abilities.

"Should I select different toys for boys and girls?"

For many decades now, researchers have been studying sex differences in children's play. In 1933, Mildred Parten observed that during free play time, boys tended to push trucks around the room while girls cooked and washed dishes for their dolls.[4] Does this seem much different from what occurs in an early childhood classroom today? Are these preferences inborn or are they due to the ways adults interact with boys and girls? From many years of research on this topic, it has become clear that preferences are due to social experiences rather than genes.

At about age 12 months, some families—and even child care professionals—become uncomfortable if a boy likes "feminine" toys and a girl prefers "masculine" ones. These adults steer children toward toys that they feel are more gender appropriate. If your goal, however, is to help children become comfortable with a variety of roles and to feel capable of having any career they choose, then it's up to you to discuss your views with parents and seek their ideas as well. When you put together your inventory, select toys without concern for gender. And then respect a child's decision to play with any and all of these toys.

"How can I be sure a toy is safe for the children?"

As noted in Chapter 7, safety must be a first consideration when you are selecting toys for children. Ask these questions about each and every toy.

❖ Is it solid, without breakable parts, sharp or jagged edges, or exposed nails, wires, pins, or splinters?

❖ Is it made of washable nontoxic materials?

---

[4] Mildred Parten. "Social Play Among Preschool Children." *Journal of Abnormal and Social Psychology*, 28:136-147, 1933.

❖ Is it too large to be swallowed (at least 1½ inches in diameter) and free of parts that might break off and become lodged in noses, ears, or windpipes?

❖ Are stuffed toys light enough to prevent accidental suffocation?

❖ Are plastic toys flexible?

❖ Are dolls' heads and limbs secure? Are facial features molded in, rather than sewn on?

❖ Are cords that could become wound around a child's neck shorter than 12 inches?

❖ Is it stable and free of parts that could pinch or pierce children or trap their hair or clothing?

❖ Are hinges and joints covered?

❖ If made of cloth, is it nonflammable or flame retardant (not flame resistant)?

"How should I arrange the environment so children can play with toys?"

Toys should be a natural part of the environment. Children can play with toys either on the floor or standing at a child-sized table. Place toys near soft, comfortable surfaces with enough space so children can play with toys near one another. While children younger than three may not play cooperatively, many like the experience of playing near or next to another child. Here are some suggestions for the arrangement of toys.

Place only a few toys out at a time. As children master these toys, you can rotate your inventory. However, don't remove all toys that children have mastered. Like a familiar book, children find comfort in a favorite toy.

Store toys on low shelving. If they are on the bottom ledge of a bookcase or room divider, children can take them out when they want to play with them. Leave ample space between stored toys to prevent a cluttered look and to aid children in distinguishing between toys. Avoid using toy chests. They are safety hazards as well as messy.

Make a picture label of each toy. For toddlers, make picture labels to place on containers and shelves to show them where things belong. You can draw a picture of the toy, photograph it, or cut out a picture from a catalog. Finding what they want and cleaning up becomes a matching game.

Group toys together for toddlers. This helps children locate their favorite puzzles, transportation toys, push and pull toys, and so forth. Grouping by type also teaches children how to classify objects.

Have duplicates of most toys. Children younger than three have a difficult time sharing. You can head off conflicts by providing duplicates.

Encouraging Children to Play with Toys

For infants and toddlers, much of your work is already done if you have set the stage appropriately. Creating a safe and comfortable place for children to explore the toys you select allows you to step back and watch what they do. Many times you may decide that your most valuable response is to let a child play without interruption. Here are some strategies you can use to encourage children to play with toys.

Young Infants

Probably the most important thing you can do for infants is to let them explore toys on their own. Just as an infant will let you know when he's hungry, tired, or in need of changing, so too will he let you know by his actions when he's ready for play.

Let's focus on how this works by taking a peek at some infant play. Linda, for example, creates an environment in which Julio can play with a mobile when he's ready. She hangs one mobile over Julio's crib and another over the changing table. Julio focuses his attention on these mobiles at times when he's comfortable—and not hungry, thirsty, or sleepy. Linda observes that in his enthusiastic play, Julio is learning that banging the mobile causes it to move, and that he can follow its movement with his eyes.

Janet encourages Jasmine's play by placing a mirror near the floor. Now, when Jasmine and Janet play peek-a-boo while sitting on a blanket on the floor, Jasmine can watch the action in the mirror. Here are the kinds of things Janet might say to Jasmine.

- ❖ **Describe the experience:** "There's Jasmine in the mirror."
- ❖ **Reflect feelings:** "That surprised you, didn't it!"
- ❖ **Play with the sounds of words:** "The ball goes bounce, bounce, bounce."
- ❖ **Describe actions:** "Are you patting yourself in the mirror?"

Mobile Infants

Mobile infants such as Willard and Abby, with their increased physical skills, can be introduced to a variety of toys that they can learn to use independently. For example, Grace can show Willard how to push a toy lawnmower so that it not only moves, but steadies his toddling walk. As he grows more confident in his steps, Willard will figure out on his own that the same handle he uses for pushing on the lawnmower can now be used to pull it.

Put out some toys you know will interest mobile infants and watch what happens. Take time to enjoy the child's enjoyment. Step in only when you think a child would benefit, as Brooks does. Abby is playing with vinyl blocks. She attempts to stack them, but they keep falling over. Instead of building a tower for her as a model, Brooks works with Abby to help her figure out a solution. She encourages Abby to experiment with placing the cubes. Eventually, through trial and error, Abby learns that the more fully the top cube covers the bottom one, the steadier the tower will be.

Taking time to watch and wonder what a child is experiencing gives you clues about how to respond. Here are some examples.

- **Help children observe changes** (cause and effect): "Look what happened when you dropped the ball on the floor. It bounced!"

- **Encourage children to solve problems:** "Do you think if we give your car a big push we can get it out of the mud?"

- **Build concepts such as color, size, and shape:** "Here's the circle. Where does it go?"

- **Develop children's feelings of competence:** "You put all the blocks in the bucket. Thank you."

Toddlers

Matthew, Leo, Gena, and the twins use toys with increasing purpose. As they play, they build their physical skills, learn concepts, apply thinking skills, explore the world of make-believe, and assert their independence. Here are some ways their caregiver/teacher might respond to their actions.

- **Build physical skills:** "Matthew, your big muscles are working today. Thank you for helping me carry these big blocks over to the tree."

- **Develop thinking skills:** "Can you find the picture on the shelf that matches the fire trucks?"

- **Promote social skills:** "Leo, why don't you and Rachel take the bristle blocks over to the rug so you can play together."

- **Encourage make-believe:** "What are you cooking for your baby?"

- **Promote a sense of competence:** "Look how tall your tower is!"

Playing with toys is one of the many ways children learn about the world around them and gain skills. The pure joy on a child's face as she pushes a button and watches a clown pop up, or dumps a can of blocks on the floor for the fourth time is enough to convince any adult of the value of toys.

Sharing Thoughts About Playing with Toys

Dear Families:

We all know that toys are fun. But if we take a closer look, we can appreciate how toys are also important tools for learning. When children play with toys, they learn how to move, think, communicate, and relate to others. Here are just a few of the ways that toys help your child grow and develop.

When your child does this...	Your child is learning...
bats an arm at a mobile to make it move	cause and effect
rolls a ball	about movement
puts pieces in a form board	concepts such as shape, size, color
pops plastic beads together	eye and hand coordination
takes blocks off the shelf and builds	independence

What You Can Do at Home

Here are some ideas that can help your child make the most of playing with toys at home.

❖ *Keep in mind that quantity doesn't always equal quality.* Your child doesn't need a great many toys. In fact, it's far better to have a few good toys that really challenge your child.

❖ *Choose simple toys at first.* Good toys for infants are those they can explore with all their senses—rubber animals and rattles they can grasp, squeeze, and mouth are especially good.

❖ *Select active toys as your infant grows.* Mobile infants enjoy playing with toys they can push or pull, such as plastic lawnmowers. They also like toys with parts they can move or handle—doors, knobs, big buttons, switches, and the like.

❖ *Pick toys that challenge your toddler.* Toddlers need toys that encourage development of specific skills and let them show their independence. Puzzles, blocks, lotto games, and riding toys are good choices for this group.

❖ *Find and make wonderful toys using things you already have at home.* An empty box, large empty thread spools, pots and pans, and plastic food containers are just a few of the items that will delight your child and lead to many hours of joyful play.

No matter whether you buy or make your child's toys, what's most important is that you take pleasure in watching your child play, and that you respond with enthusiasm to each new discovery.

Sincerely,

 ©1999, Teaching Strategies, Inc., Washington, DC. Permission granted to reprint, for non-commercial uses only, by programs implementing *The Creative Curriculum for Infants & Toddlers.*

Algunas ideas sobre los juguetes

Estimadas familias:

Si observamos con detenimiento los juguetes, podremos apreciar que, además de ser gratos, también son importantes instrumentos de aprendizaje. Cuando los niños juegan con juguetes aprenden a moverse, a pensar y a relacionarse con los demás. A continuación les mencionamos sólo unas cuantas formas en que los juguetes contribuyen al crecimiento y el desarrollo infantil.

Cuando su hijo(a):	**El/ella está aprendiendo:**
mueve un móvil con la mano	sobre la relación causa-efecto
hace rodar una pelota	sobre el movimiento
coloca piezas en un tablero de figuras	conceptos como forma, tamaño y color
ensarta cuentas	coordinación ojo-mano
toma bloques de un anaquel y construye con ellos	a ser independiente

Lo que ustedes pueden hacer en el hogar

Las siguientes son unas cuantas ideas que pueden ayudarle a sus hijos a aprovechar al máximo el juego en el hogar:

❖ *Mantengan presente que cantidad no siempre es igual a calidad.* Los niños no necesitan una gran cantidad de juguetes. De hecho, lo mejor es tener sólo unos cuantos juguetes que les ofrezcan retos.

❖ *Al principio, elijan juguetes sencillos.* Los mejores juguetes para los niños pequeños, son los que ellos puedan explorar con todos sus sentidos; los animales de caucho y los sonajeros que puedan agarrar, apretar y meterse en la boca son especialmente buenos.

❖ *A medida que los niños crezcan, elijan juguetes activos.* Los pequeños que ya se mueven por todos lados disfrutan enormemente los juguetes que pueden empujar o halar, como las cortadoras de pasto plásticas y les encantan los juguetes con partes que se muevan o se puedan manipular, como puertas, botones, manijas, etc.

❖ *Elijan juguetes que les ofrezcan retos a sus niños.* Los pequeños necesitan juguetes que estimulen el desarrollo de destrezas específicas y les permitan expresar su autonomía. Para este grupo, los rompecabezas, los bloques, los juegos de lotería y los juguetes para subirse en ellos constituyen una buena elección.

❖ *Encuentren y construyan juguetes maravillosos con objetos que tengan en su casa.* Una caja vacía, carretes de hilo grandes y vacíos, ollas y cacerolas, recipientes de plástico, etc., son sólo unos cuantos de los objetos que pueden conducir a muchas horas de juego placentero.

No importa si ustedes les compran o les construyen los juguetes a sus hijos, lo más importante es que, ustedes disfruten obervándolos jugar y que respondan con entusiasmo a cualquier nuevo descubrimiento.

Les saluda atentamente,

©1999, Teaching Strategies, Inc., Washington, DC. Se permite la reproducción, únicamente con fines no comerciales, a los programas que ponen en práctica *The Creative Curriculum for Infants & Toddlers*.

Dabbling in Art

— ◆ —

"Abby, are you ready to make some squishy cloud dough today?" Brooks lines up a bowl of flour along with plastic pitchers of salad oil and water on the child-sized table. Abby, who is familiar with the process, looks up at Brooks, and then uses her hands to shovel the flour out on the table as Brooks holds the bowl. Brooks then guides Abby in pouring oil and water into the mound of flour. "Me do it," says Abby, as she pushes Brooks's arm away. Brooks smiles, knowing how much Abby loves to do things on her own.

— ◆ —

When people think of children and art, many envision a child with crayons or a paint brush in hand. Coloring and painting are indeed typical art experiences for toddlers. But art experiences begin long before children are even able to grasp a crayon or paint brush. When a baby notices sunlight streaming through a window or the pattern in his mother's dress, he is beginning to appreciate beauty, which he will eventually express through more traditional art experiences such as drawing.

The art activities you offer infants and toddlers provide a range of sensorimotor experiences. Young children explore by touching different textures, squeezing and poking playdough, or moving their fingers through slippery pudding or fingerpaint. These sensory experiences provide children with opportunities to experiment. For example, they begin to explore cause and effect when they see a blue crayon leave a blue mark on paper, or observe that painting water on a fence can change the fence's color when it is wet. They discover they can have an impact on their world by covering a tray with fingerpaint. The art activities you offer mobile infants and toddlers like painting, coloring, and molding help them refine fine motor skills and develop eye-hand coordination. And, if you've ever noticed children's faces while fingerpainting, you'll see how satisfying these sensory experiences are.

Setting the Stage for Art

To plan art experiences in your program, review in your mind what you know about each of the children. What do they enjoy most? What new skills are they working on? Who enjoys messy activities? Who avoids them? This information will help you decide what materials are appropriate for your children and how to prepare the environment.

"What art materials are appropriate for young infants?"

Since exploring everyday sensory materials are art experiences for young infants, you don't have to plan very much. When you see an infant fingering the edges of her blanket and you talk about how soft it is, or you describe the bright color of a child's favorite stuffed animal, you are providing sensory-motor art experiences for infants. Allowing infants to run their fingers through cooked pudding or yogurt on a table top makes it an art experience.

You may, however, occasionally put out some materials to extend the range of sensory experiences available to infants. You can, for example, put out pieces of flannel, corduroy, satin, silk, taffeta, netting, knits, hosiery, denim, fleece, lace, fake fur, burlap, carpet remnants, and vinyl. Various types of nontoxic papers that infants can crumple, tear, shred, hold up to the light, and wave in the air, such as pieces of waxed paper, butcher paper, parchment, rice paper, and cellophane paper provide a different kind of experience.

"What art materials are appropriate for mobile infants?"

Mobile infants can begin to dabble in painting with their fingers, draw with crayons, and mold with dough.

Fingerpaint

3 cups liquid starch such as Vano™
1 tablespoon powdered tempera (any color)

Use a tongue depressor to mix all ingredients together in a bowl. Transfer to a squeezable bottle.

For painting:

- ❖ **Something to paint with:** Children's hands are naturally the best tools for fingerpainting. For painting with water, children can use stubby-handled brushes (5–6 inches long).

- ❖ **Something to paint on:** Table surfaces or trays are ideal for fingerpainting. Alternatively, you can cover a table with oilcloth or vinyl. Other surfaces for painting with water include the walls of buildings, sidewalks, blacktops, and tree trunks.

- ❖ **The paint:** Use fingerpaints or water.

For drawing:

- ❖ **Something to draw with:** Jumbo crayons, jumbo chalk, water-based markers, soap crayons, and scribble wafers.

- ❖ **Something to draw on:** Large sheets of sturdy paper are best. Children can use chalk on black-boards, sidewalks, and blacktops outdoors.

For molding:

- ❖ **Something soft and squishy:** For mobile infants, introduce doughs that are oily and easily squeezed, such as Cloud Dough or Homemade Plasticine. (See recipes next page.)

- ❖ **Something to make impressions:** Objects such as kitchen utensils, blocks of different shapes, and plastic cookie cutters can extend the molding experience.

Soap Crayons

1 cup soap flakes such as Ivory Flakes™
⅛ cup water
3 drops food coloring of choice

Grease plastic ice cube tray or popsicle molds with shortening or Pam™. Mix ingredients together in bowl. Pour into tray or molds. Allow time to harden. Pop out.

Scribble Wafers

Ingredients: Stubs of old crayons

1. Preheat oven to 350° and then turn off.
2. Sort crayon stubs by color.
3. Remove papers.
4. Place crayons by color in separate sections of a muffin tin.
5. Place muffin tin in oven.
6. When wax is completely melted, remove pan from oven and let cool.
7. Release shiny, waxed wafers.

"What art materials are appropriate for toddlers?"

In addition to the art materials suitable for mobile infants, you can introduce toddlers to painting and drawing activities, as well as to a greater variety of other types of art experiences. Here are some suggestions.

For painting:

- ❖ **Something to paint with:** Children can use flat bristled brushes (5–6 inches long) with nylon hairs and thick, stubby handles; empty deodorant bottles with rollers; and additional tools such as squeeze bottles, dishwashing pompoms, rollers, spray bottles, and cotton swabs.

- ❖ **Something to paint on:** Get a variety of papers—about 24 inches by 36 inches or larger. Big paper allows toddlers to paint by making broad pumping motions. Papers might include newsprint, computer paper, paper grocery bags, paper towels, and butcher paper of various sizes and shapes, as well as wallpaper, and paper plates. Try covering an entire table with butcher paper to give children a broad "canvas." Most toddlers prefer to paint on the floor or standing at a table, although some older toddlers are ready to paint at an easel.

Cloud Dough

6 cups flour
1 cup salad oil
water to bind (approximately 1 cup)

Knead ingredients together. Final product will feel oily and very smooth. Store in an airtight container.

Soft, Homemade Plasticine

1½ cups flour
1 cup salt
2 tablespoons vegetable oil
1½ cups warm water

Mix all ingredients together. Form into balls. Store dough on an open shelf; it does not have to be kept in a covered container.

Basic Playdough

3 cups flour
1 cup salt
1 cup water
¼ cup salad oil

Knead all ingredients together. Form into balls. Store in airtight container.

Tempera Paint for One

2½ ounces water
1 tablespoon powdered tempera (any color)
3 drops liquid dish detergent such as Ivory Snow™

Pour all ingredients into an empty juice can. Stir with tongue depressor.

For fingerpainting:

* **Something to paint on:** Toddlers can use cafeteria trays, mirrored surfaces with protected edges, and plastic wrap taped to table and floor surfaces. Of course, they can also fingerpaint directly on a table.
* **The paint:** Use fingerpaint and tempera paint in one or two colors. For fingerpainting, toddlers can also use whipped cream, nontoxic shaving cream or mud—either at room temperature or slightly warmed.

For drawing:

* **Something to draw with:** Toddlers can use all the materials already listed, plus water-based felt-tip markers.
* **Something to draw on:** For variety, offer toddlers plain and colored paper.

For molding:

* **Doughs of many colors:** Children can use an eye-dropper filled with liquid food coloring to add color to the doughs, and then work the color in with their fingers and fists.
* **Something to vary the experience:** Offer children basic props such as wooden mallets, tongue depressors, plastic rods cut to six-inch lengths, and potato mashers for pounding, poking, rolling, and stamping the dough.

Recipes for molding materials are shown on this and the opposite page.

For printing:

* **Something to print with:** Include a variety of printing tools such as rubber stamps, sponges, dominoes, corks, golf balls, and the rubber soles of old shoes. Make ink pads by fastening a piece of firm foam rubber or a sponge onto a Styrofoam™ meat tray, then pouring tempera paint into the foam or sponge.
* **Something to print on:** Collect tissue paper, butcher paper, newsprint, and a variety of colored and textured papers.

For older toddlers or those with good fine motor skills, you may want to include these additional art materials.

For collages and assemblages:

❖ **Materials to work with:** Almost any material will do. Consider pipe cleaners, wooden dowels, yarn, ribbons, papers with assorted textures and colors, magazines and catalogs, scraps of material, leaves, dried flowers and weeds, photographs, and recycled gift wrapping, greeting cards, post cards, and business cards.

❖ **Tools for putting artwork together:** Children can use library paste and, if appropriate, small, blunt-nosed scissors (4 inches and 4½ inches).

"Should I use food for art activities?"

In any discussion of children's art, the topic of using food as part of the art experience almost always comes up. You'll notice that most of the recipes on these pages contain one or more food products. Some families and educators strongly believe that it is inappropriate to use food or food products for anything other than nutrition. Other family members and educators may think that using food as a learning aid is entirely appropriate. Still others may take a neutral stand.

Because this topic is entirely personal, we suggest that you discuss this issue with your colleagues and the children's families. In most cases, if anyone has an objection, it would be best to honor that person's views. Alternatively, if no one has an objection, food can play a unique role in children's art. It is especially useful with infants who are forever putting things in their mouths. Also, researchers have found that children who have used food for art have no problem distinguishing food from inedible art materials as they grow older.

GOOP

3 cups corn starch
2 cups warm water

Gradually add water to corn starch. Mix ingredients together with hands. Goop is done when mass goes from lumpy to satiny texture.

Goop hardens in the air and turns to liquid when held. It resists punching, but a light touch causes a finger to sink in.

Baker's Clay

4 cups flour
1 cup salt
1½ cups warm water

Mix all ingredients together. Shape into a ball. Store in an airtight container.

Paintable Playdough

2 cups corn starch
1 cup baking soda
1 cup water

Mix all ingredients together and cook over medium heat. Stir constantly until mixture forms a ball. Allow to cool slightly and knead. Store in plastic wrap in the refrigerator.

"How should I arrange the environment for art experiences?"

Beginning art experiences are a part of everyday explorations for young infants. You don't really need a special place for art. Older infants and toddlers need no more than bare floor space and a child-sized table to draw, paint, print, mold, tear, cut, and paste.

Up until about age 2½, children have limited wrist control. As a result, they draw and paint using broad, up-and-down or side-to-side strokes. It is much easier for children to perform these pumplike motions on the floor or standing at a table than at an easel or while sitting at a table. On the other hand, older toddlers, who have more control over their wrist and hand motions, will enjoy working at an easel or drawing a wall mural. Therefore, as children develop new skills and you expand the variety of materials, you may want to create a special area.

Give some thought to storage of materials. You will want to place certain types of materials on higher shelves or in storage cabinets where children can't get to them. These items include materials that you need to set up (paints and collage items) and those that require close supervision (paste and scissors).

Other materials like modeling doughs, paper, crayons, and chalk can be displayed in containers on a low shelf. Then children can choose what they want. It's also a good idea to put a picture label on the shelf. Picture labels help children recognize materials by sight, provide an opportunity to match objects with symbols, and promote clean up and responsibility.

Here are some storage ideas you can try.

❖ Use egg cartons turned upside down to store scissors or paint brushes. (Tape the lids of the carton together so the cartons can be turned upside down.)

❖ Punch holes in the plastic lid of a coffee can and cover the edges of the holes with masking tape so children can't cut their fingers. Use the container to hold markers, scissors, or brushes.

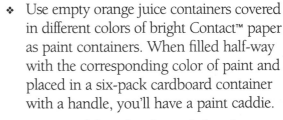

❖ Use empty orange juice containers covered in different colors of bright Contact™ paper as paint containers. When filled half-way with the corresponding color of paint and placed in a six-pack cardboard container with a handle, you'll have a paint caddie.

❖ Keep modeling doughs and clays in covered plastic containers or margarine tubs. Store library glue in squeeze bottles like ketchup and mustard containers.

❖ Use baskets or plastic containers to hold chalk and crayons.

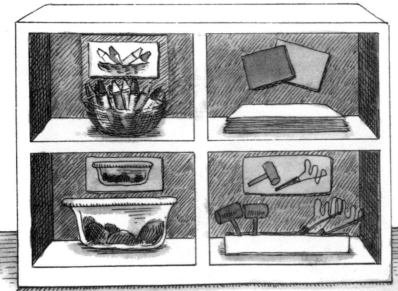

❖ Keep felt tip markers upside down in their caps. Here's one idea you can use for more permanent storage. First, pour plaster of Paris into an old jelly-roll pan or tray. When the plaster starts to set, place the marker caps upside down in it. Finally, after the plaster has hardened, return the markers to their caps.

"How can I keep mess to a minimum?"

As much as possible, you want children to be able to use art materials freely. This means preparing the environment to minimize messes while encouraging children's exploration and creativity.

To protect the floor from spills and drips, you can use an old shower curtain or a painter's drop cloth. Try to locate art activities near a water source, especially when children are fingerpainting or mixing modeling doughs. If no sink is available, you can bring buckets of water to your art area for cleaning up. It's a good idea to fill empty hand lotion or liquid soap dispensers with water for hand washing, too. Cleaning equipment such as mops, paper towels, a broom, and a dust pan should be within close reach. Squeegees used to wash windows are also helpful.

Children can wear smocks to protect themselves from messes. (Children can also wear them when cooking and doing water play activities.) You can purchase smocks or make them from old shirts or pieces of oilcloth.

"What should I do with children's work?"

Even though children are more interested in exploring what they can do with paint and other materials than in finishing a painting or drawing, you'll want to save some of their work. It's a good idea to provide a special place for hanging paintings to dry. You might buy a drying rack or use a clothesline. You can also display pieces of art where children will see them—on the bottom part of a wall or room divider, protected by clear plexiglas. When children see that you value their creations, they gain confidence and take increasing pride in their work.

Families, too, love seeing their children's artwork displayed. Think about posting a brief explanation of what you did with the children and why for parents to read while admiring their child's work. Keep some samples to put in a child's portfolio so you can note changes in a child's development.

Inviting Children to Dabble in Art

You don't have to do anything very special to encourage infants and toddlers to dabble in art; sensory-motor experiences are naturally appealing. Children love to explore and experiment with textures and colors. As they gain new skills, you can expand the types of materials and plan specific activities, especially for toddlers.

Young Infants

You probably already have many materials in your indoor and outdoor environments that infants can touch, smell, look at, and even chew on. All you need to do is allow time for infants to explore what interests them. When you hold an infant in your lap, let her feel the texture of your scarf and reach for the round cushion in the chair. Hang a mobile made of terrycloth cutouts across a crib so the infant can kick or wave at it.

See what happens when you put a dab of pudding on a child's high chair, as Janet did. She observed Jasmine's reaction to the pudding, how she used her fingers, hands, and wrists to explore its smooth texture. She noticed that Jasmine was fascinated by the patterns she made as she spread the pudding around. And characteristically, Jasmine squealed with delight, letting Janet know she was thoroughly enjoying herself.

As young infants experience the world through their senses, you can mirror their reactions of pleasure, enthusiasm, and surprise. Here is how Janet might respond:

- ❖ **Describe the sensory experience**: "That pudding feels so smooooth."
- ❖ **Describe the child's actions**: "You're making pictures in the pudding."
- ❖ **Mirror the child's feelings**: "What a good time you are having, Jasmine!"

Engaging in this experience with Jasmine gives Janet insight into her developing skills and interests and will help her in future planning.

Mobile Infants

Mobile infants like Willard and Abby will delight in squeezing and poking oily dough. They can grasp a crayon or brush, and "paint" with water on a chalkboard or fence. You can begin by offering a jumbo crayon or a homemade scribble wafer. Older infants grasp these fat, stubby crayons with their whole hand. Don't expect a child to hold the crayon with thumb and fingers, or to be able to draw using wrist movements. At this stage of development, drawing will often involve a lot of arm movement and at times movement of the whole body.

Offer the child a crayon or let him select one. He will probably be as interested in the feel, smell, and possibly the taste of the wax as he is in the crayon's color. Tape a large piece of paper (at least 24 by 36 inches) to the floor. Then, gently show the child how to use the crayon on the paper by placing his hand on the paper so he can make a mark with the crayon. Because most children have been waving their hands around since early infancy in a type of "air writing," the transition to drawing on paper is a natural one.

You can introduce older infants to painting with water in much the same way, since children go through the same developmental steps in painting as they do in drawing. Because children use their entire arms and bodies to paint, they approach painting with bold arm movements.

For molding experiences, children need nothing more than the freedom to spend time poking, pounding, and squeezing the dough. Handling molding materials is both soothing and filled with learning opportunities.

When Abby starts to play with the cloud dough they made together, Brook notices what intrigues Abby and builds on her interests. Here is what she might say:

- **Describe changes the child can observe:** "You made a big ball with the dough."

- **Help a child solve a problem:** "Looks like it's getting sticky. Should we add some more flour?"

- **Talk about a child's reaction:** "You're having a great time Abby!"

- **Comment on a child's actions:** "Abby, you sure can squeeze that cloud dough hard."

- **Build children's sense of competence:** "What a big helper you are."

Toddlers

Many of the same art experiences you offer mobile infants are appropriate for toddlers. Because their fine motor skills are more highly developed, they can begin to paint and draw with a variety of tools. Some toddlers have the muscle control to use paste and scissors; they can now try their hand at collages (pasting objects on paper) and assemblages (making three-dimensional pieces of art). Matthew, for example, proudly makes collages—in his fashion. He tears magazine pages into tiny pieces, with great concentration. When he pastes the papers, he may also paste a nearby object or get his finger stuck in his creation. For Matthew, the enjoyment is in the creative process. It makes no difference to him that his collage turns out to be a three-dimensional gob of paste with objects and the popsicle stick he used for pasting attached to it.

If you make a few simple adjustments, toddlers like Gena, who are physically challenged, can also have fun with art activities. For example, because Gena cannot fully extend her arms to reach an easel, Ivan has attached a long-handled paint brush to a Velcro™ headband. This arrangement allows her to use her head to guide the paint onto the paper. (If the child is painting at a table, tape the drawing paper onto the table and make sure the paint containers are weighted so they won't tip over.) Because Gena is very verbal for her age, she can also make use of voice-activated computer technology that allows her to use words and sounds to scribble and draw on a computer screen.[1]

Many older toddlers have developed wrist control. Because they can control their scribblings, their lines give way to curves, spirals, ovals—and eventually, to circles. These toddlers may start making patterns, repeating them, and sometimes seeing designs in what they have made. While the designs may be totally unplanned, they are thrilling for a child to discover. These experiences also impact children's thinking. For example, they learn about **predicting** (e.g., if I put this much glue on, the object sticks); about **space** (e.g., if I squeeze this much glue on, some of the glue runs off the paper); about **transformation** (e.g., if I add yellow paint to red paint, it looks different); and about **cause and effect** (e.g., if I put a lot of paint on the paper, it will drip down).

To promote a toddler's natural enthusiasm for art, you'll want to plan ahead for art activities. Here are some tips.

Preparing for an activity. As a first step, you can involve toddlers in the preparation process—making their own clays, playdoughs, fingerpaint, and GOOP. (See recipes.) You can place materials for non-messy activities, such as drawing and tearing, where children can get to them and use them on their own. For special planned activities, gather the art supplies ahead of time so you don't have to leave the children to get something.

Give some thought to preparing the environment if the activity will be messy. Floors, carpets, and children's clothing are likely to need protection. Have cleaning supplies nearby. Keep paper towels on a low, open shelf. When they are easy to find, children will readily clean up spills and splashes.

During an activity. It's fine to encourage children to draw, tear, and use molding materials on their own. However, you can work with an individual child or with groups of two or three children when they do activities that need supervision, such as painting, cutting, and pasting. Keeping groups small helps to limit confusion.

---

[1] Children and families who have been identified as eligible for receiving early intervention services under Part C of the special education law are also eligible to receive assistive technology and related services.

Interacting with children as they work. Notice what seems to interest a toddler most: "Leo, you tore the paper into so many pieces." Encourage them to reflect on their work: "Jonisha, tell me what you did with the fingerpaint." Avoid using words like "good" and "bad," words that judge children's art. When you talk about art, focus on the colors used, and the size and shape of objects created. Through positive, language-rich statements, children develop pride and ownership of their art products.

Extending Toddler's Experiences with Art

One of the best ways to enrich drawing or painting is to give children different types of papers to paint or draw on. Each different kind of paper can provide a special experience. See how children respond to:

- poster paper of differing colors, sizes, and shapes
- tissue paper of differing colors, sizes, and shapes
- crepe paper of differing colors, sizes, and shapes
- corrugated cardboard of differing colors, sizes, and shapes
- Sunday newspaper comics (for painting with water)
- fingerpainting paper coated with buttermilk, liquid starch, and sugar water (great for chalk)
- butcher paper

You can also give children different objects and tools instead of paint brushes, such as those we described earlier. Some other painting tools might include:

- feathers
- twigs or leaves
- eyedroppers
- foam rubber paint brushes
- toothbrushes
- vegetable and pastry brushes

You expose children to many science concepts when you encourage them to use paints of various textures and smells. As you prepare tempera paint, try changing its quality by adding one or more of the following items.

Adding this...	Makes paint...
flour	lumpy
Karo™ syrup	shiny and sticky
sand or sawdust	rough and gritty
Epsom salt	sparkling
liquid soap	slimy

You can also vary the experience by taking art outdoors. Natural light enriches all art experiences. Toddlers are bound to find that drawing, painting, and molding are quite different when done outside. It's also very exciting on a sunny day to "paint" the side of a building, a driveway, or a tree trunk with water, then watch the "paint" disappear before your very eyes.

Any art activity that focuses on a finished product rather than the creative process is inappropriate for infants and toddlers. Young children are not yet developmentally able to create representative art. We recommend that you avoid the following:

- using coloring books;
- using patterns (stencils, tracing paper, and so forth);
- telling a child what to draw, paint, or make;
- expecting that a child will produce anything recognizable; and
- "finishing" a child's work to make it "better."

Always keep in mind that for infants and toddlers, art activities are sensory-motor experiences that build a foundation for child's appreciating and creating beauty. It is the experience itself that is important, not what they produce.

— ◼ —

Sharing Thoughts About
Art Experiences

Dear Families:

When you think of art experiences do you imagine a child with crayons or a paint brush in hand? Painting and coloring, though, are just two of the many ways young children enjoy art. In fact, art experiences begin early in life as children notice the sunlight streaming through a window or the pattern on a mobile. As they get older, they enjoy scribbling with a crayon or squeezing playdough between their fingers. Art experiences allow children to have wonderful sensory experiences and to experiment with a variety of materials. They also help children develop thinking skills and physical abilities. Here are some examples.

When your child does this…	Your child is learning…
covers paper with paint	about spatial relationships
mixes water with dry paint	science concepts
pokes a hole in playdough	cause and effect
tears paper for a collage	eye-hand coordination
successfully learns to use paste	pride in an accomplishment

What You Can Do at Home

It's easy to provide opportunities for your child to have art experiences at home. Here are some ideas.

❖ *Keep in mind that art experiences are part of everyday life.* An art experience can be as simple as talking to your child about the color of the sky or the soft feel of a blanket.

❖ *Make art experiences fun.* Just putting some pudding on your child's highchair and letting him fingerpaint is an adventure in art.

❖ *Plan some special things to do.* You can make playdough your child can squeeze and pound, or GOOP for another wonderful sensory experience. We have several recipes we'd be glad to share with you.

❖ *Provide plenty of uninterrupted time for your child to experience art.* For young children, it is the process of creating that is important, not the finished product. They are not yet ready to draw or paint something you might recognize. They are, however, ready to express their ideas and feelings with bold strokes of crayon and splashes of paint.

Together, we can give your child the kinds of experiences that form a foundation for both appreciating and doing art.

Sincerely,

©1999, Teaching Strategies, Inc., Washington, DC. Permission granted to reprint, for non-commercial uses only, by programs implementing *The Creative Curriculum for Infants & Toddlers.*

— ❖ —
Algunas ideas sobre el juego artístico

Estimadas familias:

Cuando ustedes piensan en alguna experiencia artística, ¿se imaginan a un niño con unas crayolas o con un pincel en la mano? Pintar y colorear son sólo dos de las múltiples maneras en que sus hijos pueden disfrutar del arte. De hecho, las experiencias artísticas comienzan tempranísimo en la vida, a medida que los niños notan que la luz del sol pasa a través de una ventana, o reconocen el patrón de un móvil. A medida que crecen, ellos disfrutan al garabatear con crayolas o amasar plastilina con sus manos. El juego artístico les permite a los niños tener maravillosas experiencias sensoriales y experimentar con una diversidad de materiales. Además, les ayuda a desarrollar tanto destrezas del pensamiento como habilidades físicas. Los siguientes son unos cuantos ejemplos:

Cuando su niño(a):	**El/ella está aprendiendo:**
cubre papel con pintura	relaciones espaciales
mezcla agua con pintura seca	conceptos científicos
le hace un hoyo a la plastilina	causa-efecto
razga papel para un collage	coordinación ojo-mano
utiliza la pasta con éxito	a sentirse orgulloso por sus logros

Lo que ustedes pueden hacer en el hogar

Es sumamente fácil permitirles a sus hijos tener oportunidades artísticas en el hogar. Las siguientes son unas cuantas ideas útiles:

❖ *Mantengan presente que las experiencias artísticas hacen parte de la vida diaria.* Puede tratarse de algo tan sencillo como hablar con su niño(a) acerca del color del cielo o sobre la suavidad de una manta.

❖ *Hagan que las experiencias artísticas sean placenteras.* El mero hecho de proporcionarles a los pequeños un tazón y sentarlos en una silla alta para que "pinten" con los dedos, puede ser toda una aventura artística.

❖ *Planeen hacer algo especial.* Elaboren plastilina para que sus hijos la amasen y la golpeen y tengan una maravillosa experiencia sensorial. Si lo necesitan, contamos con varias recetas para elaborar plastilina que nos encantaría compartir con ustedes.

❖ *Ofrézcanles a sus niños suficiente tiempo para que experimenten el arte sin interrupción.* Para los pequeños, lo importante es el proceso de creación, no el producto terminado. Ellos no están listos aún para dibujar o pintar algo que ustedes puedan reconocer. Pero están listos para expresar sus percepciones, ideas y sentimientos mediante los trazos bruscos con las crayolas y la salpicadura de pintura.

Juntos, podremos ofrecerle a sus hijos las clases de experiencias que constituyen la base para apreciar y producir el arte.

Les saluda atentamente,

©1999, Teaching Strategies, Inc., Washington, DC. Se permite la reproducción, únicamente con fines no comerciales, a los programas que ponen en práctica *The Creative Curriculum for Infants & Toddlers*.

Imitating and Pretending

— ◈ —

Valisha bites her lip in concentration as she walks around the outside of the playhouse that Reggie, La Toya's husband, built in the backyard for the children. "Let's see here," she says placing one hand on her hip just as Reggie does when he is contemplating a new project. "I need a hammer." She picks up a small rock and "hammers" a spot under the window in the front. A few minutes later, she moves her hand back and forth across the same spot in a sawing motion as she makes a "chhhh, chhhh, chhhh" sound. Looking up, she sees Reggie walking out the back door. "Look," she calls to him. "I fixed it!"

— ◈ —

Pretend play—also called make-believe play, symbolic play, and dramatic play—is one of the ways that young children come to understand the world around them. While true pretend play emerges between ages one and two, its foundation is established during early infancy. As infants become increasingly aware of the world around them, they begin to imitate what they see. They actively explore objects to find out what they can do. As they interact with significant people in their lives, they build the understandings they will need to engage in pretend play. While examples of imitating and pretending are woven throughout *The Creative Curriculum*, pretend play is so essential to children's healthy development, it deserves a chapter unto itself.

When toddlers engage in pretend play, they use symbols and make believe to replay events or actions they have observed and experienced. Using symbols involves the ability to use one thing to represent or stand for something else. Children represent an object (when they use a rectangular block as a car), a person or living being (when they pretend to be a dog or a mother), or an event (when they crawl in a cardboard box and pretend to be driving a car).

Pretend play helps children become able to think abstractly. For example, to imagine that a block of wood is really a car, a child must be able to recall what a car looks like, how it moves, what sounds it might make, and then "infuse" these properties into a block of wood. This is the same skill the child will use one day to understand and use letters and numbers. For this reason, pretend play is critical to children's language and their cognitive development.

Research tells us that children who have good dramatic play skills—who know how to pretend about situations, use props in imaginative ways, and interact with peers in their play—are more likely to be successful learners than those who do not have these skills. The skills used in dramatic play prepare children to think logically, solve problems, and take turns.[1] The ability to pretend about events and experiences also helps children to cope with fears and uncertainties.

Setting the Stage for Imitation and Pretend Play

Although children imitate and pretend naturally, they will not develop high level dramatic play skills unless adults encourage this type of activity. During the first three years, you build a foundation for dramatic play by developing a responsive relationship with each child and creating an environment that promotes exploration.

"Do I need to set up a special place for pretend play?"

Young and mobile infants don't require a separate space to engage in imitation and pretend play. If you work with toddlers, however, there are advantages to creating a special place for pretend play. Here you can keep the objects and props you know toddlers will enjoy. Since they are most likely to pretend about family life, a simple house corner is an ideal setting. A small table and chairs, a doll bed, carriage, and perhaps a sink and stove create a "stage" that toddlers can use to replay scenes they know.

"What materials should I provide for young infants?"

Young infants do not require special materials. Your daily interactions will intrigue and fascinate infants more than any toy or prop.

You can, however, provide soft dolls that infants can grasp and hold. Dolls should be washable and have simple facial features with no moveable pieces or detachable parts. Young infants are attracted to bright colors and particularly enjoy dolls and stuffed animals that have rattles inside and make noise when shaken.

Nonbreakable mirrors that are securely attached to a wall or crib are another good choice for young infants. They are amused by facial expressions—their own and those of others. Seeing themselves in a mirror increases their self-awareness.

---

[1] J.E. Johnson. "The Role of Play in Cognitive Development." In E. Klugman & S. Smilansky, Eds. *Children's Play and Learning: Perspectives and Policy Implications.* New York: Teachers College Press, 1990.

"What materials will encourage mobile infants to engage in imitation?"

The active exploration of mobile infants—pushing, pulling, emptying, filling, climbing in and out, around and on top of furniture—provide experiences that build the skills they will use later in pretend play. Therefore, any of the toys discussed in Chapter 16, Playing with Toys, are also appropriate for promoting imitation and pretend play.

Realistic materials are good choices for this age group. Mobile infants show a preference for life-like dolls of vinyl or rubber that they can carry around, bathe, and "feed." Other popular objects related to real life include:

> ❖ carts to push, a baby carriage, and other wheeled toys;
> ❖ doll bottles, baby blankets, and a cradle;
> ❖ play telephones or real ones; and
> ❖ pots, pans, and plastic dishes.

Mobile infants like to put on hats and admire themselves in a full length mirror. Pocketbooks and baby carriages are ideal containers for their collections of pegs, pop beads, and small blocks.

Transportation toys like cars, buses, trucks, and trains need not be fancy or detailed. In fact, the simpler the design the better. Plastic, rubber, or wooden toys are safer than and preferable to those made of metal. Mobile infants enjoy pushing these toys across the floor and filling them with plastic animals and people.

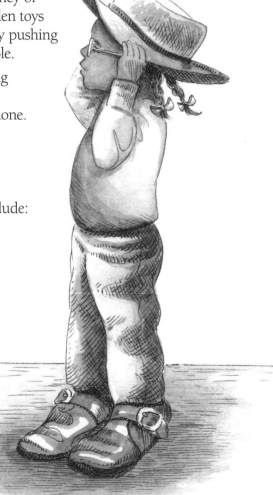

These early explorations with representations of real objects and living things sometimes inspire mobile infants to pick up a cup and pretend to drink, or hold a toy telephone to their ear and imitate an adult on the phone.

"What materials will inspire pretend play in toddlers?"

Toddlers will enjoy a variety of props to extend their play. These may include:

> ❖ dress-up clothes such as jackets, hats, and dresses;
> ❖ work-related props such as boots, firefighter hats, work gloves, stethoscope;
> ❖ suitcases, pocketbooks, lunch boxes;
> ❖ cloth bags, small briefcases; and
> ❖ ride-on toys.

While details in toys and props are not important to infants, they are very important to toddlers. Toddlers are intrigued by small cars with doors that open and shut, trucks with moveable parts, and dolls with painted features. Jonisha and Valisha are especially fond of dolls that look like real babies with movable arms and legs, hair, and fine features. They can handle simple doll clothes, removing them and replacing them. (To promote acceptance of differences, select dolls that reflect cultural diversity.)

Toddlers are developing the small muscle coordination needed to set up play scenes and move objects around. Mercedes has noticed that Matthew can play for long periods of time arranging people and animal figures inside and outside of a toy barn, talking to them as he plays. She regularly rotates the props she makes available to nurture and extend his interest.

Remember to resist the urge to display too many things at once. Toddlers can easily become overwhelmed and play often disintegrates when there are too many choices.

Encouraging Imitation and Pretend Play

You promote imitation and pretend play by developing responsive relationships with children and providing opportunities for them to explore and learn about the world. As mobile infants begin to imitate events they have experienced, and toddlers begin to pretend, you can extend their skills by becoming a partner in play. This means being ready to follow a child's lead, expanding on what a child says and does, and being sensitive about not taking over.

Some toddlers need more encouragement than others to participate in pretend play. This is especially true for children with developmental delays, who are also likely to have delayed language skills. Your careful observations will help you to pick up on a child's cues and make good decisions about when to step in and when to hold back.

Young Infants

The roots of imitation and pretend play are nourished by the trusting relationships you develop with young infants. Their trust in you leads infants to engage with the world around them, a world that soon beckons them to explore. These explorations become increasingly purposeful. Julio, for example, will explore objects in his grasp by taking them directly into his mouth, while Jasmine, at nine months, is more directed in her explorations. She also picks up a rattle, but rather than mouth it, she looks at it carefully, turns it over to examine it from different angles, and then shakes it vigorously.

The responsive interactions caregivers/teachers have with infants teaches them about imitating and pretending.

Examples:

Linda watches Julio lying in his crib carefully examining his hands in front of his face. She says, "Your hands. Look at your hands." Julio looks at her, looks back at his hands, and then back to Linda. She smiles and nods saying, "Julio discovered his hands!"

Janet is holding Jasmine as her mom, Charmaine, says good-bye. Waving her hand, Janet says, "Bye-bye mommy. Can you wave bye-bye Jasmine? Bye-bye. There goes mommy in the car. Bye car." Reaching for a toy car, she hands it to Jasmine saying, "Here's a car for Jasmine. Let's make the car go bye-bye."

Mobile Infants

Your observations of mobile infants as they explore objects tells you that they have learned to distinguish different properties. For example, when Brooks hands Abby a wooden spoon, Abby smiles and bangs it on the table, knowing that it will make noise. When given a cloth doll, however, Abby strokes it gently. This prompts Brooks to say, "You're taking good care of your baby."

Mobile infants also begin using materials in playful ways. For example, Willard takes a hat, puts it on his foot, and looks at Grace with an impish grin. Grace shakes her head, smiles, and says, "No, not there." Willard continues the game, putting the hat on different parts of his body and waiting for Grace's reaction, until he finally puts it on his head.

Grace has learned that Willard, who tends to be feisty and active, loves games that have an element of pretend. Peek-a-boo is a game Willard now initiates himself by covering his own face and re-emerging with squeals of laughter. He is learning to play Hide-and-Seek with Grace, but his favorite game is Drop-and-Fetch. In this game Willard is learning about the give and take of relationships. He looks at Grace as he drops an object, then waits for her to pick it up, and laughs when she says, "Here it is!"

Have you ever noticed how mobile infants intently watch and then imitate your actions? Imitation is the first stage of real pretend play. Mobile infants imitate events they have experienced first hand. When you describe their actions, you help them become aware of what they are doing. Your attention encourages this behavior. Here are some examples.

You see a child...	You might say...
Lying across a pillow during play time.	"Oh, is this a tired baby?"
Pick up an empty cup and pretend to drink.	"Hmm, I bet that tastes good!"
Crawl around on all fours barking.	"What a nice doggy. Are you barking because you're hungry?"
Push a doll in a plastic shopping cart.	"Are you and your baby shopping for dinner?

Toddlers

In contrast to mobile infants who imitate actions with real objects, toddlers are developing the ability to use objects for pretend. Matthew can transform a block into a car, a paper towel roll into a hose, or an empty carton into a bus. Jonisha and Valisha are able to pretend even without objects. For example, La Toya noticed Valisha holding her hand to her ear and pretending to talk on the phone. This shows a high level of ability to pretend.

Toddlers also begin planning their play episodes and combining different actions. For example, a toddler may gather together several items needed to "play baby," and then hold the doll, feed it, and put it to bed. Toddlers can transform themselves into different characters: a scary monster, a favorite person in a story they love, or an animal. Sometimes they get so immersed in the character, they won't respond when you call them by name. Gena tells Ivan, "I'm not Gena. I'm Pooh Bear." Knowing that Gena loves animals, Ivan plays along: "OK, Pooh Bear. It's time to eat your honey."

In the play of young toddlers, you can see elements of both imitation and true pretend play. Here are some signs that true pretend play is taking place:[2]

- ❖ **Performing simple actions on people or toys.** Matthew combs a doll's hair and hands a toy phone to Mercedes.

- ❖ **Substituting a toy object for the real object.** Valisha uses a ring from a stacking toy as a doughnut or a cylinder block as a baby bottle to feed her doll. (The object must bear some resemblance in size and shape to the one it represents.)

- ❖ **Pretending to do things adults do.** Jonisha pretends to put on lipstick or picks up a book and pretends to read.

- ❖ **Performing several actions in appropriate order.** Matthew replays familiar events such as lying down to sleep, getting up and dressing, or carrying a briefcase and going out to work.

- ❖ **Pretending to be another person.** Pretending to be Pooh Bear, Gena repeats familiar phrases from the stories she has heard over and over again.

- ❖ **Giving dolls or stuffed animals an active role.** Matthew places a toy animal in front of a bowl and says, "Eat!"

Older toddlers, whose pretend play has been encouraged, often show a higher level of skills than those with fewer play experiences. Here are some signs to look for if you work with children two-and-a-half to three years old.

- ❖ **Acting out less familiar scenes.** A child replays going to the doctor or grocery store, thus moving beyond the more familiar family themes.

- ❖ **Pretending with an object that is not similar to the one it represents.** A child may put on a firefighter's hat, pick up a piece of string, pretend it is a hose and use it to squirt water on an imaginary fire, and then put the string on a chair, sit down and pretend to drive off. This is an important achievement

---

[2] Based on Elaine Weitzman, *Learning Language and Loving It, A Guide to Promoting Children's Social and Language Development in Early Childhood Settings.* Toronto, Ontario: The Hanen Centre, 1992.

and shows the child is able to imagine the object in his or her mind without relying on a concrete representation.

- ❖ **Using imaginary objects**. A child holds an imaginary doll and pretends to rock it, pets an imaginary dog, or holds her hand to her ear and talks on the phone. The ability to pretend without using concrete objects is another indication that a child is able to create symbols or pictures in his or her mind.

As toddlers become increasingly aware of their world, they typically develop fears—of loud noises, big animals, being separated from their parents, and many other scary things. Pretend play is one way they gain a sense of control over these fears.

When Leo stamps around the room growling and swiping the air with his arms, he is assuming the role of the scary monster he most fears. By becoming the monster, he can control what the monster does, and therefore experience some power over that which he fears. Similarly, when Jonisha plays her mother going off to work and leaving her "baby" at child care, she is working through her own unhappy feelings about her own mother leaving her. When Barbara and La Toya see these kinds of play, they describe what the child is doing to support their efforts to deal with feelings.

Examples:

"What a scary monster! I bet that monster is hungry. Do you need something to eat, Mr. Monster?"

"Are you going to work, Mommy? Don't forget to kiss your baby good-bye. We'll keep her safe until you come and pick her up."

By accepting this type of play, verbalizing what you think a child is feeling, and joining in, you can help toddlers work through fears that they cannot put into words. For this reason, pretend play is as important to a child's emotional development as it is to cognitive and social development.

Encouraging Pretend Play During Other Activities

Opportunities to promote pretend play emerge all the time. By observing children and reflecting on what they are experiencing, you can make the most of these opportunities. Here are some examples.

> While rolling out some playdough, Leo says, "Apple." Barbara responds, "Wow, that apple looks so good. May I have a bite?" When Leo nods his head, Barbara picks up the piece of dough and pretends to take a bite and chew. "Mmm. What a good apple."

> Outside in the play yard, Willard climbs into a cardboard box. Knowing how Willard loves cars, Grace sits next to him and asks. "Are you driving your car?" He looks at her and smiles. She moves her hands as if she were steering a car and makes the sounds of the engine. Willard watches and laughs. He joins her in "beep, beep, beeping" the horn.

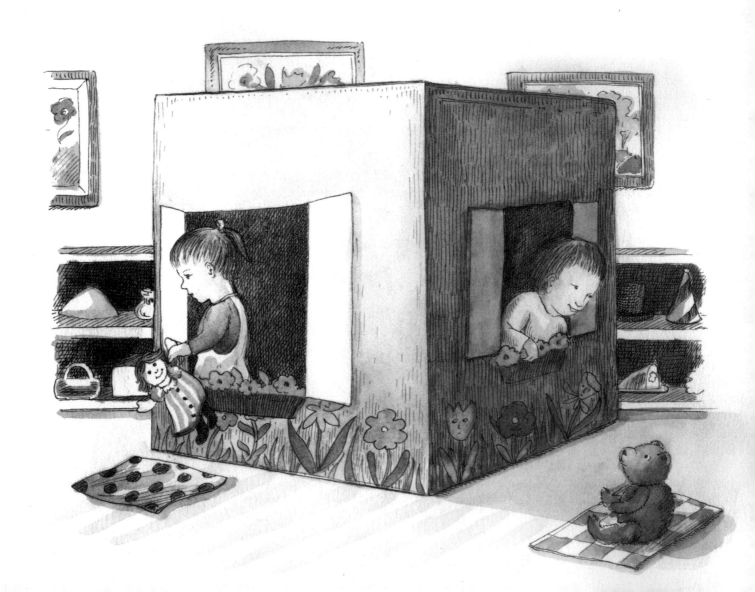

From across the room, Ivan sees Gena reaching out to touch the head of another child who is pretending to be a horse. He stays where he is and lets the children play without interruption.

As Brooks and Abby come indoors from a walk in the snow, Abby pulls off her hat and Brooks says, "Hello, Abby's head." In a minute or two, Brooks pulls off Abby's boot, looks down, and says, "Hello, Abby's toes." Abby laughs with delight and wiggles her toes.

As Mercedes and Matthew prepare grilled cheese sandwiches for lunch, they sing a silly song about taking crunchy bites of toasty, cheesy bread. Between verses, they pretend to take big crunchy bites.

Young children are most likely to use real life experiences as the content of their play. A book such as *Peekaboo, Baby!* (Denise Lewis Patrick, 1995), can encourage such play. Favorite stories can also inspire pretend play, especially with your encouragement. For example, books such as *I Am a Little Cat, I Am a Little Dog, I Am a Little Lion, I Am a Little Elephant* (Helmut Spanner, 1983), *Moo, Baa, La-la-la* (Sandra Boynton, 1984), and *Have You Seen My Duckling?* (Nancy Tafuri, 1984), can set the stage for children pretending to be animals. Books such as *I Can Build a House* (Shigeo Watanabe, 1982), *When We Went to the Park* (Shirley Hughes, 1985), and *Happy Birthday, Sam* (Pat Hutchins, 1978) can help stretch children's play beyond more common everyday events such as food preparation, going to work, and shopping.

Using **prop boxes** also promotes children's play. A prop box is a collection of various pretend play materials, usually organized around a theme. The props inspire children to replay familiar scenes. For example, older toddlers may replay first-hand experiences at the doctor's when they pull a stethoscope and bandages out of the medical box. A set of cardboard coins and empty food containers in your grocery store box can lead children to play going shopping.

Yet always remember that, while props can be very helpful in extending pretend play, the most effective strategy for encouraging this skill is your interest in what children do and your ability to follow their lead in pretending.

Sharing Thoughts About
Imitating and Pretend Play

Dear Families:

Imitation and pretend play are among the most important ways that children learn about the world. The foundation for this type of play begins when young infants explore their surroundings and build relationships with the important people in their lives. Soon, they start to imitate those around them and to make believe with real items. For example, a child might feed a doll with a spoon, or rock a doll to sleep. As they become toddlers, children develop the ability to use objects to stand for real things. For example, when a child imagines that a block is a car, the child must be able to recall what a car looks like, how it moves, what sounds it might make—and then transfer these understandings to the block.

This ability to think abstractly is the same skill your child will need one day to understand and use letters and numbers. In fact, research shows that children who have developed pretend play skills are more likely to be successful learners than those who lack these skills.

Being able to pretend also helps children cope with fears and deal with uncertainties in their lives. For these reasons—and also because children enjoy imitating and pretending—we encourage these activities every day in our program.

What You Can Do at Home

Because imitation and pretend play are so important to every child's development and eventual success in school, we hope you will try some of these activities at home.

* *Encourage your child to explore.* The more children learn about objects and people in their world, the more information they have on which to base their pretend play.

* *Provide props that inspire pretend play.* Dolls, doll blankets, a cradle, telephones (play or real), pots, pans, and plastic dishes will inspire your child to replay the roles of important people. Other useful props include rubber people and animals, and transportation toys such as cars, trucks, and boats.

* *Let your child dress up.* You can encourage your child's ability to pretend by providing dress-up clothes, work-related props such as firefighter hats, work gloves, and a stethoscope, and various ride-on toys. Remember not to confuse your child by putting out too many things at once.

* *Play make-believe with your child.* This is one of the best ways to encourage your child to pretend. You can also encourage pretend play by asking questions, offering a new prop, and taking on a role yourself.

Together we can help your child use pretend play as an important way to learn.

Sincerely,

©1999, Teaching Strategies, Inc., Washington, DC. Permission granted to reprint, for non-commercial uses only, by programs implementing *The Creative Curriculum for Infants & Toddlers*.

Enjoying Stories
and Books

— ■ —

"It's time for us to go outside," Mercedes announces. With Kara in the baby carrier,
Mercedes reaches out her left hand towards Matthew. No sooner has Matthew
grabbed her hand than he drops it. *"Books, my books,"* he says, with great urgency
in his voice. *"Of course you can take your books,"* Mercedes tells him. Matthew goes
to the coffee table and picks up the photo album of his family. He also chooses two
picture books of animals displayed on a low shelf. *"Let's go find a comfortable, shady
spot where we can read your books together,"* Mercedes suggests.

— ■ —

Infants and toddlers find books interesting and engaging. Even young infants Julio's age,
who don't yet understand the messages found in books, learn from exposure to them.
Feeling the warmth of Linda's body as she nestles with him in a rocking chair and
enthusiastically reads aloud from Margot Griego's *Tortillitas Para Mamma: And Other Spanish
Nursery Rhymes* creates enjoyable associations with books and reading. When Jasmine spends
the night at Janet's home and she reads the same stories Jasmine's mother reads, Janet helps
Jasmine build a connection to home.

As children grow older they begin to relate to pictures and stories of familiar places and
events. When Brooks and Abby read *Someone Special Just Like You* (T. Brown), they talk about
a family similar to Abby's. Gena sees herself when Ivan reads Rochelle Bunnett's *Friends at
School*, which features children of all abilities. And Jonisha and Valisha take great pleasure
in knowing that the identical twins in Valerie Flournoy's *The Twins Strike Back* have had
experiences similar to theirs.

Sharing stories and books are opportunities for you and children to enjoy one another,
the sound of words, the illustrations, and story lines. As you do so, you are literally impact-
ing the development of children's brains. During the first three years of life, the brain is
especially receptive to acquiring language. The sounds of words fascinate babies and in fact
determine "wiring" in their brains. Research shows that children who are read to often and
from a very early age, enter school with more advanced language and better listening skills
than those who have not had these experiences.

Setting the Stage for Books

The books you make available should reflect children's interests and life experiences. Your decisions about which books to select, where to keep them, and what types of book-related experiences to offer, will allow children to take full advantage of this rich and enjoyable resource.

"Which books should I be using with young infants?"

Books themselves are not of much interest for very young infants. Yet, there may be times an infant will be interested in looking at a simple, bold illustration on the page of a stiff cardboard book placed nearby on the floor or on the side of her crib. Be sure, however, that you situate the book so the baby can turn away if the colors are too much or something else catches her interest. Once a baby can support her head (at about three months), sitting on your lap as you read becomes a warm, shared experience.

As babies grow and begin to coo and grasp, they become more active partners in reading and storytelling. For the four-to-six month old, reading is sometimes book chewing, shaking, banging, sniffing, and observing. Infants this age need durable books that they can explore freely—cloth books, books with soft vinyl or oilcloth covers, and books with cloth or laminated edges. These very young children seem to prefer books with large, clear, colorful illustrations.

Infants like Jasmine, who are between six and eight months are likely to enjoy turning a book's pages. To encourage this important first step in learning to read, select board books—those with thick cardboard pages infants can easily grasp. Look for books with coated pages. These are easy for infants to turn and allow you to wash off sticky fingerprints.

Books for young infants should focus on familiar things—bottles and food, clothes, toys, pets, and people. Books should represent the diversity of the world, so that every child can identify with what he or she sees. Stories should be simple, rhythmic, or even wordless.

Here are some titles to consider when choosing books for young infants.

- *Animal Sounds for Baby* (Cheryl Willis Hudson)
- *Babies; I See;* and *I Touch* (Rachel Isadora)
- *Baby's First Picture Book* (George Ford)
- *Baby's Friends; Baby's Home; Grandma and Me; Grandpa and Me;* and *Mommy and Me* (Neil Ricklin)
- *Babytalk* (Erika Stone)
- *First Snow* (Emily Arnold McCully)
- *I'm a Baby* (Phoebe Dunn)
- *My Toys* (Dick Bruna)
- *The Pudgy Where Is Your Nose? Book* (Laura Rader)
- *What Is It?* (Tana Hoban)
- *Word Sign* (Debbie Slier)

Algunas ideas sobre el juego
de imitar y pretender

Estimadas familias:

Jugar a imitar y a representar se encuentra entre las maneras más importantes en que sus hijos aprenden acerca del mundo. La base de esta clase de juego comienza cuando los pequeños exploran sus alrededores y construyen relaciones con las personas importantes en sus vidas. Muy pronto, ellos comienzan a imitar a aquellos a su alrededor y a pretender que son alguien más, haciendo uso de objetos reales. Por ejemplo, una pequeña puede alimentar a su muñeca con una cuchara, o mecerla para que se duerma. A medida que crecen, los niños desarrollan la capacidad de emplear objetos para representar a otros.

Esta misma capacidad para pensar de manera abstracta, es la misma destreza que sus hijos necesitarán más adelante para comprender y utilizar las letras y los números. De hecho, los niños que desarrollan las destrezas del juego de pretender —o juego imaginario— muy proba blemente serán aprendices más exitosos que aquellos que carecen de tales destrezas. Pretender también les ayuda a los niños a enfrentar sus temores y a bregar con la incertidumbre en sus vidas. Por estas razones —y también porque los niños lo difrutan— nosotros estimulamos estas actividades en nuestro programa diariamente.

Lo que ustedes pueden hacer en el hogar

Debido a que el juego de imitar y pretender es de gran importancia en el desarrollo infantil y para el eventual éxito escolar, esperamos que ustedes pongan en práctica en sus hogares, algunas de estas actividades.

❖ *Animen a sus hijos a explorar.* Entre más aprendan los niños sobre los objetos y las personas en su mundo, más información tendrán sobre la cual basar su juego imaginario.

❖ *Provéanles accesorios que los inspiren a jugar a pretender.* Las muñecas, mantas, cunas, teléfonos (de juguete o reales), ollas, cacerolas y platos de plástico, inpirarán a sus hijos a recrear los papeles de las personas importantes en sus vidas. Otros accesorios útiles incluyen gente y animales de plástico, y juguetes tales como autos, camiones y botes.

❖ *Permitan que los niños se disfracen.* Ustedes pueden estimular la capacidad de sus niños de pretender, ofreciéndoles ropa para disfrazarse, accesorios relacionados con ciertos trabajos, como gorras, guantes, estetoscopios y diversos juguetes para subirse y conducirlos. Mantengan presente no sacar demasiados a la vez, para no confundir a los pequeños.

❖ *Jueguen imaginariamente con sus hijos.* Esta es una de las mejores maneras de animar a sus hijos a jugar a pretender. Mediante la formulación de preguntas, ofreciéndoles un accesorio nuevo y —asumiendo ustedes mismos— un papel imaginario.

Juntos, podremos ayudar a sus hijos a hacer uso del juego de pretender —o juego imaginario— como una importante herramienta de aprendizaje.

©1999, Teaching Strategies, Inc., Washington, DC. Se permite la reproducción, únicamente con fines no comerciales, a los programas que ponen en práctica *The Creative Curriculum for Infants & Toddlers*.

"Which books are appropriate for mobile infants?"

Willard and other infants who are 9 to 12 months old enjoy books with objects they can recognize easily. They begin to select books on the basis of content. Willard loves a book Grace made for him of animal photos.

Older mobile infants like Abby enjoy simple, to-the-point themes and messages in picture books. They also enjoy books with repetition, rhyming verses, and nonsense syllables.

Here are some suggested titles.

* *Baby Has a Boo-Boo* and *Happy Babies* (Wendy Lewison)
* *Big Friend, Little Friend* and *My Doll, Keshia* (Eloise Greenfield)
* *Brothers; Sisters; My Dad; My Mom; Shoes; Hats;* and *Clothes* (Debbie Bailey/Susan Huszar)
* *Busy People* and *Making Faces* (Nick Butterworth)
* *Clap Hands; Dressing; Family; Friends*; and *I See* (Helen Oxenbury)
* *Goodnight Moon* (Margaret Wise Brown)
* *Max's Bath; Max's Bedtime; Max's First Word;* and *Max's Toys* (Rosemary Wells)
* *Spot At Play* (Eric Hill)
* *Trucks* (Donald Crews)

"What books should I read to toddlers?"

Toddlers like Leo, Gena, Jonisha, and Valisha love to follow the simple plots in storybooks. They especially like to hear stories about children and animals whose daily lives are similar to their own. Toddlers easily identify with mice who have grandmothers, or with children who learn to use the potty. From books, children can begin to learn values, explore their feelings, and gain insight about growing up.

Toddlers enjoy the whole process of listening to a story read aloud. They like books with pages they can turn, illustrations they can point to as you ask questions, and phrases that sound silly and are repeated predictably. For toddlers, books open up the world.

Here are some recommended titles of books for the toddlers in your program.

* *All Fall Down; The Checkup;* and *Tickle, Tickle* (Helen Oxenbury)
* *Best Word Book Ever* (Richard Scarry)
* *Bright Eyes, Brown Skin* (Cheryl Willis Hudson and Bernette G. Ford)
* *The Chocolate-Covered-Cookie Tantrum* (Deborah Blumenthal)
* *Fuzzy Yellow Ducklings* (Matthew Van Fleet)
* *Gobble, Growl, Grunt: A Book of Animal Sounds* (Peter Spier)
* *Holes and Peeks* and *When You Were A Baby* (Ann Jonas)
* *I Love You Sun, I Love You Moon* (Karen Pandell)
* *Moonlight and Sunshine* (Jan Omerod)
* *My Very First Mother Goose* (Iona Opie/Rosemary Wells)
* *Once Upon a Potty* (Alona Frankel)
* *Owl Babies* and *When The Teddy Bears Come* (Martin Waddell)

- ❖ *Sheep in a Jeep* (Nancy Shaw)
- ❖ *The Tub People* (Pam Conrad)
- ❖ *Train Leaves the Station* and *You Be Good and I'll Be Night* (Eve Merriam)
- ❖ *Will You Come Back for Me?* (Ann Tompert)

How can you keep up with the constant flow of new books for infants and toddlers? One useful way is to check with your local children's librarian from time to time. You can also use annotated lists to guide you in selecting appropriate titles. Two fine resources are: *The New York Times Parent's Guide to the Best Books for Children* (Eden Ross Lipson); and *Books to Grow By* (Bob Keeshan).

"Should I make books for the children?"

Older infants and toddlers love books about themselves. Knowing this may inspire you to try your hand at making books that describe or show something about each child's life.

For infants, you can make a "feelie" book similar to *Pat The Bunny* (Dorothy Kunhardt). You can use real-life objects, such as a baby's rattle or a spoon.

Older infants and toddlers love listening to stories and looking at pictures of themselves and their families. You can title such books *Me and My Family* or *My Day*. To make books, take photos of the people and important objects in the children's lives, paste the photos on cardboard, then laminate each page or cover with clear Contact™ paper. Punch holes in the pages and tie the book together with yarn.

And why not ask parents to record their child's favorite books, nursery rhymes, and stories on tape? Children find it very comforting to hear a parent's voice. You can also work with parents to record favorite stories in languages other than English. This, too, provides a natural link between home and the program for children whose first language is not English.

"How should I display books?"

It isn't hard to make books a regular part of your program. All you need are the books themselves and a comfortable place for children to look at books and read with you. To begin, you'll probably want to display just a few books—about five to eight for young and mobile infants and eight to twelve for toddlers. While you don't want to overwhelm children with too many choices, you do want to expose them to several different titles. When you provide a variety, children have a chance to develop favorites.

For infants, one effective way to store books is in wall pockets made of heavy-duty fabric and clear vinyl. A book pocket looks something like a shoe bag with one book in each pocket. The clear vinyl pocket not only protects the books, but also allows children to see their covers. As a result, children can learn to connect a book cover with the story being read to them. You can buy book pockets commercially or make them yourself.

For infants to be able to explore the books up close, you can remove them from the pockets and stand them in the crib or on the floor. Thick, cardboard books work best.

While book pockets can also be used with older infants and toddlers, many people prefer to display books by simply fanning them out on low, open shelves. This arrangement allows children to identify and reach for their favorites. As noted earlier with Matthew, a free-standing display encourages children to pick up a book themselves whenever they are interested.

Looking at books is something children can do anywhere in your program. You'll want to encourage children to look at books in their cribs, on the floor, and in a shady area outdoors. In addition, near the book display, you'll want to have soft, welcoming places for reading. An overstuffed pillow, covered mattress, carpeted risers, or a rocking chair make cozy "book nooks." Your space should be appropriate for reading with a small group of children as well as reading with one child at a time. You'll also want to provide an inviting area where a child can sink into a pillow or rock on a child-sized rocker to read a book by himself. Solitary experiences such as gnawing on a vinyl book cover or "reading" out loud while holding a book upside down are important foundations for literacy.

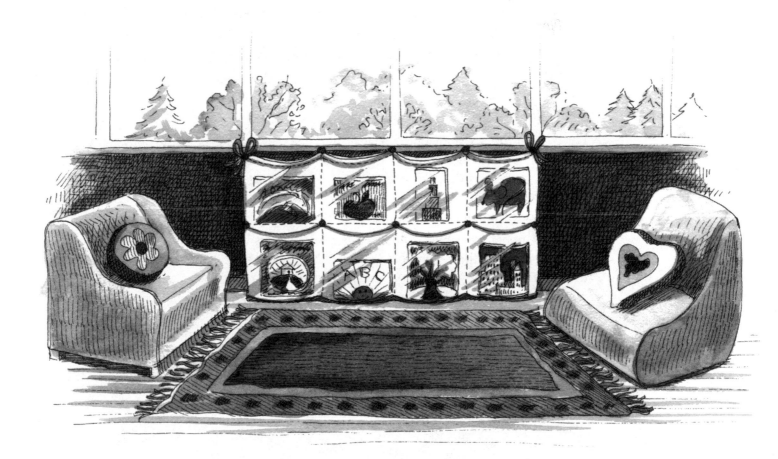

Enjoying Stories and Books
with Children

Many caregivers/teachers consider one-on-one reading experiences among the most treasured times in their day. The warmth and closeness of sharing a book with a child forges a special bond. Reading with an individual child offers a chance to become close to each other as you explore books together.

Shared (or paired) reading is a variation of one-on-one reading. Shared reading occurs when two children share a book, with one child reading to the other. If you have children of mixed ages in your group, you'll discover the benefits of having an older child "read" to a younger one. The older child usually is pleased and proud to take on your role; the younger child enjoys having the full attention of the older one.

Another variation of paired reading takes place when children "read" a book to a doll or puppet. In these situations, children are more likely to be retelling a story they have heard many times or making up a story based on a book's illustrations.

Group reading times often occur spontaneously when a child brings you a book to read or joins in to listen to a book you have been reading with another child. Books that have word play or repeated responses are especially good for these small group times. Older children love to shout out a predictable response together, or to hear how silly a funny word sounds when everyone says it at the same time. These noisy and happy reading experiences can provide lifetime associations between reading and pleasure.

Here are some suggestions for enjoying stories and books with the children in your program.

Young Infants

For young infants, the joy of language is their first step towards enjoying books and stories. The rhythm, patterns, and tone of your voice as you talk with them throughout the day, encourages their natural desire and ability to communicate. Even though they won't understand what you are saying, they will enjoy the experience of your reading to them, singing songs, and telling stories and rhymes.

Make books available for infants to explore. Infants who have learned grasping skills enjoy turning the thick, cardboard pages of board books. They need time to do this on their own and with you. When you sit down to read a book with a child, choose a time when you have the child's attention——but don't expect that attention to last! Jasmine will let you know when she's lost interest by fidgeting, slamming the book shut, or crawling down from your lap. A page or two may be as much reading as an infant feels like doing at one time. Yet, no matter how long it lasts, the time you spend together looking at words and pictures and pointing out familiar objects teaches children a lot about the pleasure of books and reading.

Mobile Infants

Older infants like Abby are beginning to be able to follow simple stories and can often listen longer—at least for a few pages! You can even try reading to children in a group of two or three. These experiences will be successful as long as you have realistic expectations and don't demand more of the children than is developmentally appropriate. To make reading most effective, keep these pointers in mind.

❖ **Wait until you have children's attention before starting:** "Let's look at this book together."

❖ **Encourage children to follow the illustrations as you read the text:** "Can you find Spot in the picture? Point to the doggie."

❖ **Take communication cues from the children's gestures, sounds, or words:** "Yes, that is a baby—just like you."

❖ **Ask simple questions.** These can help children reflect on what is being read. Even nonverbal children can respond by pointing to a picture or making a

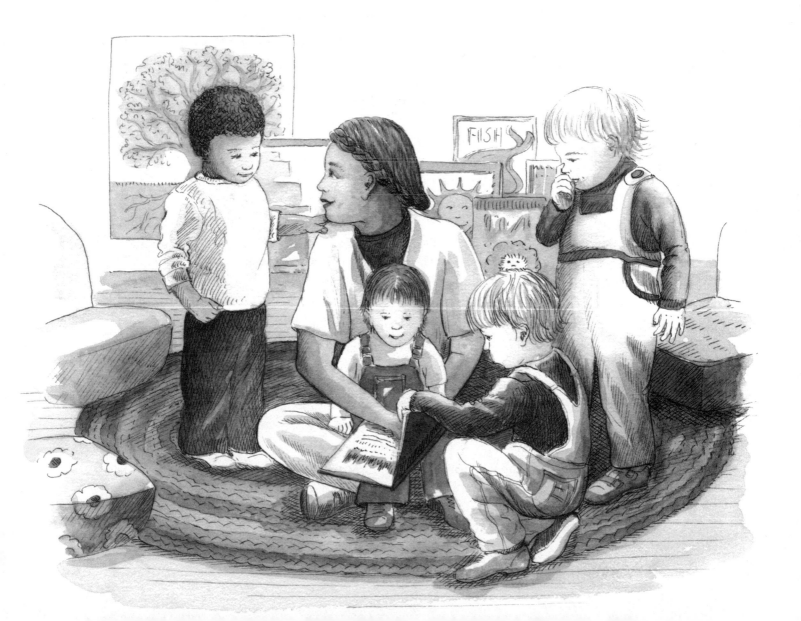

sound in response. "They're going bye-bye, aren't they? Can you wave bye-bye like the mommy in the story?"

❖ **Be prepared to stop at any point.** Lost interest is your cue that the reading activity needs to be concluded. You can pick up the book again when a child shows interest.

Toddlers

Reading with toddlers becomes a much more interactive experience. Toddlers love to look at books on their own and make up stories as they turn the pages. Valisha and Jonisha can even recite word-for-word the texts of their favorite books that their parents and La Toya have read and reread to them.

While Matthew loves curling up on Mercedes' lap to read a book one-on-one, he and other toddlers will at times enjoy hearing a story with a small group of two or three other children. Here are some simple tips to help you make the most of reading experiences.

❖ **Make sure that everyone is comfortable (including you).** Every child you are reading to should be able to see the book clearly.

❖ **Encourage children to use the illustrations to describe what is going on.** "Where are the children now?" "What do you think will happen to the little girl now that it's started to rain?"

❖ **Pause in the reading and allow children time to anticipate the next words.** This works especially well when you're reading familiar rhymes or stories with words and phrases that are used many times. Toddlers love word play and being involved with the story.

❖ **Skip an expected phrase or part of a familiar story from time to time.** Toddlers love correcting you and making you read the story "right." You'll get the same reaction if you switch words or play with words in silly ways.

❖ **Respond to the children's verbal and nonverbal cues about the illustrations.** Ask questions such as: "What's that you're pointing to? What do you think their Mommy will have to say about the spaghetti in the baby's hair?"

❖ **Relate the story to the children's own lives.** "Gena, do you go interesting places in your wheelchair like the girl in this story does?"

❖ **If children are responsive, try reading a book all the way through.** Children can become caught up in the rhythm of the words and the flow of the plot. You'll soon learn which books capture the children's attention and which children are ready to sit through an entire story.

❖ **Encourage children to reflect on the story.** "Did you ever see a monkey like George?" "Does everyone go to the potty?"

❖ **Be prepared to read the same story over and over again.** Children have favorites and they never tire of hearing those stories every day.

Perhaps most of all, book experiences lend themselves to the daily routines in a child's life. If you are having difficulty settling a child down for a nap, you might recite goodnight messages to the objects in your environment, just as in Margaret Wise Brown's *Goodnight Moon*. If you want to help children feel more independent about dressing themselves, you might recall the advise given in *How Do I Put It on?* (Shigo Watanabe).

Reading books and sharing your pleasure in language and stories is one of the most important gifts you can give infants and toddlers. Children who are regularly read to develop a foundation for literacy which helps them succeed in school. Their love for books will last throughout their lives, enriching their experiences and stretching their imaginations and dreams.

❖   ❖   ❖

— ■ —

Sharing Thoughts About Stories and Books

Dear Families:

Everyone agrees that books are a necessary part of a child's education. But do you realize that it's never too early to introduce a child to books? Long before children learn to read, they need to know what language sounds like, how a story flows, and how books "work."

Research tells us that even the youngest infants benefit from having stories read to them! Looking at books and hearing an adult read stimulates an infant's brain development in critically important ways. Children who learn to love books from an early age are more likely to become successful learners and lifelong readers. In our program, we offer your child a wide variety of good books and we read together every day.

What You Can Do at Home

The most important thing you can do is to read and tell stories together every day. The words are important. So, too, are a book's pictures. But most of all, spending time with you as you read and tell stories aloud lets your child know how much you value this activity. What's more, these times together—whether part of a bedtime ritual or a lazy weekend moment—can be treasured memories for both of you.

Here are some suggestions of things to do as you read.

- *Pick a story you yourself enjoy. Share rhymes, chants, songs, and stories from your childhood.* Your interest and enthusiasm will become contagious. Start by talking about the book's cover or simply reading. This helps you get your child's attention.

- *Encourage your child to follow the illustrations as you read. You can use the illustrations to ask questions:* "Where is the dog's bone?" You can also take cues from your child's gestures, sounds, or words: "Yes, that's the baby's Grandma—just like Nona Maria."

- *Be prepared to stop at any point.* You don't want to force a child to be still while you read. Sometimes, children would rather do something more active. Stop when your child seems no longer interested. Alternatively, be prepared to read a story over and over again.

- *We'd be glad to share with you the titles of the books your child enjoys here.* You can help us, too. Let us know your child's current favorite books, stories, and rhymes at home so we can get copies for our program. We'd also love to have you make a tape as you read your child's favorite story or nursery rhyme so we can play it for your child here. We'll be glad to help you with the taping.

Together, we can help prepare your child to be a lifelong reader.

Sincerely,

©1999, Teaching Strategies, Inc., Washington, DC. Permission granted to reprint, for non-commercial uses only, by programs implementing *The Creative Curriculum for Infants & Toddlers*.

Algunas ideas sobre el placer
de las historias y los libros

Estimadas familias:

Todo el mundo está de acuerdo con que los libros son esenciales en la educación infantil. Pero, ¿saben ustedes que nunca es demasiado pronto para presentarles libros a los niños? Mucho antes de que ellos aprendan a leer, necesitan saber cómo son los sonidos del lenguaje, como se encadena una historia y cómo "funcionan" los libros.

¡Incluso los niños más pequeños se benefician a partir de las historias que se les leen! Los niños que aprenden a amar los libros desde temprana edad, muy probablemente se convertirán en aprendices exitosos y en ávidos lectores por el resto de sus vidas. En nuestro programa, tenemos libros maravillosos y leemos con ellos diariamente.

Lo que ustedes pueden hacer en el hogar

Lo más importante que ustedes puede hacer para que sus hijos desarrollen el gusto por los libros, es leer junto con ellos todos los días. Aunque las palabras que les lean sean importantes, tal como lo son la historia y las ilustraciones, lo más importante, es destinar tiempo a leerles en voz alta a sus hijos, pues les demuestra cuánto valoran ustedes esta actividad. Más aún, estos momentos juntos —o bien como parte de un ritual a la hora de dormir, o un momento de pereza el fin de semana— pueden constituir valiosos recuerdos para ambos.

Las siguientes son unas cuantas sugerencias de lo que podrían hacer cuando lean:

* *Esperen hasta captar la atención del niño para comenzar.* Así estimularán la concentración en las palabras y las ilustraciones.

* *Animen a los niños a seguir las imágenes a medida que les lean.* Ustedes pueden emplear las ilustraciones para formularles preguntas: "¿Adónde está el hueso del perro?" Además, podrían basarse en los gestos, sonidos y palabras de sus hijos: "Si,esa es la abuelita del bebé, como la nona María".

* *Estén preparados para detenerse en cualquier momento.* No se debe forzar a los niños a permanecer quietos mientras se les lee. A veces, los pequeños prefieren hacer algo más activo. Cuando los niños parezcan no estar interesados, es mejor detenerse.

A nosotros nos encantaría recomendarles algunos libros que sus hijos podrían disfrutar. (También podrían consultar en la biblioteca local para que les ayuden a escoger). Permítannos saber cuáles prefieren sus hijos para que podamos obtener copias. Y, nos encantaría que grabaran una cinta cuando les lean sus historias favoritas para que, después, ellos puedan escucharlas aquí. Déjennos saber si podemos ayudarles con la grabación.

Juntos, podremos ayudar a sus hijos para que se conviertan en ávidos lectores por el resto de su vida.

Les saluda atentamente,

©1999, Teaching Strategies, Inc., Washington, DC. Se permite la reproducción, únicamente con fines no comerciales, a los programas que ponen en práctica *The Creative Curriculum for Infants & Toddlers*.

Tasting and Preparing Food

— ◼ —

"We're going to having an exciting snack today," announces La Toya to the children in her family child care home. "We have carrots right from our garden! After we scrub them clean, we can taste our home-grown snack." La Toya asks Valisha to help her set out vegetable brushes and water bowls on the trays in front of each child. She then lets each child take two carrots to scrub. As Jonisha displays her carrot for all the children to see how clean it is, La Toya raises her hand to give Jonisha a "high five."

— ◼ —

When you invite children to explore or taste a new food or, like La Toya, include them in helping you prepare a snack, you are nourishing their bodies—and so much more. Food and related conversation and activities are nurturing to the mind as well. They evoke feelings of security, family, and home. In addition, they provide a wealth of sensory experiences guaranteed to delight a curious child and to promote the development of fine motor skills and eye-hand coordination.

Tasting and preparing food are part of everyday living with infants and toddlers. Children become aware of the tastes and textures of different cereals, fruits, and vegetables as you and their families gradually introduce them to new foods. They begin to express their personal preferences and soon start to learn the names of different foods. At first, they are primarily interested in squishing, mashing, and smearing food. But before long, they become eager and able to help prepare some of the foods they eat. Whether it's scrubbing a carrot or dipping a slice of apple in melted cheese, children will enjoy and feel proud to help you with a necessary "real-life" task.

Setting the Stage for Tasting and Preparing Food

To prepare for experiences with food, make whatever changes are necessary to ensure children's health and safety. Think about the children you care for, and adjustments you might make to the environment to minimize waiting and confusion and maximize children's sense of competence and accomplishment.

"What safety measures should I be taking?"

Food preparation experiences that involve using adult utensils, gadgets, and appliances require close supervision. Some preventive measures will, however, eliminate many potential problems. For example, by choosing nonbreakable materials, you guard against accidents becoming dangerous. A plastic bowl, for example, may make a mess if its contents fall on the floor. However, plastic will not cut a child or get in food the way glass and ceramic shards might. Storing adult items—egg beaters, or anything with an electrical plug—out of reach or in a locked cupboard also makes sense.

Another preventive measure is to "childproof" the area where you will be cooking, especially if it is a kitchen. Cover outlets when not in use, and cover or lock the controls on the stove. Hide or remove electrical wires. (Consult Chapter 8, Ensuring Children's Safety, for more detailed information on checking the environment for safety considerations.)

Finally, in any tasting and food preparation experience with children, there is always the possibility that despite every precaution, a child may suddenly gag or choke. Since it's often difficult to think clearly in an emergency, it makes sense to post the guidelines for giving first aid for choking in the area where you will be cooking with children.

"Are there health issues I need to consider?"

According to the Centers for Disease Control, every year one in ten Americans has a bout of foodborne illness (usually vomiting, diarrhea, and fever). Therefore, you must pay careful attention to food safety when planning food experiences for infants and toddlers. This means refrigerating all perishable foods (meat, poultry, fish, milk products, eggs, mayonnaise) and not leaving them out for more than an hour; washing hands well before preparing food; not returning your tasting spoon to the bowl; avoiding the use of raw eggs (e.g., in cookie/cake batter); and washing hands, utensils, and cutting boards after touching raw meat/poultry/eggs. In cooking experiences with young children, it's best not to let them touch raw meat/poultry/eggs. Be sure to familiarize yourself with the health considerations outlined in Chapter 9, Promoting Children's Health.

In introducing children to new foods, follow the guidelines in Chapter 13, Eating and Mealtimes. Involve parents and introduce new foods gradually. Children need time (five days is usually recommended) to get used to the taste and feel of new foods and to be sure that they aren't showing signs of allergic reactions.

"What changes do I need to make to the environment to include food activities in my program?"

For tasting experiences, you shouldn't need to make any changes to your program's environment, since eating is already a part of your daily routines. For special food activities, you may wish to make some adjustments. However, you needn't be concerned if you don't have access to a kitchen. In many ways it's easier to create your own space for cooking, since you'll want everything to be safe and accessible to children. For example, if an oven is not available, a toaster oven, an electric frying pan, or a wok will do nicely. Here are some considerations for setting up your program for food activities.

Have available a child-sized table and chairs. To enjoy the food preparation experience fully, children need to be able to work, move about, and observe freely. A child-sized table can be used as a work station as well as for eating. Chairs enable children to sit while someone else is at work, thus making the activity more orderly. You can include infants by bringing their high chairs over to the table.

Select and use utensils that children can explore and use on their own. As much as possible, start children using real utensils and appliances rather than toy ones. Real gadgets and utensils not only make the experience more authentic, but are less frustrating to use than toy ones that are often not intended to do real work. For safety's sake, use plastic, rubber, and non-breakable tools. Utensils that children can learn to use include wooden spoons, plastic measuring cups, vegetable brushes, and potato mashers. Any potentially dangerous utensils or appliances you might use in leading a special cooking project should be stored out of the children's reach.

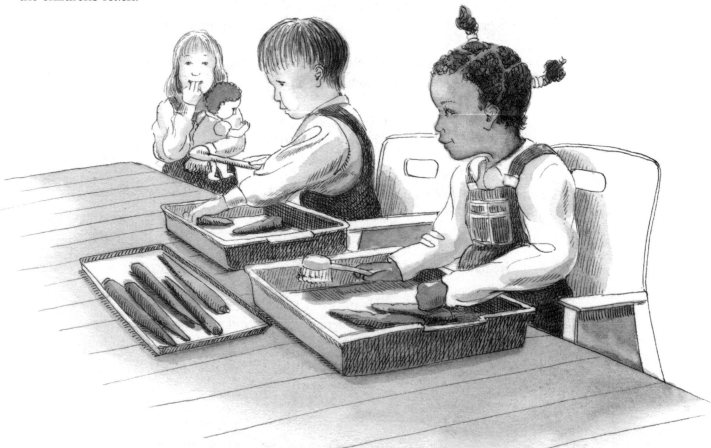

Store the safe cooking gadgets and utensils in low cabinets. If materials are stored on low shelves, children can get what they need on their own. Picture labels can show children where these materials belong so that they can help clean up.

Keep duplicates of the utensils children use for preparing food available for pretend play. This avoids waiting and allows children to recreate and extend their cooking experiences.

Have smocks available for the cooks to use. In this way children are free to be creative without fear of getting themselves or their clothes stained. If you don't have smocks, you or a parent can easily make them from old shirts or pieces of oilcloth.

Store cleaning supplies nearby so you can reach them easily. Invite children to help you wipe up the spills that are sure to occur.

"How can I make food preparation with mobile infants and toddlers a successful experience?"

Mobile infants and toddlers are by definition active "hands-on" people. This can be challenging when you are trying to organize a food preparation activity. Here are some suggestions to help minimize confusion for children—and for you.

Limit the number of children. Invite one child or a small group of no more than three or four to cook with you. This will minimize confusion and assure everyone has a chance to participate. If cooking is a regular activity, and only one of many options available, children will soon learn that if they don't cook today, they can do so tomorrow.

Have all the ingredients and utensils assembled ahead of time. This will free you to focus on the children, which is where your attention should be.

Keep waiting time as brief as possible. You can cut down on waiting time by making sure children always have a task. For instance, if one child is stirring, another child can hold the bowl steady.

Communicate rules clearly, in positive terms. For example, say, "Wooden spoons are for stirring." Gently but firmly remind a child of the rule when she uses her spoon to poke another child instead of stirring the zucchini muffin batter.

Make picture cards for older toddlers to use. To give children a beginning foundation for literacy, use pictures to demonstrate the cooking steps they are following. Pictures pasted on index cards or chart paper and laminated can help children visualize the one or two steps they will take during the cooking experience. For instance, one card might show a picture of hands being washed. The second card can show a butter knife spreading apple butter on a cracker. Children can also use these picture cards to review and relive the cooking experiences they've had.

Inviting Children to Taste and Prepare Food

Food experiences are a part of everyday life in the child care setting. Your role is to highlight them in ways that build upon what you observe about children's interest and capabilities. You won't have to work hard to encourage children's participation. Food is interesting, it usually tastes good, and perhaps most important of all, it brings people together to laugh, talk, taste, and enjoy each other's company.

Young Infants

Food experiences with young infants are primarily tasting and relationship building experiences that naturally occur throughout the day when a child eats. When Linda holds Julio and feeds him his bottle, he tastes his milk, and more importantly, he feels safe and secure.

Janet gives Jasmine the opportunity to explore her food and talks with her about what is happening. She sometimes takes advantage of the opportunity to build on Jasmine's apparent interest in new words by introducing the names of food and utensils. For example, she might say:

> "You're having a hard time picking up the applesauce because it's so slippery."

> "You like the taste of that squishy banana, don't you?"

Young infants will also enjoy being included as you "cook" with older children. Depending on their age and skill level, they can enjoy the sights, smells, and sounds of food preparation activities from a back pack, your lap, or a highchair and may be able to begin to participate in some of the activities we have listed in the next section.

Mobile Infants

In addition to tasting experiences, mobile infants enjoy being involved in the preparation of their own snacks and meals. Appropriate experiences for this age group include *shaking, dabbing, dipping, stirring,* and *mashing.* Some examples include:

- shaking grated cheese on macaroni or vegetable purees (squash, green beans, peas, carrots, beets, cauliflower, or zucchini)
- dropping cheese cubes onto rice or mashed potatoes
- dabbing apple butter on bread or toasted bagel
- shaking cinnamon on cottage cheese, yogurt, cooked cereal, or apple sauce
- dipping banana chunks, steamed apple, or pear wedges into yogurt
- mixing cottage cheese with macaroni, or kasha (roasted buckwheat) with noodle bow ties
- mixing dips for snacks using grated cheese or spices (such as powdered cinnamon and nutmeg) with sour cream, yogurt, or mashed chick peas

Talking with mobile infants about what they are experiencing builds your relationship, enhances their language development, and can stretch their thinking.

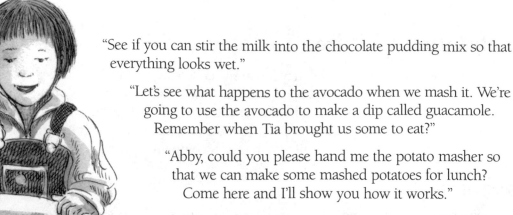

"See if you can stir the milk into the chocolate pudding mix so that everything looks wet."

"Let's see what happens to the avocado when we mash it. We're going to use the avocado to make a dip called guacamole. Remember when Tia brought us some to eat?"

"Abby, could you please hand me the potato masher so that we can make some mashed potatoes for lunch? Come here and I'll show you how it works."

Toddlers

Toddlers can take an active role in preparing their food. Based on individual children's interests and abilities, you can plan activities that involve *spreading, pouring, slicing, whisking, squeezing,* and *garnishing,* such as:

❖ preparing finger food snacks using cucumber slices, toast strips, or crackers for the base, and cheese, cottage cheese, or fruit wedges for toppings

❖ using a plastic knife or a small icing spatula to spread apple butter (or other fruit butters) on crackers, bread, or toast

❖ stirring together the ingredients for hot cereal, and pouring milk or maple syrup into the finished dish

❖ scrambling eggs in a bowl

❖ dipping bread slices in beaten eggs, cinnamon, and milk to make french toast

❖ scrubbing potatoes or yams; mashing the cooked potatoes or yams

❖ mixing gelatin in water to make gelatin jigglers and wigglers

❖ squeezing lemons, oranges, and limes for fruit drinks

❖ snapping ends off of green beans

❖ shelling peas

❖ arranging foods decoratively on a plate, tray, or table

Barbara, Mercedes, Ivan, and La Toya extend toddlers' food experiences by asking questions that cause them to reflect on the process. Consider these examples.

"How does this mashed banana look different from this whole banana?"

"Can you remember what else we baked on this cookie sheet?"

"How do you think we can open this pea pod?"

"What was the best part about making snack?"

Getting Ideas for Cooking Activities

Where can you get ideas for food preparation activities? Start with the meals and snacks you serve the children. Then think about how you might involve the children in preparing them. Preparations that have a limited number of steps and require only beginning physical skills such as dipping, shaking or mashing are good starters. More complex skills such as pouring, spreading, and squeezing can be added as children's mastery of fine motor skills improves.

For special projects, you might want to consult some of the published books for cooking with children. Here are a few.

 ❖ *Cup Cooking: Individual Child-Portion Picture Recipes* (Barbara Johnson)
 ❖ *Learning Through Cooking* (Amy Houts)
 ❖ *Learning Through Cooking: A Cooking Program for Children Two to Ten* (N.J. Ferreira)

One word of caution, though. Most children's cookbooks on the market are intended for use with preschoolers and older children. Moreover, even some that claim to be for infants and toddlers are often too difficult for young cooks or include preparing foods that are nutritionally inappropriate. To use cookbooks effectively with infants and toddlers, you'll need to rethink the recipes in terms of children's skills and any special dietary requirements.

Families are also an ideal resource for cooking ideas. Invite parents to share recipes for foods they prepare for their children at home. By recreating these foods at meals and snacks, you strengthen the bond between home and the program. Including family recipes is one way for your program to acknowledge the cultural backgrounds of the children and families you serve.

You'll find that most children are eager to participate in experiences involving food. With some thoughtful planning, you can make these experiences ongoing learning opportunities.

❖ ❖ ❖

Sharing Thoughts About Tasting and Preparing Food

Dear Families:

Perhaps the idea of children so young participating in food preparation activities seems strange to you. Yet one of the reasons preparing food appeals to children is that it is a grown-up activity. To participate in these activities—the ones your child observes you doing day in and day out—is both exciting and motivating.

In our program, we build on this natural interest in food experiences. There are so many concepts and skills children can learn. For example, what do you think your child might learn from doing a simple task such as snapping the ends off green beans? Did you include these things?

shape	eye-hand coordination
color	part and whole
cause and effect	fine motor skill development
pride in completing a task	

As you can see, preparing food is educational as well as practical and fun!

What You Can Do at Home

The most natural laboratory for involving your child in food preparation activities is at home. Here are some ideas:

❖ *Let your child participate.* Because you probably already cook at home, it's easy for you to involve your child. You can even include a young infant. Let him or her sit in a high chair as you discuss what's going on. Older infants and toddlers can be active participants. When your child helps you prepare or serve foods, you're showing that you value his or her contributions to keeping your family healthy and happy.

❖ *Talk about what's going on.* Here are some topics you might discuss as you prepare and taste foods together.
  • the names of different foods, and how they look, smell, feel, and taste
  • what different utensils do and where you keep them in the kitchen
  • why you serve a variety of foods with each meal

❖ *Maybe you'd like to do some cooking activities with the children at our program.* We'd love you to supply a recipe or help the children make their snack. Also, please send us your ideas for food preparation activities. We especially welcome your own family favorites or recipes that reflect your family's heritage. We want your child to have wonderful food-related experiences both here and at home.

Sincerely,

©1999, Teaching Strategies, Inc., Washington, DC. Permission granted to reprint, for non-commercial uses only, by programs implementing *The Creative Curriculum for Infants & Toddlers*.

Algunas ideas acerca de
preparar y probar los alimentos

Estimadas familias:

Quizá a algunos de ustedes les sorprenda que los niños tan pequeños participen en actividades culinarias. Sin embargo, una de las razones por las cuales a los pequeños les llama la atención la preparación de alimentos es porque es una actividad de los adultos. Para ellos, participar en en esta clase de actividad —que los han observado a ustedes llevando a cabo diariamente— les fascina y motiva.

En nuestro programa nosotros construimos sobre la base de este interés natural en las experiencias alimenticias. Existe una gran cantidad de conceptos y de destrezas que los niños pueden aprender a partir de actividades de esta naturaleza. Por ejemplo, ¿se imaginan qué podrían aprender sus niños a partir de una tarea tan sencilla como cortarle los extremos a las habichuelas verdes? ¿Incluyeron lo siguiente?

coordinación ojo-mano	parte y todo
forma	desarrollo de la motricidad fina
color	orgullo por completar una tarea
causa-efecto	

Como pueden ver, preparar alimentos es —además de educativo— algo práctico y placentero.

Lo que ustedes pueden hacer en el hogar

❖ *Permitan que sus hijos participen.* Dado que es probable que ustedes cocinen en su hogar, les será fácil involucrar en ello a sus hijos, incluso a los más pequeños. Permítanles sentarse en una silla alta y comenten lo que hacen. Cuando sus hijos les ayudan a preparar o a servir los alimentos, ustedes les demuestran que valoran sus contribuciones para mantener a la familia saludable y feliz.

❖ *Hablen con los niños sobre lo que sucede.* Los siguientes son unos cuantos temas que ustedes podrían comentar, a medida que preparen y prueben alimentos juntos.
  • los nombres de los diferentes alimentos, su apariencia, olor, sabor y textura
  • lo que se puede hacer con los diferentes utensilios y adónde se guardan en la cocina
  • por qué ustedes sirven una variedad de alimentos en cada comida

❖ *Es posible que estedes deseen llevar a cabo algunas actividades culinarias con los niños de nuestro programa.* Nos encantaría que ustedes prepararan alguna receta o que les ayudaran a los niños con la merienda. Especialmente, las recetas favoritas de su familia o una que refleje su herencia cultural. Ya que, deseamos que sus hijos tengan experiencias maravillosas relacionadas con los alimentos, tanto en nuestro programa, como en sus hogares.

Les saluda atentamente,

©1999, Teaching Strategies, Inc., Washington, DC. Se permite la reproducción, únicamente con fines no comerciales, a los programas que ponen en práctica *The Creative Curriculum for Infants & Toddlers*.

Exploring
Sand and Water

— ✦ —

"Your dinosaur is looking mighty clean, Willard," says Grace, as Willard waves the washed animal in front of her. "Look how shiny it is when it's wet." "Mmmm," says Willard in an insistent tone, as he climbs to a standing position. "I bet you want another animal to wash," says Grace to a beaming Willard.

— ✦ —

Infants and toddlers are naturally attracted to sand and water play. There's something about the cool splash of water and the magical sensation of sand sifting through fingers that almost everyone finds appealing. Even as an adult, there may be times when you crave a warm bath or a walk on a beach. Sand and water remain soothing and relaxing throughout life.

In addition to its calming nature, sand and water play introduces children to basic concepts such as wet and dry, full and empty, and heavy and light as they play. You can see this happening when, for example, Matthew adds water to dry sand and creates a wet mixture that he then dribbles across the sandbox. Or when Abby dumps cupfuls of sand into a bucket filling it up, then pours the sand out, holds the empty bucket up, and peers into it.

Sand and water also offer opportunities for spontaneous art and dramatic play experiences. Barbara knows that Leo, whose behavior can be hard to predict, will happily spend 20 minutes combing flowing designs in the sand. Stop by La Toya's backyard and the twins will likely serve you tea—a cup of water and plate of molded sand biscuit.

Setting the Stage for Exploring Sand and Water

It does require some advance planning to ensure children's health and safety, keep mess to a minimum, and gather props and tools to enhance the experience. But as you plan, remember, sharing your pleasure in these materials is the most important thing you can do to encourage children's exploration of them.

"What safety and health considerations should I be concerned about?"

There are a few small precautions you need to take so children can play safely with sand and water. While you don't have to hover over the children's every move, infants and toddlers do depend on your constant supervision.

For water play, individual basins are better than a communal table to avoid the spread of diarrheal disease. Sprinklers are also a safe and healthy way to offer water play. Begin with no more than a tray full of water for infants. As children grow, you can progress up to two or three inches. (However, children have been known to drown in less than an inch of water. As remote as it may seem, you need to know mouth to mouth resuscitation procedures should an incident occur.)

Remember to empty the water after each use. Standing water not only poses a drowning hazard, but is a growth medium for bacteria.

If you're using a sink for water play, you'll need to check that the water temperature has been adjusted and that faucets do not easily turn on when touched. You'll also want to be sure that if children use a step stool, it is protected by rubber slats. Remove all electrical appliances (such as hair dryers) and cover the outlets so that the children's wet hands won't accidentally come into contact with electricity.

For sand play, sterilized, fine grained sand (purchased from lumber yards) is best for health reasons and because it holds its shape. While not toxic, eating it (as babies often do) is hardly recommended. Therefore, sand play activities are best left for older infants and toddlers. To avoid slips and falls, be sure to sweep sand off of sidewalks and walking/running/riding areas.

For a different texture experience, consider using rice, cornmeal, or oatmeal as an alternative to sand. (Keep in mind though, that for some individuals, using food in this way is offensive. Talk with families before deciding to do this.) Avoid Styrofoam™ "peanuts" as they pose a choking hazard.

For both sand and water play, use individual trays or tubs to reduce the spread of infections. Sanitize the tubs each day using a bleach solution. Remember to cover outdoor sand areas while not in use to prevent cats and dogs from leaving droppings in them.

Props, too, need daily cleaning with bleach solution. Sponges—although great fun to play with—should be avoided, since they are a breeding ground for germs.

"How can I keep mess to a minimum?"

If you feel that sand and water play are simply too messy to deal with, you are not alone. You may ask yourself, aren't there less difficult ways of providing children with meaningful learning experiences?

Of course there are less messy activities such as looking at books and playing with toys. However, because children learn in a variety of ways and through a variety of experiences, the broader the array of experiences you provide, the more opportunities there are for exploring and learning.

With a little planning on your part, sand and water play can be an activity that is manageable and fun. Here are some suggestions.

Start doing sand and water play activities outdoors. The best place to start is outdoors, where making a mess is not really a concern. A bare spot of ground and a puddle are nature's sand and water "tubs." Sandboxes and wading pools are also ready starting points. You can bring out dish tubs, specially designed sand and water tables, or use an old tire or inner tube as a sandbox frame. In warm climates, many centers use sand as their outdoor ground cover. This makes the entire outdoor area a giant sandbox.

Choose your indoor spaces carefully. To keep messes in check indoors, think about where clean up will be easiest. For family child care providers, the bathroom or kitchen are likely choices. Each of these rooms has a sink where you can do water play, and floors that are designed to be mopped. In a center, an uncarpeted area is the logical choice. However, even if all your floors are carpeted, you can still conduct sand and water play successfully, if you spread an old plastic tablecloth, shower curtain, or crib sheet on the floor.

Prepare for spills. You can wipe up spills easily and carry the sand outdoors to be emptied if you use a dropcloth. For further protection, spread old towels or newspapers on top of the plastic. Some caregivers put individual tubs inside a plastic wading pool. The pool catches the splashed water or spilled sand.

Protect children's clothing. Protecting the children is a matter of either covering or uncovering them. In warm weather, you might find it easiest to let children play with sand and water wearing just their diapers or pants. Clean up is a breeze when there are no outfits to protect. Smocks can be commercially purchased or fashioned from old shirts, aprons, or heavy duty trash bags with holes cut in them to make ponchos. Another option is to have children play with water dressed in their raincoats and boots. In any event, it's always wise to have a fresh change of clothes on hand for each child—just in case!

Keep group size small. Limit the number of children playing with sand and water to no more than three or four at a time. If you offer other interesting options of things to do, this won't be an issue. Small groups are easier for children to handle and permit you to interact with each child.

Keep clean-up supplies handy. Keep supplies—paper towels and child-sized brooms, dust pans, and mops—close at hand so that the older children can assist you in clean up. When clean up becomes a part of the play experience rather than a chore you have to attend to afterwards, sand and water play is a more inviting experience for all of you.

Determine the best time to make sand and water play available. Of course you want to let children choose whether or not to play in sand and water, but it is up to you to decide when to make these options available. We suggest you choose a time of day when there is adequate time for set up, play, and clean up. Many caregivers/teachers find the late morning to be a good time.

"What supplies and props do I need to encourage children to explore with sand and water?"

To hold the sand and water, you can make use of cafeteria-style trays or shallow dish tubs. Individual trays or tubs allow each child to play in a defined area. Toddlers, who enjoy the company of other children, will enjoy playing at a child-sized water or sand table.

Young infants do not need props for water play. Exploring water alone is satisfying for them.

Mobile infants enjoy sensory exploration too. Props you make available will help them stretch their skills and imaginations. Here are some props to consider:

- rubber/plastic animals or people figures
- balls
- floating toys, such as boats
- small shovels and pails
- rakes

- nesting cups (plastic measuring cups)
- funnels
- colanders
- sprinkling/watering can

For toddlers, any of the props listed previously are appropriate. You may want to add some of the following:

- wire whisks
- sieves
- water/sand mills
- plastic cookie cutters
- slotted spoons
- squeeze bottles
- pie tins (with and without bottom holes)
- ladles
- scoops
- muffin tins
- straws
- bubble blowing supplies
- large shells

Selected props are best stored on low, open shelves where children can get at them on their own. Picture labels make it easy for children to know where the wire whisk or squeeze bottle should be returned. However, avoid storing props in the tub or on the table. This is not only messy and unsanitary, but discourages children from deciding what they want to play with.

Inviting Children to Explore Sand and Water

For infants and toddlers exploring sand and water is a wonderful sensory experience that introduces basic concepts and promotes their creativity in natural ways. At the same time, sand and water explorations develop fine motor skills, eye-hand coordination, and balance. Here are some ways to make these experiences enjoyable and encourage children's curiosity and wonder about the world.

Young Infants

Many infants love exploring water. The feel of water on their cheeks, tickling their feet, and dripping down their tummies makes them squeal with delight. As babies sit in your lap, allow them time to splash water in a plastic tub. Just watching water jump when it's hit and feeling its coolness when it splatters on their skin provides infants with many sensory experiences.

Observe to see children's responses. If they are pleased and interested, make time to play with water a regular activity.

Talk with infants about what they are experiencing.

- ❖ **Describe the experience:** "I bet the water is tickling your toes."
- ❖ **Help a child feel safe:** "I'm holding you in the water. Doesn't it feel good?"
- ❖ **Talk about their actions:** "You splashed the water!"
- ❖ **Mirror an infant's emotions:** "That splash on your cheek surprised you, didn't it?"

Mobile Infants

Mobile infants, who are more likely to play with sand than to eat it, can enjoy exploring both sand and water. They like using their hands as well as simple props such as funnels and sifters. Introduce props gradually and one at a time. Measuring cups and colanders, for example, open up a whole new world of play. Floating toys add another dimension to water play, as do a shovel and pail to a sandbox. Observe to discover what props children enjoy. Make them available so children have many opportunities to play with them. Remember, however, that too many props can be distracting.

As we mentioned earlier, some children will be entranced by these activities and want to do them. Others like Abby, who has a slight sensitivity to touch, may be more reluctant. Invite these children to explore sand and water by sharing your interest and pleasure in these activities, but never, never force a child.

When you offer sand and water activities to mobile infants, here are some ways to interact with them to promote their learning.

- ❖ **Describe changes the child can observe:** "The sand turned wet and dark when we added water."
- ❖ **Encourage children to appreciate designs:** "You made all those wavy lines in the sand with the rake."
- ❖ **Help children become aware of their emotions:** "Playing in the water can be so relaxing."
- ❖ **Provide children with vocabulary for their explorations:** "If we turn on the faucet, the cold water will come out."

Toddlers

With their ever-developing thinking and physical skills, toddlers explore sand and water with zeal. Leo can now use a vegetable brush to scrub a rock. Valisha can "cook" mudpies to serve La Toya, and Jonisha can wash her own hands as well as those of her doll.

In exploring water and sand, toddlers may observe that some objects float on water and that sifted sand forms a mound. They notice how sand and water drift through holes in a colander, and can spend long periods of time filling and dumping containers. Toddlers find great enjoyment in burying their feet and making imprints in the sand. Sand and water are excellent laboratories for finding answers to the many "Why?" questions toddlers like to ask.

To tap into the toddler's natural enthusiasm for sand and water play, talk with them in ways that help them reflect on what they are doing.

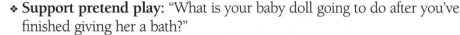

❖ **Point out cause and effect relationships:** "What happened to the sand when you poured it in the colander?"

❖ **Encourage children to solve problems:** "How can we get this sand into the bucket?"

❖ **Challenge children to make predictions:** "What do you think will happen if we drop the block in the water tub?"

❖ **Support pretend play:** "What is your baby doll going to do after you've finished giving her a bath?"

Props expand toddlers' thinking by helping them explore and experiment with sand and water in new ways. When Valisha uses a whisk in the water tray, she makes bubbles that pop when she pokes at them. Likewise, she sees that sand falls through a colander and stays in her cup. Each interaction teaches her new concepts.

As with younger children, introduce props gradually, making sure that toddlers have ample time to test and try them out. One all-time favorite for many is blowing bubbles into the wind. (A recipe for making long-lasting bubbles is shown below.)

Bubble Solution

2/3 cup of liquid detergent
  (Joy™ or Dawn™ work best)
1 quart of water
1/3 cup of glycerin

Dip empty frames into the solution to make large bubbles. To make foamy bubbles, use empty shampoo bottles.

Give older toddlers a variety of frames to dip into the bubble solution and then blow or wave them through the air. Empty eyeglass frames or plastic berry baskets make wonderful bubbles. Show children that bubble blowing works best when their hands and the frames are both completely wet. (A dry surface causes bubbles to burst on contact.)

Other special activities you might wish to try with toddlers include:

❖ "painting" a building, sidewalk, or tree with water;

❖ playing mood music to set the tone for children's sand and water play; and

❖ telling stories, for example, about jumping in a puddle or the bulldozer you spotted at a nearby construction site on a walk.

Though it takes some planning and supervision on your part, exploring sand and water is a natural and enjoyable experience that happens to be filled with rich learning opportunities for infants and toddlers.

❖   ❖   ❖

Sharing Thoughts About
Exploring Sand and Water

Dear Families:

Sand and water play is messy, no doubt about that. But children love it, and they learn from it, too. When an infant splashes at water, he learns that swinging his arm makes the water move (cause and effect). When a toddler pours a cup of sand into a bucket, she begins to learn about size, shape, and quantity. At the same time, these children are developing muscle skills and are learning to express themselves.

Here at the program, the children play with sand and water both indoors and outdoors. Infants splash at water in a tray. Older infants wash dolls and rubber toys; they practice digging and pouring sand. Toddlers squirt water through basters and blow bubbles into the breeze; they make designs in the sand with combs and cookie cutters. We encourage all children to explore sand and water.

What You Can Do at Home

Because sand and water play offers your child many different kinds of experiences, you'll probably want to do some activities at home. Here are some suggestions to consider.

❖ *Fill a tray or plastic tub with an inch or so of water.* A small amount of water is all your child needs to have fun. Place the tub on the floor, on top of some towels, and then let your child just splash away! If you have an older infant or toddler, you can provide plastic measuring cups, squeeze bottles, a funnel, or a sieve.

❖ *Talk with your child while you bathe him or her.* Ask questions to encourage observation and thinking: "What do you think will happen if you drop your big rubber froggie in the water?"

❖ *Fill a dishpan with clean sand.* In this way your child can play with sand either indoors or out. The container forms the boundaries for the sand and allows your child to control the area of play. To vary the experience, add a shovel, funnel, scoop, small plastic animals, or a variety of kitchen utensils.

❖ *Add a bit of water to the sand to make mud.* Invite your child to make mudpies for a pretend party.

We have many more ideas for creative sand and water play. We'd love to share them with you. Even more importantly, we hope you'll give us your ideas for sand and water activities your child especially likes.

Sincerely,

©1999, Teaching Strategies, Inc., Washington, DC. Permission granted to reprint, for non-commercial uses only, by programs implementing *The Creative Curriculum for Infants & Toddlers.*

Algunas ideas sobre el juego
con arena y agua

Estimadas familias:

Es indiscutible que el juego con arena y agua ocasiona suciedad. Pero, a los pequeños les fascina y pueden aprender del mismo. Cuando un(a) pequeño(a) chapotea agua, aprende que al mecer su mano ocasiona que el agua se mueva (causa-efecto) y cuando vierte una taza de arena en un balde aprende sobre los tamaños, formas y cantidades. Al mismo tiempo, estos niños están desarrollando sus destrezas musculares y aprendiendo a expresarse.

En nuestro programa, los niños juegan con arena y agua, tanto dentro como fuera del salón. Los pequeños chapotean agua en bandejas y los mayorcitos bañan a sus muñecas y juguetes de plástico. Excavan y vacian arena; filtran agua a través de cedazos y soplan burbujas al viento; hacen diseños en la arena con peines y con moldes para galletas. Nosotros animamos a todos los niños a explorar la arena y el agua.

Lo que ustedes pueden hacer en el hogar

Dado que el juego con arena y agua les ofrece a los niños una variedad de experiencias, es probable que ustedes deseen llevar a cabo algunas de estas actividades en sus hogares. Tengan en cuenta las siguientes recomendaciones:

❖ *Llenen una bañera o una bandeja plástica con una pulgada de agua.* Lo único que necesitan sus hijos para disfrutarlo es un poco de agua. Coloquen la bañera en el suelo, sobre unas cuantas toallas y permítanles chapotear el agua. Si tienen otro(a) hijo(a) mayorcito(a) provéanles tazas plásticas para medir, envases que se puedan apretar, un embudo o un tamiz.

❖ *Hablen con su hijo(a) mientras el/ella se baña.* Formulen preguntas con el fin de estimular la observación y el pensamiento: "Mira cómo salen burbujas con el champú".

❖ *Llenen un platón de arena.* Así los niños podrán jugar adentro o afuera. El recipiente le pone límites a la arena y les permite a los niños controlar el área de juego. Para variar la experiencia, añada una pala, un embudo, una cuchara, animales de plástico pequeños u otros utensilios de cocina.

❖ *Añádanle un poco de agua a la arena para producir lodo.* Inviten a sus hijos a hacer pasteles para una fiesta imaginaria.

Nosotros contamos con otra serie de ideas para el juego creativo con arena y agua y nos encantaría compartirlas con ustedes. Esperamos que nos ofrezcan sus ideas acerca de las actividades con arena y agua preferidas por su niño(a).

Les saluda atentamente,

©1999, Teaching Strategies, Inc., Washington, DC. Se permite la reproducción, únicamente con fines no comerciales, a los programas que ponen en práctica *The Creative Curriculum for Infants & Toddlers.*

Having Fun with Music and Movement

— ◼ —

After starting a tape for the older children to dance to, Janet notices Jasmine sitting on the floor bouncing to the music. "It looks like you want to dance too," Janet says. Janet sits on the floor next to Jasmine and moves her head and body to the beat. They smile at one another. Then Janet holds out her arms and asks, "Do you want me to pick you up to dance?" When Jasmine reaches toward her, Janet picks her up and begins dancing across the room holding Jasmine in her arms. Jasmine smiles, then shrieks with pleasure.

— ◼ —

Music and movement are a natural part of children's lives. As newborns, they can often be comforted by the rhythmic sound of a parent's heartbeat as the parent holds them close, or by being rocked or gently bounced to a steady beat. By the time they can sit, they may bounce up and down or move their arms to music. Toddlers often have favorite songs. They love making "music" by hitting a spoon on a pot and they enjoy moving to different tempos and rhythms.

Music and movement also contribute to children's overall development. Indeed, research indicates that listening to and making music in early childhood helps wire children's brains in ways required for understanding mathematics, science, and engineering. In addition, music and movement provide opportunities to explore feelings, relationships, and learn concepts and skills. These experiences also promote the development of listening and speaking skills, motor skills, creativity, and aesthetic appreciation. For example, when Abby does "The Itsy Bitsy Spider" with Brooks, she not only enjoys being with Brooks, but learns about up and down, and sharpens her fine motor skills as her fingers become the spider, rain, and sun. When Jonisha dances with other children to a calypso tape she brought to La Toya's, she feels full of energy and connected to home. As she moves in different ways to the music, she stretches both her body and her imagination. And for Gena, learning the words to a new song makes her feel proud and able to participate in singing with other children.

Setting the Stage for Music and Movement

In providing music and movement activities, you'll have many decisions to make. These include how to set up the environment, what kinds of music to play, what kinds of instruments you need, what types of activities are most appropriate for infants and toddlers, and how accomplished you need to be as a singer or dancer. Each topic is discussed below.

"How should I set up the environment for music and movement activities?"

It is likely you have already done what you need to do. Simply be sure you have a safe open space for dancing and moving. The space should be big enough so that children won't bump into anything or each other. Of course, it's often a good idea to use a carpeted floor space. Young children like to fall down, and they may not be wearing shoes for movement activities.

If you have a radio, tape recorder, or compact disc player, be sure to locate it—and any wires used to connect it to an electric outlet—out of children's reach.

"What kinds of music do infants and toddlers enjoy?"

Young children seem to prefer music and songs that have a strong rhythm, repetition, and nonsense syllables; evoke a mood (such as calm or lively); suggest different movements; and tell a story.[1] You can make up simple songs about the children themselves and about familiar things and people in their lives. For example, Gena loves to hear Ivan sing "Here come Gena and Franklin" when she and Franklin, her stuffed lamb, arrive in the morning. Children also enjoy songs you make up about the sounds of things—such as bells that "ding," horns that "honk," and trains that go "choo choo." You can, of course, also have fun singing old favorites such as "Old MacDonald Had a Farm" and "Wheels on the Bus."

In addition, there are many good recordings for young children. Examples include *Let's Sing Fingerplays* and *Activity and Game Songs* (Tom Glazer), *This-a-Way, That-a-Way* (Ella Jenkins), *Singin' and Swingin'* (Sharon, Lois, and Bram) and *Singable Songs for the Very Young* and *More Singable Songs for the Very Young* (Raffi).

You don't have to limit your music choices to selections recorded for children. Look over your own collection for music to share with children. Like you, children enjoy listening and moving to a variety of sounds: folk songs, jazz, classical music, popular music, and music from different cultures. Many public libraries have selections of children's records as well as other types of music children enjoy. Families can also be a rich source of music that reflects their individual tastes and cultures.

---

[1] Joan P. Isenberg and Mary Renck Jalongo. *Creative Expression and Play in the Early Childhood Curriculum.* New York: Macmillan Publishing Company, 1993.

"Do I need instruments? If so, what kinds?"

Simple rhythm instruments such as drums, xylophones, bells, clackers, rattles and shakers, tambourines, maracas, cymbals, wood blocks, and pots and pans with wooden spoons will allow children to create and respond to music as they bang, ring, swish, and click. You can make many of these instruments as well as buy them. For example, you can make drums from oatmeal boxes, cymbals from pie pans, and rattles and shakers by filling containers with rice, macaroni, or buttons, and fastening them securely.

If you—or any parents—play instruments, bring them in and play for children. Don't be surprised if toddlers join you for a jam session by strumming on a cardboard block as you play your guitar, or blowing through a funnel or cardboard tube as you play your recorder.

"What types of music and movement experiences are most appropriate for infants and toddlers?"

Music and movement are already a natural part of children's day. Here are five types of music and movement experiences that children under three will especially enjoy throughout the day—with you and on their own.

Listening to sounds and music. Sounds are everywhere. When you call children's attention to the "pop" of snaps as you change their clothes, the "crunch" of the apple in the fruit salad they helped prepare, and the "honking" of horns during a neighborhood walk, you help children become even more aware of their world and promote the skill of listening.

Listening to music can occur any time during the day. You may already play soft music for children to listen to at naptime or sing to them during routines such as dressing, diapering, and toileting. In Janet's home, children have been listening to a waltz tape that one family brought in. You can promote children's concentration and listening skills when you play music selectively and invite a child or two to listen with you. By choosing to play music at certain times, you prevent it from becoming background sound and tell children it is something to pay attention to and enjoy.

Making sounds and singing. Older infants and toddlers enjoy making sounds—of animals, vehicles, and anything else in their environment—and will do so without prompting. You can build on this interest by encouraging them to imitate repeated sounds in stories that you read or to make sounds during pretend play. As for singing, most children enjoy it. Focus on the fun of singing together. Children—and adults—differ in their abilities to carry a tune and sing words. Invite children to copy your rhythms, rhymes, and gestures. And, have fun copying theirs!

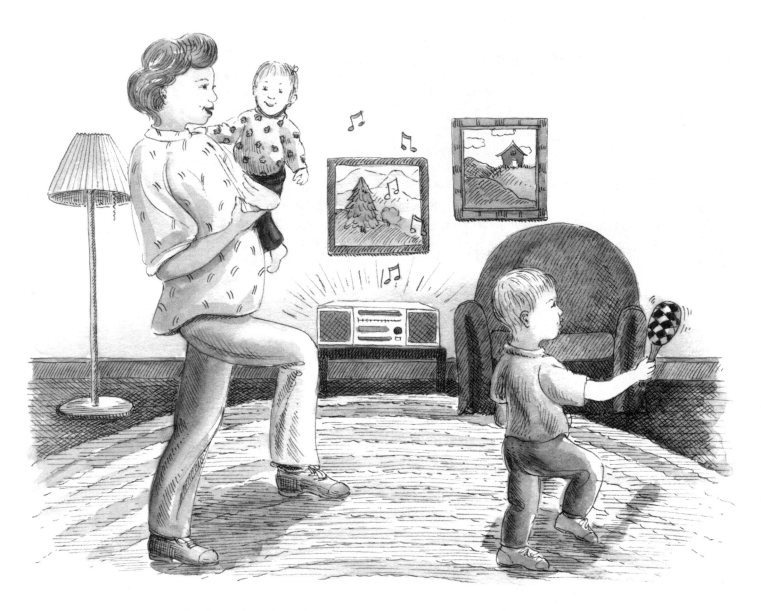

Dancing and moving. Movement is a natural partner of music. Even the youngest infants enjoy being held in your arms as you dance. Mobile infants will bounce and sway to music. They may like to sit in your lap facing you and play musical games such as "Row, Row, Row Your Boat," while holding hands and rocking back and forth. As they grow more steady on their feet, many children enjoy "Ring Around the Rosie." Toddlers often like to imitate the movement of various animals such as an elephant, butterfly, wiggly worm, or a road runner. As they move, they explore various concepts, such as when you suggest "Let's wiggle our fingers *silently*," or "Let's stamp our feet as *loudly* as we can." Over time, children learn how they can move their legs, feet, arms, and hands quickly and slowly, up and down, in and out, and over and under. As they become more comfortable with moving to music, you may want to offer them simple props such as feathers, scarves, or ribbons.

Fingerplays. Adding finger movements to classics like "The Itsy Bitsy Spider," "Two Little Blackbirds," and "Open Shut Them" gives children the opportunity to practice fine motor skills and coordination as they sing familiar songs. While some children may be able to get their fingers moving while they sing, others will participate by doing one or the other. Fingerplays also provide times to enjoy being together as you sit face to face with one child or with a small group. An "Itsy Bitsy Spider" fingerplay can lead to conversations about spiders, rain, and sunny days. A fingerplay to "Two Little Blackbirds" can end up in a conversation about hellos and good-byes as your fingers form blackbirds that fly away and come back again. You may enjoy browsing through books of fingerplays, such as *Fingerplays and Action Chants* (Tonja Weimer) and *Fingerfrolics* (Liz Cromwell and Dick Hibner).

Playing rhythm instruments. Mobile infants and toddlers enjoy the pleasure and satisfaction of creating their own music. You can encourage children to create rhythms by clapping or stomping quickly, slowly, softly, and loudly. Later, introduce some simple instruments. (Provide duplicates to avoid fights, and be ready to step in to prevent children from using instruments as weapons.) Allow plenty of time for children to explore instruments. As with singing, place your emphasis on the pleasure of creating sounds and being together rather than on performing.

"Do I need to be able to sing and dance to do music and movement experiences with children?"

While some adults are accomplished singers and dancers, most of us are not. Don't worry. You can share music and movement with young children even if you can't carry a tune or do the *Macarena*.

Much more important than any music or dance skills you may—or may not—have is your ability to share with children your pleasure in and appreciation of music and movement. This is an important way to encourage children's interest and participation.

Sharing Music and Movement with Children

As with all activities, take time to observe the children carefully so you can respond in ways that make each experience fun and meaningful for them. No matter how much you may want to share the beauty and pleasure of music and movement with children, remember that the key idea is that these activities should be fun. At no time should you force children to listen to music or to move and dance. At the same time, you should be aware of children's interest in one or more of various musical experiences. When necessary, you can step in to prevent the over-stimulation that can turn a music or movement activity into noise and chaos.

Here are some strategies you can use to promote children's exploration and enjoyment of music and movement.

Young Infants

Young infants like Julio and Jasmine may respond to sounds and music by turning their heads, smiling, laughing, or moving an arm or leg. They are generally soothed and calmed by soft, rhythmic sounds, such as a lullaby and the voice of a familiar caregiver. They tend to respond in more lively ways when music is peppy. Some infants are more sensitive than others to sounds and may cry at an unexpected or loud sound. Others are curious and attentive but may show fear when they hear certain sounds, such as the vacuum cleaner or garbage disposal.

For infants, as with older children, movement is the natural extension of music. Infants tend to respond to music with their entire bodies. Jasmine, for instance, bounces up and down and sways back and forth when Janet plays the new tape her older son brought home last week.

One of the most important ways to encourage infants' enjoyment of music and movement is to highlight and build on experiences that occur naturally in the course of daily life. Let's see how this works by looking in on Julio and Jasmine with their caregivers.

When Julio gets fussy, Linda picks him up and sings softly to him as she rocks with him in the rocking chair. He quiets down and gazes at her. She smiles and says, "You are feeling better, aren't you? Do you want to sing some more?" As Linda continues rocking and singing, she gives Julio a positive experience with music and movement.

Each afternoon, Janet and the children she cares for go outside into her backyard. While some of the older children play, Janet sits on a blanket with Jasmine. "Listen," she says, "do you hear the birds singing in the trees?" After a pause so Jasmine can listen, she whistles, copying their song. "Can you sing like a bird?" she asks. Janet is helping Jasmine understand that listening is an important skill. Over time, Jasmine will learn to distinguish among different sounds, rhythms, and volumes.

To encourage children's exploration of music and movement, you can talk with them about what they are experiencing. Always be sure, as Janet was, not to talk so much that you interfere with the sound and flow of the music. Here are some examples of what you might say.

- **Describe the experience:** "We're moving to the music. Back and forth. Side to side."

- **Help them feel safe:** "Let's sit and rock in this chair and I'll sing to you."

- **Mirror the infant's emotions**: "You like to dance with me, don't you?"

- **Describe interesting sounding language**: "That's a tuba you hear playing. It makes a deep sound."

Mobile Infants

Willard and Abby also enjoy the sounds and music that are part of their daily lives. For example, each morning Willard waits for Grace to push the button of the blender to mix orange juice and happily joins in the "whirring." Abby beams with pleasure when Brooks sings, 'Abby, Abby, where is little Abby?" to the tune of "Alouette."

To respond to children's increasing skills, you can introduce music and movement activities to individual children or to small groups. These activities may include singing, playing rhythm instruments, and dancing during daily routines and playtime. For example, sing a song when changing a child's diaper. Encourage children to take "giant" steps when taking a walk around the neighborhood or playing outdoors.

As their language skills improve, some mobile infants may join you in a song. Sometimes they may repeat a sound over and over again, such as "B-B-B-B" or "DADADADADADA." They may half-babble half-talk, and even sing through a familiar song such as "Happy Birthday." With their increasing physical coordination and body awareness, they also enjoy playing simple rhythm instruments and moving to the music.

As you interact with mobile infants, you can promote both their pleasure in and learning from music and movement. Here are some ideas of ways to help children focus on their experiences.

- ❖ **Describe what they are doing:** "You are singing a song to the teddy bear."
- ❖ **Encourage children to respond to music with their bodies:** "You are moving slowly to this slow music."
- ❖ **Ask children to identify familiar sounds:** "Do you hear the clock ticking?"
- ❖ **Point out different sounds:** "The drum is beating in this marching music. It goes 'boom, boom, boom.'"
- ❖ **Build relationships** around music and movement: "Let's hold hands and stomp through the leaves together."

Toddlers

Over the years, Leo, Matthew, Gena, and the twins have had many experiences with music and movement. They have discovered songs that they particularly like. They have learned to discriminate among certain sounds, and like some toddlers, can identify the sound of a specific instrument. They sometimes hum and sing as they play. Their increased fine and gross motor skills give them more control as they do fingerplays and move their arms and legs. And their growing imaginations open the way for different kinds of movement. Here are some ways to interact with toddlers to support these new learnings.

- ❖ **Encourage toddlers' enjoyment of songs:** "Shall we play the animal song you like so much?"
- ❖ **Help them discriminate among different sounds:** "Listen carefully. Do you know what instrument this is that makes such high notes?"
- ❖ **Encourage toddlers to sing familiar songs:** "Is today your baby's birthday? Are you going to sing 'Happy Birthday' to him?"

❖ **Focus attention on how their bodies move:** "Can you move quickly like the beat of this drum?"

❖ **Stimulate toddlers' imaginations:** "Let's pretend we are pancakes 'flip flopping' in the pan."

Music and movement are all around us. By including them in your program each day, you are opening the door to experiences that children can enjoy for the rest of their lives.

■   ■   ■

Sharing Thoughts About Music and Movement

Dear Families:

The pleasures of listening to music and moving their bodies are natural and important parts of children's lives. Newborns are naturally comforted when they are rocked or gently bounced to a steady rhythm. Older infants and toddlers may have favorite songs, or may even make music by banging a spoon on a pot. In addition to the pleasures of listening and moving to music, these activities are important to children's overall development. Here are some examples.

When your child does this…	Your child is learning…
holds hands and dances with another child	about relationships
plays a rhythm instrument	being a "music maker"
stomps around the room to a march	to respond to musical patterns
claps slowly, then quickly	concepts of slow and fast
enjoys singing and dancing with others	the pleasure of music and moving

What You Can Do at Home

It's easy and fun to make music and movement a part of your child's life. Here are some suggestions for things you can do at home.

- *Notice everyday sounds with your child.* Point out the clock ticking or the birds singing. Encourage your child to point out different sounds to you.

- *Sing with your child. You can make up songs about your child and familiar people and events.* To start, use a familiar tune and just substitute the name of a person or an event: "Sarah had a little doll, little doll, little doll…" We'll be happy to share with you the songs we sing and we'd love to learn some of your "home" songs.

- *Move and dance together.* It's fun to take giant steps, then tiny steps during a walk. You can even try to hop like a frog or wiggle like a worm!

- *Offer your child simple rhythm instruments.* You can make drums from oatmeal boxes, cymbals from pie pans, and shakers by filling containers with rice or buttons and fastening them securely.

It doesn't matter if you can't carry a tune or play an instrument. What does matter is that you share your enjoyment of music and movement with your child. With that thought in mind, we can open the door to experiences your child will enjoy for the rest of his or her life.

Sincerely,

©1999, Teaching Strategies, Inc., Washington, DC. Permission granted to reprint, for non-commercial uses only, by programs implementing *The Creative Curriculum for Infants & Toddlers*.

Algunas ideas sobre el placer de la música y el movimiento

Estimadas familias:

Escuchar música y mover el cuerpo son aspectos naturales, placenteros e importantes en la vida de los niños. Los recién nacidos se sientes reconfortados cuando se les mece con delicadeza y a un ritmo continuo. Los mayorcitos pueden tener canciones favoritas o, incluso, producir música al golpear una olla con una cuchara. Además de los placeres de escuchar música y moverse al son de la misma, estas actividades son de gran importancia para el desarrollo general de los niños. Los siguientes son unos cuantos ejemplos:

Cuando su hijo(a):
se toma de las manos y baila con otro(a) niño(a)
toca un instrumento rítmico
aplaude lentamente y luego rápido
disfruta el cantar y bailar con otros

El/ella aprende:
sobre las relaciones sociales
a ser un(a) "productor(a) de música"
a responder a la música
los placeres de la música y el movimiento

Lo que ustedes pueden hacer en el hogar

Es sumamente fácil y grato convertir la música y el movimiento en parte de la vida de sus hijos. Las siguientes son unas cuantas sugerencias que podrían poner en práctica en su hogar.

❖ *Noten los sonidos diarios con sus hijos.* Hagan notar el sonido del reloj o el canto de los pájaros. Anímenlos a señalarles a ustedes los diferentes sonidos.

❖ *Canten con sus hijos.* Ustedes pueden inventar canciones sobre sus hijos, parientes y eventos familiares. Para comenzar, elijan una melodía conocida y sustituyan el nombre de una persona o de un evento: "María tiene una pequeña muñeca, pequeña muñeca, pequeña muñeca…" Nos encantaría compartir con ustedes nuestras canciones y aprender algunas de las "hogareñas".

❖ *Muévanse y bailen juntos.* Durante una salida a caminar, es muy agradable dar pasos gigantescos y, luego, pasos pequeños. Ustedes podrían tratar, incluso, de saltar como las ranas o de deslizarse como los gusanos.

❖ *Ofrézcanles a los niños instrumentos rítmicos sencillos.* Ustedes pueden construir tambores con tarros de avena, timbales con los moldes para hornear y maracas con recipientes llenos de arroz o de botones, sellados en forma segura.

No se preocupen si no pueden cantar ni tocar ningún instrumento. En realidad no importa. Lo importante es que compartan con sus niños su gusto por la música y el movimiento. Así, podremos brindarle a sus hijos la oportunidad de gozar experiencias que disfrutarán por el resto de sus vidas.

Les saluda atentamente,

©1999, Teaching Strategies, Inc., Washington, DC. Se permite la reproducción, únicamente con fines no comerciales, a los programas que ponen en práctica *The Creative Curriculum for Infants & Toddlers*.

Going Outdoors

— ◼ —

"Look Gena, our lettuce will be ready to eat in a few days," Ivan says as he and Gena study the first crop in the wheelbarrow garden. "Do you think our garden needs a little more sun?" "Yes," agrees Gena as she observes the garden from her adaptive stroller. She watches as Ivan pushes the portable garden into a sunny corner of the Crane School's play yard. Gena turns her attention to the grassy spot under the tree. There children are chasing bubbles a teacher is blowing. "Do you want to go over and help blow bubbles?" asks Ivan. Gena nods and Ivan pushes her over to join the other children.

— ◼ —

Going outdoors is joyful for children. It gives them—and you—a chance to stretch large muscles, breathe fresh air, take in the sunshine (or the rain or snow), and enjoy the freedom of open spaces. Young infants like the touch of a soft, warm breeze on their cheeks or the sight of light filtering through the leaves as they look up from their carriage during a walk. By the time they are mobile, they enjoy splashing in a bin of water and crawling over a path you can create by adding blankets, tires, and floor mats to the natural textures that exist in your outdoor play space. As toddlers, they cannot resist the challenge of running in open space, climbing over tree trunks, chasing soap bubbles you blow, and propelling themselves on riding toys.

In addition, outdoor play can contribute to children's overall development by giving them a chance to explore with all their senses, practice fine and gross motor skills, develop social skills, and begin to appreciate and respect other living things. For example, when Jasmine touches and pulls on the grass in Janet's backyard, she is exploring with her senses and using fine motor skills. For Leo, being outdoors is a time to use his big muscles as he runs and climbs in the center's yard. Outdoor play also allows children to experience the bigger world in which people are going about their everyday lives. When Leo walks with Barbara, he loves to stop in at the grocery store to visit Ben, who is sometimes sweeping or putting things on the shelves.

Infants and toddlers should go outdoors every day, unless the weather is extreme. Going outdoors is important for their mental and physical health—and for yours.

Setting the Stage for Outdoor Play

When you go outdoors with the children, you need to make several decisions. These include which health and safety factors to consider, how to make the most out of the space you have, and what types of activities are most appropriate for infants and toddlers.[1]

"How do I create a safe and healthy outdoor environment?"

The keys to safe and healthy outdoor play are a safe environment, safety rules, and supervision.

Adult supervision. An adult needs to be able to see the entire play area at all times. If you are in a setting with more than one adult, each person can supervise an area, always being sure someone has a picture of the whole scene. Of course, everyone needs to be flexible and ready to step in if help is needed.

Nontoxic landscape. Soil should be analyzed for lead content initially and for toxic chemicals or other substances where there is reason to believe a problem may exist. Be sure all vegetation is non-poisonous in case a curious child takes a taste. Be on the lookout for mushrooms which can sprout up overnight. Check with your Regional Poison Control Center or Cooperative Extension Service for complete information.

Preventing drowning. According to the *National Health and Safety Performance Standards*, drowning is the third leading cause of unintentional injury in children younger than five. In some states, it is the leading cause of death. To prevent drowning, outside play areas should not include unprotected swimming and wading pools, ditches, quarries, canals, excavations in which water can collect, fish ponds, and other bodies of water.

The layout. The layout of your play area can make it more manageable, interesting, and safe. Defined areas with clear pathways not only provide a traffic pattern, but also help children make choices about what they want to do. All fixed play equipment should be arranged so that children playing on one piece of equipment will not interfere with children playing on or running to another piece of equipment. Locating swings and riding toys away from areas where children run can help prevent children from accidentally wandering into them and getting hurt.

Preventing unnecessary conflicts and crowding. You can reduce hitting, pushing, and biting incidents by offering plenty of interesting things to do. Provide duplicates of favorite outdoor toys such as balls, buckets and shovels, and riding toys. Be alert and ready to step in when necessary.

---

[1] The section is based on Jim Greenman and Anne Stonehouse, *Prime Times: A Handbook for Excellence in Infant and Toddler Programs*. St. Paul, MN: Redleaf Press, 1996, pp. 226–233; American Public Health Association and the American Academy of Pediatrics, *National Health and Safety Standards: Guidelines for Out-of-Home Child Care Programs*. Arlington, VA: National Center for Education in Maternal and Child Health, 1992, pp. 183–192; and Karen Miller, *The Outside Play and Learning Book*. Beltsville, MD: Gryphon House, 1989, pp.13–19; 23–26; 156; 159; 212.

Developmentally appropriate equipment. Equipment should be designed to match the size and skills of infants and toddlers. A general rule of thumb is one foot for every year of age (e.g., a two year old should be on equipment no higher than two feet). Choose equipment based on what you know about children's developmental abilities. (See Chapter 7, Creating a Welcoming Environment.)

Safe equipment. All equipment must meet all *Consumer Product Safety Standards* in regard to exposed surfaces, spacing, design, and location. All playground equipment should be installed so that an average-sized adult cannot cause a structure to wobble or tip. (See the *Safety Checklist* in Appendix C.)

Daily monitoring and maintenance. Outdoor play areas should be checked daily for broken glass, trash, and other hazardous materials such as animal feces, garden chemicals, or housepaint.

Monthly monitoring and maintenance. Check for the following once a month:

* visible cracks, bending or warping, rusting or breakage of any equipment;
* faulty or broken open hooks, rings, links, etc.;
* worn swing hangers and chains;
* missing, damaged, or loose swing seats;
* broken supports or anchors;
* cement support footings that are exposed, cracked, or loose in the ground;
* accessible sharp edges or points;
* exposed ends of tubing that require covering with caps or plugs;
* protruding bolt ends that have lost caps or covers;
* loose bolts, nuts, and screws that require tightening;
* splintered, cracked, or otherwise deteriorating wood;
* lack of lubrication on moving parts;
* broken or missing rails, steps, rungs, or seats;
* worn or scattered surfacing material;
* hard surfaces, especially under swings and slides, where resilient materials have shifted;
* chipped or peeling paint; and
* pinch or crush points, exposed mechanisms, and moving parts.

You may want to use items from this list and the checklists in Appendix C to create a checklist for tracking ongoing monitoring and maintenance of your program's outdoor play space.

Shock-absorbent materials. Any surface higher than 18–24 inches should be on 8–12 inches of shock-absorbent material that meets *Consumer Product Safety Guidelines*. Avoid using rubber, sand, pea-gravel, or wood chips that children might choke on.

Protection from exposure to the sun. Encourage families to supply sunhats, sunglasses, and sunscreen for their children. Offer children water on very hot days. If you do not have a naturally occurring shady spot where children can get out of the sun, you can create one. Drape a sheet from a fence, put up a tent, or use an awning.

"My outdoor space—and my budget—are limited. How can I make the most of what I have?"

Money and space for outdoor play areas are often in short supply. But don't despair. With thought and careful planning, you can offer children safe and valuable outdoor experiences. Here are some suggestions to help you make the most of your space.

Build on what nature has to offer. Take advantage of soft grass for sitting and playing on, tree stumps for climbing, wildlife, and various textures and sounds. Though we do suggest bringing toys and activities outdoors, don't get so busy lugging things and planning games that you forget to take time to watch a squirrel climbing a tree or to roll down a grassy hill with the children.

Think in terms of flexibility. Your space and what children can do in it naturally change with changes in the weather and the seasons. In addition, you can transform your space and add variety to children's experiences with props such as planks, boxes, rubber tires, and balls.

Make going outdoors manageable. You'll most likely take children outdoors frequently and enthusiastically if you can reduce related hassles. For example, you may not look forward to putting on snowsuits or searching for missing boots, but it helps to understand that dressing is a valuable learning experience in itself. For days when you take a walk, pack a shoulder bag or backpack with sunscreen, tissues, and a first-aid kit that contains emergency phone numbers and money for a pay phone. Add a container of bubble-blowing solution, and you will always have an engaging activity at hand.

Adapt your environment as necessary for children with special needs. According to the Americans with Disabilities Act (ADA), your outdoor play space should ensure that children with special needs can have the same or an equivalent experience as other children. Many adaptations are simply a matter of common sense and easy to do. For example, a ramp can make getting strollers and/or a wheelchair in and out easier. Consider using wagons for going outdoors and on field trips. Take special care to remove equipment that is easily overturned if a child pulls herself up on it or leans heavily against it. If more extensive adaptations are necessary, look into options for funding sources, including civic organizations and local businesses. Some programs may be eligible for a tax credit or deduction under the ADA to make structural adaptations.

Visit and talk with colleagues for other ideas. You never know what you might learn. Ivan, for example, heard about wheelbarrow gardens at a conference he attended last spring.

"Should I divide my outdoor space into different areas?"

Ideally, outdoor play space for infants and toddlers should include three areas: a shaded, grassy area for infants, an area with something to climb on and swings, and an area for riding toys that also has a place to play with sand and water. These three areas allow for a variety of experiences that children under three will enjoy.

In addition, think of areas in your community where children can visit. For example, children may enjoy playing in a neighborhood park, taking "field trips" to the corner market, or walking down the street to the large tree to collect and run through the falling leaves.

"What kinds of outdoor experiences should I offer infants and toddlers?"

Outdoor play should be a regular part of your daily schedule. (When possible, plan outdoor times in the mornings and afternoons.) There are three types of outdoor experiences children under three will especially enjoy: sensory exploration; gross motor play; and fine motor play.

Sensory exploration

With the sounds of singing birds and honking horns, the varied textures of grass, tree bark, and sand, and the bright colors of sky, flowers, and leaves, outdoors is perfect for sensory exploration. To build on what nature has to offer, consider the following ideas.

Create interesting patterns of light. Hang colored plexiglas or a crystal from a tree branch or a fence. You can also hang large pieces of bright fabric to let the sun shine through and to create temporary shade.

Make effects of the wind visible and audible. Hang fabrics, banners, parachutes, pie tins, and wind chimes on a fence. Encourage children to watch, listen, and reach for items.

Become aware of smells. With older infants and toddlers, you can plant flowers and herbs. Call children's attention to the smell of grass, dried leaves, and the rain.

Grow foods for snacks. Plant lettuce, peas, carrots, and herbs for children to taste.

Take a texture walk. Call the attention of older infants and toddlers to rough bark on a tree, prickly sticky pine cones, and a smooth hard rock. Children will enjoy collecting some of these items in buckets.

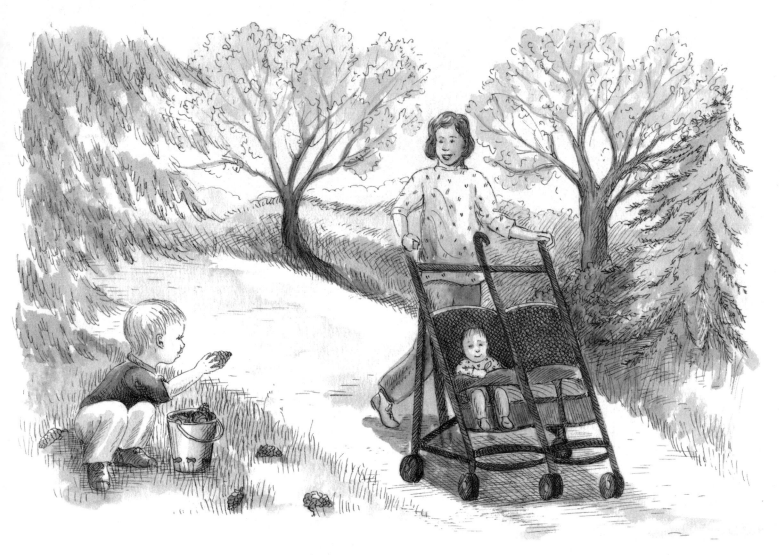

Eat outdoors. Spread out a blanket and enjoy a picnic together.

Take a magnifying glass outside. Older toddlers will enjoy looking at the magnified leaves and flowers under the glass.

Go out—even if it is raining or snowing lightly. Many older infants and toddlers love jumping in puddles. If warmly dressed, they often enjoy feeling snowflakes on their cheeks or making footprints in light snow. On days when the weather is too severe to go outdoors, bring some of the outdoors in. For example, invite children to poke and dig in bins of snow.

Gross Motor Play

Moving their bodies comes naturally to infants and toddlers. To promote gross motor play, consider some of these ideas.

Create safe places for young infants. A blanket spread out on the grass away from the traffic patterns of older children provides a safe place for an infant to stretch, reach for a toy, and practice rolling over. Some infants may enjoy spending some time on the grass, while others will protest and tell you they do not like the feel. You can place an infant on his tummy on a blanket and take him for a "ride" by pulling the blanket around.

Encourage crawlers to move by creating interesting places to go. You may, for example, decide to bring some equipment outdoors, such as cardboard boxes, cloth tunnels, covered ramps, or a table covered with a blanket to create places for children to go in, under, and through.

Give newly mobile infants something to hold on to. Show children how to hold on to a fence or low bench. Consider building a low rail 8–12 inches off the ground to encourage mobile infants to cruise.

Provide safe places for children to climb. A "climber" need be no higher than 18 inches off the ground. Low wide steps should lead to a platform large enough for two or three children at a time, with cushioning material underneath. There should be handholds for children to grab when they need to steady their balance.

Provide wheel toys for toddlers. Riding toys, wagons, wheelbarrows, and doll carriages give toddlers a variety of ways to move themselves, their dolls, and assorted objects from place to place.

Play movement games with older mobile infants and toddlers. Invite children to flutter like butterflies, wiggle like worms, or pretend to be baby birds who fly away and come home to the nest. Show children how to make their shadows move. Play "Follow the Leader" or "Can You Do What I Do?"

Invent games that promote the development of gross motor skills. You can create a "balancing path" by laying a scarf or piece of rope across the ground for children to walk on. Set up a bowling game where children try to knock down empty food boxes or plastic soda bottles using a beach ball. Challenge older toddlers to throw a beach ball into a laundry basket or large box. Invite mobile infants and toddlers to chase bubbles that you blow.

Fine Motor Play

Outdoor play gives children many opportunities to use their fine motor skills. Here are some examples.

Collecting small natural objects. Mobile infants and toddlers love collecting leaves, pine cones, maple seeds, or small sticks in wagons, buckets, or other containers with handles. They may want to keep their items for a time or may enjoy transporting them to a different place, then dumping them out.

Sand play. Many activities discussed in Chapter 21, Exploring Sand and Water, can be done outside without worry about spilling sand on the floor. Remember to cover sand boxes (always popular with cats) when they are not in use.

Water play. Toddlers often enjoy painting a fence, sidewalk, or wall with water. On a hot day, most infants like to splash in a shallow bin of water. (Be sure to empty, clean, and disinfect the basin afterwards.) Mobile infants and toddlers can have fun as they run through a sprinkler.

Art. For toddlers, painting and pounding on dough are different experiences in the great outdoors. Encourage children to create "nature sculptures" by adding natural items to their dough. Children can collect and paint with twigs, stones, and leaves.

Reading. Sit together under a tree and read books about the outdoors. Make a texture book by gluing leaves, moss, twigs, and small stones to pages made of cardboard.

Pretend play. Offer toddlers props such as toy rubber people and animals, and plastic vehicles for the sandbox. Encourage children to think where each toy may be going and what each is doing.

Inviting Children to Explore Outdoors

It can be tempting to equate going outdoors with taking a break. While a change of scene is usually refreshing, children need you to remain "on duty" observing, interacting, and sometimes playing with them. This doesn't mean you can't sit down for a moment or talk to a colleague. It does mean that children are depending on you outdoors—just as they do indoors—to keep them safe and to respond in ways that make their experience fun and meaningful. Here are some strategies you can use.

Young Infants

Young infants like Julio and Jasmine usually enjoy outdoor sights and sounds. For them, being outdoors is not only a change of scene, but an interesting experience in itself. While Julio may fall asleep, many infants Jasmine's age may enjoy watching other children, sitting and playing on a blanket, crawling through the grass, and joining an adult in reading a story or singing a song.

To enhance children's pleasure and exploration of the outdoors, talk with them about what they are experiencing. Here are some examples of what you might say.

- ❖ **Describe the experience:** "Doesn't the breeze blowing your hair feel good?"
- ❖ **Help them feel safe:** "I'm going to hold you in my arms so you can see all the children."
- ❖ **Mirror an infant's emotions:** "You like to touch the grass, don't you?"
- ❖ **Encourage their explorations:** "You are finding all sorts of interesting things in the grass to look at today."
- ❖ **Enjoy interesting sounds together:** "Do you hear the wind chimes clinking? Cling-clang, cling-clang."

Mobile Infants

Willard and Abby love going outdoors. Each morning, Willard looks up eagerly when Grace asks if he is ready to go outside. Abby sometimes asks Brooks, "Out?" and goes over to her stroller.

Mobile infants need little encouragement to take off crawling, cruising, and climbing. Some may join in simple movement games. Almost all enjoy digging in the sand, playing with water, pushing wheel toys, and dumping and filling.

As you interact with mobile infants, you can talk to them to enhance their fun and learning.

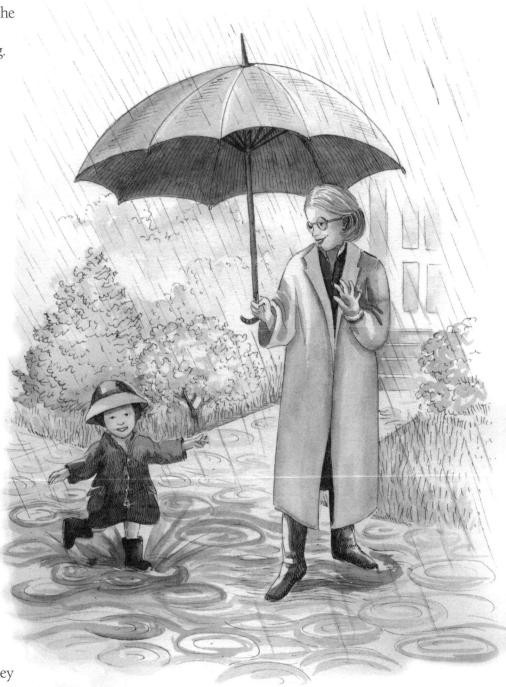

- ❖ **Encourage appreciation and respect for nature:** "Let's sit here and watch the squirrel climbing in the tree."
- ❖ **Promote feelings of competence:** "You popped all the bubbles!"
- ❖ **Describe and identify familiar sounds:** "Do you hear the wind blowing in the leaves?"
- ❖ **Note differences in the natural environment:** "It is colder today than yesterday. Maybe it will snow."
- ❖ **Promote positive social interactions:** "Let's roll the ball to Lianna now."

Toddlers

Leo, Matthew, Gena, and the twins have spent lots of time outdoors over the months and years. Through their experiences they have learned new vocabulary and concepts. Their developing gross and fine motor skills give them more control as they explore and play. Their growing imaginations open the door to more complex pretend play. The following are some ways to interact with toddlers to support these new learnings.

- ❖ **Encourage toddlers' growing vocabulary about the outdoors:** "These maple tree seeds remind me of little helicopters as they fall to the ground."

- ❖ **Explain new concepts:** "The ants are crawling into their home under the ground."

- ❖ **Encourage toddlers' moving and exploring:** "Can you jump like the grasshopper?"

- ❖ **Promote use of fine motor skills:** "Can you bury this pine cone in the pile of leaves?"

- ❖ **Stimulate toddlers' imaginations:** "What do you think the bird is saying to us when it goes, 'chirp, chirp'?"

The outdoors offers unique opportunities for children to explore and learn. By making going outdoors part of daily life in your program, you are opening the door to a world children can enjoy for the rest of their lives.

❈   ❈   ❈

— ■ —
Sharing Thoughts About Going Outdoors

Dear Families:

Going outdoors is fun for children. It gives them—and you—a chance to stretch large muscles, breathe fresh air, take in the sunshine (or the rain or snow), and enjoy the freedom of space.

Going outdoors contributes to children's overall development:

When your child does this…	Your child is learning…
crawls through the grass	to explore with all senses
climbs over a tree stump	to use gross motor skills
picks up a pine cone to put in a bucket	to use fine motor skills
watches a squirrel climb a tree	to appreciate nature
rolls a ball to another child	social skills

What You Can Do at Home

Here are some activities you might want to try next time you go outdoors with your child. Some of these you probably do already. Others, we hope, will give you some new ideas:

❖ *Enjoy nature.* Talk about the breeze touching your cheeks. Roll down a grassy hill together. Plant a garden—in your yard, a window box, or in a wheelbarrow you can move into the sun. Take a bucket so your child can collect things such as pine cones, acorns, leaves.

❖ *Take a texture walk.* Call your child's attention to soft sand, pine cones, and a smooth, hard boulder.

❖ *Invent games to play.* Create a "balancing path" by laying a piece of rope across the ground for your child to walk on. Play "catch and toss." Set up a bowling game in which your child tries to knock down empty food boxes by rolling a beach ball.

❖ *Take some "inside" activities outdoors.* Sit together under a tree and read a book. Give your child a paintbrush and water to paint the side of your house.

By working together, we can introduce your child to the fun and the wonders of the outdoors.

Sincerely,

©1999, Teaching Strategies, Inc., Washington, DC. Permission granted to reprint, for non-commercial uses only, by programs implementing *The Creative Curriculum for Infants & Toddlers*.

Algunas ideas sobre el juego
al aire libre

Estimadas familias:

Estar al aire libre es sumamente agradable para los niños. Además, les brinda —tanto a ellos como a ustedes— la oportunidad de estirar los músculos, respirar aire fresco, recibir sol (o disfrutar de la lluvia o la nieve) y gozar de la libertad del espacio abierto.

Jugar al aire libre contribuye al crecimiento de los niños en varias formas:

Cuando él/ella:	**Su hijo(a) aprende:**
gatea sobre el pasto	a explorar con todos sus sentidos
se trepa sobre el tronco de un árbol cortado	a hacer uso de su motricidad gruesa
recoge una bellota y la coloca en una canasta	a hacer uso de su motricidad fina
observa a una ardilla que trepa a un árbol	a apreciar la naturaleza
hace rodar una pelota y la dirige a otro(a)	destrezas sociales niño(a)

Lo que ustedes pueden hacer en el hogar

Las siguientes son unas cuantas actividades que ustedes podrían poner en práctica la próxima vez que salgan con sus hijos. Probablemente, algunas ustedes ya las practican. Otras, esperamos que les sirvan de inspiración:

❖ *Disfruten de la naturaleza.* Hablen sobre la brisa que toca sus mejillas. Rueden juntos por una pendiente. Planten un jardín en su patio, en materas, o en una carreta que puedan mover y poner al sol. Lleven un balde para que los pequeños puedan recolectar bellotas, hojas, piedrecillas, etc.

❖ *Vayan a caminar y noten texturas.* Háganles notar a los niños la suavidad de la arena, la dureza de las bellotas y la suavidad y firmeza de algunas piedras.

❖ *Inventen juegos.* Creen un "sendero de equilibrio" mediante un lazo puesto sobre el terreno y sobre el que puedan caminar los niños. Jueguen a "lanzar y atrapar". Organicen un juego de "bolos" en el que los pequeños traten de derribar cajas vacías con una pelota.

❖ *Lleven al exterior, algunas de las actividades que siempre realizan adentro.* Lean un libro sentados bajo la sombra de un árbol. Permítanles "pintar" una pared exterior con una brocha y agua.

Trabajando juntos, podremos hacer que sus hijos disfruten de las maravillas del mundo al aire libre.

Les saluda atentamente,

©1999, Teaching Strategies, Inc., Washington, DC. Se permite la reproducción, únicamente con fines no comerciales, a los programas que ponen en práctica *The Creative Curriculum for Infants & Toddlers*.

Part
V Appendices

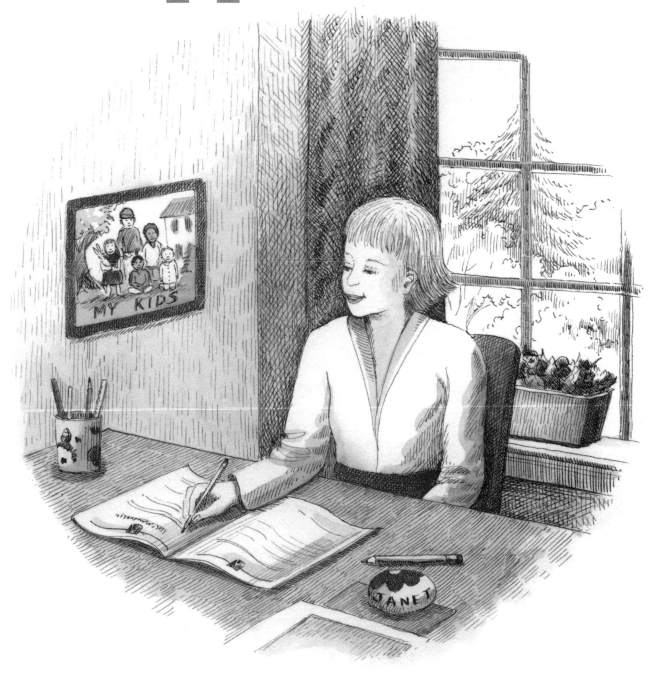

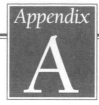

Self-Assessment

Goals and Objectives for Caregivers/Teachers

Caregiver/Teacher: _____ **Date completed:** _____

Directions: Read each goal, its objectives, and the examples. To rate yourself on each objective, write **X** in the appropriately numbered box. On the lines following the word *Comments,* give examples that explain your rating or that describe how you can improve.

Goal 1: To build responsive relationships

Objective: To form positive, trusting relationships with each child over time

RATING
5 HIGH
4
3
2
1 LOW

Examples:
❖ Feed, change, and offer naps to infants on demand
❖ Offer consistency in caregiving from day to day so each child forms social attachments
❖ Mirror children's emotions and feelings (e.g., show excitement when a child makes a discovery or accomplishes a task; respond sympathetically if a child is upset)

Comments: _____
_____
_____
_____
_____

Objective: To form positive relationships with families to support children's growth and development

RATING
5 HIGH
4
3
2
1 LOW

Examples:
❖ Interact daily with families in a positive manner, answering questions and discussing children's progress
❖ Recognize that parents' values must be addressed by the program (e.g., consult with parents about dietary concerns; discuss approach to handling challenging behaviors)
❖ Encourage parents to participate regularly in program activities, conferences/home visits, and to join in on field trips

Comments: _____
_____
_____
_____
_____

©1999, Teaching Strategies, Inc., Washington, DC. Permission granted to reprint, for non-commercial uses only, by programs implementing *The Creative Curriculum for Infants & Toddlers.*

Goal 1: To build responsive relationships (continued)

Objective: To work with colleagues and community representatives to support children and families

RATING
5 HIGH
4
3
2
1 LOW

Examples:
- Collaborate with specialists and refer children with disabilities to community services
- Consult with colleagues and community representatives to develop procedures for reporting suspected child abuse
- Maintain a "yellow pages" of community resources and the services they provide, including contact persons and phone numbers

Comments: _____
_____
_____
_____
_____

Goal 2: To plan and manage a developmentally appropriate program

Objective: To plan and evaluate a program that meets the needs of the children and families served

RATING
5 HIGH
4
3
2
1 LOW

Examples:
- Specify long-range and short-term goals and objectives for the program
- Develop a daily schedule that allows for individual and small group activities, balances quiet and active times, and is responsive to children's needs and interests
- Assess plans continually for effectiveness and make adjustments as indicated

Comments: _____
_____
_____
_____
_____

Objective: To observe children regularly and individualize the program based on these observations

RATING
5 HIGH
4
3
2
1 LOW

Examples:
- Observe children regularly to learn about their special characteristics, temperament, and learning styles
- Complete the *Individualizing Goals and Objectives for Children* form and the *Planning Form for Individualizing* on each child at least three times a year
- Specify curricular goals and objectives for each child based on the child's observed skills and needs

Comments: _____
_____
_____
_____
_____

©1999, Teaching Strategies, Inc., Washington, DC. Permission granted to reprint, for non-commercial uses only, by programs implementing *The Creative Curriculum for Infants & Toddlers*.

Goal 2: To plan and manage a developmentally appropriate program
(continued)

Objective: To create a warm and welcoming environment that supports children's growth and development

Examples:

RATING
5 HIGH
4
3
2
1 LOW

- Create an environment that fosters trust and security (e.g., spaces for crawling and snuggling; soft, cuddly textures; safe and clean materials)
- Provide materials and toys that stimulate children's senses, build on developing skills, and are adaptable, if necessary, for a child with special needs
- Provide an outdoor environment in which children can safely play and explore

Comments: _____
_____
_____
_____
_____

Objective: To ensure the safety of children in the program

Examples:

RATING
5 HIGH
4
3
2
1 LOW

- Use the *Safety Checklist* form regularly to ensure that preventive measures are in place to reduce chances of injuries
- Have emergency procedures available in case of sudden emergencies and natural disasters
- Balance children's need for safety with their need to explore

Comments: _____
_____
_____
_____
_____

Objective: To promote the health of children in the program

Examples:

RATING
5 HIGH
4
3
2
1 LOW

- Have procedures in place for responding to health emergencies
- Follow proper sanitation and hygiene procedures to prevent the spread of disease
- Provide well-balanced meals and snacks that meet children's nutritional requirements

Comments: _____
_____
_____
_____
_____

Objective: To guide children's behavior in positive ways

Examples:

RATING
5 HIGH
4
3
2
1 LOW

- Set up the environment to eliminate potential behavior problems (e.g., provide duplicates of favorite toys, remove breakables, offer soothing activities)
- Work with families to provide children with consistent messages at home and at the program
- Develop strategies for helping children deal with frustration and anger in positive rather than negative ways (e.g., through words or pretend play rather than by hitting or biting)

Comments: _____
_____
_____
_____
_____

©1999, Teaching Strategies, Inc., Washington, DC. Permission granted to reprint, for non-commercial uses only, by programs implementing *The Creative Curriculum for Infants & Toddlers.*

Goal 3: To promote children's development and learning

Objective: To use routines as opportunities for growth and learning

RATING
5 HIGH
4
3
2
1 LOW

Examples:
* Respond and repeat sounds infants make; talk, sing, and play word games while feeding, changing, and dressing children
* Offer toys to children to stimulate play during routines
* Explain what is being done during a routine and ask questions, even to nonverbal children

Comments: _____
_____
_____
_____

Objective: To provide activities that will facilitate children's growth and development

RATING
5 HIGH
4
3
2
1 LOW

Examples:
* Offer children toys and materials that can be mouthed, shaken, cuddled, and explored with all the senses
* Plan daily activities for children—art, outdoor play, food experiences, and so forth—increasing activity periods as children mature
* Introduce activities as a natural part of the child's day

Comments: _____
_____
_____
_____

Goal 4: To continue learning about children, families, and the field of early childhood education

Objective: To participate in training to expand skills and knowledge

RATING
5 HIGH
4
3
2
1 LOW

Examples:
* Seek training opportunities offered by professional organizations
* Ask colleagues, supervisors, and families for assistance in acquiring new skills
* Identify areas where additional training would improve job performance

Comments: _____
_____
_____
_____

Objective: To participate in professional early childhood education organizations

RATING
5 HIGH
4
3
2
1 LOW

Examples:
* Read books and journals on young children published by professional organizations (e.g., *Young Children, Child Development, Child Care Information Exchange, Zero to Three*)
* Attend local, state, and national conferences sponsored by professional organizations
* Conduct workshops or present papers on topics of interest

Comments: _____
_____
_____

©1999, Teaching Strategies, Inc., Washington, DC. Permission granted to reprint, for non-commercial uses only, by programs implementing *The Creative Curriculum for Infants & Toddlers*.

Goal 4: To continue learning about children, families, and the field of early childhood education (continued)

Objective: To observe colleagues to learn new successful techniques and approaches

RATING

5 HIGH
4
3
2
1 LOW

Examples:

❖ Visit and observe colleagues and other programs

❖ Ask colleagues and/or supervisors to model particular teaching skills or interactions with children

❖ Work as a member of a team; develop a system of mutual support with colleagues

Comments: _____

_____

_____

_____

_____

Goal 5: To maintain professional standards

Objective: To be ethical in all dealings with children, families, and community representatives

RATING

5 HIGH
4
3
2
1 LOW

Examples:

❖ Be honest, reliable, and dependable; come to work each day and notify families of program policies (e.g., vacations, absences—yours and children's)

❖ Act conscientiously in performing routines (e.g., change children when they are wet; do not allow children to sit indoors with coats on; comfort crying children)

❖ Follow all regulations concerning health and safety standards, group size and ratios, and child abuse reporting procedures

Comments: _____

_____

_____

_____

_____

Objective: To respect the privacy and confidentiality of children and parents

RATING

5 HIGH
4
3
2
1 LOW

Examples:

❖ Share children's records only with their family and professionals who have a "need to know"

❖ Keep children's records—including observations—in a secure place

❖ Do not discuss children and families in public and/or with colleagues (unless there is a programming reason to do so)

Comments: _____

_____

_____

_____

TEACHING STRATEGIES ©1999, Teaching Strategies, Inc., Washington, DC. Permission granted to reprint, for non-commercial uses only, by programs implementing *The Creative Curriculum for Infants & Toddlers.*

Goal 5: To maintain professional standards (continued)

Objective: To demonstrate respect for all children and families

RATING

5 HIGH
4
3
2
1 LOW

Examples:

- ❖ Learn ways to communicate successfully with all families (e.g., learn at least a few words in each family's home language, make home visits)
- ❖ Schedule meetings and conferences to meet an individual family's needs
- ❖ Seek input from families about home culture

Comments: _____

_____

_____

_____

_____

Goal 6: To be an advocate in support of children and families

Objective: To educate others about the need for high standards and quality programs

RATING

5 HIGH
4
3
2
1 LOW

Examples:

- ❖ Introduce families to *The Creative Curriculum for Infants & Toddlers*; distribute and discuss *Letters to Families*
- ❖ Use meetings and workshops with parents and colleagues to stress the importance of a quality program for infants and toddlers
- ❖ Provide research and evaluation reports to program policy makers and parents

Comments: _____

_____

_____

_____

_____

Objective: To work with community agencies in support of children and families

RATING

5 HIGH
4
3
2
1 LOW

Examples:

- ❖ Support organizations working to improve salaries and benefits for early childhood educators
- ❖ Campaign to elect public officials who support child and family issues; lobby elected officials to pass laws supportive of child and family issues
- ❖ Invite representatives of the community to visit the program to observe what is being done in support of children and families

Comments: _____

_____

_____

_____

_____

©1999, Teaching Strategies, Inc., Washington, DC. Permission granted to reprint, for non-commercial uses only, by programs implementing *The Creative Curriculum for Infants & Toddlers*.

Planning and Individualizing Forms

The following blank forms to help you plan your program and individualize for children and families are included in this Appendix:

Weekly Planning Form

Target goals/objectives: _____

_____

Week of: _____

Changes to the Environment

Special Activities I Plan to Offer This Week

	Monday	Tuesday	Wednesday	Thursday	Friday
Indoor Opportunities to Explore and Discover					
Outdoor Opportunities to Explore and Discover					

Changes to Daily Routines

Family Involvement

To Do

©1999, Teaching Strategies, Inc., Washington, DC. Permission granted to reprint, for non-commercial uses only, by programs implementing *The Creative Curriculum for Infants & Toddlers.*

Individualizing Goals and Objectives for Young Infants
(0–8 months)

Name of child:_____   **Caregiver/Teacher:**_____

Date of birth:_____

Goal 1: To learn about themselves	
Objectives	**Notes (Date each entry)**
To feel valued and secure in their relationships Examples: ❖ smiles and shows pleasure when talked to ❖ moves body towards caregiver when she approaches ❖ enjoys games with others like "Where Is Your Nose?"	
To feel competent and proud about what they can do Examples: ❖ kicks a mobile and smiles ❖ squeezes a rubber toy and shows pleasure at its squeak ❖ drops a ball and laughs as it bounces	
To express their independence Examples: ❖ pushes away bottle ❖ pulls at diaper when being changed ❖ grabs for spoon when being fed	

Goal 2: To learn about their feelings	
To communicate a broad range of emotions through gestures, sounds, and—eventually—words Examples: ❖ cries when hears sudden loud noises ❖ coos and smiles when being rocked and sung to ❖ laughs aloud when playing peek-a-boo	
To express their feelings in appropriate ways Examples: ❖ while crying, lifts arms up to indicate need to be picked up and comforted ❖ bounces to get adult to continue a knee ride ❖ looks to familiar adult when a stranger approaches	

©1999, Teaching Strategies, Inc., Washington, DC. Permission granted to reprint for non-commercial uses only, by programs implementing *The Creative Curriculum for Infants & Toddlers.*

Goal 3: To learn about others

Objectives	Notes (Date each entry)
To develop trusting relationships with nurturing adults **Examples:** ❖ listens attentively to adult when being fed or changed ❖ kicks legs and squeals when familiar adult appears ❖ looks to adult for attention or help	
To show interest in peers **Examples:** ❖ watches other children ❖ reaches out to touch another infant's face ❖ grabs for toy another infant is holding	
To demonstrate caring and cooperation **Examples:** ❖ hugs doll ❖ pats adult on back when being held ❖ lifts bottom, in response to caregiver's actions, when being changed	
To try out roles and relationships through imitation and pretend play **Examples:** ❖ smiles at self in the mirror ❖ plays peek-a-boo ❖ pretends to feed familiar adult	

Goal 4: To learn about communicating

Objectives	Notes (Date each entry)
To express needs and thoughts without using words **Examples:** ❖ smiles to invite an adult to interact ❖ fidgets or cries when uncomfortable or bored ❖ holds rattle up for adult to shake	
To identify with a home language **Examples:** ❖ listens to conversations ❖ recognizes and begins imitating sounds of home language ❖ understands names of familiar objects in home language	

©1999, Teaching Strategies, Inc., Washington, DC. Permission granted to reprint for non-commercial uses only, by programs implementing *The Creative Curriculum for Infants & Toddlers*.

Goal 4: To learn about communicating (continued)

Objectives	Notes (Date each entry)
To respond to verbal and nonverbal commands Examples: ❖ looks up when called by name ❖ opens mouth as adult opens her mouth and offers a spoonful of food ❖ touches mirror when adult asks, "Where's the baby?"	
To communicate through language Examples: ❖ vocalizes to self and others ❖ begins babbling ❖ imitates tones and inflection	

Goal 5: To learn about moving and doing

To develop gross motor skills Examples: ❖ holds head up without support ❖ rolls over and sits alone ❖ begins creeping and crawling	
To develop fine motor skills Examples: ❖ scoops up piece of banana and eats it ❖ pulls large pegs out of pegboard ❖ transfers objects from hand to hand	
To coordinate eye and hand movements Examples: ❖ follows toy with eyes as adult slowly moves it ❖ looks at hand ❖ reaches for and grasps a rattle	
To develop self-help skills Examples: ❖ begins to hold own bottle ❖ begins to feed self finger foods ❖ pulls off socks	

©1999, Teaching Strategies, Inc., Washington, DC. Permission granted to reprint for non-commercial uses only, by programs implementing *The Creative Curriculum for Infants & Toddlers*.

Goal 6: To acquire thinking skills

Objectives	Notes (Date each entry)
To gain an understanding of basic concepts and relationships **Examples:** ❖ picks up pacifier and sucks on it ❖ drops spoon and watches it fall to the floor ❖ closes eyes as adult pulls shirt over his head	
To apply knowledge to new situations **Examples:** ❖ shakes stuffed animal in same way as rattle to hear noise ❖ kicks new crib toy to see if it will move ❖ squeezes and tastes new finger food	
To develop strategies for solving problems **Examples:** ❖ uses hand to steady self when sitting up ❖ reaches for a toy that has rolled away ❖ raises bottle as level of milk drops	

©1999, Teaching Strategies, Inc., Washington, DC. Permission granted to reprint for non-commercial uses only, by programs implementing *The Creative Curriculum for Infants & Toddlers*.

Individualizing Goals and Objectives for Mobile Infants
(8–18 months)

Name of child:_____   **Caregiver/Teacher:**_____

Date of birth:_____

Goal 1: To learn about themselves	
Objectives	**Notes (Date each entry)**
To feel valued and secure in their relationships Examples: ❖ looks at, goes over to touch familiar adults while playing ❖ imitates parent(s) and caregiver(s) ❖ points to pictures of family	
To feel competent and proud about what they can do Examples: ❖ fits a triangle into shape box and claps ❖ climbs up the slide and proudly looks around for caregiver ❖ chooses slice of pear at snacktime and smiles as she takes a bite	
To express their independence Examples: ❖ moves away the hand of an adult who is helping with a puzzle ❖ insists on choosing what shirt to wear ❖ says "Me do!" when adult offers help in dressing	

Goal 2: To learn about their feelings	
To communicate a broad range of emotions through gestures, sounds, and—eventually—words Examples: ❖ watches self making happy, sad, or angry faces in the mirror ❖ pushes aside unwanted food ❖ clings to parents as they say good-bye	
To express their feelings in appropriate ways Examples: ❖ helps caregiver comfort a crying child ❖ says "No!", instead of hitting when another child takes his toy ❖ looks to an adult for help when frustrated	

©1999, Teaching Strategies, Inc., Washington, DC. Permission granted to reprint for non-commercial uses only, by programs implementing *The Creative Curriculum for Infants & Toddlers*.

Goal 3: To learn about others

Objectives	Notes (Date each entry)
To develop trusting relationships with nurturing adults Examples: ❖ brings adult a book to read ❖ enjoys helping with chores (e.g., carrying paper towels into the bathroom) ❖ grabs onto caregiver's hand or leg when frightened	
To show interest in peers Examples: ❖ identifies the family members and possessions of other children ❖ joins other children in rocking wooden rowboat ❖ knows names of other children	
To demonstrate caring and cooperation Examples: ❖ helps caregiver hold young infant's bottle ❖ joins in search for a child's missing sweater ❖ gives adult a big hug	
To try out roles and relationships through imitation and pretend play Examples: ❖ enacts familiar events (e.g., puts on hat and looks in the mirror) ❖ scribbles on a shopping list adult is writing and says "Milk" ❖ pretends to call parents on the phone	

Goal 4: To learn about communicating

Objectives	Notes (Date each entry)
To express needs and thoughts without using words Examples: ❖ points to ask for an out-of-reach toy ❖ shakes head "No" when asked if hungry ❖ catches eye of an adult to ask for help	
To identify with a home language Examples: ❖ looks at a doll on hearing the word *doll* in the home language ❖ uses same sounds and intonations as parents do ❖ says several words in home language clearly	

©1999, Teaching Strategies, Inc., Washington, DC. Permission granted to reprint for non-commercial uses only, by programs implementing *The Creative Curriculum for Infants & Toddlers.*

Goal 4: To learn about communicating (continued)

Objectives	Notes (Date each entry)
To respond to verbal and nonverbal commands Examples: ❖ reacts to facial expressions of adult ❖ follows simple directions such as, "Bring the book to me, please?" ❖ pushes foot into boot as adult pulls it up	
To communicate through language Examples: ❖ creates long babble sentences ❖ repeats familiar words ❖ calls caregiver by name	

Goal 5: To learn about moving and doing

To develop gross motor skills Examples: ❖ pulls self up and cruises around furniture ❖ walks ❖ seats self in small chair	
To develop fine motor skills Examples: ❖ scribbles with a crayon ❖ turns pages of a book, often two or three at a time ❖ stacks several blocks, one on top of the other	
To coordinate eye and hand movements Examples: ❖ stirs ingredients when helping to make playdough ❖ puts toy in a bucket ❖ peels a half of a banana	
To develop self-help skills Examples: ❖ uses spoon and cup, but may spill ❖ pushes arm through jacket sleeve ❖ undresses self	

©1999, Teaching Strategies, Inc., Washington, DC. Permission granted to reprint for non-commercial uses only, by programs implementing *The Creative Curriculum for Infants & Toddlers*.

Goal 6: To acquire thinking skills

Objectives	Notes (Date each entry)
To gain an understanding of basic concepts and relationships Examples: • fills bucket with pop beads and dumps them out repeatedly • asks for wooden spoon to bang on homemade drum • pretends to open door using a toy key	
To apply knowledge to new situations Examples: • blows on noodles when adult explains they are hot • spots cat and says "dog" • uses hammer instead of hand to flatten playdough	
To develop strategies for solving problems Examples: • points to picture in a storybook and looks to adult for name of that object • brings over a stool to help reach a toy • tries various pieces in shape-sorting box until one fits	

©1999, Teaching Strategies, Inc., Washington, DC. Permission granted to reprint for non-commercial uses only, by programs implementing *The Creative Curriculum for Infants & Toddlers*.

Individualizing Goals and Objectives for Toddlers
(18–36 months)

Name of child:_____   **Caregiver/Teacher:**_____

Date of birth:_____

| Goal 1: To learn about themselves ||
Objectives	**Notes (Date each entry)**
To feel valued and secure in their relationships Examples: ❖ points out family picture in a scrapbook ❖ knows which child is out for the day after seeing who is there ❖ looks to caregivers for comfort and at times may comfort caregiver	
To feel competent and proud about what they can do Examples: ❖ pours own juice at snack time and says, "I did it!" ❖ helps another child find the crayons ❖ stands on one foot and calls, "Look at me!"	
To express their independence Examples: ❖ insists on putting on own jacket ❖ willingly joins in a new activity ❖ cheerfully says "good-bye" to parents and goes to play	
Goal 2: To learn about their feelings	
To communicate a broad range of emotions through gestures, sounds, and—eventually—words Examples: ❖ says, "I did it!" after using the potty successfully ❖ hugs a doll and lovingly feeds it a bottle ❖ raises hand to make a "high five"	
To express their feelings in appropriate ways Examples: ❖ roars like a lion when angry instead of biting ❖ recognizes feelings in others (e.g., "Camilo sad") ❖ bites on a bagel when has urge to bite	

©1999, Teaching Strategies, Inc., Washington, DC. Permission granted to reprint for non-commercial uses only, by programs implementing *The Creative Curriculum for Infants & Toddlers*.

Goal 3: To learn about others

Objectives	Notes (Date each entry)
To develop trusting relationships with nurturing adults **Examples:** ❖ imitates adult activities (e.g., reading a newspaper, setting the table) ❖ eager to help with chores (e.g., preparing meals, feeding the fish) ❖ calls adult over to show an accomplishment (e.g., a painting, block structure)	
To show interest in peers **Examples:** ❖ enjoys including other children in pretend play (e.g., driving in a car or going food shopping) ❖ refers to other children by name ❖ comments on who is a girl and who is a boy	
To demonstrate caring and cooperation **Examples:** ❖ responds to emotions of other children (e.g., helps adult pat a crying child) ❖ works with another child to complete a task (e.g., putting away a puzzle) ❖ feeds and puts doll to bed	
To try out roles and relationships through imitation and pretend play **Examples:** ❖ acts out simple life scenes (e.g., making dinner, going to the doctor) ❖ puts hat on and says, "I'm going to work" ❖ uses object to represent something else (e.g., box as car, block as phone)	

Goal 4: To learn about communicating

To express needs and thoughts without using words **Examples:** ❖ uses facial expressions to show excitement ❖ catches adult's eye for attention and reassurance when needed ❖ tugs on pants to indicate need to go to bathroom	
To identify with a home language **Examples:** ❖ speaks in home language with family members and others ❖ uses main language spoken in child care with those who don't speak home language ❖ recognizes tapes of stories and songs from home culture	

TEACHING STRATEGIES ©1999, Teaching Strategies, Inc., Washington, DC. Permission granted to reprint for non-commercial uses only, by programs implementing *The Creative Curriculum for Infants & Toddlers.*

Goal 4: To learn about communicating (continued)

Objectives	Notes (Date each entry)
To respond to verbal and nonverbal commands **Examples:** ❖ follows directions such as, "Will you carry these napkins to the table, please?" ❖ responds to adult's facial expression (e.g., stops throwing blocks after a stern look) ❖ goes over to cot when lights are dimmed for naptime	
To communicate through language **Examples:** ❖ tells a story ❖ tells about what happened over the weekend ❖ talks with other children while playing together	

Goal 5: To learn about moving and doing

Objectives	Notes (Date each entry)
To develop gross motor skills **Examples:** ❖ walks up stairs ❖ throws a ball ❖ runs	
To develop fine motor skills **Examples:** ❖ threads large beads ❖ scribbles with marker or crayons ❖ pastes papers together	
To coordinate eye and hand movements **Examples:** ❖ places pieces in a simple puzzle ❖ closes Velcro™ fasteners on shoes ❖ pours juice into a cup	
To develop self-help skills **Examples:** ❖ uses the potty and washes hands ❖ pours own milk and juice from small plastic pitcher ❖ puts on own jacket and hat when going outside	

©1999, Teaching Strategies, Inc., Washington, DC. Permission granted to reprint for non-commercial uses only, by programs implementing *The Creative Curriculum for Infants & Toddlers.*

Goal 6: To acquire thinking skills

Objectives	Notes (Date each entry)
To gain an understanding of basic concepts and relationships **Examples:** ❖ experiments with mixing colors when painting ❖ tells another child, "Your mommy comes back after nap" ❖ runs to the tree and says, "I run fast"	
To apply knowledge to new situations **Examples:** ❖ sees a picture of a zebra and calls it a horse ❖ paints on side of building with water after painting at easel ❖ completes new puzzle using familiar strategy of turning pieces until they fit	
To develop strategies for solving problems **Examples:** ❖ cooperates with others in implementing a plan (e.g., carries a large pillow across the room for a jumping game) ❖ asks "Why?" questions ❖ dips paintbrush in water to clean it	

©1999, Teaching Strategies, Inc., Washington, DC. Permission granted to reprint for non-commercial uses only, by programs implementing *The Creative Curriculum for Infants & Toddlers*.

Summary of Development

Name of child:_____

Date:_____

Comment on what you learned about this child in any of the following areas of development.

What is the child learning about:

Self:

Feelings:

Others:

Communicating:

Moving and Doing:

Thinking:

©1999, Teaching Strategies, Inc., Washington, DC. Permission granted to reprint for non-commercial uses only, by programs implementing *The Creative Curriculum for Infants & Toddlers.*

Planning Form for Individualizing

Name of child:_____ Parent(s)/Guardian(s):_____

Date of birth:_____ Caregiver/Teacher:_____

Date completed:_____

This child likes

This child's temperament is

This child learns best by

This child's special needs are

To individualize for this child, I intend to make these changes:

To the environment (including equipment & materials):

To routines, transitions, and planned activities:

To the daily schedule:

To interactions:

©1999, Teaching Strategies, Inc., Washington, DC. Permission granted to reprint for non-commercial uses only, by programs implementing *The Creative Curriculum for Infants & Toddlers.*

Goals for Working with Families

Parent(s)/Guardian(s): _____   **Child:** _____

Completed by: _____

Goal 1: To build a partnership with families	
Objectives	**Notes (Date each entry)**
To involve families in the program's planning and evaluation process	
To listen to and discuss families' questions, concerns, observations, and insights about their children	
To communicate regularly with families at arrival and departure times about how things are going for their child at home and at the program	
To schedule regular conferences and/or home visits	
To discuss with families ways to handle children's challenging behaviors	
To resolve differences with families in a respectful way	
To help families gain access to community resources	

Next steps:

_____

_____

_____

_____

©1999, Teaching Strategies, Inc., Washington, DC. Permission granted to reprint for non-commercial uses only, by programs implementing *The Creative Curriculum for Infants & Toddlers.*

Goal 2: To support families in their parenting role

Objectives	Notes (Date each entry)
To demonstrate respect for a family's approach to childrearing and their feelings about sharing the care of their child	
To celebrate with families each new milestone in their child's development	
To incorporate family rituals and preferences into the daily life of the program	
To offer workshops/training on child development and other topics of interest to families	
To help families network with one another for information and support	

Next steps:

_____

_____

_____

_____

_____

©1999, Teaching Strategies, Inc., Washington, DC. Permission granted to reprint for non-commercial uses only, by programs implementing *The Creative Curriculum for Infants & Toddlers.*

Goal 3: To support families in their role as primary educators of their child

Objectives	Notes (Date each entry)
To encourage family involvement and participation in program activities	
To provide families with strategies to support children's learning at home	

Next steps:

©1999, Teaching Strategies, Inc., Washington, DC. Permission granted to reprint for non-commercial uses only, by programs implementing *The Creative Curriculum for Infants & Toddlers.*

Goal 4: To ensure that the home cultures of the children's families are reflected in the program

Objectives	Notes (Date each entry)
To support children's use of their home language	
To encourage children's awareness of and interest in home languages spoken at the program	
To seek the families' assistance in learning about the children's home culture	
To include objects and customs from the children's home culture in the program's environment, routines, and activities	
To interact with children in a style that is respectful of their home culture	

Next steps:

_____

_____

_____

_____

_____

©1999, Teaching Strategies, Inc., Washington, DC. Permission granted to reprint for non-commercial uses only, by programs implementing *The Creative Curriculum for Infants & Toddlers.*

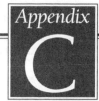
Safety and Health Checklists

Safety

This checklist identifies potential problems and describes safety measures that will reduce the chances of injuries occurring. Duplicate copies of this form and use it to identify problems in your program and note when they were corrected.

Safety Problem: Falls, Physical Injury		
Safety Measures	**Looks OK/ Not Applicable**	**Problems Identified and Date Corrected**
Furniture is in good repair, with sharp edges protected by corner or edge bumpers.		
Safety straps are used in high chairs, strollers, swings, and car seats.		
Sides of cribs are kept in a raised position; latches and locks on the drop side are fastened.		
Windows open only from the top and are kept locked when closed. Furniture children can climb up on is positioned away from windows.		
Stairs and hallways are kept free of clutter.		
Locked safety gates are placed at tops and bottoms of stairs. Gates should be at least three-fourths of children's height.		
Riding toys and trikes are used on flat surfaces only. Children wear helmets at all times.		
Steps and walks are kept free of snow and ice.		

 ©1999, Teaching Strategies, Inc., Washington, DC. Permission granted to reprint, for non-commercial uses only, by programs implementing *The Creative Curriculum for Infants & Toddlers.*

Safety Problem: Choking, Strangulation, or Suffocation

Safety Measures	Looks OK/ Not Applicable	Problems Identified and Date Corrected
Infants are held while fed. Toddlers eat meals and snacks seated and supervised.		
Rattles and/or pacifiers are not hung around children's necks.		
Crib corner posts do not exceed $1/16$ inch, so that clothing will not get caught.		
Toys are not tied to cribs.		
Venetian blind cords are secured out of children's reach or replaced with plastic rods.		
Batteries are stored and disposed of in areas out of children's reach.		
Pillows, heavy blankets, and large stuffed animals are kept out of cribs.		
Rattles and squeeze toys are removed from cribs when babies are sleeping.		
Children do not wear long scarves when climbing or jumping.		
Children do not wear hoods with drawstrings.		

Safety Problem: Fire, Burns, Scalding, Electrical Shock

Smoke alarm batteries are checked monthly.		
Emergency exits are marked, kept clear, and unlocked from the inside. Fire drills are conducted monthly.		
Heating and cooling systems are inspected regularly. Water temperature is less than 120°F.		
Water temperature in bathtubs and swimming and wading pools is between 82°F and 93°F.		
Unused electrical outlets are covered with caps.		
Small appliances are unplugged when not in use. Electrical cords are kept out of children's reach.		

continued on next page

©1999, Teaching Strategies, Inc., Washington, DC. Permission granted to reprint, for non-commercial uses only, by programs implementing *The Creative Curriculum for Infants & Toddlers.*

Safety Problem: Fire, Burns, Scalding, Electrical Shock (continued)

Safety Measures	Looks OK/ Not Applicable	Problems Identified and Date Corrected
Matches, lighters, gasoline, and cleaning fluids are stored in locked cabinets.		
Heaters, fireplaces, and radiators have screens or safety guards; pipes are covered or insulated.		
Outdoor metal slides and other play equipment are covered in hot weather when not in use so they don't overheat.		
Temperature of infant formula and children's food and drink is checked before being offered. Microwave ovens are not used to heat baby bottles (heating is uneven).		
Only back burners on a stove are used; pot handles are turned inward and to the back.		
Cooking or warming foods is not done while holding an infant.		
Adults do not drink hot beverages while holding an infant or standing near children.		

Safety Problem: Poisoning

Cleaning supplies, insecticides, weed killers, and paint supplies are kept in their original, labeled containers and stored in locked cabinets.		
Medicine is kept in child-proof containers and placed in locked cabinets or the refrigerator, as indicated on labels.		
Adult handbags and briefcases (which may contain unsafe objects or materials) are stored out of children's reach.		
Empty cleaning product bottles are rinsed before being thrown away.		

©1999, Teaching Strategies, Inc., Washington, DC. Permission granted to reprint, for non-commercial uses only, by programs implementing *The Creative Curriculum for Infants & Toddlers.*

Safety Problem: Cuts, Eye Injuries

Safety Measures	Looks OK/ Not Applicable	Problems Identified and Date Corrected
Sharp objects (pins, needles, knives, adult scissors) are stored out of children's reach.		
Toys and outdoor playthings are regularly checked to see that they have not developed sharp edges and are splinter-free.		
Toys are stored on open shelves, with the heavier items placed at the bottom.		
Drawers are secured by locks.		
Wastebaskets are kept out of children's reach.		
Outdoor play area is kept free of glass, nails, and debris.		

Safety Problem: Security

Children are supervised at all times, both indoors and outdoors.		
Children do not enter or leave the program on their own.		
Children in all areas of the program are always in view.		
Injury/incident reports are completed promptly. Families are notified immediately, if appropriate.		
Vehicles used to transport children are kept locked when not in use.		

Safety Problem: Transportation

Adults wear seat belts and never hold any children in their laps in a moving vehicle.		
Children weighing less than 20 pounds are strapped in an infant carrier when being transported in a vehicle. They ride backwards in a semi-reclining position in the back seat.		

continued on next page

©1999, Teaching Strategies, Inc., Washington, DC. Permission granted to reprint, for non-commercial uses only, by programs implementing *The Creative Curriculum for Infants & Toddlers.*

Safety Problem: Transportation (continued)

Safety Measures	Looks OK/ Not Applicable	Problems Identified and Date Corrected
Children weighing 20 pounds or more (who can sit by themselves) are secured in a toddler safety seat. The seat is attached to the car with a seat belt. Children ride in the back seat, facing forward.		
Children enter and leave vehicles only on the curb side of the road or in a driveway.		
Only adults are permitted to buckle and unbuckle children at pick-up and drop-off.		
Children are kept from sticking their heads, hands, or objects out of the vehicle windows.		
Emergency evacuation procedures are practiced with children.		
Children wear identification tags when being transported (and when away from the program site).		
Children hold adult's hand when walking across streets.		
Emergency data on children and first-aid kit are taken on outings.		

Safety Problem: Drowning

Safety Measures	Looks OK/ Not Applicable	Problems Identified and Date Corrected
Children play in or near water only with an adult standing directly beside the water, not at a distance from it.		
Children play in water no deeper than two inches.		
Water tubs are emptied daily and turned upside down when not in use.		
Swimming pools and/or built-in wading pools are fenced in on four sides with a locked gate.		
Children do not use toilets and other bathroom facilities unsupervised.		

©1999, Teaching Strategies, Inc., Washington, DC. Permission granted to reprint, for non-commercial uses only, by programs implementing *The Creative Curriculum for Infants & Toddlers.*

Emergency Procedures

A list of procedures can be helpful when emergencies happen. Below is a chart that may be copied. We recommend that you display it where adults can see and use it.

Emergency Procedures List

1. **Find out what happened.** Discover who was injured, if the scene is safe, and if there are bystanders who might be of assistance.

2. **Check for life-threatening problems.** These are known as the ABC's:
   A = open the airway;
   B = check for breathing;
   C = check for circulation (pulse and bleeding).

3. **Call your local emergency medical services—911 or an ambulance—if you have any doubts about the seriousness of the problem.** In situations that are life-threatening, it may be advisable to call the emergency medical service before administering any first aid, so that the ambulance can be dispatched and on its way while you are tending to the child. Use your judgment and good common sense to decide if the child has a better chance of survival if you call for an ambulance before or after you administer emergency first aid.

4. **Check for injuries, starting at the head and working down.** You will need to give this information to medical personnel.

5. **Regroup.** Calm the other children. If the injured child needs your attention, ask a co-worker or back-up provider for assistance.

6. **Contact the child's parents or guardian** as soon as possible.

7. **Follow local procedures for filing an injury report.** Be sure families get a copy.

Above all:

- **Do not move a child,** unless it is to save the child's life. Movement may make injuries worse; and,

- **Do no harm.** Harm means both failing to do anything and making things worse.

©1999, Teaching Strategies, Inc., Washington, DC. Permission granted to reprint, for non-commercial uses only, by programs implementing *The Creative Curriculum for Infants & Toddlers.*

First Aid

A first-aid kit should contain everything you need should an emergency arise. Make a point to check your program's kits several times a year to ensure that they are fully stocked. You can use the checklist below for this purpose.

First-Aid Kit			
Items	**Date Checked**	**Date Checked**	**Date Checked**
Roll of quarters (for calling doctors or children's families from a pay phone)			
Copy of each child's emergency contacts form; *Emergency Telephone Guide*			
Index cards and pens (for writing down instructions or keeping notes to give medical staff)			
A quick reference manual (for example, *A Sigh of Relief: The First-Aid Handbook for Childhood Emergencies* by M. Green) or standard first-aid chart			
Water			
Clean washcloth and soap			
Small plastic cup			
Disposable nonporous gloves			
Flashlight with working batteries			
Thermometer (non-glass)			
Blunt tip scissors			
Tweezers			
Small plastic or metal splints			
3-ounce rubber bulb syringe (for rinsing out wounds and eyes)			
Gauze pads (one box each of nonstick, sterile 2x2 and 4x4)			

continued on next page

©1999, Teaching Strategies, Inc., Washington, DC. Permission granted to reprint, for non-commercial uses only, by programs implementing *The Creative Curriculum for Infants & Toddlers*.

First-Aid Kit (continued)

Items	Date Checked	Date Checked	Date Checked
Flexible gauze bandages (one box each of 2" and 4")			
25 1" (the most commonly used size) and 25 assorted smaller bandages			
2 triangular muslin bandages			
Bandage tape			
Syrup of ipecac (1-ounce bottle) *Before* administering, check with child's pediatrician or Poison Control Center. The vomiting induced by syrup of ipecac can cause serious harm to the esophagus if child has swallowed a poison such as lye or drain cleaner.			
Insect sting ointment			
Cold pack or plastic bags for ice packs			
Alcohol-based wipes			
Safety pins			
Additional supplies for specific health needs of children in care (e.g., antihistamine for child with severe allergies, glucose tablets for diabetic child who might experience low blood sugar)			

©1999, Teaching Strategies, Inc., Washington, DC. Permission granted to reprint, for non-commercial uses only, by programs implementing *The Creative Curriculum for Infants & Toddlers.*

Good Health Practices in Your Program

Keeping infants and toddlers healthy requires ongoing monitoring of your environment and practices. Use the checklist below to ensure that your program promotes good health and to identify practices that need your attention.

Area of Concern: Environment		
Practices	**Yes, we do this regularly**	**No, we don't practice this**
Clean all surfaces with fresh bleach solution made by mixing ¼ cup bleach with 1 gallon of water (or 1 tablespoon bleach per quart of water) according to recommended schedule.		
In programs without central air conditioning, open windows every day.		
Keep air temperature between 65° and 72°F.		
If air is dry, use a humidifier or cool air vaporizer. Clean these with bleach solution, change water, and add a mold inhibitor every day. (Steam vaporizers may be dangerous to children who get too close and should not be used.)		
If you use air conditioners, clean them weekly to remove dust and mold.		
Take children outdoors daily.		
Avoid using aerosol products.		
Place garbage in lined metal containers or in plastic containers with lids.		
Use the food preparation area only for food.		
Locate the refrigerator near the food preparation area. Check daily to make sure the refrigerator is working and that the temperature is less than 40°F.		
Locate the food preparation area near a water source.		
Locate the diapering/toileting areas near a second water source.		
Separate sleeping areas from other activities.		
Keep each child's clothes and personal belongings separate to avoid contamination.		
Don't use cribs for storage when children are not asleep.		
Wear indoor slippers or shoe coverings when walking in infant play areas.		

©1999, Teaching Strategies, Inc., Washington, DC. Permission granted to reprint, for non-commercial uses only, by programs implementing *The Creative Curriculum for Infants & Toddlers.*

Area of Concern: Toys and Play Equipment

Practices	Yes, we do this regularly	No, we don't practice this
Clean rubber, plastic, and wooden toys; infant seats and feeding tables; changing tables; and eating utensils every day with fresh bleach solution (¼ cup bleach to 1 gallon of water).		
Clean mouthed toys with fresh bleach solution after use.		
Wash stuffed toys weekly in a washing machine; wash them more frequently if soiled.		
Cover outdoor sand play areas at night to protect from animal feces.		

Area of Concern: Diapering and Toileting

Practices	Yes, we do this regularly	No, we don't practice this
Use diapering area exclusively for diapering.		
Be sure changing surface is at least 3 feet above the floor (to prevent spread of infectious diseases).		
Check that the diapering surface is nonporous (e.g., plastic with no tears or cracks).		
Clean diapering surface with fresh bleach solution after each use.		
Use disposable plastic gloves in accordance with program policy.		
Place a fresh, clean piece of paper beneath the child's buttocks so that the child's body does not directly touch the diapering surface.		
Use disposable diapers to reduce skin irritations. Cloth diapers may be used with waterproof covers that open in the front and are changed after each use.		
Seal soiled diapers in plastic bags and place them in plastic-lined containers that are equipped with a cover and foot pedal.		
Place soiled outer clothing in plastic bags, stored away from child's other belongings; send bag home with parents at the end of the day.		
Clean the child's urinary and anal areas with disposable wipes or paper towel with soap and water. Wipe child front to back once with each wipe until clean, to reduce chances of urinary tract infections.		
Apply creams and lotions only with parental permission. Label products with child's name and use only with that child. Avoid using talcum powder because of danger to children's lungs.		

continued on next page

©1999, Teaching Strategies, Inc., Washington, DC. Permission granted to reprint, for non-commercial uses only, by programs implementing *The Creative Curriculum for Infants & Toddlers.*

Area of Concern: Diapering and Toileting (continued)

Practices	Yes, we do this regularly	No, we don't practice this
Wash the child's and your hands after each changing.		
Keep written records of each child's diapering times and bowel movements.		
Locate toilets in rooms separate from cooking, eating, or play areas.		
Accompany all children to and from the toileting area or bathroom.		
Check that there is a minimum of one sink and one toilet available for every 10 toddlers. In centers, be sure that fixtures are child-sized (i.e., a maximum of 11" for toilets and 22" for sinks). If child-sized equipment is not available, use modified toilet seats and step aids.		
Use bleach solution to sanitize the bathroom daily and as needed, if contaminated by feces or vomit. Keep bathroom well stocked with disposable wipes, toilet paper, paper towels, and soap.		
If your program uses potty chairs, flush contents down toilet, rinse chair in a utility sink not used for any other purpose, wash with soap and water twice using paper towels (empty rinse water into the toilet), spray with bleach solution, and allow it to air dry. (Potty chairs are only recommended if your program has a utility sink.)		
Be sure that there is at least one container with a pedal-operated lid in the toileting area. Empty the containers daily and sanitize them with bleach solution.		
Be sure you wash your hands after you use the toilet or change children's diapers. Toddlers should wash their hands after using the toilet. Use paper towels to dry hands. Turn water off with the towel. Use hand lotion to prevent drying and cracking skin.		

Area of Concern: Personal Hygiene

	Yes, we do this regularly	No, we don't practice this
Wash your hands and apply hand lotion before and after each task (e.g., before and after handling food; assisting a sick child; upon arrival; before giving a child medication or taking temperature; after sneezing, coughing, or blowing your nose; after touching your face or hair; after handling money or a pet; and after toileting or diaper changing).		
Use disposable towels to dry your hands. Don't reuse towels.		

continued on next page

©1999, Teaching Strategies, Inc., Washington, DC. Permission granted to reprint, for non-commercial uses only, by programs implementing *The Creative Curriculum for Infants & Toddlers.*

Area of Concern: Personal Hygiene (continued)

Practices	Yes, we do this regularly	No, we don't practice this
Drape a clean towel, diaper, or pad across your shoulder when you hold an infant. Don't reuse shoulder drapes.		
Label children's toothbrushes and do not permit sharing. Store brushes with bristles up. Replace brushes every three months.		
Store each child's brushes, combs, and personal items separately from those of other children.		

Area of Concern: Sleeping and Resting

Assign each child who spends more than 4 hours a day in care his or her own crib, bed, mat, or cot.		
Locate cribs away from heaters, drafts, window blinds, and hanging cords.		
Separate cribs and cots by at least 3 feet of space to discourage the spread of germs (unless you use plexiglass partitions).		
Use nonabsorbent, washable covers on mats and cots.		
At rest time, place children head to foot to reduce spread of germs.		
Place infants on backs in cribs to help prevent Sudden Infant Death Syndrome (SIDS).		
Have each child use own linens. Send linens home each week for laundering—or sooner if the linens are soiled.		
Clean crib mattresses and cots weekly and when soiled or used by another child.		
Avoid using substances of animal origin as bedding. Wool and feathers may cause allergic reactions. Cotton is best.		
Avoid using pillows, fluffy blankets, and bumper guards to reduce the chances of suffocation or SIDS.		
Avoid crib gyms, once an infant is pushing up.		

©1999, Teaching Strategies, Inc., Washington, DC. Permission granted to reprint, for non-commercial uses only, by programs implementing *The Creative Curriculum for Infants & Toddlers*.

Area of Concern: Feeding and Eating

Practices	Yes, we do this regularly	No, we don't practice this
Be sure that individual feeding supplies are available and that children use their own bottles, bowls, and utensils.		
Post information on children's food allergies and special nutritional needs in the food preparation area and eating areas.		
Label and date food brought from home. Store perishable foods (such as expressed milk) in the refrigerator or freezer.		
Prepare formula according to written instructions from parent or health professional and store it in refrigerator until used. Discard any unused portion within 48 hours. Once a child has stopped drinking at feeding time, do not save the bottle to give to the child later in the day.		
Hold infants being bottle fed; do not prop bottles.		
Introduce semi-solid foods (such as rice cereal) when infants are between 4 and 6 months old, or as directed by a health care professional. Observe a 5-day "watch and see" period before introducing another food.		
Transfer baby food to a bowl, rather than feeding infants from a jar, which is unsanitary.		
Introduce solid foods such as fruits and vegetables when infants are between 6 and 8 months old, or as directed by a health care professional. Observe a 5-day "watch and see" period before introducing another food. Introduce wheat products only after children are at least 7 months old because many younger infants are allergic to them.		
Introduce food with lumps, such as mashed potatoes, at 8 to 9 months, or as directed by a health care professional. Introduce these foods one at a time. Observe a 5-day "watch and see" period before introducing another food.		
Serve a complete meal to children who eat finger food and table foods. Encourage children to eat foods of their own choosing.		
Introduce cow's milk when children are 12 months old, or as directed by a health care professional. Don't introduce low-fat milk until 24 months (or later, if so directed) because children need the extra calories and contents of whole milk for nerve and brain development.		
Keep records for each child of the time, type of feeding, and, for young infants, amount of food consumed.		

©1999, Teaching Strategies, Inc., Washington, DC. Permission granted to reprint, for non-commercial uses only, by programs implementing *The Creative Curriculum for Infants & Toddlers.*

Area of Concern: Management of Illness

Practices	Yes, we do this regularly	No, we don't practice this
Verify that policies regarding exclusion of children and staff, isolation requirements, administration of medicine, emergency contacts, and long-term care are in place.		
Make daily health checks of each child for the following signs of illness: severe coughing, difficulty in breathing, sore throat, yellowish skin or eyes, pinkeye (tearing, red or pus-filled eyes), infected skin patches, nausea or vomiting, diarrhea, loss of appetite, rashes, lice, oozing insect bites or sores, bruises, and unusual behavior.		
Send ill children home until they are well enough to participate in activities and until such time as they are no longer considered contagious.		
When a sick child needs to be sent home, provide a comfortable, quiet area to rest until a parent or guardian arrives and supervise the child closely.		
Wash your hands after assisting a sick child.		
Wash and disinfect a crib or cot used by a sick child; launder bed linens.		
Send written notes to notify families of children exposed to communicable diseases as soon as possible, so families can watch for symptoms.		
Administer both prescription and nonprescription drugs only following training and with written instructions of a parent or health care professional. Keep all drugs in the original child-proof medication dispensers, which specify the schedule, dose, route, and duration of treatment. Maintain documentation of the time and amount given. Store the medication out of children's reach.		
Take universal precautions for blood. These include using nonporous disposable gloves when in contact with blood, body fluids, or tissue discharges containing blood. Following exposure, discard gloves immediately and wash hands with soap. Use bleach solution to disinfect blood-contaminated surfaces and mops used in cleaning.		

©1999, Teaching Strategies, Inc., Washington, DC. Permission granted to reprint, for non-commercial uses only, by programs implementing *The Creative Curriculum for Infants & Toddlers.*

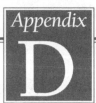

Appendix
D

Intervention Resources

Contact Information for the Central Directory of Early Intervention Services, Resources, and Experts

Available in the States and Jurisdictions
Participating in the Part C Program*

Alabama
Department of Rehabilitation Services
Division of Early Intervention
2129 East South Boulevard
PO Box 11586
Montgomery, AL 36111-0586
(800) 543-3098 (voice/TDD)

Alaska
Alaskans Information Line
The AKINFO Network
United Way of Alaska
1057 West Fireweed Lane, Suite 101
Anchorage, AK 99503-1736
(800) 478-2221
(voice/TDD, AK only)
http://www.ak.org

American Samoa
Part C Program
Department of Health
Government of American Samoa
Pago Pago, AS 96799
(684) 633-4929 or 2697

Arizona
Children's Information Center
Department of Health Services
1740 West Avenue, Room 200
Phoenix, AZ 85008
(800) 232-1676
(voice/TDD, AZ only)

Arkansas
Division of Developmental Disabilities
Department of Human Services
PO Box 1437, Slot 2520
Little Rock, AR 72203-1437
(800) 643-8258 (voice/TDD)

California
Department of Developmental Services
Prevention and Children Services Branch
Early Start Program
1600 9th Street, Room 310
Sacramento, CA 95814
(800) 515-BABY (voice, CA only)
(916) 654-2054 (TDD)
http://www.dds.cahwnet.gov/
services.htm

Colorado
Special Education Division
Department of Education
201 East Colfax, Room 305
Denver, CO 80203
(800) 288-3444
(voice/TDD, CO only)
http://www.dooronline.org

Commonwealth of Northern Mariana Islands
Early Childhood/Special Education Programs
CNMI Public School System
PO Box 1370 CK
Saipan, MP 96950
(670) 322-9956

Connecticut
Birth to Three INFOLINE
United Way of Connecticut
1344 Silas Deane Highway
Rocky Hill, CT 06067
(800) 505-7000
(voice/TDD, CT only)
http://www.birth23.org

Delaware
Birth to Three Early Intervention System
Department of Health and Social Services
1901 North DuPont Highway
New Castle, DE 19720
(800) 464-4357
(voice/TDD, Helpline I&R, DE only)
(800) 273-9500
(voice/TDD, Helpline I&R, outside DE)

District of Columbia
DC EIP Services
Office of Early Childhood Development
609 H Street NE
Washington, DC 20002
(202) 727-8300 (voice, ChildFind)
(202) 727-2114 (TDD)

Florida
Directory of Early Childhood Services
2807 Remington Green Circle
Tallahassee, FL 32308
(850) 921-5444 (voice/TDD)
(800) 654-4440 (voice)
http://www.centraldirectory.org

---

* Compiled by the National Early Childhood Technical Assistance System (NEC*TAS). Because this information changes frequently, readers are encouraged to refer to the NEC*TAS site on the World Wide Web for current information: http://www.nectas.unc.edu/. NEC*TAS is supported through cooperative agreement number H024A60001 with the Office of Special Education Programs of the U.S. Department of Education. For more information about NEC*TAS and the resources it offers, please contact NEC*TAS at: 137 East Franklin Street, Suite 500, Chapel Hill, NC 27514; (919) 962-2001 (voice); (919) 966-4041 (TDD); (919) 966-7463 (fax); E-mail: nectas@unc.edu; World Wide Web: http://www.nectas.unc.edu/.

Georgia
Babies Can't Wait Directory
Parent-to-Parent of Georgia, Inc.
2900 Woodcock Boulevard, Suite 240
Atlanta, GA 30341
(800) 229-2038
(voice/TDD, GA only)
info@parentotparentofga.org
http://www.parenttoparentofga.org

Guam
Department of Education
Division of Special Education
PO Box DE
Agana, GU 96932
(617) 475-0549

Hawaii
H-KISS
Zero to Three Hawaii Project
1600 Kapiolani Boulevard, Suite 1401
Honolulu, HI 96814
(808) 955-7273
(voice/TDD, Oahu only)
(800) 235-5477
(voice/TDD, other islands)

Idaho
Idaho CareLine
Idaho Infant/Toddler Program
450 West State Street
Boise, ID 83720-0036
(800) 926-2588
(English voice, ID only)
(800) 677-1848
(Spanish voice, ID only)
(208) 332-7205 (TDD)

Illinois
Help Me Grow Hotline
Department of Human Services
2501 North Dirksen Parkway
Springfield, IL 62702
(800) 323-4769 (voice, IL only)
(800) 547-0466 (TDD)

Indiana
Indiana Parent Information Network
4755 Kingsway Drive, Suite 105
Indianapolis, IN 46205
(800) 964-IPIN (voice/TDD, IN only)
ipin@indy.net

Iowa
Iowa COMPASS
Information and Referral for Iowans
with Disabilities and Their Families
University Hospital School
100 Hawkins Drive, Room S277
Iowa City, IA 52242-1011
1 (800) 779-2001 (voice/TDD)
(319) 353-8777 (voice/TDD)
iowa-compass@uiowa.edu
http://www.medicine.uiowa.edu/
iowacompass/

Kansas
Make a Difference Information Network
Department of Health and Environment
900 Southwest Jackson, LSOB, 10th Floor
Topeka, KS 66612-1290
(800) 332-6262
(voice/TDD, KS only)

Kentucky
First Steps, Kentucky's Early Intervention System
275 East Main Street
Frankfort, KY 40621
(800) 442-0087 (voice)
(800) 648-6057 (TDD)
http://www.iglou.com/katsnet/
first_steps/home.htm

Louisiana
ChildNet Information and Referral
Disabilities Information Access Line
(DIAL)
Developmental Disabilities Council
PO Box 3455
Baton Rouge, LA 70821-3455
(800) 922-DIAL (voice)
(800) 256-1633 (TDD)

Maine
Child Development Services
State House Station #146
Augusta, ME 04333
(207) 287-3272 (voice)
(207) 287-2550 (TDD)

Maryland
Maryland Infants and Toddlers Program
Division of Special Education
Department of Education
200 West Baltimore Street, 4th Floor
Baltimore, MD 21201
(800) 535-0182 (voice, MD only)
(800) 735-2258 (TDD)

Massachusetts
Family TIES of Massachusetts
Department of Public Health
250 Washington Street, 4th Floor,
DCSHCN
Boston, MA 02108-4619
(800) 905-TIES (voice, MA only)
(617) 624-5992 (TDD)
division.cshcn@state.ma.us

Michigan
Early On
Michigan 4C Association
2875 Northwind Drive, Suite 200
East Lansing, MI 48823
Intake: (800) EARLY-ON (voice/TDD)
earlyon@earlyon-mi.org
http://www.earlyon-mi.org

Minnesota
Children with Special Health Needs
Division of Family Health
Department of Health
85 East 7th Place, #400
Minneapolis, MN 55101
(800) 728-5420 (voice/TDD, MN only)
http://www.health.state.mn.us/
divs/fh/mcshn/iandr.htm

Mississippi
First Steps Early Intervention Program
Department of Health
2423 North State Street
PO Box 1700
Jackson, MS 39215-1700
(800) 451-3903 (voice, MS only)

Missouri
Early Childhood Special Education Section
Department of Elementary and
Secondary Education
PO Box 480
Jefferson City, MO 65102-0480
(573) 751-0187 (voice)
(800) 735-2966 (TDD)

Montana
Parents Let's Unite for Kids (PLUK)
516 North 32nd Street
Billings, MT 59101-6003
(800) 222-7585
(voice/TDD, MT only)
plukmt@aol.com
http://www.pluk.org

Nebraska
ChildFind Information and Referral for Children and Their Families
Assistive Technology Project
Department of Education
301 Centennial Mall South
PO Box 94987
Lincoln, NE 68509-4987
(800) 742-7594 (voice/TDD, NE only)
atp@nde4.nde.state.ne.us
http://www.nde.state.ne.us/ATP/
TECHome.html

Nevada
Project ASSIST
Nevada Early Childhood Association for
Special Children
PO Box 70247
Reno, NV 89570-0247
(800) 522-0066 (voice, NV only)
(775) 688-2818 (TDD)

New Hampshire
Family Resource Connection
New Hampshire State Library
20 Park Street
Concord, NH 03301
(800) 298-4321 (voice, NH only)
(800) 735-2964 (TDD)
http://www.state.nh.us/nhsl/frc

New Jersey
Resources
Developmental Disabilities Council
PO Box 700
20 West State Street
Trenton, NJ 08625-0700
(800) 792-8858 (voice)
(609) 777-3238 (TDD)

New Mexico
Information Center for New Mexicans with Disabilities/Babynet
435 Saint Michael's Drive, Building D
Santa Fe, NM 87505
(800) 552-8195 (voice/TDD, NM only)

New York
Office of Advocate for Persons with Disablities
One Empire State Plaza, Suite 1001
Albany, NY 12223-1150
(800) 522-4369 (voice/TDD, NY only)
information@oapwd.state.ny.us
http://www.state.ny.us/
disabledadvocate

North Carolina
Family Support Network of North Carolina
University of North Carolina, CB#7340
Chapel Hill, NC 27599-7340
(800) 852-0042 (voice/TDD)
http://www.med.unc.edu/
commedu/familysu

North Dakota
Developmental Disabilities Unit
Department of Human Services
600 South 2nd Street, Suite 1A
Bismarck, ND 58504-5729
(800) 755-8529 (voice/TDD, ND only)

Ohio
Help-Me-Grow Helpline
Department of Health
246 North High Street
Columbus, OH 43215
(800) 755-GROW (voice/TDD, OH only)

Oklahoma
Oklahoma Areawide Services Information System (OASIS)
Oklahoma University Health Sciences Center
4545 North Lincoln Boulevard, Suite 284
Oklahoma City, OK 73105-3414
(800) 426-2747 (voice/TDD)
oasisok@juno.com
http://oasis.ouhsc.edu

Oregon
Office of Special Education
Department of Education
225 Capitol Street NE
Salem, OR 97310
(503) 378-3598, ext. 651
(voice, TDD available upon request)

Republic of Palau
Special Education
Department of Education
PO Box 189
Koror, PW 96940
(680) 488-2537

Pennsylvania
CONNECT Information Service
150 South Progress Avenue
Harrisburg, PA 17109
(800) 692-7288 (voice/TDD, PA only)
connect@southstar.org

Puerto Rico
Primeros Pasos
Programa de Intervención Temprana
División de Servicios de Habilitación
Secretaría Auxiliar de Promoción y Protección de la Salud
Departamento de Salud
PO Box 70184
San Juan, PR 00936-8184
(787) 763-4665
(800) 981-8492

Rhode Island
Rhode Island Parent Information Network (RIPIN)
175 Main Street
Pawtucket, RI 02860-6260
(800) 464-3399 (voice, RI only)
(401) 727-4151 (TDD)

South Carolina
BabyNet Central Directory
South Carolina Services Information System (SCSIS)
Center for Disability Resources
University of South Carolina School of Medicine
Columbia, SC 29208
(800) 922-1107 (voice/TDD)
http://www.cdd.sc.edu/scsis

South Dakota
Office of Special Education
Department of Education and Cultural Affairs
700 Governors Drive
Pierre, SD 57501
(800) 529-5000 (voice/TDD, SD only)

Tennessee
Division for Special Education
Department of Education
710 James Robertson Parkway
Nashville, TN 37243-0380
(800) 852-7157 (voice, TN only)

Texas
Early Childhood Intervention (ECI) Program
ECI Care Line
4900 North Lamar
Austin, TX 78751-2399
(800) 250-2246 (voice)
(800) 735-2989 (TDD)
http://www.eci.state.tx.us/

Utah
Access Utah Network
555 East 300 South, Suite 201
Salt Lake City, UT 84102
(800) 333-UTAH (voice/TDD)
accessut@state.ut.us
http://www.accessut.state.ut.us

Vermont
Agency of Human Services
Department of Health
Children with Special Health Needs
PO Box 70
Burlington, VT 05402
(802) 863-7338 (voice/TDD)
(800) 660-4427
(voice/TDD, VT only)

Virgin Islands
Guide to Services for the Disabled in the USVI
Infant and Toddler Program
Department of Health
Elaine Co Complex
St. Thomas, VI 00803
(809) 777-8804 (voice)

Virginia
Babies Can't Wait—First Steps
United Way Information and Referral Center
224 East Broad Street
PO Box 12209
Richmond, VA 23241-0209
(800) 234-1448 (voice/TDD)

Washington
Healthy Mothers, Healthy Babies Coalition of Washington
300 Elliott Avenue West, Suite 300
Seattle, WA 98119-4118
(800) 322-2588 (voice/TDD, WA only)
(800) 833-6388 (TDD)

West Virginia
Family Matters
PO Box 1831
Clarksburg, WV 26302-1831
(888) 983-2645 (voice/TDD)
wvfamily@msys.net
http://www.msys.net/wvfamily

Wisconsin
First Step
Lutheran Hospital-Lacrosse
1910 South Avenue
Lacrosse, WI 54601
(800) 642-7837 (voice/TDD)

Wyoming
Governor's Planning Council on Developmental Disabilities
122 West 25th Street
Herschler Building, 1st Floor West
Cheyenne, WY 82002
(800) 438-5791 (voice/TDD)
http://wind.uwyo.edu/pathways/
index.htm

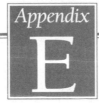

Supplemental Resources

General References

The following resources offer additional insight about developing quality programs for infants and toddlers. Write or phone for further information.

Caring for Infants & Toddlers in Groups: Developmentally Appropriate Practice
J. Ronald Lally, Abbey Griffin, Emily Fenichel, Marilyn Segal, Eleanor Szanton, and Bernice Weissbourd (1995). This book is a guide to the special knowledge and program design necessary to address the unique developmental characteristics of children in the first three years of life. (Available from ZERO TO THREE: National Center for Infants, Toddlers and Families, 734 15th Street NW, Suite 1000, Washington, DC 20005-1013, 800-899-4301.)

Developmentally Appropriate Practice in Early Childhood Programs, Revised Edition
Sue Bredekamp and Carol Copple (Eds.) (1997). This revised edition of the industry standard on appropriate practices devotes a chapter to exploring the needs and appropriate caregiving responses to children from birth through age three. (Available from NAEYC, 1509 16th Street NW, Washington, DC 20036-1426, 800-424-2460.)

Infants, Toddlers, and Caregivers
Janet Gonzalez-Mena and Dianne Widmeyer Eyer (1997). This book gives a wonderful overview of infant-toddler development and quality infant-toddler child care. It emphasizes respect for the individual child and helps caregivers focus on the relationships they build with children. It addresses multicultural issues facing caregivers, such as bilingual communication and culturally appropriate curriculum. (Available from Mayfield Publishing Company, 1280 Villa Street, Mountain View, CA 94041, 800-433-1279.)

Prime Times: A Handbook for Excellence in Infant and Toddler Programs
Jim Greenman and Anne Stonehouse (1996). This book helps readers understand the needs of children under three, and their families and caregivers, and how to use this information to create a quality program. (Available from Redleaf Press, 450 N. Syndicate, Suite 5, St. Paul, MN 55104-4125, 800-423-8309.)

1,2,3… The Toddler Years: A Practical Guide for Parents and Caregivers
Irene Van der Zande (Second Edition, 1993). Written with the staff of the Santa Cruz Toddler Care Center, this easy-to-read, practical book gives readers a clear picture of the characteristics of toddlers and strategies for ways to live and work with them. (Available from Santa Cruz Toddler Care Center, 1738 16th Avenue, Santa Cruz, CA 95060, 831-476-4120.)

Topic-Related References

The following resources are recommended to readers who wish to know more about specific topics explored in *The Creative Curriculum for Infants & Toddlers.*

Knowing Children's Families

Getting Men Involved: Strategies for Early Childhood Programs
James A. Levine, Dennis T. Murphy, and Sherill Wilson (1993). This book offers practical suggestions for ways to welcome and involve the men in the lives of the children in your program. (Available from Families and Work Institute, 330 Seventh Aveune, 14th Floor, New York, NY 10001, 212-465-2044.)

The Six Stages of Parenthood
Ellen Galinsky (1987). As it describes the stages of parenthood, this book reminds readers that parents are growing and developing too. (Available from Families and Work Institute, 330 Seventh Aveune, 14th Floor, New York, NY 10001, 212-465-2044.)

Communities: Building a Network of Support

Community Mobilization: Strategies to Support Young Children and Their Families
Amy Laura Dombro, Nina Sazer O'Donnell, Ellen Galinsky, Sarah Gilkeson Melcher, and Abby Farber (1996). This guide includes detailed descriptions of hundreds of community collaborations throughout the country that have as their goal improving the lives of young children and their families. It takes the reader through the practical steps of creating change and offers tips and lessons learned, thus allowing communities to build on what others have done. (Available from Families and Work Institute, 330 Seventh Avenue, 14th Floor, New York, NY 10001, 212-465-2044.)

Promoting Health and Safety

American Red Cross Child Care Course: Health and Safety Units
The American National Red Cross and the American Academy of Pediatrics (1990). This multi-media package provides in-depth training for caregivers on infant and child care first aid, as well as preventing childhood injuries. (Available from local Red Cross chapters, stock # 654300.)

The Consumer Reports Guide to Baby Products (Sixth Edition, 1999).
This report provides ratings of thoroughly tested childproofing products and child gates. It includes warnings on products judged not acceptable. (Available from Consumer Reports Books, PO Box 10637, Des Moines, IA 50336, 515-237-4903.)

First Aid for Children Fast

The Johns Hopkins Children's Center (1995). This user-friendly manual gives step by step instructions that are easy to understand and follow. Color photographs illustrate each step. This book is an excellent resource for preparing emergency plans. (Available from Johns Hopkins Children's Center, 111 Market Place, Suite 901, Baltimore, MD 21202, 410-223-1724.)

Healthy Young Children: A Manual for Programs

Abby Shapiro Kendrick, Roxanne Kaufmann, and Katherine P. Messinger (Eds.) (1995). This resource focuses on ways to promote the health and well-being of young children in group programs. The research-based information covers safety, first aid, emergency procedures, and other topics. The manual represents a cooperative effort by the following groups: the Administration for Children, Youth, and Families (ACYF); the Division of Maternal and Child Health, U.S. Department of Health and Human Services (HHS); Georgetown University Child Development Center; the Massachusetts Department of Public Health; and the National Association for the Education of Young Children (NAEYC). (Available from NAEYC, 1509 16th Street NW, Washington, DC 20036-1426, 800-424-2460.)

Caring for Our Children, National Health and Safety Performance Standards: Guidelines for Out-of-Home Child Care Programs

American Public Health Association and the American Academy of Pediatrics (Second Edition, in press 2000). This definitive statement on safety standards can serve well as a reference in every infant and toddler program. (For information, contact the National Resource Center for Health and Safety in Child Care, Campus Box C288, 4200 E. 9th Avenue, Denver, CO 80262, 800-598-5437.)

Starting Point: How To Open Your Program (and Your Heart) to Children with Special Health Needs

Division of Maternal and Child Health, Graduate School of Public Health, San Diego State University (1993). This helpful manual provides guidance on providing services for children with health and/or physical challenges, developing culturally competent services, ensuring confidentiality, preventing childhood injuries, preventing the spread of communicable diseases, providing play experiences, and dealing with challenging behaviors. A Spanish version, *Punto de Partido*, is available. (Available from California Child Care Health Program, 6505 Alvarado Road, Suite 108, San Diego, CA 92120, 619-594-3728.)

Creating a Welcoming Environment

Caring Spaces, Learning Places: Children's Environments That Work

Jim Greenman (1988). This excellent book shows how to create environments that make use of space creatively, with attention to children's developmental needs. A separate chapter on infant and toddler environments includes wonderful ideas illustrated with photographs and diagrams of indoor and outdoor spaces. (Available from Exchange Press, Inc., PO Box 3249, Redmond, WA 98073-3249, 800-221-2864.)

Landscapes for Learning: Designing Group Care Environments for Infants, Toddlers, and Two Year Olds
> Louis Torelli and Charles Durrett (1996). This excellent handbook on designing developmentally appropriate learning environments for infants and toddlers merges the principles of child development with architectural design. (Available from Torelli-Durrett, 1250 Addison Street, Suite 113, Berkeley, CA 94702.)

Learning Through Routines and Activities

Anti-Bias Curriculum: Tools for Empowering Young Children
> Louise Derman-Sparks and the A.B.C. Task Force (1989). This classic on the subject of multiculturalism provides guidance on selecting materials for children that eliminate barriers based on race, culture, gender, age, or ability. (Available from NAEYC, 1509 16th Street NW, Washington, DC 20036-1426, 800-424-2460.)

Behavior Guidance for Infants and Toddlers
> Alice S. Honig (1996). In simple and vivid language, this book offers caregivers and parents positive discipline techniques that are appropriate for infants and toddlers. Tips for thinking about fusses and "disobedience" will be useful for adults puzzled by such behaviors. (Available from Southern Early Childhood Association, PO Box 55930, Little Rock, AR 72215, 501-663-0353.)

Creative Art for the Developing Child
> Clare Cherry (1990). This useful text takes a developmental approach to children's explorations with art. The book is filled with teaching suggestions and strategies. (Available from Frank Schaffer Publications, PO Box 2853, Torrance, CA 90509, 800-421-5533.)

Creative Expression and Play in Early Childhood
> Joan P. Isenberg and Mary Renck Jalongo (Second Edition, 1996). Grounded in the authors' experiences teaching teachers, this book offers strategies and activities to stimulate readers' ideas of ways to promote the play and creativity of young children. (Available from Prentice Hall, PO Box 11071, Des Moines, IA 50336-1071, 800-643-5506.)

Emerging Literacy: Linking Social Competence and Learning
> Derry Koralek for Aspen Systems Corporation (1997). This excellent guide, targeted to teachers and other educators, provides background information and training ideas on making children partners in conversation, the magic world of reading, and setting the stage for literacy. (Available from the Head Start Publications Management Center (HSPMC), PO Box 26417, Alexandria, VA 22313-0417, 202-737-1030.)

Much More Than the ABCs: The Early Stages of Reading and Writing
> Judith A. Schickendanz (Second Edition, 1999). This standard in the field traces the development of literacy skills which begin at birth. It describes ways to maximize the reading experience for children throughout the early childhood years. (Available from NAEYC, 1509 16th Street NW, Washington, DC 20036-1426, 800-424-2460.)

The Outside Play and Learning Book: Activities for Young Children
  Karen Miller (1989). This comprehensive and extremely creative collection of outdoor activities includes a separate chapter on "Infants and Toddlers Outside." In addition, many of the ideas in other sections of the book are appropriate or can be adapted for infants and toddlers. (Available from Gryphon House, PO Box 207, Beltsville, MD 20704, 800-638-0928.)

Play Is a Child's World: A Lekotek Resource Guide on Play for Children with Disabilities for Families, Friends, and Professionals
  The National Lekotek Center (n.d.). The 51 Lekotek Centers throughout the United States provide support, resources, and toys to families of children with disabilities. This guide and the companion manual, *Lekotek Play Guide for Children with Disabilities*, focus on using appropriate adaptive toys for children with disabilities. (Available from National Lekotek Center, 2100 Ridge Avenue, Evanston, IL 60201, 800-366-7529.)

The Right Stuff for Children Birth to 8: Selecting Play Materials to Support Development
  Martha B. Bronson (1995). This comprehensive manual is an excellent resource for selecting toys to match the developmental skills of children. Careful consideration is given to safety issues. (Available from NAEYC, 1509 16th Street NW, Washington, DC 20036-1426, 800-424-2460.)

Talking with Your Baby: Family as the First School
  Alice S. Honig and Holly E. Brophy (1996). Caregivers and parents will appreciate the ideas for using "turn-talking-talk" to enhance their daily interactions with very young children. Many photos illustrate how tuned-in talk can enrich affectionate relationships and promote early learning. Diapering, bath time, shopping trips, and other ordinary routines become opportunities to increase language power. (Available from Syracuse University Press, 1600 Jamesville Avenue, Syracuse, NY 13244, 315-443-2597.)

Index

About the Authors

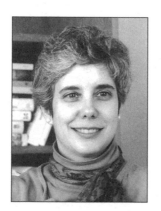

Amy Laura Dombro, M.S., is the author of numerous articles and books on infant/toddler and family child care. She has extensive experience training Head Start and child care staff and consults for national organizations. Her newest book is *The Power of Observation* (with Judy Jablon and Margo Dichtelmiller). Amy was a member of the Advisory Committee on Services for Families with Infants and Toddlers that guided the design of the new Early Head Start program. She began her professional career by serving for eight years as the director of the Bank Street Infant and Family Center.

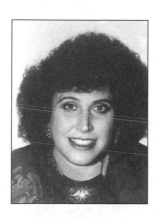

Laura J. Colker, Ed.D., is the author of more than 90 articles and numerous books on early childhood education. She has designed curriculum, training materials, and videos for teachers and supervisory staff, and story books, videos, software, and videodiscs for children. Laura conducts training and teaches courses on child development issues throughout the United States, Europe, and Asia.

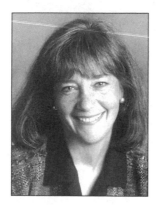

Diane Trister Dodge, M.S., founder and president of Teaching Strategies, Inc., is the author of more than 30 books on early childhood education. Her 35 years of experience working with teachers and administrators have taught her the value of curriculum and training materials that articulate a clear philosophy and practical approach to meaningful learning. Diane served on the Governing Board of the National Association for the Education of Young Children (NAEYC), and is currently a Board member of the Center for the Child Care Workforce.

— Notes —

— Notes —

— Notes —

— Notes —

✦ Infant/Toddler Resources ✦

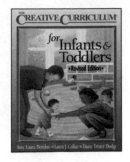

The Creative Curriculum® for Infants & Toddlers, Revised Edition
A comprehensive yet easy-to-use framework for planning and implementing infant and toddler programs in center-based and family child care settings. It emphasizes that the focus of curriculum for infants and toddlers is all about caregivers/teachers building responsive relationships with children and their families.
#CB0052, **$34.95**

Also available in Spanish, fall 2000: #CB0029, **$34.95**

A Trainer's Guide to The Creative Curriculum® for Infants & Toddlers
A complete roadmap for fully implementing the Curriculum and transforming it into a living and breathing part of your program. Includes 12 workshop series, forms for individualizing staff development, and dozens of reproducible handouts. It also shows you how to use the Journal as part of your staff development program.
#CB0049, **$27.95**

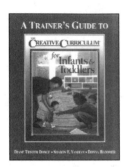

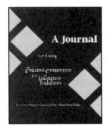

A Journal for Using The Creative Curriculum® for Infants & Toddlers
A companion to *The Creative Curriculum® for Infants & Toddlers,* for use as a personal guidebook for understanding and applying the Curriculum. A perfect tool for ongoing staff development, group meetings, and personal reflection.
#CB0053, **$5.00**

A Parent's Guide to Infant/Toddler Programs
Shows parents how warm and responsive care helps shape the development of infants and toddlers and their ability to learn.
#CB0033, **$22.50** (set of 10)
Also available in Spanish: #CB0034, **$22.50** (set of 10)

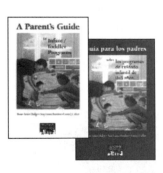

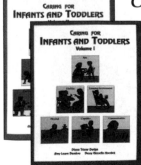

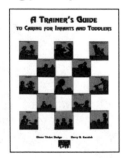

Caring for Infants and Toddlers
A two-volume set comprised of 13 modules that correspond to the Child Development Associate (CDA) functional areas. The perfect tool for staff working towards their CDA credential.
Volume 1: #CB0082A, **$34.95**
Volume 2: #CB0082B, **$34.95**
Trainer's Guide: #CB0083, **$23.95**

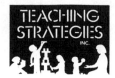

Book & Video Order Form

Please type or print clearly.

4 Ways to Order

Order by phone
800-637-3652
Washington, D.C. area:
202-362-7543
9 a.m.–5 p.m. EST

Order by fax
202-364-7273
24 hours a day

Order online
www.TeachingStrategies.com
24 hours a day

Order by mail
Teaching Strategies, Inc.
P.O. Box 42243
Washington, DC 20015

Ship to:

NAME

ORGANIZATION

ADDRESS

CITY	STATE	ZIP

PHONE	FAX

E-MAIL

Bill to:

NAME

ORGANIZATION

ADDRESS

CITY	STATE	ZIP

PHONE	FAX

Order:

ITEM #	QTY	DESCRIPTION	UNIT PRICE	TOTAL
			$	$
			$	$
			$	$
			$	$
			$	$
			$	$
			$	$
			$	$
			$	$
			$	$

Please call for information on quantity discounts.

SUBTOTAL	$
SALES TAX DC Residents only add 5.75%	$

SHIPPING
United States: Orders up to $60.00—$5.00;
Orders over $60.00—9% of total.
International/U.S. Territories: $20.00 (first book)
+ $7.00 for each additional book.
Rush Delivery: Call for shipping charges.

	$
TOTAL	$

Method of payment

All orders must be accompanied by payment, P.O. number, or credit card information. Customers with an established credit history are welcome to use P.O. numbers.
First-time customers must enclose pre-payment with order.

❏ Check (payable to Teaching Strategies)   ❏ Money order

❏ Purchase order (indicate P.O. # below)   ❏ Visa   ❏ MasterCard

CREDIT CARD OR PURCHASE ORDER NUMBER   EXPIRATION DATE

SIGNATURE OF CARD HOLDER

❏ Yes, I would like to receive occasional e-mail notifications about new Teaching Strategies products and special offers. I understand that TSI will not share or sell my e-mail address with any other individual, company, or organization.

❏ Please send me more information about the Center for the Child Care Workforce (CCW) and its Worthy Wage Campaign.

Guarantee: Teaching Strategies guarantees your complete satisfaction. If you are not thoroughly delighted with the printed materials you order, return the item(s) in sellable condition within 30 days for a full refund. However, all video tape sales are final.

Prices subject to change without notice. Infant/Toddler CB

Thank you for your order.

✦ OTHER RESOURCES ✦

CURRICULUM RESOURCES

The Creative Curriculum® for Early Childhood, 3rd Ed.

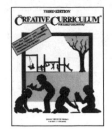

Shows how teachers build curriculum for preschool and kindergarten children around the environment using ten interest areas: Blocks, House Corner, Table Toys, Art, Sand and Water, Library, Music and Movement, Cooking, Computers, and Outdoors.
#CB0071, **$39.95**
Also available in Spanish: #CB0074, **$39.95**

Connecting Content, Teaching, and Learning

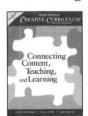

This supplement to *The Creative Curriculum®* includes revised *Curriculum* goals and objectives; a new Developmental Continuum that shows the specific developmental sequence for each objective; and overviews of key components of standards as they apply to preschool in each subject area—literacy, math, science, social studies, the arts, and technology.
CB0032, **$9.95**

The Creative Curriculum® for Family Child Care

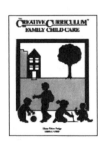

Helps you design a developmentally appropriate program in your home for each age group—infants, toddlers, preschoolers, and school-age children.
#CB0084, **$29.95**

RESOURCES FOR PARENTS

A Parent's Guide to Early Childhood Education

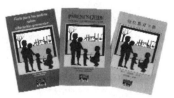

Explains what happens in a developmentally appropriate early childhood program and the important role parents play in helping their children succeed in school and in life.
#CB0075, **$22.50** (set of 10)
#CB0089, **$22.50** (set of 10) (Spanish edition)
#CB0060, **$22.50** (set of 10) (Chinese edition)

OBSERVATION

The Power of Observation

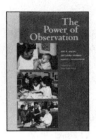

Explores the vital connection between observing and effective teaching. This book offers both specific guidelines for effective observation and the inspiration to get started with observing.
#CB0035, **$19.95**

VIDEOS

The Creative Curriculum®

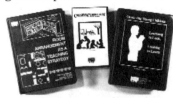

A 37-minute, award-winning videotape that shows how children learn in each interest area and how teachers set the stage and encourage their learning.
#CB0072, **$99.50**
Also available with Spanish subtitles:
#CB0014, **$99.50**

Observing Young Children: Learning to Look, Looking to Learn

This 30-minute videotape illustrates how staff can use ongoing observation to learn about each child, measure children's progress, and evaluate their program.
#CB0054, **$55.00**

The NEW Room Arrangement as a Teaching Strategy

A 15-minute slide/videotape. Presents concrete ideas for arranging early childhood classrooms to support positive behavior and learning.
#CB0076, **$35.00**
Also available in Spanish: #CB0010, **$35.00**

Caring and Learning

This 23-minute, award-winning videotape shows four exceptional family child care providers in action using the activity areas described in *The Creative Curriculum®* for *Family Child Care*.
#CB0087, **$42.00**

Order online at our web site, www.TeachingStrategies.com, or call 800-637-3652 or 202-362-7543